Classification of Nursing Diagnoses

Proceedings of the Seventh Conference

Classification of Nursing Diagnoses

Proceedings of the Seventh Conference

**North American
Nursing Diagnosis Association**

Edited by

Audrey M. McLane, Ph.D., R.N.

Professor, College of Nursing
Marquette University
Milwaukee, Wisconsin

with 26 illustrations

The C. V. Mosby Company

ST. LOUIS • WASHINGTON, D.C. • TORONTO   1987

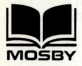

A TRADITION OF PUBLISHING EXCELLENCE

Editor: Barbara Ellen Norwitz
Developmental editor: Sally Adkisson
Project editor: Kathleen L. Teal
Editing, Production: Editing, Design & Production, Inc.
Design: Staff

The C.V. Mosby Company
11830 Westline Industrial Drive, St. Louis, Missouri 63146

Library of Congress Cataloging-in-Publication Data

Classification of nursing diagnoses.
  Proceedings of the Seventh Conference on the Classification
of Nursing Diagnoses, held in St. Louis, Mo.,
March 9-13, 1986.
  Includes bibliographies and index.
  1. Diagnosis—Congresses. 2. Nursing—Congresses.
3. Diagnosis—Classification—Congresses. I. McLane,
Audrey M. II. North American Nursing Diagnosis Association.
III. Conference on the Classification of Nursing
Diagnoses (7th: 1986: St. Louis, Mo.) [DNLM: 1. Nursing
Assessment—Congresses. WY 100 C614 1986]
RT48.C5542   1987   610.73   87-5564

ISBN 0-8016-3847-X

AC/VH/VH 9 8 7 6 5 4 3 2 1   02/D/231

Contributors

Gordon A. Allen, PhD
Miami University,
Oxford, Ohio

Beth Anderson, RN
Miami Valley Hospital,
Dayton, Ohio

Virginia Aukamp, MS, RN
Millikin University,
Decatur, Illinois

Myrtle Aydelotte, PhD, RN, FAAN
University of Iowa,
Iowa City, Iowa

Linda S. Baas, RN, MSN, CCRN
University Hospital,
Cincinnati, Ohio

Carol Baer, MS, RN
New England Deaconess Hospital,
Boston, Massachusetts

Toni Balistrieri, MSN, RN
Clement J. Zablocki V.A. Hospital,
Wood, Wisconsin

Jean K. Bartek, MSN, MS, RN
University of Nebraska and University of
   Nebraska Medical Center,
Omaha, Nebraska

Mary Beibel, RN
Columbia Hospital,
Milwaukee, Wisconsin

Adele M. Beiting, MSN, RN, CIC
University Hospital,
Cincinnati, Ohio

Suzanne Beyea, MSN, RN
St. Anselm's College,
Manchester, New Hampshire

Kathleen Beyerman, MSN, RN
The Cambridge Hospital,
Cambridge, Massachussets

Genee Brukwitzki, MSN, RN
Alverno College,
Milwaukee, Wisconsin

Catherine Burns, MN, RN, PNP
Oregon Health Science University
Portland, Oregon

Carol J. Cattaneo, MN, RN, ET
Johnson County Community College,
Overland Park, Kansas

Pat Chambers, RN
Miami Valley Hospital,
Dayton, Ohio

Mary T. Champagne, PhD, RN

University of North Carolina,
Chapel Hill, North Carolina

Kenneth L. Cianfrani, PhD, RN

University of Health Sciences/Chicago Medical
School,
North Chicago, Illinois

Marga Coler, EdD, RN, CS

University of Connecticut,
Storrs, Connecticut

Ann Fass Collard, MS, RN, ANP

Brandeis University,
Waltham, Massachusetts

Kathleen Connors, BSN, RN

Brigham and Women's Hospital,
Boston, Massachusetts

Susan Copeland-Owen, BSN, RN

Kent State University
Kent, Ohio

Cynthia P. Coviak, MSN, RN

Michigan State University,
East Lansing, Michigan

Nancy Creason, PhD, RN

Parkland College/University of Illinois,
Champaign/Urbana, Illinois

Frances Stevralia Crosby, MS, RN

V.A. Medical Center,
Buffalo, New York

Janet Cuddigan, MSN, RN

Creighton University,
Omaha, Nebraska

Lynne Ann Dapice, MS, RN, CEN

The University of Vermont,
Burlington, Vermont

Gail C. Davis, EdD, RN

Texas Christian University,
Fort Worth, Texas

Anayis Derdiarian, DNSc, RN

University of California—Los Angeles,
Los Angeles, California

Pat deSilva, MSN, RN

University of Texas at Austin,
Austin, Texas

Theresa DiBenedetto, BSN, RN

Kent State University
Kent, Ohio

Carol Dickel, RN

Mercy Hospital,
Davenport, Iowa

Geri Dickson, MSN, RN

University of Wisconsin—Milwaukee,
Milwaukee, Wisconsin

Pauline T. Dion, MS, RN

Williamstown, Massachusetts

Cynthia M. Dougherty, MA, RN

University of Washington,
Seattle, Washington

Therese T. Dowd, MS, RN

University of Nebraska Medical Center,
Lincoln, Nebraska

Joan Dolce Dunn, MS, RN

Niagra University,
Niagra Falls, New York

Teresa Fadden, MSN, RN

St. Joseph's Hospital,
Milwaukee, Wisconsin

Nancy Falconer, MS, RN

Alverno College,
Milwaukee, Wisconsin

Richard J. Fehring, DNSc, RN

Marquette University,
Milwaukee, Wisconsin

Ann Fitzgerald, MS, RN

University of Nebraska and University of
 Nebraska Medical Center,
Omaha, Nebraska

Joan Fitzmaurice, PhD, RN, FAAN

Institute of Health Professions,
Massachussetts General Hospital,
Boston, Massachusetts

Joyce J. Fitzpatrick, PhD, RN, FAAN

Case Western Reserve University,
Cleveland, Ohio

Ann M. Frank, BSN, RN

Midwest Arthritis Treatment Center,
Columbia Hospital,
Milwaukee, Wisconsin

Sheila L. Fredette, EdD, RN

Fitchburg State College,
Fitchburg, Massachusetts

Cecilia Freeman, MSN, RN

University of Wisconsin—Milwaukee,
Milwaukee, Wisconsin

Marilyn Frenn, MSN, RN

Marquette University,
Milwaukee, Wisconsin

Gail Furney, BSN, RN

Kent State University,
Kent, Ohio

Katherine L. Garthe, MSN, RN

Leelanau Memorial Hospital,
Northport, Michigan

Kristine M. Gebbie, MSN, RN

Oregon State Health Division,
Portland, Oregon

Jill Gershan, MSN, RN, CCRN

Marquette University,
Milwaukee, Wisconsin

Barbara Gibb, BSN, RN

Columbia Hospital,
Milwaukee, Wisconsin

Mary Ann Glynn, MBA, RN

Brigham and Women's Hospital,
Boston, Massachusetts

Adelita Gonzales, MS, RN

Martin Luther King, Jr. Health Center,
Dallas, Texas

Marjory Gordon, PhD, RN, FAAN

Boston College,
Chestnut Hill, Massachusetts

Davina Gosnell, PhD, RN

Kent State University,
Kent, Ohio

Angelynn M. Grabau, MSN, RN

University of Nebraska Medical Center,
Lincoln, Nebraska

Jessee Greene, BSN, RN

Clemson University,
Clemson, South Carolina

Kay Greenlee, MSN, RN, CCRN

St. Joseph's Hospital,
Milwaukee, Wisconsin

Edward D. Halloran, PhD, RN, FAAN

University Hospitals of Cleveland and Case
 Western Reserve University,
Cleveland, Ohio

Mary V. Hanley, MA, RN

Consultant,
Boston, Massachusetts

Jane H. Hawks, MSN, RN

University of Nebraska and University of
 Nebraska Medical Center,
Omaha, Nebraska

Steven C. Hayes, PhD

University of Nevada,
Reno, Nevada

Elizabeth Hiltunen, MS, RN

Boston College,
Chestnut Hill, Massachusetts

Adrienne Hitchock, BSN, RN

Memorial Hospital,
Cambridge, Minnesota

Martha Horst, BSN, RN

Kent State University,
Kent, Ohio

Elinore Howard, MS, RN

Brockton Hospital,
Brockton, Massachusetts

Carol Jacobs, MSN, RN

University of Wisconsin—Milwaukee,
Milwaukee, Wisconsin

Janice K. Janken, PhD, RN

Rhode Island Hospital,
Providence, Rhode Island

Mary K. Jiricka, MSN, RN, CCRN
Milwaukee County Medical Center,
Milwaukee, Wisconsin

Dorothy A. Jones, PhD, RNC, FAAN

Boston College,
Chestnut Hill, Massachusetts

Sherrie L. Goldsberry Justice, MA, RN

Medical College of Ohio,
Toledo, Ohio

Annette Kaminsky, RN

Columbia Hospital,
Milwaukee, Wisconsin

Mary Ann Kelly, EdD, RN

Clemson University,
Clemson, South Carolina

Sheila Kelly-Knox, BSN, RN

Kent State University,
Kent, Ohio

Eileen Kenkel-Rossi, MSN, RN

St. Joseph's Hospital,
Milwaukee, Wisconsin

Mary E. Kerr, MNEd, RN

West Pennsylvania Hospital School of Nursing,
Pittsburgh, Pennsylvania

Marylou Kiley, PhD, RN

University Hospitals of Cleveland and Case
 Western Reserve University,
Cleveland, Ohio

Mary Kolbe, MSN, RN

University of Nebraska Medical Center,
Lincoln, Nebraska

Barbara Krainovich, MS, RN

Teacher's College, Columbia University,
New York, New York

Patricia Kraynick, RN

Columbia Hospital,
Milwaukee, Wisconsin

Mary Kunes-Connell, MSN, RN

Creighton University,
Omaha, Nebraska

Nancy R. Lackey, PhD, RN

University of Kansas,
Kansas City, Kansas

Susan S. Lampe, MS, RN

Creative Nursing Management, Inc.,
Minneapolis, Minnesota

Paul F. Langlois, MSN, RN

Rush University,
Chicago, Illinois

Linda L. Lazure, MSN, RN

Creighton University,
Omaha, Nebraska

Helena Lee, MSN, RN

Milwaukee County Mental Health Complex,
Milwaukee, Wisconsin

Cindy Lessow, BSN, RN

Nursing Care Specialists, Inc.,
Phoenix, Arizona

Rona Levin, PhD, RN

Adelphi University,
Garden City, New York

Myra Levine, MSN, RN, FAAN

University of Illinois,
Chicago, Illinois

Marlene G. Lindeman, MSN, RN

University of Nebraska and University of
    Nebraska Medical Center,
Omaha, Nebraska

Lou Ann Madson, RN

Columbia Hospital,
Milwaukee, Wisconsin

Mary Marcello, BSN, RN

Kent State University,
Kent, Ohio

Karen Martin, MSN, RN

Visiting Nurse Association of Omaha,
Omaha, Nebraska

Nancy Matulich, MSN, RNC

West Jefferson General Hospital,
Marrero, Louisiana

Barbara W. McCabe, PhD, RN

University of Nebraska Medical Center,
Lincoln, Nebraska

Eleanor S. McConnell, MSN, RN

University of North Carolina,
Chapel Hill, North Carolina

Gertrude K. McFarland, PhD, RN

Health Resources & Services Administration,
USPHS—USDHHA,
Rockville, Maryland

Rosemary J. McKeighen, PhD, RN, FAAN

University of Iowa,
Iowa City, Iowa

Audrey M. McLane, PhD, RN

Marquette University,
Milwaukee, Wisconsin

Peg Mehmert, BA, RNC

Mercy Hospital,
Davenport, Iowa

Karen L. Metzger, MS, RN

Mercy Hospital,
Portland, Maine

Karen Miller, MSN, RN

St. Mary's Hospital,
Milwaukee, Wisconsin

Mary Molitor, BSN, RN

Columbia Hospital,
Milwaukee, Wisconsin

Marilyn Morgenstern-Stanovich, BSN, RN

Kent State University,
Kent, Ohio

Dawneane K. Munn, MSN, RN

University of Nebraska Medical Center,
Lincoln, Nebraska

Margaret A. Murphy, MS, RNC

Boston College,
Chestnut Hill, Massachusetts

Judith L. Myers, MSN, RN

St. Louis University,
St. Louis, Missouri

Charlotte E. Naschinski, MS, RN

St. Elizabeth Hospital,
Washington, D.C.

Virginia Neelon, PhD, RN

University of North Carolina,
Chapel Hill, North Carolina

Margaret A. Newman, PhD, RN

University of Minnesota,
Minneapolis, Minnesota

Marian Newton, MN, RN

University of Nebraska and University of
  Nebraska Medical Center,
Omaha, Nebraska

Joan Norris, PhD, RN

Creighton University
Omaha, Nebraska

Laura J. Nosek, MSN, RN

University Hospitals of Cleveland and Case
  Western Reserve University
Cleveland, Ohio

Karen P. Padrick, MN, RN

Oregon Health Sciences University,
Portland, Oregon

Deborah Peters, MSN, RN

Manchester Health Department,
Manchester, New Hampshire

Kathryn Hope Peterson, BSN, RN

University of Washington,
Seattle, Washington

Janice Smith Pigg, BSN, RN

Midwest Arthritis Treatment Center,
Columbia Hospital,
Milwaukee, Wisconsin

Carol Pontius, BSN, RN

Kent State University,
Kent, Ohio

Eileen Jones Porter, MA, RN

University of Wisconsin—Oshkosh,
Oshkosh, Wisconsin

Devamma Purushotham, EdD

University of Windsor,
Windsor, Ontario

Dee-J Putzier, PhD, RN

Oregon Health Sciences University,
Portland, Oregon

Linda S. Rabinowitz, MS, RN

Preston-Hollow-Dallas School District,
Dallas, Texas

Marlene Reimer, MN, RN

University of Calgary,
Calgary, Alberta

Betty Ann Reynolds, MS, RN

Rhode Island Hospital,
Providence, Rhode Island

Elvi N. Rigby, MSN, RN, CS

Brockton Hospital,
Brockton, Massachusetts

Mary P. Riordan, MS, RN

Bunker Hill Community College,
Charlestown, Massachusetts

Laura Rossi, MS, RN

Brigham & Women's Hospital,
Boston, Massachusetts

Laurie Rufolo, MS, RN

Long Island College Hospital,
Brooklyn, New York

Wanda B. Ruthven, MS, RNC, PHN

Nurse Practitioner,
Fremont, California

Sheila Ryan, PhD, RN

Creighton University,
Omaha, Nebraska

Monica Sanger, MSN, RN

St. Joseph's Hospital,
Milwaukee, Wisconsin

**Renee Semonin-Holleran, MSN, RN, CCRN, CS,
 CEN**

University of Cincinnati,
Cincinnati, Ohio

Rebecca Shaw, MS, RN

Bradley University,
Peoria, Illinois

Kathleen Sheppard, MSN, RN, CCRN

M.D. Anderson Hospital,
Houston, Texas

Eileen Sjoberg-O'Neill

Fitchburg State College,
Fitchburg, Massachusetts

Carol Smejkal, MSN, RN, CCRN

University of Wisconsin—Milwaukee,
Milwaukee, Wisconsin

Deborah Ann Smith, BSN, RN

Columbia Hospital,
Milwaukee, Wisconsin

Donna R. Smith, MS, RN

University of Nebraska Medical Center,
Lincoln, Nebraska

Carol A. Soares-O'Hearn, PhD, RN

Stonehill College,
North Easton, Massachusetts

Marilyn Sawyer Sommers, MA, RN, CCRN

University Hospital,
Cincinnati, Ohio

Martha M. Spies, MSN, RN

Deaconess College School of Nursing,
St. Louis, Missouri

Judith Spilker, BSN, RN, CNRN

University of Cincinnati Medical Center,
Cincinnati, Ohio

Drue Steele, MSN, RN

Kettering Medical Center,
Kettering, Ohio

Maribeth Stein, MN, RN

Swedish Hospital Medical Center,
Seattle, Washington

Kathleen A. Strong, MS, RN

Moraine Park Technical Institute and
 Mount Scenario College,
West Bend, Wisconsin

Christine Tanner, PhD, RN

Oregon Health Sciences University,
Portland, Oregon

Joyce Waterman Taylor, MS, RN

San Francisco General Hospital,
San Francisco, California

Mary Kathryn Thompson, MN, RN, FNP

The Oregon Health Sciences University,
Portland, Oregon

Marita Titler, MA, RN

University of Iowa Hospitals and Clinics,
Iowa City, Iowa

Beatrice B. Turkowski, MS, RN

University of Wisconsin—Milwaukee,
Milwaukee, Wisconsin

Karen Vincent, MSN, RN, CS

Coastal Community Counseling Center,
Braintree, Massachusetts

Anne M. Voith, BSN, RN

Compcare Health Services Insurance Corp.,
Milwaukee, Wisconsin

Cathy R. Ward, MSN, RN

UCLA Center for the Health Sciences,
Los Angeles, California

Judi Weatherall, MS, RN

Parkland College/University of Illinois,
Champaign/Urbana, Illinois

Harriet H. Werley, PhD, RN, FAAN

University of Wisconsin—Milwaukee,
Milwaukee, Wisconsin

Una E. Westfall, MSN, RN

Oregon Health Sciences University,
Portland, Oregon

Joy Wong, MS, RN

Bedford Veterans Administration Hospital,
Bedford, Massachusetts

Karen A. York, MSN, RN

Miami Valley Hospital,
Dayton, Ohio

Pamela J. Youngbauer, BSN, RN

Columbia Hospital,
Milwaukee, Wisconsin

Preface

The Seventh Conference on Classification of Nursing Diagnoses was held in St. Louis, Missouri, from March 9 to 13, 1986 under the auspices of the North American Nursing Diagnosis Association, Inc. (NANDA). Leadership for the conference was provided by NANDA's program committee, A.M. McLane (chairperson), A. Becker, M.A. Kelly, M.J. Kim, and L. Rossi; NANDA's board of directors; the taxonomy and diagnostic review committees chaired by P. Kritek; the research committee chaired by G.K. McFarland; and K. Murphy, NANDA's executive administrator. A total of 615 nurses (clinicians, educators, clinical researchers, administrators, consultants, and students) from the United States and Canada attended the conference.

Highlights of the Seventh conference and these proceedings include: invited papers from 11 distinguished scholars and clinicians; 47 scientific papers and 27 abstracts from the paper and poster presentations; formal endorsement of NANDA Taxonomy I; 21 new nursing diagnoses; and use of numerical codes from NANDA Taxonomy I with the diagnostic labels for purposes of ordering the approved diagnoses.

The substantive issues addressed by the invited speakers (Section I) provided a solid understructure for the conference consistent with NANDA's goals as an organization. Taxonomic issues were discussed by M. Aydelotte in her state-of-the-art keynote address and by M. Levine. In a related paper,

M. Newman shared her conceptualizations of nursing's emerging paradigm. The continuing concern of nurse scholars and NANDA with the issue of etiology was portrayed by J. Fitzpatrick, while the practical relevance of etiology was delineated by A. Derdiarian. Economic issues and their impact on fee-based reimbursement were described by K. Gebbie. H. Werley reported on the development of the Nursing Minimum Data Set (NMDS), the diagnosis component within the NMDS, and the research potential of the NMDS. In a paper presentation followed by a workshop, S. Hayes (clinical psychologist/researcher) described the use of research strategies to evaluate on-line clinical interventions to treat/validate nursing diagnoses and to build a scientific base for a practice discipline. Clinical concerns were also addressed by two nurse clinicians who demonstrated the use of functional health patterns (L. Rossi) and conservation principles (J. Taylor) to organize data for nursing diagnosis. NANDA's president, M. Gordon, reflected on several of the issues surrounding nursing diagnosis, identified some of the current disputes and debates, and reviewed issues requiring discussion and resolution in the future.

Since all papers and posters selected for presentation at the Seventh conference were data-based, the manuscripts and abstracts were categorized to illuminate the quality and quantity of scholarly development in each category. The largest number of studies was in the diagnostic validation category (Section II A, B, and C) with manuscripts submitted from 7 paper and 17 poster presentations. Thirteen presenters of validation papers or posters elected to submit abstracts rather than a completed manuscript. The paucity of epidemiologic studies discussed by M. Gordon is reflected in that category (Section II D, E, and F) with only two manuscripts from poster presentations and four abstracts. Studies categorized as diagnostic reasoning (Section III A, B and C) fared somewhat better with manuscripts from five paper and one poster presentation, plus four abstracts. The category of nursing process (Section III D and E), comprised of assessment, prioritization, documentation, and intervention studies, includes seven manuscripts submitted from poster presentation and one abstract. The utilization category (Section IV A, B, and C) begins with Halloran's nursing complexity, DRG, and length of stay paper, followed by manuscripts from four posters and three abstracts. The few studies in the education category (Section IV D, E, and F), manuscripts from one paper and four poster presentations, and one abstract, is somewhat surprising given nursing's long affiliation with education. Placement of studies within a given category was not always intuitively obvious from the title or from the abstract. Decisions were made on the basis of stated purposes and substantive contents of manuscripts.

The process for review of proposed new diagnoses was implemented for the first time at the Seventh conference. Debate and discussion of 22 proposed diagnoses by the General Assembly was lead by P. Kritek, assisted by members of NANDA's Diagnostic Review Committee (DRC). Recommendations from the General Assembly were implemented by the DRC prior to submission to NANDA's membership for voting by mail ballot. The 21 approved new diagnoses (Section V-1) were placed in the appropriate

Human Response Patterns by the Taxonomy Committee. Guidelines for development/submission of new diagnoses (Section V-2) and a description of the diagnosis review cycle (Section V-3) are included in these proceedings to encourage further development and use of nursing diagnoses.

An historic document, NANDA Taxonomy I (Section VI), represents the culmination of more than a decade of effort by NANDA members and their associates in the profession. The tentativeness of such a document was emphasized by P. Kritek, chairperson of the Taxonomy Committee, who expects the next version of the taxonomy to be ready by the Eighth conference. In addition to NANDA Taxonomy I (Section VI-3), this section includes some of the taxonomy committee's observations about the taxonomy and definitions of diagnosis qualifiers (Section VI-2 and 3).

Section VII contains two documents, the list of approved diagnostic labels and the approved nursing diagnoses. The numerical codes and Human Response Patterns from NANDA Taxonomy I were used to prepare the List of Approved Diagnostic Labels (Section VII A). New diagnoses are marked with a (+) sign for easy recognition. The format developed for new diagnoses by the Diagnosis Review Committee was used by the editor to reformat diagnoses approved at previous conferences. The numerical codes from NANDA Taxonomy I were used with the diagnostic labels for purposes of ordering the Approved Nursing Diagnoses (Section VII B). Multiple diagnoses (e.g., self-care deficits) required special attention, because each deficit has been assigned a different numerical code. In the case of self-care deficits, sufficient work had been completed on each deficit to warrant their separation into unique diagnoses. Rape-trauma syndrome was also amenable to separation into discrete diagnoses. Sensory/perceptual alterations and tissue perfusion were left as multiple diagnoses with a caveat to use the appropriate numerical code to designate the specific sense (sensory/perceptual) or tissue (tissue perfusion).

The appendices (Section VIII) include: (A) NANDA officers, board of directors, and committee chairpersons; (B) NANDA's business meeting, committee reports and motions approved; (C) summary of the Awards Ceremony; (D) summary and future directions; (E) summary of regional group meetings; (F) special interest group reports; (G) other acknowledgements; (H) NANDA bylaws; and (I) list of Seventh conference participants.

The editor wishes to express appreciation to NANDA's Board of Directors and the Publications Committee for the opportunity to edit these proceedings; to Karen Murphy, Executive Director of NANDA, for providing and verifying information; to the invited speakers and paper and poster presenters for responding to editorial queries and for their scholarly contributions to this publication. A special thanks is extended to L. Rossi and M.A. Kelly, organizers of the Regional and Special Interest Group Meetings respectively, the group leaders, and recorders who shared the difficult task of providing a forum for individual members. The summaries of their meetings are an important part of the networking function of the biennial conferences and they provide valuable feedback to NANDA's officers, board of directors, and committees. Finally, I am grateful to Marquette University, Milwaukee, Wisconsin for granting me a sabbatical leave which facilitated completion of this endeavor in a timely manner.

Audrey M. McLane, Ph.D., R.N.
Professor, Marquette University,
Milwaukee, Wisconsin

Contents

Welcome Address

MARJORY GORDON, Ph.D., R.N., F.A.A.N

President, North American Nursing Diagnosis Association

On behalf of the officers and directors of the North American Nursing Diagnosis Association, I would like to welcome you to the Seventh Conference on Classification of Nursing Diagnoses. Interest in nursing diagnosis has increased considerably since the 1970's when a conference such as this would attract 100 to 200 nurses. What has been maintained is the blend of ideas from practitioners, educators, researchers, and theorists and the sharing of those ideas with the hope of improving our nursing care services to individuals, families, and communities.

Nursing diagnosis is the gateway to scientific practice. It provides a structure for knowledge development within nursing science, a focus for clinical research, and a language to clearly communicate to legislators, third-part payors, administrators, and consumers the need for access to nursing care.

Nursing diagnosis, as the gateway to scientific practice, does not deny nursing diagnosis as a gateway to expressing humanistic concern. In fact, what could be more appropriate to patients concerned with "Will I be able to. . .?" than a nurse's focus on the patient's experience of immobility, impaired home maintenance management, and anticipatory anxiety? Many have commented on our technologically oriented health care system, a system that encourages us to frequently place disease-related care before human responses, respect cure-at-any-cost versus quality of life and prevention of illness and disability. We are asked to think about "production units" instead of people. Diagnosis-based nursing practice permits us to reach out to the person experiencing a problem, focus our treatment, and help people to improve the quality of their lives.

As have previous conferences, this Seventh conference will further shape developments in nursing practice. I welcome you to join in the examination of the ideas and research to be presented and to reflect on these with your colleagues from many states of the United States and provinces in Canada. Have a happy and stimulating conference.

CHAPTER 1

Keynote address: nursing taxonomies—state of the art

MYRTLE K. AYDELOTTE, Ph.D., F.A.A.N.
KATHRYN HOPE PETERSON, B.S.N., R.N.

The development of a knowledge base for nursing practice has been of particular concern for those who view nursing as a practice profession essential to the care of the ill and to the improvement of the health of people. The recognition that *practice* is central to nursing has accelerated a trend away from an emphasis upon educational technology and has placed more emphasis upon the identification, analysis, and refinement of the content upon which practice is based. The concept of *nursing diagnosis* has been the primary instrument in the refinement of that content. Although the idea of nursing diagnosis continues to be unacceptable to some nurses, its use, nevertheless, is gaining acceptance. The need for *taxonomy*, a classification system in nursing and a nomenclature for the system, is increasingly recognized.

To address the topic *Nursing Taxonomies: State of the Art* is a formidable task. It requires exploration of such matters as the domains of nursing knowledge, the definitions and criteria of taxonomy and classification, current practices in the construction of taxonomy and classification systems, and the nursing perspective. To focus my remarks for this presentation, I have chosen to address four questions:

- What is the historical development of nursing knowledge, its domains, its classification, and its language?
- What do we mean when we discuss taxonomy? Does it differ from classification systems of schemes?
- What are the current nursing taxonomies?
- What are the difficulties that confront us as we proceed on the task of developing our discipline?

DEVELOPMENT OF NURSING KNOWLEDGE AND ITS LANGUAGE

The historical development of *nursing diagnosis*, as a concept, is intimately related to the growth of nursing knowledge and recognition of nursing as a discipline. The idea of nursing diagnosis followed or emerged concurrently with the development and inclusion of a number of highly important ideas.

Although the general purpose of nursing has held constant since the writings of Florence Nightingale (Aydelotte, 1977; Rothrock, 1984), the growth of knowledge required for the execution of that purpose has been steady and spectacular. If one examines the development of nursing knowledge, three major periods are identified:

- Period of Transition—1920 to 1950
- Period of Enlightenment—1950 to 1970
- Period of Refinement—1970 to present

As Kathryn Peterson, my research assistant, and I were searching the early history of nursing practice, she examined a microfiche of the writings of Bertha Harmer, titled *Methods and Principles of Teaching the Principles and Practice of Nursing,* published in 1926. Harmer proposed what she called "the correct and most fruitful relation between the basic sciences, medicine and nursing. That is, while medicine draws directly from and is dependent upon the basic sciences, and nursing draws from medicine, should not nursing also derive its facts, principles, methods, spirit, and imagination directly from science?" She continued, "the problem then . . . was to find out, by study and experiment, whether this scientific method could be applied to nursing and whether by doing so a definite organized content of nursing knowledge could be built up as had resulted in medicine and other fields."

This remarkable woman continued her discussion to outline the approach to study, identifying the steps in problem solving: stating the problem; gathering all facts from various sources which would help solve the problem; reflecting upon what the facts revealed, "analyzing, weighing, comparing, making inferences, associated cause and effect; and selecting facts useful in solving the problem. The fourth step would be to draw conclusions and formulate a plan of care. . . ." The fifth step would be to apply and test out the plan. She referred to this as the scientific method of study and proposed that, by using it, a definite, organized body of knowledge could be developed.

Later in the book she raised the question, "Should not nurses prescribe nursing care

for each patient as doctors prescribe medical care?" To prescribe means simply "to write before" or "to designate in writing." Harmer proposed "nursing treatments," the collection of records indicating their use, and analysis of the data. By studying these, she proposed to "organize knowledge—the process of making science." Further, in the *Outline of Case Study,* she used the term *diagnosis,* modifying the word by social, but defined it further by "that is what the immediate problem seems to be."

I cannot help but wonder, where would we be in the development of nursing knowledge if Harmer's proposals had been closely followed?

The *Period of Discovery* (the first period, 1920–1950) is characterized by common knowledge drawn from the physical and medical sciences. Much of this knowledge was stated as facts and principles underlying procedures and tasks performed by nurses. The terms *nursing needs* and *health needs* appeared increasingly in the 1940's, and the "ability to think critically, relating facts and principles, and interpreting data in light of them" was given as essential to the nurse's performance. Problem solving was stressed, but it was not directed toward making a nursing diagnosis or planning action. In a footnote appearing in *Nursing for the Future,* Esther Lucile Brown (1948, p. 138) stated that faculty should "cultivate in students a far greater skill in the use of words and conceptual thinking than has been undertaken as yet." Nursing was, in large part, viewed as dependent upon medicine, although independent functions were recognized. The independent functions were achieved by carrying out nursing procedures, which were carefully described and taught. The early textbooks and procedure books emphasized personal attributes, adherence to procedures and techniques, careful observation, and reporting of medical signs and symptoms and changes in these. There was little emphasis placed upon the development of clinical judgment and independence and nursing's own language.

The year 1947 is highly significant. In the first edition of *Legal Aspects of Nursing*, Lesnick and Anderson, in a lengthy footnote (1947, p. 157), discussed the word *diagnosis*. They stated:

Although diagnosis has been long regarded as the province of the physician, there is current belief, and support for that belief, that this province warrants clarification insofar as the activities of nursing are concerned.

Approached basically, diagnosis involves the utilization of intelligence in interpreting known facts. The decision is the result of interpretation. Certainly the utilization of intelligence is not the exclusive province of the physician, insofar as this inseparable aspect of the science of diagnosis is concerned. A definition of nursing which embraces the functions of symptoms and reactions assumes that aspect of diagnosis which requires the exercise of intelligence.

This statement is a precursor of the writings by McManus and Fry (1953), in which they used the term *nursing diagnosis*. McManus' personal papers (1950) suggest that others were also using the term, for example, Leino, Reiter, and Abdellah. During the 1950's and 1960's, the term *nursing diagnosis* underwent many interpretations but has gradually emerged with a meaning which is gaining acceptance, although stated definitions vary.

The second period, *Period of Exploration*, 1950–1970, was precipitated by the recognition that nurses used their intelligence in making decisions about the clinical conditions of their patients. In this period, major events bearing upon nursing practice took place:
- The study of nursing functions which described in major categories the activities of nurses in different settings (Hughes, *et al.*, 1958).
- The development of the concept that practitioners use logic in their practice. The logic has been called *nursing process*. The term *nursing process* appeared a few years after the term *nursing diagnosis* (Douglas and Murphy, 1981), but its evolution parallels and intertwines with nursing process. Since its introduction, nursing process has been described by many authors who disagree about the number of steps in the process and what they are properly called (Mitchell and Walter, 1976; Brodt, 1978; Stelzer and Becker, 1982; Henderson, 1978; Bulechek and McCloskey, 1985).
- A classification of nursing problems (Abdellah and others, 1959; Heidgerken, 1959).
- Introduction of the problem-oriented medical record (Carnevali, 1976).
- Concept development, clarification, and some clinical testing (Norris, 1982).
- Development of nursing theories and methodologies for clinical nursing research.

The interplay of these various ideas gave rise to the need for the development of a standard taxonomy, a classification system, and nomenclature for nursing practice. The definitions of critical terms in nursing were confused, and consequently, terms were misused (Bloch, 1974).

The refinement of language, synthesis of ideas, and the development of a classification system based on nursing diagnosis characterizes the third period, the *Period of Refinement*.

The nursing literature of 1984 emphasizes the need for refinement of knowledge related to the nursing diagnosis. A search for a single approach or conceptual framework for the classification of the phenomena of nursing is apparent. The inductive method, used by the National Conferences (Gebbie and Lavin, 1975; Kim and Moritz, 1982; Kim, McFarland, and McLane, 1984), involves the development of nursing diagnoses from individual practice experiences. This has resulted in an eclectic approach to the categorization of diagnoses ranging from a pathophysiological to a biopsychosocial focus. The need for a deductive approach that utilizes a conceptual framework to generate nursing diagnoses has led to the adoption of Martha Roger's concept of *unitary man* by the National Conference (Roy, 1984). However, the need to refine this work has been identified. Issues, such as definition of terms, levels of abstraction, pattern characteristics and congruence with the principles of classification and development of a taxonomy must be addressed. Many individuals have contributed to this period. Six major national meetings have been held by the National Conference on the Classification of Nursing Diagnoses since 1973. At the fifth conference, 1982, a new name, North American Nursing Diagnosis Association (NANDA), was adopted to mark the inclusion of nurses from Canada. The articles and books on the subject are numerous. Regional and local groups are meeting to pursue the problem. The surge of activity is remarkable.

With this brief history of nursing knowledge development as background, I now wish to turn to a more particular discussion of the development of knowledge and the language used in its description and communication. It is not my intent to discuss theory and its development. I wish to make only two points. The first deals with the importance of language in the development and use of knowledge. Knowledge is a complicated type of symbolism, expressed through language. Symbols (language as labels) are used to convey the interpretation of our experience gained through perception or intuition. Second, knowledge is structured by the mind. It is the result of thinking, by which we select experiences and interpret those experiences. The social inheritance of language is highly important, for through its use, a conceptual interpretation of experiences is handed down. The individual does not create the world in which he lives, but each determines it to the extent of individual selections and interpretation (Lee, 1973). In nursing, by our use of language and by our selection of experiences and the interpretation of them to ourselves and others, we determine the nursing world, for we see the world through a nursing perspective (Smirvov, 1970).

Knowledge development evolves through seven stages (Tavanec, 1970):

- Observation of phenomena and collection of observations by use of established protocols
- Analysis of those observations and discovery of empirical connections between elements
- Discovery of the behavior of the system of connections, or of the relation of one characteristic to another, leading to prediction
- Elaboration of the basic ideas and the discovery of fundamental relations, basic to explanation and to the construction of a theory
- Formulation of a theory
- Explanation of scientific facts, that is, through empirical testing
- Discovery of empirical connections through theoretical descriptions

These seven stages are very similar to the four levels of theory building in nursing, as proposed by Dickoff and James (1968) and to those referred to in the papers by Kritek (1978, 1979), Jacox (1974), and Kim (1973).

Examining these stages, one can see that knowledge evolves, changes, reforms, and gradually becomes more certain. It may become common knowledge. It moves from its early formation to that of being well structured knowledge with distinct boundaries, well developed generalizations, precise language, established predictions, programmed decisions, and easy communication.

What, then, is nursing's subject matter?

What is its knowledge base? The subject matter of the discipline is the concepts and the links between the concepts. The structure of the knowledge includes the pattern of the relationships between these concepts, the logic of the relationships, and the methodological approaches used in the study of the discipline; that is, how we look at reality. The "goodness" of the structure is estimated by the degree to which information is simplified for its use by members of the profession, to the extent that it leads to the generation of new propositions, and the utility of the concepts and prescriptions in practice. If the theory explains and predicts empirical phenomena, thus generating knowledge and guidelines for practitioners, it is useful.

The concepts may be one of two kinds: those that are property concepts which express the state of things, a description of phenomena such as patient states; or process concepts, the way to make things happen, for example, nursing interventions or treatments. The gathering of concepts into bundles results in three types of knowledge. The first two, explanatory and descriptive knowledge, lead to prediction (that is, what will happen) and the third, prescriptive knowledge, indicates what kind of action is prescribed to make things happen. Prescriptive knowledge is that knowledge drawn upon by practicing professions. Dickoff and James (1968), Kim (1983), and Kritek (1978) have stressed this point. The other types of knowledge are used primarily by those who study the discipline in order to eventually generate prescriptive knowledge or to teach practitioners.

Knowledge is organized through thinking and it is systematized under master concepts called categories. Categories or classes are related to each other by inclusion or exclusion, made explicit in their definitions. The logical formulation places the categories or classes in a structure of delineated and articulated relationships, derived from the process of analysis, generalization, and abstraction. The intent of the logical sorting out and placing of concepts into major categories is to introduce order in the real world into the experience of the individual. As a result of the placement, one can coherently relate and assimilate the concepts into the rest of one's experience. Lee (1973, p. 233) states that "a critical categorical scheme produces a well-ordered experience and yields understanding. Understanding is achieved when it is shown how each part or aspect of experience is related to all other parts or aspects." Of course, no category is absolute, for these major concepts will change over time with each new discovery, be that discovery by empirical testing or new insight. This construction of a critical categorical scheme is the business to which we are currently attending. The design of a taxonomy and a classification scheme has been the primary goal of the North American Nursing Diagnosis Association.

The basic criterion for organization of nursing knowledge is, of course, the nursing perspective. It is appropriate, then, for me to share with you my nursing perspective. To me, nursing is a practicing profession. Its central focus is the patient or client, be that an individual, a group, or a community. The intent of nursing is to enable an individual or individuals in groups and communities to function with the least amount of nursing assistance possible. Nursing is practiced in an environment. The practice requires the use of nursing tools and technology. It requires that the individual practicing hold certain beliefs, values, and attitudes about practice, the social worth of what is done for clients, and the social worth of the client. Nursing practice involves the use of diagnoses, interventions, and outcomes. Interventions are intrusions into the person, life, or environment of individuals that are intended to bring about or maintain beneficial changes for those involved (Thomas, 1984).

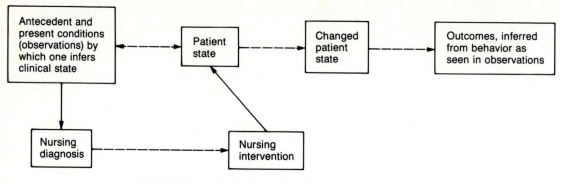

FIGURE 1 Patient states and nursing intervention

The schematic model I have used (Fig. 1) sets forth these ideas (Aydelotte, 1977).

NURSING TAXONOMY: A GENERAL DEFINITION

The word *taxonomy* is derived from two Greek words meaning *arrangement* or *order* and *distribution*. The word was defined in 1893 as follows:

Taxonomy is that branch of botany which has as its object the combination of all our observations on plants so as to form a system of classification (The Oxford Dictionary, 1933, p. 122).

Implied in this early definition and the words of its origin are two ideas: that of *classification* and *order*, the latter based upon principles of distribution which lead to an arrangement of categories.

Sokol makes distinctions between taxonomy and classification. He defines *classification* as a process during which objects (or phenomena) "are ordered into groups or sets on the basis of their relationships" (Sokol, 1974, p. 1116). Classification systems are the products of this process. Taxonomy is the science of how to classify and identify. Identification is the allocation or assignment of additional unidentified objects to the correct class, once such classes have been established by prior classification.

In my paper today, I will choose to use these distinctions which are also referred to

in the writings of Woods (1984), Douglas and Murphy (1981), Bircher, (1975, 1978), Lunney (1984), and Gordon (1983). I will attempt to keep in my use of language a clear distinction between process, product, and science. I will discuss in the next section of this paper current classification schemes which make use of the second meaning of the word *taxonomy*.

The writings pertaining to the science of taxonomy contain general ideas that are applicable to the nursing field, both the product and classification and the process itself. The general purposes of engaging in classification are well known: to establish a system that enables us to economically summarize information; to make it easy for us to use it; to enable us to retrieve information quickly; to describe relationships between the parts of it, leading to generalizations; and to generate hypotheses. Regardless of the field under study, these are the general purposes for which we engage in classification.

Principles of classification, included in the science of taxonomy, relate to the criteria by which objects are grouped, the relationship between names given to classes of entities and their objective definitions, and the perception of similarity. Sokol (1974) and others (Schenk and McMasters, 1956; Sokol and Sneath, 1963) discuss these in detail and I will attempt a brief summary. Sokol does not discuss the development of objective definitions and the labelling of the object itself, a task in which we are currently engaged in the development of nursing diagnoses. In other words, he and others do not offer advice on how to clearly identify, with observer reliability, that what we see, as Henry James, the novelist, uses the term in his writings. Sokol does not propose how scholars and practitioners in a field should view their objects. Inferred in his writings and others is the idea that those who are making the classification have established the boundaries of the domain under study and have worked through the problems of the perspective by which objects are to be identified.

There are two major principles in classificatory theory. The principle of monothetic classification proposes that the established classes must differ by at least one property or characteristic that is common to the members of each class. An example of an application of this principle in the nursing field is the classification of nursing personnel in the occupation. Registered nurses are one class, practical nurses another, and nursing assistants, still another. Each class has a single property all share in common (that is, licensure) and which differentiates it from the other classes. Other properties may be similar to those in other classes, such as age, marital status, and so forth.

The second principle of classificatory theory is called polythetic classification. In application of this principle, "groups of individuals or objects share a large portion of their properties but do not necessarily agree on any one property" (Sokol, 1974, p. 1117). This principle has been used in the development of classes in patient classification systems based upon activity. Patients in Class IV may share certain characteristics, but any one characteristic will not necessarily be observed in all members of the class. Sokol points out that "many properties may be necessary to classify objects" (Sokol, 1974, p. 1117).

The development of classifications may be arrived at by different methods. Taxonomy suggests the arrangement of properties of objects by use of pairing, clustering, ordination, use of graphs and trees, evolutionary analysis, and complex arithmetic formulae. Techniques grow increasingly sophisticated. The problems in classification are, then, related to making a decision as to which principle is to be used in the establishment of classes and how similarities and dissimilarities are to be handled.

I have been puzzling over what is entailed in taxonomy development. Taxonomy, the science of classification, often emerges after the process of classification has been instituted. It appears to me that, to say we have a science of taxonomy, we need to minimally meet at least these few conditions:

- The purposes for the classification are clear and widely accepted by the profession.
- The procedures and rules for describing and naming properties (defining characteristics of phenomena) have been adopted and implemented. The parameters of the domain have been established.
- The principles and rules of ordering by which nursing diagnoses are placed into classes have been adopted.
- Criteria for classes and subclasses have been identified. These classes and subclasses have been defined and their definitions and labels convey a relationship which is logical and has meaning to the user. The relationship may be a serial relationship or an equivalence relation. The classes are exhaustive and mutually exclusive.
- The format or structure of the system has been selected and shows a relationship between classes and subclasses.

The result of classifying is a classification scheme or system, which is often the second meaning of the word taxonomy. Gebbie (1984, p. 4) says that, "In a taxonomy, diagnoses are associated in hierarchial schemes that present general classes of diagnoses, specific sub-groups or clusters and specific conditions." Kritek (1984, p. 77) enlarges slightly upon this idea: "Classification is the systematic arrangement of entities or categories according to their relevant features or properties. It assumes recognition of similarities as a basis of grouping or clustering and assigning entities into categories."

How does one judge the value of a classification scheme or system? A classification scheme, or a taxonomy, using the second meaning of the term, is judged by its general adequacy for the field under discussion, in other words, how well it provides an organized account of the discipline. I propose that the usefulness of a classification system for nursing depends on the following (Rudner, 1966; Kerlinger, 1973; Roy, 1975; Lunney, 1984; Woods, 1984):

- The degree to which definitions systematize the knowledge in the field, and lead to a standardized nomenclature
- The degree to which simplicity (economy) characterizes the system
- The power of the system—its range of application, its usefulness to practitioners in the field as well as to scholars and theorists
- The degree to which it clarifies the knowledge of the field—the validity and verifiability of the content included in the system, its internal consistency, it relation to the real world, and its focus on the nursing domain
- The degree to which it is relevant to other systems with which nursing deals
- The degree to which it stimulates and accommodates the discovery of new knowledge

CURRENT NURSING TAXONOMIES

This leads me to a discussion of current taxonomies. Using the first definition, that is, the science of taxonomy, and applying the criteria in the previous section, I suggest that a taxonomy for nursing diagnosis is emerging. My reply is based on the following argument.

A review of the literature indicates that the purposes for classifying nursing knowledge by diagnosis are gaining acceptance. There has been objection to the use of nursing diagnosis (Hagey and McDonough, 1984; Shamansky and Yanni, 1982) but the rebuttal of the objection has been immediate and powerful (Letters, *Nursing Outlook*, 1984; Kritek, 1985). Support for the use of nursing diagnoses and their classification is reflected in writings in a diverse set of publications. There has been a long history of recognition of the need for the development of nursing knowledge.

Second, procedures have been instituted for initiating the identification, documentation, labelling, and the review by expert task forces and the adoption of diagnoses by the North American Nursing Diagnosis Association (undated). The procedures, though they state four definitions of the term *diagnosis*, are clear. Dissemination of information is more consistent.

Unfortunately, some elements of the taxonomy and procedure are missing. The nomenclature is not yet standardized. Words continue to be used interchangeably and their meanings are sometimes ambiguous. In the literature, words such as characteristics, clues, signs, symptoms, and etiology appear without reference to their meaning or whether they are the same or different. Nursing action, intervention, and treatment are used interchangeably, but are the meanings of all interchangeable? Pattern and cluster, likewise, present the same difficulty. The reports of the Minimum Data Set Conference, called by Werley and Lang, which was held May 15–17, 1985, have not yet been disseminated. That group may be addressing the further problem of uniformity of language and its meaning as Werley and

Grier did in their earlier publication (1981). The importance of the establishment of a standard nomenclature prior to classification cannot be overemphasized.

No principle for ordering of classes has yet been established, other than an alphabetical listing, and perhaps the greatest drawback is that there is not yet full agreement on the nursing perspective. We still see the domain of practice in different frameworks and have not yet negotiated an unambiguous field for viewing. These are problems being addressed by the various task forces of the North American Nursing Diagnosis Association.

What about the second meaning of *taxonomy?* Do we have classification systems? Nurses have always engaged in classification, although our efforts may be somewhat unsophisticated and have resulted in a "folk taxonomy." When we consider classification systems in nursing, we examine the systems or schemes developing in all domains—practice, settings, patients and clients, personnel, technology, and tools. I will describe the state of the art of classification in only a few of these before I turn to the major subject, nursing diagnosis.

For years, nurses have been classifying patients. We have always recognized that some patients are more acutely ill and require more care than others. Attempts to operationalize the categorization of patients have been reported in the literature during the last 50 years.

Patient classification methodologies can be defined as "the systematic identification and assessment of the nursing care requirements of a group of patients" resulting in the placing of patients into categories with similar time requirements for care and, in some cases, with similar aspects of care. The earlier systems were very subjective, casting individual patients into global types, but modern, highly sophisticated systems make use of more precise measurement of both aspects of care and time required to perform aspects of care.

It is interesting, and worth one's time, to review the evolution of these systems. In doing so, one can identify over different periods of time themes of concern about their use and one can also examine the implications of the use of the systems. Questions remain about their future development and application.

Currently, a number of systems for classification of patients are in use in medicine and in nursing. Hartley and McKibbin (1984) state that the present day systems are based on the type of information used for classification, the factors selected to develop categories. Hartley and McKibbin describe five types: procedure based; acuity based; disease based; those that combine disease, procedures, and complications; and intensity plus disease based. They indicate that, for the most part, the nursing classification systems fall within the acuity-based grouping. The other groups are essentially medical systems. The differences between medical and nursing patient classification systems relate to the variety of information contributing to the categories; the range and diversity of that information; and the scope and depth of the information.

In their recent book on nursing staff, Lewis and Corini (1984) identify three basic styles of patient classification systems used in nursing: the descriptive style, which is highly subjective; the checklist style, which provides a description of care by activities and uses value units and estimated time for each activity; and time or relative value unit style, which uses direct care measurement obtained through time and motion studies.

Patient classification systems in nursing are used as part of the nursing management information system. They serve to predict basic staffing needs, for planning variable staffing, and for cost-accounting nursing services. Two elements are gradually being introduced into patient classification systems and nursing staffing methodologies that may, in the future, modify the approach to patient classification systems. As nursing theories develop, the descriptors under consideration may change, and as nursing diagnosis and interventions become more precise these may be built into the system in place of the current aspects and procedural practices. The patient care descriptors used at Virginia Mason Hospital, Oncology Unit, reflect the Roy Adaptation Model (DeLeon, 1983). Halloran, who has compared nursing diagnosis and medical diagnosis as predictors of nursing workload and found differences, is continuing the use of nursing diagnosis as the basis for classification of patients.

The knowledge and skill of both engineering and nursing have been brought to bear upon the development of patient classification schemes and staffing methodology. As nursing continues to develop its scientific base and sets forth with more precision, nursing diagnoses and interventions, new patient classification systems will emerge. These will be similar to the diagnostic-related groups (DRGs) of medicine and will accurately depict nursing work load. It will also give us a standardized patient classification system for nursing, one that will be consistent among various nursing units and institutions.

In the conclusion of the review of the literature pertaining to staffing methodologies, I recommended that patient classification schemes be built around nurses' perceptions of care (Aydelotte, 1973). These should be constructed and tested. One sentence reads, "It should be based on data used by nurses in assessing patient care requirements" (Aydelotte, 1973, p. 65). I still believe the statement.

Classification schemes have not yet been developed for nursing interventions, treatments, or actions. As I stated, these terms have been used interchangeably. Lists of what a nurse can perform for patients or clients appear with the report of a nursing diagnosis but these appear as tasks or acts. But how do we classify these tasks or acts?

Neither have we classified those we serve and their environments. Reference is made to clients, patients, individuals, families, significant others, units, and physical settings. Imprecise descriptors are attached to these various terms.

We are today most concerned about the classification schemes for nursing diagnosis. Numerous principles of ordering classification systems are being introduced into the literature, but none of the systems is yet well developed. A review of the literature for the last 5 years reveals several frameworks for the study and development of nursing diagnosis and proposals for classifying diagnoses. At the Fifth National Conference on Classification of Nursing Diagnoses (1984), Kritek identified a number of organizing principles in the then existing classification systems. I have noted at least ten different frameworks appearing in the literature and influencing classification. These range in complexity, and some draw upon the work of different theorists. The frameworks, including a few phrases to enlarge upon their descriptions are:

- Patterns of unitary man (Roy, 1984)
  Health pattern in point of time/space
  Interactional patterns between man/environment
- Adaptation (Johnson, 1984)
  Adaptive dimensions, adopted from Gordon's functional health pattern
  Sequence across time dimension
- Health risks (Muecke, 1984)
  Epidemiological approach
- Child and youth taxonomy (Burns and Thompson, 1984)
  V.N.A. taxonomy
  Plus medical domain
- Self-care (applications of Orem's theory; Greenfield and Pace, 1984)
  Universal

Health-deviated

Developmental

- Functional health patterns (Hauck and Roth, 1984)

    Adaptation of Gordon's functional health patterns

- Body systems (Thompson, *et al.*, 1986)

    Related to nursing diagnosis

- Disequilibrium (response to stress; Wiens, 1985)

- Task *x* competencies required of client/family (Pridham and Schutz, 1985)

- Daily living, environment, functional health status, age, developmental tasks, and pathology (Carnevali, *et al.*, 1984)

- Alterations (appreciation of Krug's theory; Moulton, 1984)

Suggested in these frameworks is the idea that nurses are using "overlapping maps" to identify data from which decisions regarding diagnosis are made. These "maps" are drawn from the knowledge domains of human development and normal and abnormal human functioning, drawing upon physiology, psychology, sociology, and pathology. The boundaries are vague since the knowledge domains overlap.

The review of literature reveals that the classes for placement of nursing diagnoses are not well defined. The list of diagnoses prepared and adopted by the North American Nursing Diagnosis Association are reflected in many articles on the subject. Reference is made to major diagnoses, and the resultant subgroups are stated as variations, alterations, deficits, impairments, imbalance, and intolerance. The diagnostic data are called *attributes, characteristics, behaviors, cues, indicators, factors, signs, symptoms* and *etiology*. A great deal of data is being collected in relation to each diagnosis, but there is little evidence that it is critically and clinically relevant.

PROBLEMS AND ISSUES

A number of problems and issues are apparent from the review of the literature. Stan-

dardization of nomenclature is sadly lacking, presenting much semantic difficulty. The development of a consistent nomenclature precedes the development of classification. There is inconsistency in the labelling of diagnoses, less so since the publishing of the list of diagnoses approved by the North American Nursing Diagnosis Association. Classes of data have not been defined and labelled consistently.

One of the most serious problems, however, is the absence of isolated, defined, clinically validated, and reliable diagnostic data that are associated with a particular diagnosis. Although Gordon and Sweeney (1979) have addressed how these methodological problems can be handled, there have been few studies identifying and validating what data are needed to make a specific diagnosis and differentiating that diagnosis from others (McLane and Fehring, 1984). The tendency is to collect as much information as possible about a particular problem or response or health state of a patient or client which nurses have the knowledge and skill to treat (Grier, 1981).

Gordon's (1985) review of the research of nursing diagnosis is an excellent one. She points out the paucity of clinical research to identify and validate nursing diagnostic concepts. In her review of research from 1953–1983, Gordon found that the studies lacked consistency in concept labels, definitions, and diagnostic labels and presented variations in estimates of reliability and validity. Gordon concluded that the pressing problems or needs, are six-fold: to refine concepts; to identify predictor variables; to identify co-occurrence of nursing diagnoses; to determine the influence on the practice setting, specialty, and level of care; to carry out epidemiological studies; and to conduct studies of clinical validity and reliability.

Problems evident from the review of publications relate to perception of the matter under study, the complexity of the phenomena with which nursing deals, and its scope, variety, and range (Webster, 1984). Our unwillingness to establish boundaries for the domain of nursing practice make it exceedingly difficult to identify and simplify the data which are clinically relevant and manageable. Our perception of nursing varies greatly. This is a result of the great diversity of practitioners in the field, the diversity of the populations we serve, and our inability to accept the expertise of our nursing colleagues. We have not yet demonstrated confidence in those of our colleagues who are experts.

This review of the state of the art on nursing taxonomies finds us at a point where we are gathering the basic information regarding our objects, the diagnoses themselves. Unfortunately, we see and describe these objects from varying vantage points, from our individual perspectives. We also describe them in our individual terms. Fortunately, we are moving toward a common perspective and, in time, a common language.

We are struggling to find a means of classifying objects in a vast field. Medicine has adopted more than one major parameter or axis for its classification of diseases (Levy, 1981; World Health Organization, 1977; Thomas and Hayden, 1952). What will be nursing's axes or parameters? So far, we have not found an answer to our dilemma, but I am confident the answer will be found. This is no time to be discouraged or impatient. We are at an embryonic stage in this development. The task forces on taxonomy have been struggling with this very difficult task. They are to be commended on their effort. We must remember that there is no simple, quick answer and we must be steady in our search and patient with each other.

CONCLUSION

This assessment of the state of the art of nursing taxonomies may appear harsh. This was not my intent. My purpose has been to describe where we are at this point in time. We need also to look back to discover how far we have come. Let me review for you a little of our recent past.

The first national conference was held in 1973. Since that time, the number of nurses who are committed and involved in the development of nursing diagnoses and their classification is in the thousands. The writings on the subject are numerous and burgeoning.

Examples of how the concept of nursing diagnosis is being implemented in practice settings appear in the literature (Yoder, 1984; Mackie, *et al.*, 1984; Adams, 1984; Davidson, 1984; Hickey, 1984; Novotony-Dinsdale, 1985; Rantz, *et al.*, 1985; Cleary, 1985). Nurses are also reporting the development of individual nursing diagnoses and the interventions associated with them (Boss, 1984; Engelking and Steel, 1984; Fredette, 1984; Howers, 1984; Carpenito, 1985; Cregger and Strickland, 1985; Dalton, 1985; Dougherty, 1985; Taylor, 1985; Bulecheck and McCloskey, 1985). Many of these draw upon the guidelines and approved set of diagnoses of the North American Nursing Diagnosis Association. A few are examining the relation of medical and nursing diagnoses, an unresolved problem to date (Soares, 1978; Taylor, 1985; Hickey, 1984).

The quality of the content is vastly improved. Clinical nursing studies are beginning to appear, and many are more aware of the nature of the research that needs to be done.

Through conferences and publications, the nature and purpose of taxonomy, classification, and nomenclature are being introduced to a wide audience. A coalition of educators, theorists, clinicians, and administrators has been brought together to bring about a move to get knowledge about diagnoses into the minds of all. As a result of this effort, the base is being built for the acceptance of the work being done.

One must not forget that the present generation of students are the ones who will accept or reject the product of our current effort to classify. Highly influential in the acceptance or rejection of new knowledge and new language are those who influence the practice settings, nurse-administrators. I propose that these individuals be well educated in new practice trends, nursing theories, the use of nursing diagnoses, the idea of treatment, and the need for classification and nursing diagnostic systems. Such a proposal is timely. Forward-looking administrators see a relation between nursing diagnoses, the use of diagnostic-related groups, and payment of services.

A question to which no reference has been made in my reading is: Who is qualified to make a nursing diagnosis? By inference, it falls within the purview of the professional nurse. Given nursing's tendency to give away or readily share the content of its practice, I pose this sticky question: Who is qualified to make the diagnosis? As diagnoses are ordered by level of abstraction, is there a level at which decision making will be accorded to support personnel? Since we have not yet achieved a structure for the occupation, will we be befuddled on this decision regarding nursing diagnosis? Will certain diagnoses be made by selected categories of nursing personnel? You may say that to raise this question is premature; I argue it is not. Nursing has tended to operate by egalitarian principles rather than by rational reasoning. Experience has shown that, all too often, authority is allowed to be assumed by others before the matter is fixed.

Another prickly question centers on the legitimization of the work being done in classification. At what point does the leadership group seek endorsement of its efforts from the professional and nursing organizations? The American Nurses' Association's action has been to legitimize nursing diagnosis through *Nursing: A Social Policy Statement* (1980), through types of legislation, and liaison. When will the approach to classification of the North American Nursing Diagnosis Association be officially endorsed? Likewise, when will the official endorsement of the several nursing specialty groups be sought? The political problem is not simple, and it is not too soon to plan a strategy. Our experience with the credentialling of nurses should teach us a number of important lessons.

The leaders of this group have brought about a movement greatly needed in nursing, and the excitement is wonderful to behold. I congratulate you all, but more than that, I thank this conference for refocusing nursing on its subject matter, its practice, and the need to structure it, to standardize our nomenclature, and to do research. You are making Bertha Harmer's dream a reality. And as one who has been engaged in executive work in nursing for many years, I can say, you are fulfilling a long-standing wish of my own.

REFERENCES

Abdellah, F.G., Beland, I.L., Martin, A., and others: Patient centered approaches to nursing, New York, 1959, Macmillan.

Adams, C.E.: Nursing diagnosis in patient care planning, Milit. Med. **149**(4):202-204, 1984.

American Nurses' Association: Nursing: a social policy statement, Kansas City, MO, The Association.

Aydelotte, M.K.: Nurse staffing methodology: a review and critique of selected literature, D.H.E.W. Pub. No. NIH73-433. U.S.H.E.W., P.H.S., N.I.H. Bureau of Health Manpower Education, Div. Nursing, Washington, D.C., 1973.

Aydelotte, M.K.: Clinical nursing investigation and the structure of knowledge. In Miller, M.H. and Flynn, B.C. editors: Current perspectives in nursing: social issues and trends, St. Louis, 1977, The C.V. Mosby Co.

Bircher, A.U.: On the development and classification of nursing diagnoses, Nurs. Forum **14**(11):10-29, 1975.

Bircher, A.U.: The concept of nursing diagnosis. In Kim, M.J. and Moritz, D.A. editors: Classification of nursing diagnoses: proceedings of the third and fourth national conferences, New York, 1978, McGraw-Hill.

Bloch, D.: Some crucial terms in nursing: what do they really mean? Nurs. Outlook 22(11):689-694, 1974.

Boss, B.J.: Dysphasia, dyspraxia, and dysarthria: distinguishing features, Part II, J. Neurosurg. Nurs. 16(4):211-216, 1984.

Brodt, D.E.: The nursing process. In Chaska, N.L. editor: The nursing profession: views through the mist, New York, 1978, McGraw-Hill.

Brown, E.L.: Nursing for the future, New York, 1948, Russell Sage Foundation.

Bulechek, G.M., and McCloskey, J.C., editors: Nursing interventions: treatments for nursing diagnoses, Philadelphia, 1985, W.B. Saunders Co.

Burns, C.E., and Thompson, M.K.: Developing a nursing classification system for P.N.P.'s, Ped. Nurs. 10(6):411-414, 1984.

Carnevali, D.: Nursing process: a problem-oriented system. In Walter, J.B., Pardee, G.P., and Molbo, D.M. editors: Dynamics of problem-oriented approaches: patient care and documentation, Philadelphia, 1976, J.B. Lippincott Co.

Carnevali, D.: Nursing care planning: diagnoses and management, Philadelphia, 1983, J.B. Lippincott Co.

Carnevali, D., Mitchell, P.H., Woods, N.F., and others: Diagnostic reasoning in nursing, Philadelphia, 1984, J.B. Lippincott Co.

Carpenito, L.J.: Diagnosing nutrition problems, Am. J. Nurs. 85(5):584, 1985.

Cleary, M.J.: Integration of the nursing diagnostic process in the clinical setting, Crit. Care Nurse 5(1):28-30, 1985.

Cregger, N.J., and Strickland, C.C.: Selecting a nursing diagnosis for change in consciousness, Dim. Crit. Care Nurs. 4(3):156-163, 1985.

Dalton, J.: A descriptive study: defining characteristics of the nursing diagnosis, cardiac output, alterations in: decreased, Image 17(4):113-117, 1985.

Davidson, S.B.: Nursing diagnosis: its application in the acute care setting, Topics Clin. Nurs. 5(4):50-56, 1984.

DeLeon, T.M.: The development of an oncological patient classification system using the Roy adaptation model. In Nursing staffing based on patient classification: an examination of case studies. Chicago, 1983, American Hospital Association.

Dickoff, J., and James, P.: A theory of theories: a position paper, Nurs. Res. 17(3):197-203, 1968.

Dickoff, J., and James, P.: Researching research's role in theory development, Nurs. Res. 17(3):204-206, 1968.

Dougherty, C., editor: Symposium on nursing diagnoses, Nurs. Clin. North Am. 20(4):787-799, 1985.

Douglas, D.J., and Murphy, E.K.: Nursing process, nursing diagnosis, and emerging taxonomies. In McCloskey, J.C. and Grace, H.K. editors: Current issues in nursing, Boston, 1981, Blackwell.

Engelking, C.H., and Steele, N.E.: A model of pretreatment assessment of patients receiving cancer chemotherapy, Cancer Nurs. 7(3):203-212, 1984.

Fredette, S.L.: When the liver fails, Am. J. Nurs. 84(1):64-67, 1984.

Fry, V.S.: The creative approach to nursing, Am. J. Nurs. 53(3):301-302, 1953.

Gebbie, K.M.: Development of a taxonomy of nursing diagnosis. In Walter, J.B., Pardee, G.P., and Molbo, D.M. editors: Dynamics of problem oriented approaches: patient care and documentation, Philadelphia, 1976, J.B. Lippincott Co.

Gebbie, K.M., and Levin, M.A., editors: Classification of nursing diagnosis: proceedings of the first national conference, St. Louis, 1975, The C.V. Mosby Co.

Gordon, M.: Nursing diagnosis and the diagnostic process. In Chaska, N.L. editor: The nursing profession: views through the mist, New York, 1978, McGraw Hill.

Gordon, M.: Diagnostic category development. In McCloskey, J.C. and Grace, H.K., editors: Current issues in nursing, ed. 2, Boston, 1985, Blackwell.

Gordon, M.: Nursing diagnosis. In Werley, H.H. and Fitzpatrick, J.J. editors: Annual review of nursing research, vol. 3, New York, 1985, Springer Verlag.

Gordon, M. and Sweeney, M.A.: Methodological problems and issues in identifying and standardizing nursing diagnoses, Advan. Nurs. Sci. 2:1-5, 1979.

Greenfield, E., and Pace, J.C.: Orem's self-care theory of nursing: practical application to the end-stage renal disease (ESRD) patient, J. Nephrol. Nurs. 2(4):187-193, 1985.

Grier, M.R.: The need for data in making nursing decisions. In Werley, H.H. and Grier, M.R. editors: Nursing information systems, New York, 1981, Springer Verlag.

Hagey, R., and McDonough, P.: The problem of professional labeling, Nurs. Outlook 32(3):151-157, 1984.

Halloran, E.J.: Nursing diagnosis for patient classification in the development of a process-oriented nurse staffing methodology. In Werley, H.H., and Grier, M.R. editors: Nursing information systems, New York, 1981, Springer Verlag.

Hardy, J.A.: A patient classification system for home health patients, Caring 3(9):26-27, 1984.

Harmer, B.: Methods and principles of teaching the practice of nursing, New York, 1926, MacMillan.

Hartley, S.S., and McKibbin, R.C.: Hospital payment mechanisms, patient classification systems and nursing: relationships and implications, Kansas City, MO, 1983, American Nurses Association.

Hauck, M.R., and Roth, D.: Application of nursing diagnoses in a pediatric clinic, Ped. Nurs. 10(1):49-52, 1984.

Heiderken, L.E., editor: Improvement of nursing through research, Proceedings of the workshop on improvement of nursing through research, Catholic University of America, June 14-24, 1958, Washington, D.C., 1959, Catholic University of America Press.

Henderson, R: Nursing diagnosis: theory and practice, Advances Nurs. Sci. 1(1):75-83, 1978.

Hickey, M.: Nursing diagnosis in the critical care unit, Dimen. Crit. Care Nurs. 3(2):91-97, 1984.

Howes, A.C.: Nursing diagnosis and care plans for ambulatory care patients with AIDS, Topics Clin. Nurs. 6(2):61-66, 1984.

Hughes, E.C., Hughes, H.M., and Deutscher, I.: Twenty thousand nurses tell their story, Philadelphia, 1958, J.B. Lippincott Co.

Jacox, A.: Theory construction in nursing: an overview, Nurs. Res. 23(1):4-13, 1974.

Johnson, M.N.: Theoretical basis for nursing diagnosis in mental health, Issues Mental Health Nurs. 6(1-2):53-71, 1984.

Kerlinger, F.N.: Foundations for behavioral research, New York, 1973, Holt, Rinehart & Winston.

Kim, H.S.: The nature of theoretical thinking in nursing, Norwalk, CT, 1983, Appleton-Century Crofts.

Kim, M.J., MacFarland, G.K., and McLane, A.M., editors: Classification of nursing diagnoses: proceedings of the fifth national conference, St. Louis, 1984, The C.V. Mosby Co.

Kim, M.J., and Moritz, D.A., editors: Classification of nursing diagnoses: proceedings of the third and fourth national conferences, New York, 1982, McGraw-Hill.

Kritek, P.: Commentary: development of nursing diagnosis and theory, Adv. Nurs. Sci. 2(1):73-79, 1979.

Kritek, P.: Generation and classification of nursing diagnosis: toward a theory of nursing, Image 10:33-40, 1978.

Kritek, P.: Current nomenclature and classification systems: Pertinent issues. In Kim, M.J. McFarland, G.K. and McLane, A.M. editors: Classification of nursing diagnoses: proceedings of the fifth national conference, St. Louis, 1984, The C.V. Mosby Co.

Kritek, P.: Nursing diagnosis in perspective: response to a critique, Image 17(1):3-8, 1985.

Kritek, P.: Nursing diagnosis: theoretical foundations, Occ. Health Nurs. 33(8):393-396, 1985.

Lee, H.N.: Precepts, concepts and theoretic knowledge, Memphis, 1973, Memphis State University.

Lesnick, M.J., and Anderson, B.E.: Legal aspects of nursing, Philadelphia, 1947, J.B. Lippincott Co.

Levy, R.: The new language of psychiatry: learning and using DSM-III, Boston, 1981, Little, Brown & Co.

Lewis, E.N., and Carini, P.V.: Nurse staffing and patient classification, Rockville, MD, 1984, Aspen Systems Corp.

Lunney, M: A framework to analyze a taxonomy of nursing diagnosis. In Kim, M.J. McFarland, G.K. and McLane, A.M. editors: Classification of nursing diagnoses: proceedings of the fifth national conference, St. Louis, 1984, The C.V. Mosby Co.

Mackie, R., Peddie, R., and Pendleton, R.: Perioperative care plan guides: putting nursing diagnoses to work. AORN J. 40(2):192-201, 1984.

McLane, A.M., and Fehring, R.J.: Nursing diagnosis: a review of the literature. In Kim, M.J., McFarland, G.K., and McLane, A.M., editors: Classification of nursing diagnoses: proceedings of the fifth national conference (pp. 525-540), St. Louis, 1984, The C.V. Mosby Co.

McManus, R.: Personal papers, citations, publications, Hist. Nurs. Arch., Ser. 5, R. McManus Collection, Fiche 3205, 24:1, 1950.

McManus, R.: Series VIII. Personal papers, citations, publications. Series 5, R.L. McManus Collection. Hist. of Nurs. Arch., Fiche 3206, 24:1, 1950.

Mitchell, P., and Walter, J.B.: A conceptual framework. In Walter, J.B. Pardee, G.P. and Molbo, D.M. editors: Dynamics of problem oriented approaches: patient care and documentation, Philadelphia, 1976, J.B. Lippincott Co.

Moulton, P.J.: Chronic illness, grief, and the family, J. Commun. Health Nurs. 1(2):75-88, 1984.

Muecke, M.: Community health diagnosis in nursing, Pub. Health Nurs. 1(1):23-35, 1984.

Norris, C.M.: Concept clarification in nursing, Rockville, MD, 1982, Aspen Systems Corp.

North American Nursing Diagnosis Association. Development/submission guidelines for proposed new nursing diagnoses. Undated.

Novotony-Dinsdale, V.: Implementation of nursing diagnoses in one emergency department, J. Emerg. Nurs. 11(3):140-144, 1985.

Pridham, K.F., and Shutz, M.E.: Rationale for a language for naming problems from a nursing perspective, Image 17(4):122-127, 1985.

Rantz, M., Miller, T., and Jacobs, C.: Nursing diagnoses in long term care, Am. J. of Nurs. 85(8):916-917, 926, 1985.

Rothrock, J.C.: Nursing diagnosis: in the days of Florence Nightingale, AORN J. 40(2):189-190, 1984.

Roy, C.A.: A diagnostic classification system for nursing, Nurs. Outlook, 74(2):90-94, 1975.

Roy, C.A.: Framework for classification systems development: progress and issues. In Kim, M.J. McFarland, G.K. and McLane, A.M. editors: Classification of nursing diagnoses: proceedings of the fifth national conference, St. Louis, 1984, The C.V. Mosby Co.

Rudner, R.S.: Philosophy of social science, Englewood Cliffs, NJ, 1966, Prentice-Hall.

Schenk, E.T., and McMasters, J.H.: Procedure in taxonomy, ed. 3, Stanford, 1956, Stanford University Press.

Shamansky, S.L., and Yanni, C.R.: In opposition to nursing diagnosis: a minority opinion, Image **25**(2):47-50, 1983.

Smirvov, V.A.: Levels and stages of knowledge. In Tavanec P.V., editor: Problems in the logic of scientific knowledge, Dordrecht, Holland, 1970, D. Reidel.

Soares, C.A.: Nursing and medical diagnoses: a comparison of variant and essential features. In Chaska N.L. editor: The nursing profession: views through the mist, New York, 1978, McGraw-Hill.

Sokol, R.R.: Classification, principles, prospects, Science **185**:1115, 1974.

Sokol, R.R., and Sneath, P.H.A.: Principles of numerical taxonomy, San Francisco, 1963, W.H. Freeman & Co.

Stelzer, F.K., and Becker, A.M.: Historical development of nursing diagnosis. In Carlson, J.H. Craft, C.A. and McGuire, A.D.: Nursing diagnosis, Philadelphia, 1982, W.B. Saunders.

Tavanec, P.V.: Problems in the logic of scientific knowledge, Dordrecht, Holland, 1970, D. Reidel Publishing Co.

Taylor, J.W.: Nursing management of stroke: acute care—Part 1, Cardiovasc. Nurs. **21**(1):1-5, 1985.

Taylor, J.W.: Nursing management of stroke: acute care—Part 2, Cardiovasc. Nurs. **21**(2):7-12, 1985.

The Oxford English Dictionary: Vol. XI, T-U: Oxford, 1933, Clarendon Press.

Thomas, E.J.: Designing interventions for the helping professions, Beverly Hills, 1984, Sage Publications.

Thompson, E.T., and Hayden, A.C.: Standard nomenclature of diseases and operations, ed. 4, New York, 1952, McGraw-Hill.

Thompson, J.M., McFarland, G.K., Hirsch, J.E., and others: Clinical nursing, St. Louis, 1968, The C.V. Mosby Co.

Webster, G.A.: Nomenclature and classification system development. In Kim, M.J. McFarland, G.K. and McLane, A.M. editors: Classification of nursing diagnoses: proceedings of the fifth national conference (pp. 14-25), St. Louis, 1984, The C.V. Mosby Co.

Werley, H., and Grier, M.R.: Nursing information systems, New York, 1981, Springer Verlag.

Wiens, A.G.: Rehabilitation assessment—a nursing perspective, Rehab. Nurs. **10**(2):25-27, 1985.

Woods, N.F.: Toward a taxonomy of nursing phenomena. In Carnevali, D.L. Mitchell, P.H. Woods, N.F. and others: Diagnostic reasoning in nursing, Philadelphia, 1984, J.B. Lippincott Co.

World Health Organization. International classification of diseases: manual of the international statistical classification of disease, injuries and causes of death (Vol. 1). Geneva, 1977, The Organization.

Yoder, M.E.: Nursing diagnosis: application in perioperative practice, AORN J. **40**(2):183-188, 1984.

CHAPTER 2

Issues in nursing diagnosis

MARJORY GORDON, Ph.D., R.N., F.A.A.N

When one reflects on the issues surrounding nursing diagnosis and the definition of the term, discussions, debates, and disputes should come to mind. There is a profusion of issues in the area of nursing diagnosis, and a number generate much debate. The purpose of this paper is to lay to rest some issues from the 1970's, to recognize some current debates and disputes, and to review some issues that will require discussion for the rest of this decade and, no doubt, beyond.

We may lay to rest one question: *Do nurses diagnose?*

This aspect of nursing practice has been sanctioned by state laws, professional policy statements, and standards for professional nursing practice. It is a rare textbook that does not include nursing diagnoses. In addition, journals have published many articles on the subject, and four have devoted entire issues to nursing diagnosis. A related proposition that bears mention and burial is: *If nurses diagnose, physicians will get upset.* Most physicians welcome the care that patients receive with diagnosis-based interventions, and most professional nurses have learned to tolerate "upset" physicians. This is not to play down our colleagues' concern and responses to nurses seeking reimbursement for nursing services and private practice.

Debates and disputes around the conceptual focus of nursing diagnosis are still with us. Two issues insure lively interactions.

First, we have the much publicized issue surrounding "physiological" diagnoses. The question for debate can be framed as: *Should nursing diagnoses be created to describe all of nursing practice or only that segment of practice that is the unique, independent area of nursing expertise?* The answer does not lie in what nurses *do* in practice. All would agree on the realities: some problems are totally within the area of nursing expertise; others require medical diagnosis and treatment with the major aspects of treatment carried out and monitored by nurses until patients can manage on their own. The underlying issue is twofold: *What should be the broad conceptual focus of nursing diagnoses, that is, what class of health-related problems should nursing diagnoses describe?* and *When a health-related condition is referred to as a* nursing *diagnosis, what consequent responsibility and accountability for practice and research does this imply?*

The second issue that has received some attention is the lack of health-related or strengths-oriented nursing diagnoses. Reframing aspects of the previous questions demonstrates the relation of the two issues: *What should be the broad conceptual focus of nursing diagnoses? Should the concept be limited to problems and potential problems or should it also include healthy states and strengths?*

It is argued that we should not just identify problems. Most nurses would concur. The point is not, shall we identify strengths and help patients and families to use these strengths to solve problems or facilitate their growth, but rather shall strengths be called nursing diagnoses? Strengths are used in care planning but are not the focus of the plan. Health diagnoses are a different issue. They suggest a focus for intervention because through a desire or potential for growth the individual or family can reach higher levels of wellness than those described by health norms for populations. Concern is expressed that an "alterations-focused" classification system has no room for describing potential for growth beyond the accepted norms. Having mentioned the prominent areas for debate and dispute, let us now turn to issues currently under discussion.

VALIDITY AND RELIABILITY OF CATEGORIES

Validity of a diagnostic category describes the extent to which the cluster of defining characteristics represents a clinical reality. Reliability refers to the precision of defining characteristics. If a cluster of characteristics defining a category is reliable, it can be expected that there will be interdiagnostician agreement. This is similar to the measurement of inter-rater reliability.

Very few of the current diagnostic categories were developed from studies of patients. The majority were derived from nurses' recall of the signs and symptoms manifested when the problems were encountered. Some consensual validity was assumed when participants voted to accept categories proposed at biennial conferences, but no claim to representative sampling of nurses, settings, or regions can be made. Reliability of defining characteristics is a neglected area of research, although lack of agreement between clinicians in practice settings can occur and result in discrepancies in treatment.

Diagnostic categories began to be identified in 1973, but by 1981 only five studies were published in which data gave an indication that the phenomena described by these categories existed (Leslie, 1981; Jones and Jakob, 1981; Jones and Jakob, 1980; Halloran, 1980; Campbell, 1978; Gebbie, 1976). For the most part, these studies reported diagnostic labels; few were designed to provide validity and reliability estimates of defining characteristics.

In recent years studies have increased in number. Fifty-nine reports, stating that one or more nursing diagnoses were the focus of the study, were published between 1981 and early 1986. The majority are contained in publications of the North American Nursing Diagnosis Association (Hurley, 1986; Nursing Clinics of North America, 1985; Kim, McFarland, and McLane, 1984; Gould, 1983; Kim and Moritz, 1982; Avant, 1979; Guzzetta and Forsythe, 1979). Forty-three of these studies reported on defining characteristics or critical characteristics of diagnostic categories. Thirty-three different diagnoses were studied, 28 of which were listed by the North American Nursing Diagnosis Association (NANDA). Twenty of the studies were based on patient observations and 22 employed nurse consensus.

EPIDEMIOLOGICAL STUDIES

Investigators have studied the epidemiology of nursing diagnoses but not to the extent recommended by Brown (1974). Most studies have described nursing diagnoses in medical-surgical populations (Campbell, 1978; Gebbie, 1976; Gould, 1983; Halloran, 1980; Jones and Jakob, 1980; Leslie, 1980; Hoskins, McFarlane, Rubenfeld, and others, 1986). There has been one report from an obstetrical-gynecological area (McKeehan and Gordon, 1980) and one from community health (Simmons, 1980), neither of which provided full reports on the incidence of each diagnosis.

The knowledge gained from epidemiological studies is important for early case-finding and prevention and to increase nurses' cue-sensitivity when caring for populations in which the likelihood of certain diagnoses is high. These studies are necessary for the identification of age-related, cultural, or setting predispositions. In addition, knowledge about the co-occurrence of nursing diagnoses with specific medical diagnostic populations or DRG populations is important if changes are to be made in prospective reimbursement programs. The Halloran and Halloran study (1985) and Gould's (1983) small study of nursing diagnoses co-occurring with multiple sclerosis are examples of epidemiological studies focusing on medical disease populations. Also, identification of high-incidence nursing diagnoses can contribute to the refinement of patient classification tools when diagnoses are used as a basis for predicting nurse workload (Halloran, 1980).

FUTURE DIRECTION AND NEED

Explicit guidelines for the application of qualitative and quantitative research methodology in nursing diagnosis research are needed to stimulate studies in this area. Part of the reason for the dearth of research on diagnostic categories since identification began in 1973 is the lack of models for the design of clinical research in this area. Two articles (Fehring, 1986; Gordon and Sweeney, 1979) begin to meet this need, but research texts have ignored this critical area of nursing research. In addition to the need for the type of studies described above, research on the diagnostic process and on diagnostic errors is critical to accurate clinical implementation of nursing diagnosis. No studies of diagnostic errors have been reported, yet this type of study may suggest categories that need more precision in their definition and structure. Cross-cultural studies have not been done. This type of research is possible; nursing diag-

nosis is being used in parts of Nigeria, Japan, Australia, and South America. No investigators have studied the ethical issues that may arise in nursing diagnosis and treatment. Yet, nurses often comment that they do not have time for a nursing-based assessment and nursing diagnosis. This should be associated with ethical problems related to the allocation of resources.

Research and diagnostic category development has not kept pace with implementation in practice and incorporation of nursing diagnoses into the curricula of professional schools. For example, nursing diagnoses are being used as a basis for writing outcome and process standards (American Nurses' Association-American Association of Neuroscience Nurses, 1985) and in health-care agencies for quality assurance. A number of hospitals and community health agencies have computerized information systems that include nursing diagnoses, and many are contemplating a move in this direction. One hospital is studying a system for establishing nursing costs on the basis of nursing diagnoses (Halloran and Halloran, 1985). In addition, as nurses move toward reimbursement for their health care services, there will be a need for precise, reliable diagnostic categories that are correlated with nurses' time or patient visits.

It will also be necessary to examine the possibility of consolidating the work on classification by various groups. Nursing diagnoses have been identified in community health (Simmons, 1980), in large studies (Jones and Jakob, 1980), and by various specialty groups. Both similarities and dissimilarities with the NANDA-accepted diagnoses have to be examined. This is imperative for comparisons across settings, age groups, and DRGs. The profession should speak with one language.

The issue of one language to describe actual and potential problems of concern to nurses in their practice has arisen because of recent professional developments. The

President of the American Nurses' Association has written to the World Health Organization's Division on Classification requesting nursing participation in the next revision of the International Classification of Diseases. It may be possible to add fields containing nursing diagnoses to this often-used format for statistical reports. A second professional development is the work of the conference group on a nursing minimum data set; Werley's report of this work is included in these proceedings. The recommended nursing minimum data set (NMDS) for reporting health statistics includes nursing diagnoses, interventions, outcomes, an acuity or intensity factor, and demographic variables. Each datum within the set has to be based on a standardized classification. For example, an agency's nursing statistics report would have to use a standardized classification of nursing diagnoses in summarizing patient care activities for third party payors or for government reports. The NANDA classifications were viewed as most promising for this purpose. There is a need to consolidate existing classification systems and to increase the precision of diagnostic categories. The prospect of an international classification of nursing diagnoses and the work on the minimum data set for nursing suggest that research on diagnostic categories has to increase in scope and amount. Interest in this type of research has to be stimulated, and models for the design of research have to be developed and disseminated to interested investigators. These needs are urgent to the immediate future of nursing diagnosis.

REFERENCES

American Nurses' Association—American Association of Neuroscience Nurses: Standards for neuroscience nursing practice based on nursing diagnoses, Kansas City, MO, 1985, American Nurses' Association.

Avant, K.: Nursing diagnosis: maternal attachment, Ad. Nurs. Sci. **2:**45-55, 1979.

Brown, M.: The epidemiological approach to the study of clinical nursing diagnoses, Nurs. Forum **13:**346-359, 1974.

Campbell, C.: Nursing diagnosis and intervention in nursing practice, New York, 1978, John Wiley & Sons.

Fehring, R.J.: Validating diagnostic labels: standardized methodology. In Hurley, M. editor: Classification of nursing diagnoses: proceedings of the sixth conference, St. Louis, 1986, The C.V. Mosby Co.

Gebbie, K.M.: Research project. In Gebbie, K.M. editor: Classification of nursing diagnoses: summary of the second national conference, St. Louis, 1976, National Group for Classification of Nursing Diagnoses.

Gordon, M. and Sweeney, M.A.: Methodological problems and issues in identifying and standardizing nursing diagnoses, Adv. Nurs. Sci. **2:**1-15, 1979.

Gould, M.: Nursing diagnoses co-occurring with multiple sclerosis, J. Neurosurg. Nurs. **15:**339-345, 1983.

Guzzetta, C.E. and Forsythe, G.L.: Nursing diagnostic pilot study: psychophysiological stress, Adv. Nurs. Sci. **2:**27-44, 1979.

Halloran, E.: Analysis of variation in nursing workload by patient medical and nursing condition, doctoral dissertation, Chicago, 1980, University of Illinois.

Hoskins, L.M., McFarlane, E.A., Rubenfeld, M.G., and others: Nursing diagnoses in the chronically ill: methodology for clinical validation, Adv. Nurs. Sci. **8:**80-89, 1986.

Hurley, M.: Classification of nursing diagnoses: proceedings of the sixth conference, St. Louis, 1986, The C.V. Mosby Co.

Jones, P. and Jakob, D.: The definition of nursing diagnoses: phase 3, unpublished manuscript, Toronto, 1980, University of Toronto, Faculty of Nursing.

Jones, P. and Jakob, D.: Nursing diagnosis: differentiating fear and anxiety. Nurs. Papers **14:**20-29, 1981.

Kim, M.J., McFarland, G., and McLane, A.: Classification of nursing diagnoses: proceedings of the fifth national conference, St. Louis, 1984, The C.V. Mosby Co.

Kim, M.J. and Moritz, D.A.: Classification of nursing diagnoses: proceedings of the third and fourth national conferences, New York, 1982, McGraw-Hill.

Leslie, F.M.: Nursing diagnosis: use in long-term care, Am. J. Nurs. **81:**1012-1014, 1981.

McKeehan, K. and Gordon, M.: Utilization of accepted diagnoses. In Kim, M.J. and Moritz, D.A. Classification of nursing diagnoses: proceedings of the fifth national conference, New York, 1982, McGraw-Hill.

Nursing Clinics of North America: Nursing diagnosis, New York, 12(4), Saunders.

Simmons, D.A.: Classification scheme for client problems in community health, Rockville, MD, 1983, U.S. Government Printing Office.

CHAPTER 3

Nursing diagnosis and the nursing minimum data set*

HARRIET H. WERLEY, Ph.D., R.N., F.A.A.N.

I have been asked to speak on the subject of nursing diagnosis and the nursing minimum data set (NMDS). I am going to place the emphasis on the content of the latter, the NMDS, for two reasons. First, I assume most of the conferees present are familiar with matters pertaining to nursing diagnosis, want to learn more about that subject from those directly involved in work of this type, and wish to share with one another what each can contribute. Second, the development of the NMDS will be a relatively new subject for many in attendance, with whom I wish to share a development that has the potential to contribute to the advancement of nursing generally and to the nursing-diagnosis movement in particular.

I have organized my paper so that I may cover the following, broadly: (1) some recognized advances in the nursing diagnosis movement that I noted have taken place since 1973, when Gebbie and Lavin (1975) planned and conducted the first national conference on nursing diagnosis; (2) the identification and development of the NMDS; (3) postconference follow-up work; (4) gaining acceptance of the NMDS; (5) potential benefits of implementing the NMDS; and (6) implications for nursing, the nursing diagnosis group, and individual nurses. In my explication of this matter, I will touch also on: background related to uniform minimum health data sets; the NMDS conference; the postconference task force effort; the NMDS elements; testing and refining the NMDS; seeking review of the NMDS by the Health Information Council of the U.S. Department of Health and Human Services; suggestions of possible ways nurses can disperse more widely the nursing-diagnosis and nursing-intervention movements, thus, helping to make a difference in nursing; and nursing's opportunity to become involved in the ICD–10 revision.

SOME RECOGNIZED ADVANCES IN THE NURSING DIAGNOSIS MOVEMENT

There appears to have been a steadily increasing interest in nursing diagnosis on the part of nurses in both clinical and academic

*Appreciation is expressed to my Wisconsin colleagues—Rita M. Beck, Jacqueline F. Clinton, Suzanne M. Falco, Janet M. Kraegel, Phyllis B. Kritek, Norma M. Lang, and Susan K. Westlake, who met with me periodically for a number of months to discuss the idea of developing a Nursing Minimum Data Set (NMDS) and then served as the planning committee for the NMDS Conference; also to Regina M. Maibusch, Carol A. Manternach, and Betty K. Mitsunaga, who joined the group during and after the Conference for Postconference planning, and to Elizabeth C. Devine who joined us to help move forward the pilot testing of the NMDS.

settings. However on occasion one also hears that relatively few nurses have implemented nursing diagnosis in their practice. If one pursues this question further, to learn just how widely nursing diagnoses have been implemented in nursing service settings, it soon becomes evident that the answer is not really known. This is clearly a researchable question that should be investigated, and in the interest of having the leaders of this North American Nursing Diagnosis Association (NANDA) be informed on the status of nursing diagnosis implementation locally, regionally, and nationally, periodic surveys should be part of NANDA's research program. Such periodic surveys, conducted with an appropriately planned questionnaire, also could result in additional information needed to guide the Association's leadership as they plan for advances in many aspects of the nursing diagnosis movement.

It is evident to the ordinary reader of nursing literature that there are increasing numbers of articles and books on nursing diagnosis. A measure of to what extent this literature is research-based would also be valuable for NANDA, so that the Association could keep abreast of the number of diagnoses that have been tested and validated and keep abreast of the kinds of issues related to nursing diagnosis that are being investigated or are left unstudied. In this age of computerization, NANDA should be able to call up all this up-to-date information readily so that such status reports could serve as bases for further work and action.

In the nursing diagnosis literature I was delighted to see that Lash (1978) acknowledged Dr. R. Louise McManus' influence in the nursing diagnosis movement. She pointed out that a quarter of a century had passed since, in 1950, the term *nursing diagnosis* was used by McManus (1951) to describe a unique nursing function. I can recall conversations with Dr. McManus about nursing diagnosis as a 1950–1951 graduate student at Teachers College, Columbia University. But more meaningful to me, and valuable, were later conversations and discussions on the subject when Dr. McManus was a member of the Office of Defense Advisory Committee on Women in the Service and, later, a consultant to us in the Department of Nursing Research at the Walter Reed Army Institute of Research. Dorothy Smith (1968) earlier also referred to Dr. McManus' views on nursing diagnosis, as Smith was struggling to develop a clinical nursing tool that would be useful in diagnosing patients' problems.

The classification of the nursing diagnosis, is, of course, getting more attention in both book chapters and journal articles, for example, Kritek's (1985) article on the theoretical foundations and Gordon's (1985) chapter on diagnostic category development. Gordon's (1982, Appendix B, pp. 327–328) earlier Grouping of Currently Accepted Diagnoses Under Functional Health Pattern Areas has been well received by a number of nurses working in the nursing diagnosis area; the research on its wide application should be pulled together and reported. Halloran and his associates have continued their research, in which they examined the influence of nursing diagnosis on nursing work load (Halloran, 1985), as well as on identification of severity of condition and resource use (Halloran, Kiley, and Madzam, in press).

With a nursing diagnosis movement ongoing, there must follow a nursing intervention movement, and I think that movement has been started. Some of you will recall that 2 years ago at this conference, when someone stated that nursing was not ready to move on several fronts until certain things were established, I spoke in opposition to that restrictive thinking, calling to the audience's attention that I had just seen at one of the book vendor's stand the mock-up volume, or flyer, on nursing interventions by Bulechek and McClosky (1985). And, I expressed the belief that if certain individuals were ready to move with different aspects of this total nursing diagnosis enterprise, I believed we should wish them well and support them. In the interim, I have seen increasing activity in the intervention area and, in fact, learned recently of a second book on nursing interventions, by Snyder (1985). In addition, I recently examined a nursing-standards document produced by the neuroscience nurse group that dealt with nursing diagnosis and interventions (American Nurses' Association & American Association of Neuroscience Nurses, 1985). I am pleased to know that nurses increasingly are examining the status of nursing interventions, or nursing actions, for as Bulechek and McClosky stated even in their book title, these are the treatments for nursing diagnoses. Later as I speak on the NMDS, it will become even more clear why I am pleased to know that there also is an intervention movement getting started; the two go together—nursing diagnoses and nursing interventions—even if, to date, more work has been done on the former.

It is good also to see that nurse educators are beginning to study how they can use the nursing diagnosis framework to assess student competence (DeBack, 1981; Lee and Strong, 1985). Efforts like this should help the nursing-diagnosis movement by having new generations of nurses prepared and ready to practice from the nursing-diagnosis standpoint.

I know that much has been done organizationally within NANDA to develop mechanisms to facilitate the review and addition of new diagnoses, and this is a plus for the organization. I trust that through the professionally mature way in which this matter is being handled, nursing can avoid territorial or philosophical splits and instead see ways to handle, in a cohesive way, diversity and the richness that it fosters. One might ask, what overtures are being made to groups of nurses who are developing new nursing diagnosis outside of NANDA?

It is good that, from the beginning of the national conferences on classification of nursing diagnosis, an effort was made to keep a record of progress of the nursing-diagnosis movement through the published volumes of proceedings, and, I am pleased that real efforts have been made to have these volumes presented in a scholarly manner (Kim and Moritz, 1982; Kim, McFarland, and McLane, 1984). I trust this scholarly recording of the nursing-diagnosis movement and development will continue. However, it should be remembered that, to date, chapters in proceedings, generally, are not indexed as retrievable literature, so, these writings do not show up on electronic data bases. This is particularly important in the case of studies of nursing diagnoses that are reported in these proceedings. Investigators should be urged to report their research in the open professional and scientific literature, preferably in refereed journals. And, it should be recognized that journal editors usually do not wish to publish studies after they have been reported in proceedings. It is all right to include research abstracts in proceedings, but the research articles should then appear in refereed journals. It also is all right, on occasion, to reprint a published research article in proceedings.

From an examination of the previous proceedings, it becomes evident that the nursing-diagnosis conference groups have grappled with many issues related to advancing the nursing diagnosis movement; have sought consultation and presentations from authorities on some of the issues; have raised research questions or offered research suggestions; and have shared references pertinent to the respective diagnoses. Of the research questions and suggestions, one might raise the question: What are the Association leaders doing about research programs? Maybe a Vice President for Research is needed, an expert in clinical judgment and nursing diagnosis, a fully research-prepared and actively research-productive person, who has a track record in obtaining research grants. (I have for years been aware of the work of the Vice President for Research of the American Cancer Society, because I have known the incumbents as former Army officers who were excellent researchers and research administrators. The American Cancer Society has certainly done well in developing its research programs.) With vision, nursing could develop an organizational mechanism within NANDA to develop, support, and obtain financial support for research programs pertaining to nursing diagnoses. This year's program again includes presentations and discussion sessions on content essential to advancing the nursing diagnosis movement, or content that is timely in terms of happenings in the health care field that have a bearing on nursing. I look forward to learning much from the sessions of this year's program, as well as from my contacts during the Conference.

IDENTIFICATION AND DEVELOPMENT OF THE NURSING MINIMUM DATA SET

I want to clarify from the beginning that I am not speaking about a *series* of minimum data sets for various aspects of nursing for which nurses may identify needed data and then plan for the collection, processing, storage, and retrieval of such data needed for clinical decision-making in various areas of nursing. I am speaking of those elements of the NMDS that could be national or international in scope, to provide clues about trends in nursing and nursing-resources allocation, that nurses and others might investigate further by using the more detailed data accumulated in computerized nursing information systems (NISs). These NISs *should*

be in existence at the institutional or facility level, where through relational data-base systems, the nursing data could be related to, or articulated with, other health-related information systems.

The conference mode of identifying the NMDS

This work on the NMDS is, in essence, a follow-through on some of my earlier work done while I was at the University of Illinois College of Nursing. During that time I was involved in reviewing research proposals for the National Center for Health Services Research, Health Care Technology Study Section. This was the group that reviewed the research proposals for all those medical and hospital information systems that today are the big, well-recognized systems, such as those led by Barnette, Warner, Weed, and so on. Because of my concern that nurses were not submitting proposals to draw on the millions of dollars available then, despite my urgings in many other ways, I developed and conducted a Nursing Information Systems Conference, inviting Margaret Grier to join me as co-director. In that conference, which I hoped would stimulate nurses to move toward computerization, we had a small-group problem on identifying basic sets of nursing data. The group did well, considering the time we could allot for group work in that conference, as reflected in the Werley and Grier (1981) volume on *Nursing Information Systems* and as later assessed by one of the officials of the National Center for Health Statistics. But, despite my urging, no one seemed to follow through on the idea of a basic nursing data set, so when I moved to the University of Wisconsin, I opened the subject with Dean Norma Lang, who was encouraging me and who helped me identify some people mainly faculty—who might meet with me periodically to discuss what could be done in the area.

In our initial discussions (locally) of what

should be included in the NMDS, we went through stages of sharing material, brainstorming, and wanting to include everything. However, we kept reminding ourselves of the fact that this was to be an NMDS in the tradition of earlier work on uniform minimum health data sets (UMHDSs). For guidance we looked to historical and more recent precedents.

Florence Nightingale can be credited as one of the earliest proponents of uniform minimum health data. In the mid-19th century, she devised a system of gathering uniform hospital statistics about events, such as admissions, discharges, lengths of stay, recoveries, and deaths, in the hope that particular methods of medical and surgical treatments could be evaluated. Although Nightingale's idea of gathering uniform statistics was clearly a good one, it was far ahead of its time and was not then put into general practice (Cohen, 1984).

Later some health data sets were developed through the National Center for Health Statistics, so, we held before us the concept of the minimum data set (MDS) as described by Murnaghan (1976, 1978) and later included in the federal government's Health Information Policy Council (HIPC), (1983) Background Paper. There were precedents and guidelines to follow as a result of the development of these earlier health-related MDSs, such as the 1980 version of the Long-Term Health-Care Minimum Data Set, the 1980 version of the Uniform Hospital Discharge Minimum Data Set, and the 1981 version of the Uniform Ambulatory Medical Care Minimum Data Set (National Committee on Vital and Health Statistics [NCVHS], 1980a, 1980b, 1981).

We believed that, if we accepted the general concept and definition of a UMHDS, we could more readily define what is meant by an NMDS. According to the HIPC (1983), a UMHDS is "a minimum set of items of information with uniform definitions and categories, concerning a specific aspect or dimension of the health care system, which meets the essential needs of multiple data users" (p. 3). By the above definition, an NMDS is a minimum set of items of information with uniform definitions and categories concerning the specific dimension of professional nursing, which meets the information needs of multiple data users in the health care system. Presumably, the NMDS would include those items of information that are used on a regular basis by the majority of nurses in delivering nursing care, keeping in mind the emphasis on "minimum."

Following the precedents of format (Murnaghan, 1973, 1976; Murnaghan and White, 1970) used to develop the earlier UMHDSs (NCVHS, 1980a, 1980b, 1981), I proposed that the conference mode be used to identify the NMDS, and I obtained a grant from the Hospital Corporation of America (HCA) Foundation to support the effort. The local Milwaukee group, mainly faculty, who had been meeting periodically for a number of months to discuss the potential NMDS, became the planning group, and I invited Norma Lang to join me as co-director of the conference.

Objectives. The objectives identified for the NMDS Conference were:

1. To discuss the philosophical and pragmatic issues involved in generating a NMDS and to assess the potential impact of this development on health care delivery and health policy development.

2. To establish comparability of nursing data across clinical populations, settings, geographic areas, and time, through consensual agreement on data categories, variables, and uniform definitions for these in nursing's clinical, educational, administrative, and research endeavors.

3. To discuss the issues that may facili-

tate or impede the delineation and implementation of an NMDS and the possible subsequent establishment of specialty care supplementary data sets.

4. To develop the NMDS in accordance with established professional standards of practice.
5. To analyze the processes previously used in developing health-related minimum data sets and in obtaining their approval and acceptance for governmental health policy implementation.
6. To explore and develop strategies to promote research and testing of the NMDS in a variety of settings.

Format and process. The NMDS Conference, sponsored by the University of Wisconsin-Milwaukee School of Nursing, was a 3-day national invitational working conference conducted May 15–17, 1985 in Milwaukee, Wisconsin. Sixty-five individuals were invited to deliberate issues involved in the development, implementation, and evaluation of the NMDS and to generate such an initial set. Participants included nurse-clinicians, administrators, educators, and researchers. Among these nurses were experts in clinical nursing practice, patient classification, nursing diagnosis, quality assurance, nursing information systems, nursing resources allocation, and professional standards. Also included were public and private health policy spokespersons, information systems experts, a health records specialist, and individuals knowledgeable in the historical development and current status of existing UMHDSs.

Thirty participants were commissioned to prepare papers to address issues relevant to developing an NMDS, as viewed from their individual perspectives and in keeping with the objectives of the conference. The commissioned papers were not presented at the conference, but they were distributed to all participants several months prior to the conference, so that everyone had time to

study and review them critically and come to the conference prepared to contribute to the discussions and the work to be done. On the first day of the conference, seven discussants presented reviews of groups of the papers. Their charge was to summarize, synthesize, and highlight the issues raised by the authors, and to lead the total conference group in discussion of their particular group of papers.

On the second and third days of the conference, the conferees were assigned to one of six small task forces to work on developing the NMDS content in the following areas: Nursing Assessment, Nursing Diagnosis, Nursing Interventions, Nursing Outcomes, Nursing Acuity or Intensity, and Demographics. These areas had been identified tentatively by the planning group prior to the conference as the key categories for the NMDS and were accepted by the conference membership as an initial working organizational structure for the data set. The categories were viewed as being grounded in the nursing process and were believed to be congruent with nurses' efforts to practice nursing in the real world.

The charge to members of the task forces was to generate the NMDS content in their respective category through a process of (a) initially identifying the data elements appropriate to that category; (b) seeking consensus within the task force and among the total conference membership regarding these elements; (c) developing the definitions of the category and the elements within, as well as possibly identifying some of the measures for the elements, if time permitted; and (d) seeking consensus on the definitions and any measures. As indicated by the progress of the working task forces, general sessions were called occasionally to get consensus on the work of the smaller groups, so that an initial NMDS could be generated by the end of the conference. Each of the six task forces was provided with a personal computer, a printer, and software from IBM Corporation Academic Information Systems, so that the NMDS content could be entered as it was developed and then revised as needed as consensus was reached. A copy machine was available to provide individual copies of the content under review.

POSTCONFERENCE FOLLOW-UP WORK
Postconference task force effort

An 11-person, 1-day postconference task force meeting, part of the original conference planning, was held September 16, 1985, at the Chicago airport; postconference task force members were individuals who were participants in the May conference. Originally it had been thought that the job of this Postconference Task Force would be to refine the initial NMDS as produced by the May conference group. However, because of the shortage of conference time and the differential difficulties experienced by some of the six task forces, there were other tasks to be addressed, including the development of a number of the needed definitions that were not completed. The project staff attempted to identify gaps, raise questions, and suggest definitions for scrutiny by the task force. After the local planning group reacted to these materials, they were forwarded to the Postconference Task Force in advance, so the members might prepare for the September 16 meeting.

A major focus of discussion that day was how the nursing information flow should be structured, and there was concern also that an appropriate number of nursing items be included in the NMDS, to do nursing justice. A three-level pyramid model, as shown in Fig. 1, was considered. At the base, would be the narrative or computerized record of care, where format and content are specific to the institution or facility, and the standards for information content are set broadly by general professional standards. At the middle level, would be a clinical nursing abstract (CNA), possibly represented as a nursing cover, or face sheet, which would function as the standardized professional data base. It would include the following data: assessment, diagnosis, intervention, outcome, selected demographics, and intensity or resource consumption. This information would remain within the facility, be available for research purposes, and be coded in machine-readable form. The CNA conceivably could be mandated by an accrediting body, such as the Joint Commission on the Accreditation of Hospitals (JCAH). At the top level would be the more abstract NMDS, a subset of the CNA data. The group then debated exactly what information should go up from the CNA to the NMDS.

The proceedings of the Postconference Task Force meeting and the tentative NMDS of this latter effort were sent to Postconference Task Force members for reaction, to be certain staff captured the essence and decisions of the complex discussion on that busy day. In February 1986 these materials were shared with all of the May 1985 conference participants.

Examples of other uniform minimum health data set elements

In case you are unfamiliar with other UMHDSs, I brought a handout (Table 1) that shows the comparison of the data elements for three of them—Hospital Discharge, Ambulatory Medical Care, and Long-Term Health Care. Note that these three sets have 14, 18, and 24 elements, respectively (and, it is said that the latter is too long). Where possible, if the needed data already are collected for one set, those elements can be drawn upon for another minimum data set through relational data-base systems, provided they are defined in the same way, so the data will be comparable. Seeing these minimum data set examples will help you to better understand the NMDS.

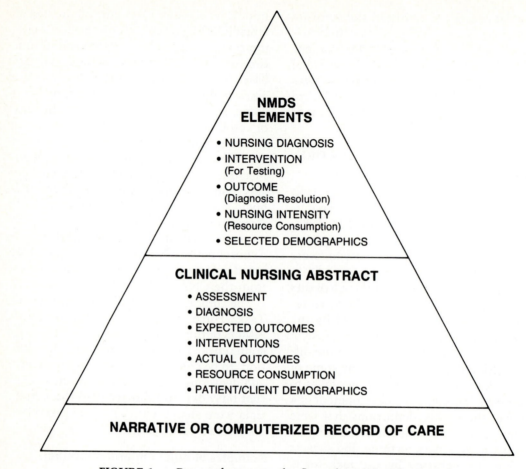

FIGURE 1   Proposed structure for flow of nursing information.

The nursing minimum data set elements

The NMDS includes three broad categories of items: nursing care, demographics, and service elements or items. The following NMDS items, or elements, were generated by the six task force groups at the May 15–17, 1985, NMDS Conference. Later (Sept. 16, 1985), they were refined by an 11-member Postconference Task Force, selected from the original conferees, and are recommended as the content for the NMDS. Elements included in the previously mentioned UHDDS (HIPC, 1985; NCVHS, 1980b) are indicated by an asterisk (*). Elements, or items, comparable to those already being collected need not be duplicated in situations where they can be obtained through relational data-base systems.

Nursing care elements
1. Nursing diagnosis
2. Nursing intervention (for pilot testing
3. Nursing outcome
4. Intensity of nursing care

Patient or client demographic elements
*5. Personal identification

Table 1: Comparison of minimum health data sets

Hospital discharge[a]	Ambulatory medical care[b]	Long-term health care[c]
	Demographic data	
Unique ID#	Name and unique ID#	Unique ID#
Residence	Residence	(as below)
Sex	Sex	Sex
Date of birth	Date of birth	Date of birth
Race/ethnicity	Race/ethnicity	Race/ethnicity
		Marital status
		Living arrangements: type/location
		Court-ordered constraints
	Health status data	
Principal and other DXs	Principal and other DXs	Principal and other DXs
	Patient's reason for encounter	Vision
		Hearing
		Communication
		ADLs
		Mobility
		Adaptive tasks
		Behavior problems
		Memory impairment
		Disturbance of mood
	Service/administrative data	
Hospital ID		Agency ID
Attending physician ID	Provider ID	
Operating physician ID		
	Provider location	Agency location
	Type of practice	Agency type
	Profession	
		Last provider ID
Admission date	Encounter date	Admission date
Discharge date		Discharge date
		Disposition
Principal procedures and dates	Diagnosis services	Direct services (15 categories)
	Therapeutic services	
	Preventive services	
Disposition	Disposition	(as above)
Source of payment	Source of payment	Source of payment
	Charges	Charges

a. Health Information Policy Council: 1984 Revision of the uniform hospital discharge data set, Hyattsville, MD, DHHS, Public Health Service. (Unpublished revision.)
b. National Committee on Vital and Health Statistics: Uniform ambulatory medical care: minimum data set, U.S. Department of Health and Human Services Pub. No. PHS-81-1161, Washington, D.C., 1981, U.S. Government Printing Office.
c. National Committee on Vital and Health Statistics: Long-term health care: Minimum data set, U.S. Department of Health and Human Services, Pub. No. PHS 80-1158, Washington, D.C., 1980, U.S. Government Printing Office.

*6. Date of birth
*7. Sex
*8. Race and ethnicity
*9. Residence
Service elements
*10. Unique facility or service agency number
11. Unique health record number of patient or client
12. Unique number of principal registered nurse provider
*13. Episode admission or encounter date
*14. Discharge or termination date
*15. Disposition of patient or client
*16. Expected payer for most of this bill (anticipated financial guarantor for services)

Nursing Intervention will be included in the NMDS during the pilot testing period, so that the feasibility of adding it as an NMDS element may be assessed. The value of including intervention data in the NMDS was acknowledged by the NMDS Conference and Postconference Task Force participants, but there must be an acceptable, exhaustive, and mutually exclusive coding scheme for categorizing nursing intervention phenomena. During the pilot testing, two proposed coding schemes originally developed by the NMDS Conference Nursing Intervention Task Force will be evaluated.

Some members of the audience who were members of the NMDS Conference and the Postconference Task Force may note the slight changes in several elements, or items, drawn from the UHDDS (those with *). This is because we updated these elements according to the changes in the 1984 revision of the UHDDS, as now published in the *Federal Register* (HIPC, 1985).

The purposes of the NMDS

To date, no national data standards and guidelines have been developed for the collection of clinical nursing information and related administrative data, such as for nursing resources allocation. The implementation of the NMDS would be a first step in the effort to facilitate the collection of national comparable, uniform, minimum nursing data. The purposes of the NMDS are to: (1) establish comparability of nursing data across clinical populations, settings, geographic areas, and time; (2) describe the nursing care of patients and their families in a variety of settings; (3) demonstrate or project trends regarding care needs and allocation of nursing resources to patients or clients according to their health problems, or nursing diagnoses; and (4) stimulate nursing research through links to the detailed data existing in nursing and health-care information systems (HCISs), in both institutional and noninstitutional settings. Some of the research could pertain to the quality and outcome of nursing care, the availability and costs of nursing resources for that care, and the total use and costs of nursing services.

Sharing information. The Conference papers are being edited for publication in an NMDS volume (Werley and Lang, in press) by Springer Verlag; these papers are excellent. This volume also will include a chapter on the work of the task forces, the resultant NMDS, as well as an annotated bibliography of work published in the areas of health-related minimum data sets and computer use in nursing.

An executive summary of the Conference (Werley, Lang, and Westlake, in press) was submitted and will probably be published simultaneously in three journals about July 1986, to reach the readership of nursing management, research, and education.

Testing and refining of the NMDS. An NMDS data collection instrument has been developed recently and has been pretested on a limited basis in an inpatient and an outpatient setting to identify preliminary problems and to assess the availability of data, as well as the ease of data collection. To encourage use of the data to answer a variety of questions regarding pertinent cost-related information, the data collection instrument includes medical diagnoses and the diagnostic related group (DRG) assignments, in addition to the NMDS elements. The instrument is being refined further for use in a pilot test of the NMDS.

Approval of the human-subjects protocol has been obtained from the University of Wisconsin-Milwaukee Institutional Review Board. And, we have scheduled meetings with personnel in several types of settings to work through their system of approval and to negotiate how we may work with them on data collection. It is essential to do some testing in a variety of settings (acute inpatient, long-term care, outpatient care, and home care) to see if the nursing data are, in fact, collectable. A number of individuals have expressed interest and willingness for their agencies to be considered as test sites, but currently, because of funding problems, we are using local facilities for pilot work. This pilot work is essential, if later we are to be ready for larger-scale national testing. Federal representatives have continued to encourage testing and refining of the NMDS.

The testing, of course, has implications that include exploring whether nursing services have developed their computerized Nursing Information Systems (NISs), so that in the testing it can be shown that the data are being collected at the institution level, or that there is intention of moving in that direction shortly. Given that nursing is committed to identifying, systematizing, and computerizing data for decision making in nursing, there will be great opportunities for research in nursing, some of which may be given impetus from the trends indicated from the NMDS data collected regionally or nationally, depending on the acceptance and implementation of the data set at the health policy level. Parenthetically, the American Nurses' Association (ANA) Council on Computer Applications in Nursing is sub-

mitting a resolution to the ANA House of Delegates at the Convention in June, urging encouragement and support to nursing services to develop computerized NISs. Be on the lookout for this resolution and speak up favorably from all your respective states.

GAIN ACCEPTANCE OF THE NMDS
At the professional level

In the early planning for the identification of an NMDS, an effort was made to move this work forward in accordance with the profession's standards of practice. In addition, many of the participants in the NMDS Conference and Postconference Task Force were nurses at the forefront of helping to advance nursing practice, administration, research, and education. It is believed, therefore, that there will be professional support of the NMDS movement, its testing and implementation. Promoting the implementation of the NMDS will involve looking back at the needed NISs at the institutional and noninstitutional areas of nursing practice, if the more detailed research is to be done to follow up on trends revealed through the NMDS. Through the standards developed by nurses in various groups within the ANA and published by the ANA, as well as through the standard guidelines used by Joint Commission on Accreditation of Hospitals (JCAH), there is hope of communicating the need and benefits of having nurses' colleagues support and accept the NMDS movement.

At the federal health policy level

The goal of achieving implementation of the NMDS at the federal health policy level can be reached only through systematic testing and review. U.S. Deputy Surgeon General and Chief Nurse Officer, United States Public Health Service, Faye G. Abdellah (in press), outlined the steps in the process in the closing paper on future direction that she delivered at the May NMDS Conference.

She advised that we begin by pilot testing the NMDS on a small scale in a variety of settings and follow this with a letter to the Health Information Policy Council, requesting review of the data set. We now have submitted that letter to the Acting Assistant Secretary for Health, who is also chairperson of the Health Information Policy Council. I proceeded, having been in touch with Faye Abdellah along the way. I also got suggestions from Reginal McPhilips and Margaret Sovie. We are awaiting word of the Secretary's willingness to meet us to discuss the NMDS and to pursue continued development of the NMDS. We asked that an appointed review group include representation from the nursing profession, the Health Care Financing Administration, and the U.S. Public Health Service.

POTENTIAL BENEFITS OF IMPLEMENTING THE NMDS

The benefits of implementing an NMDS will be far reaching, ranging from being an impetus to getting nursing's information systems in place to rounding out health-care information systems (HCISs) that were heretofore incomplete to the extent that they consisted only of HISs (hospital information systems) and MISs (medical information systems), that is, they omitted NISs.

To the nursing profession

Because of the various trends that can be observed locally, regionally, and nationally across clinical populations and settings through an NMDS, questions requiring nursing research will abound. To investigate these questions will require that a data audit trail be traceable to local institution or agency NISs. This will serve as an impetus to fuller use, and improvement of, these NISs where they exist and to their establishment in institutions or agencies without them. Many needed studies should emerge, and both nursing care practitioners and adminis-

trators should begin to see that they can base their decision making on data-based information. Patients or clients with various types of diagnoses (medical and nursing) can be studied from the standpoint of nursing interventions that are planned, implemented, and evaluated. The research from this kind of investigative nursing practice will be the basis for further development of nursing knowledge and will lead to accumulating a list of validated nursing diagnoses and tested nursing interventions. From research of this type, nurses will develop greater insights as to what data are needed in NISs; as a consequence there will be modifications and refinement of NISs. Nursing care planning can be improved as documentation improves and evaluation can be done more readily; the result will be improved care.

Nursing administrators will be looking for data to help them to "cost" nursing resources used to make research-based decisions about the nursing services for which they are responsible. With appropriate NISs in place, the trends revealed through the NMDS data can be investigated, with the results serving as research-based information on which administrators can make their decisions about the operations and quality of their services.

Nursing education, too, can benefit from the development and implementation of an NMDS, because education for any given nursing level can then be more research based.

To the health care delivery system

The total health-care delivery system benefits as each care-provider group improves its documentation and quality of care. In addition, as the respective professionals' data complement, supplement, and articulate with the total HCISs, the various professionals benefit, because one group can draw on another group's data. Nurses, in their caring function, have long been concerned about the psychosocial aspects of patient or client care and have collected pertinent data, but for too long without support to have these data entered into an organized, retrievable information system. This must and can be changed through research and development of appropriate NISs, some of the appropriateness possibly stemming from research questions raised as trends are revealed through the use of a NMDS.

To health policy development

Those who develop health policy, private or public, should be concerned that, as they do, they consider the *complete* health-care delivery picture. For too long the data being used to develop health policy have not included nursing data; therefore, health policy pertaining to the care of patients might be questioned. If nurses are concerned about correcting this situation, there must be a concerted movement to help test and conduct research on the NMDS, so it may move forward, hopefully, to be implemented at the federal health policy level, where data can be collected on Medicare and Medicaid cases, for example, as well as on other health-care programs. Multiple benefits will thus accrue to the federal government as well as to nursing and the health-care delivery system, generally.

To third party payers

Third party payers will profit by the availability of nursing documentation in the form of comparable data about nursing care provided, the resources allocated, and the cost of nursing services. Conceivably such documentation will be of value in assessing nursing care in relation to the higher cost of physicians' care. Clear, precise nursing-care documentation also will be useful in assessing quality of care. Through improved comparable documentation of nursing diagnosis, interventions, and outcomes, studies can be done on numerous types of cases locally, regionally, and nationally, that will demonstrate that nursing care is an identifiable, autonomous provider service worthy of reimbursement.

IMPLICATIONS FOR NURSING AND NURSES
Continued support of the nursing diagnosis movement

It is very important for nurses to support and help put into effect nursing care that is based on sound clinical judgment and results in making a nursing diagnosis, thus leading to the nursing actions, or interventions, to be taken on the patient's behalf. As was pointed out by Bulechek and McCloskey (1985), this is the professional model of nursing, and as stated by Aydelotte (1985) in the foreword of the Bulechek and McClosky book, it reflects a domain of practice that belongs to nurses, independent of physicians' prescriptions. For this nursing diagnosis movement to come about more fully, will require hard work on the part of all nurses, irrespective of functional area—in clinical nursing practice, administration, research, and education.

It will be important for nurses to show a united front in promoting and using nursing diagnoses, if nurses are to convince federal officials who make health information policy that they should review the NMDS favorably as one of the family of UMHDSs, support its being field tested nationally, and then implement it in a variety of their health care programs, such as Medicare and Medicaid. This type of mandated implementation at the national level would for the first time provide our profession with a national accumulation of comparable nursing-care and nursing-resources data. In the letter to the Assistant Secretary of Health and Chairperson of the Health Information Policy Council, we enumerated nine examples of potential benefits of the NMDS to the federal government. This list was not meant to be exhaustive, but it pointed up clearly a broad range of benefits.

In order for nurses to have a united front regarding the nursing diagnosis implementation in practice, this group may need to consider more fully how you will handle the diversity of approaches. Certainly, coming to grips with a beginning nursing-diagnosis classification scheme will be a major step in this direction. What will be your approaches to groups outside of NANDA, to invite them into the fold, as it were? What efforts will be made to have this large powerful NANDA group collaborate with nursing's professional society, the ANA? How will this be done, and on what matters will there be such joint work?

As a growing force in nursing, how will the nursing diagnosis group work to encourage and support further the more neophyte nursing interventions movement? I think some of the things that are being done, as for example this year's scheduled program presentation by Steven Hayes and the workshop on nursing interventions, are moving in the right direction. What more should be done, especially since you meet only every second year?

Promoting nursing diagnosis research programs

What can be done about moving further in the direction of promoting nursing diagnosis research programs? What can be done about facilitating funding for research on nursing diagnosis? With all the rejections potential investigators have had from the U.S. DHHS Division of Nursing, has any official group from NANDA made an effort to explore with Division of Nursing personnel what problems cause nursing-diagnosis proposals to fare so badly? Is there something more to it than weaknesses in the proposals? I think this should be explored because, without approved proposals for nursing-diagnosis re-

search, how is nursing education to be built on research-based content? Does some of it stem from the fact that many of the investigators may be viewed by the proposal reviewers as not sufficiently research prepared? If so, what is being done to attract more fully research-prepared nurses to this very rich area of nursing that virtually begs for research to be done? Should an approach be made to the ANA Council of Nurse Researchers to have a joint discussion on the matter? And, what is being done about teaming up excellent clinicians with excellently prepared and productive researchers to develop research proposals jointly, so the clinicians and researchers can work together to develop the area. I will not repeat here some of the other examples of needed research I mentioned earlier.

Nursing's inclusion in the ICD-10 revision

Is the Nursing Diagnosis group ready to help the nursing profession put its best foot forward to insure that nursing is included in the International Classification of Diseases (ICD-10) Revision. The ANA Council on Computer Applications in Nursing (CCAN), of which I presently am the Chair, has a liaison relationship with the WHO Center for Classification of Diseases for North America, so we have known of the Revision Conference meetings; Dr. Virginia Saba, of the CAAN Executive Committee, is the liaison person. Through her, we have been in touch with that office and explored whether nursing could be included as a member of the Family of Classifications of the tenth, and future revisions, of the ICD. She obtained instructions on how the nursing profession should proceed to be included, but of course, this means nursing must be ready to move on classification matters with the total revision group, per the scheduled dates, when certain things must be done between now and their 1990 deadline. The Council communicated to ANA headquarters this information and an expression of belief that nursing should "go for it," even though nurses of today are not quite ready with a classification scheme. A letter required from the ANA was sent by the ANA President, committing the Association and requesting that nursing be included. If the use of nursing diagnosis reflects the professional model of nursing, in what way should NANDA be involved and helping with this matter, which is tied closely to the taxonomy efforts of this body, and what might that mean for this body? It might mean that you speed up your time schedule for accomplishing things in relation to the diagnoses and their classification. It might also mean that there should be a more concerted effort directed toward developing research programs on matters pertinent to moving the classification scheme forward.

The letter that was mailed to the WHO office from the ANA President was a nice one, mentioning nursing diagnosis, NANDA, ANA standards, the ANA Social Policy Statement, and so on. I believe that NANDA's president might want to explore what all this means for NANDA's involvement, for it has implications for NANDA program development. In the ANA letter Irma Hirsch, senior staff specialist, Practice, Policy Development, and Strategic Planning, was named contact person; she is here and she may wish to make a few comments. I do not know whether President Cole's letter of October 30, 1985, was answered by the WHO Center for Classification of Diseases for North America. I assume it has been and that committed nurses will see to it that the necessary work is done to assure that nursing is included among the Family of Classifications of the 10th and future revisions of the ICD.

REFERENCES

Abdellah, F.G.: Future directions: refining, implementing, testing, and evaluating the nursing minimum data set. In H.H. Werley, and Lang, N.M., editors: Identification of the nursing minimum data set, New York, Springer Verlag. (In press.)

American Nurses' Association and American Association of Neuroscience Nurses: Neuroscience nursing practice: process and outcome criteria for selected diagnoses, Kansas City, MO, 1985, American Nurses' Association.

Bulechek, G.M., and McClosky, J.C.: Nursing interventions: treatments for nursing diagnoses, Philadelphia, 1985, W.B. Saunders.

Cohen, I.B.: Florence Nightingale, Sci. American **250:** 128, 136, 144, 1984.

DeBack, V.: The relationship between senior nursing students' ability to formulate nursing diagnosis and the curriculum model, Advances Nurs. Sci. **3:**51, 1981.

Gebbie, K.M., and Lavin, M.A., editors: Classification of nursing diagnoses: proceedings of the first national conference, St. Louis, 1975, The C.V. Mosby Co.

Gordon, M.: Grouping of currently accepted diagnoses under functional health pattern areas. Nursing diagnosis: process and application, Appendix B, New York, 1982, McGraw-Hill.

Gordon, M.: Diagnostic category development. In McCloskey, J.C., and Grace, H.H., editors: Current issues in nursing, ed. 2, Boston, 1985, Blackwell Scientific Publications.

Halloran, E.: Nursing workload, medical diagnosis related groups, and nursing diagnoses, Res. Nurs. Health **8:**421, 1985.

Halloran, E.J., Kiley, M.L., and Nadzam, D.: Nursing diagnoses for identification of severity of nursing condition and resource use. In Hurley, M.E., editor: Classification of nursing diagnosis: proceedings of the sixth conference, St. Louis, 1986, The C.V. Mosby Co.

Health Information Policy Council. Background paper: uniform minimum health data sets, Washington, DC, U.S. Department of Health and Human Services, unpublished manuscript, 1983.

Health Information Policy Council: 1984 revision of the uniform hospital discharge data set. Federal Register. **50:**31038, July 31, 1985.

Kim, M.J., McFarland, G.K., and McLane, A.M., editors: Classification of nursing diagnosis: proceedings of the fifth national conference, St. Louis, 1984, The C.V. Mosby Co.

Kim, M.J., and Moritz, D.A., editors: Classification of nursing diagnosis: proceedings of the third and fourth national conferences, New York, 1982, McGraw-Hill.

Kritek, P.B.: Nursing diagnosis: theoretical foundations, Occ. Health Nurs. **33:**393, 1985.

Lash, A.A.: A re-examination of nursing diagnosis, Nurs. Forum **17:**333, 1978.

Lee, H.A., and Strong, K.A.: Using nursing diagnosis to describe the clinical competence of baccalaureate and associate degree graduating students: a comparative study, Image **17**:82, 1985.

McManus, R.L.: Assumptions of functions. In *Regional Planning for Nursing and Nursing Education.* Report of work conference at Plymouth, NH, June 12-23, 1950. New York, 1951, Teachers College, Columbia University.

Murnaghan, J.H., editor: Ambulatory medical care data: report of the conference on ambulatory medical care records, Med. Care **11**:(2, Suppl.), 1973.

Murnaghan, J.H., editor: Long-term, care data: report of the conference on long-term health care data, Med. Care **14**:(5, Suppl.), 1976.

Murnaghan, J.H.: Uniform basic data sets for health statistical systems, Int. J. Epidemiol. **7**:263, 1978.

Murnaghan, J.H., and White, K.L., editors: Hospital discharge data: report of the conference on hospital discharge abstracts systems, Med. Care **8**:(4, Suppl.), 1970.

National Committee on Vital and Health Statistics: Long-term health care: minimum data set, U.S. Department of Health and Human Services, Pub. No. PHS 80-1158, Washington, D.C., 1980, U.S. Government Printing Office.

National Committee on Vital and Health Statistics: Uniform hospital discharge data: minimum data set, DHEW Pub. No. PHS 80-1157, Washington, D.C., 1980, U.S. Government Printing Office.

National Committee on Vital and Health Statistics: Uniform ambulatory medical care: minimum data set, U.S. Department of Health and Human Services Pub. No. PHS 81-1161, Washington, D.C., 1981, U.S. Government Printing Office.

Smith, D.M.: A clinical nursing tool, Am. J. Nurs. **68**: 2384, 1968.

Snyder, M.: Independent nursing interventions, New York, 1985, John Wiley.

Werley, H.H., and Grier, M.R., editors: Nursing information systems, New York, 1981, Springer Verlag.

Werley, H.H., and Lang, N.M., editors: Identification of the nursing minimum data set, New York, Springer Verlag. (In press.)

Werley, H.H., Lang, N.L., and Westlake, S.K.: The nursing minimum data set conference: executive summary, Manuscript submitted for publication, 1986.

CHAPTER 4

Fee-based reimbursement using nursing diagnosis

KRISTINE M. GEBBIE, M.N., R.N.

At least one person who read the title of this paper assumed I would present a discussion of an idealized method to construct the perfect billing system for a mythical hospital in which all nursing records resemble a how-to-use-nursing-diagnosis manual. That is not my intent. I have taken as my viewpoint the context in which nursing is practiced and in which decisions about reimbursement are made. I will be discussing four general questions:

- Why hasn't reimbursement based on nursing diagnosis happened yet?
- Why is such a system sought?
- What is the potential for political support of instituting such reimbursement?
- What are the prerequisites to such a system?

I am afraid I will sound to some like a skeptic, or like a person who has no confidence in the capacity of nursing for advancement. I would be foolish if I tried to deceive you by presenting only the Pollyanna side of my world view. That side is there: I have a deep conviction in the value of the profession of nursing to the social system and in its capacity to endure and grow over long periods of social evolution. Like all of us who have made commitments to development of nursing diagnosis over the past 13 years, I am convinced of its value to the pro-

fession and to society. I am, however, a Pollyanna who is a political realist; my viewpoint is shaped in part because of the job I do in support of the public health of 2.5 million Oregonians. In that perspective, I am doubtful that nursing will achieve social status as an independent, well reimbursed profession within the next quarter to half century without major changes in the behavior patterns of most nurses. The development of a vocabulary of nursing diagnoses and the utilization of the concepts represented by that vocabulary in practice can be major contributions to that end. We who are already convinced have a long way to go in educating other critical audiences by our example.

WHY HASN'T A DIAGNOSIS-BASED REIMBURSEMENT SYSTEM HAPPENED?

There is one simple answer: Reimbursement systems are based on generally accepted practices, and nursing diagnosis is not yet generally accepted. That is not to say that it is not being used by growing numbers of nurses or that many schools of nursing are not providing at least an introductory orientation to the diagnostic process. But it is clear as you listen to "typical" nurses describe their days at work, or their relationships with patients, that the diagnostic process is not central to those days or relationships. For many nurses, diagnosing is a verbal overlay brought into play to satisfy a demand for a certain type of record keeping, or to sound current. There are many other nurses, for whom diagnosing is a central thought process, who are impatient for the development of sufficient diagnoses to encompass all of the problems they see in patients that have not yet been assigned a name. Attaching payment to diagnosing as the general experience in nursing practice will not occur until diagnosing itself is the dominant thought process applied to nursing practice.

Most of us have paid a great deal of attention to the massive changes in reimbursement patterns brought about by the advent of hospitalization insurance during the Depression and the creation of Medicare and Medicaid in the mid-1960's. We are stimulated to imagine that the proper configuration of legislators fond of nurses or impressed by nurses' voting power, or the proper configuration of the planets, could bring about a similar flow of cash to nurses. A closer look, however, reveals that there was a change in the method of directing cash only for a well-established practice, medical diagnosis and treatment. The practical impact was the intrusion of observers to verify that there was value for the investment, in that the diagnoses were consistent with symptoms, the treatment consistent with diagnoses, and the total cost not abusive. The public was convinced throughout that there was a benefit to be gained from using dollars to assure access to the desired service. We make an error if we think that the funding could be authorized first as an incentive to convert recalcitrant nurses to diagnosis-based practice, which will then become valued by the public.

Another way of describing the situation is to state that nursing diagnosis is politically irrelevant outside of nursing circles. If we wise nurses who understand diagnosing controlled the checkbook, the reimbursement could begin tomorrow. The fact is that nurses do not reimburse nurses. We are paid by our patients: directly (rarely), or indirectly by third parties (also rare) or even more indirectly, by institutions which are themselves the recipients of third-party payments. In all of these instances, nurses are defined as necessary, useful or relevant for certain activities or services. We are sometimes needed to be the custodians of patients entrusted to an institution. In that role we know where the patient is at all times, and assure that no harm comes (or if it does, that an incident report is properly completed). At times we are the assistants in procedures performed by others, as in surgery or childbirth. In other places, nurses are seen as needed because they provide very specific aids to basic hygiene and mobilization. This is not to say that the nurses providing these services perceive themselves in the manner I have just described. In fact, many nurses would see those descriptions as pejorative. But if one listens closely to the rationale given for the employment of a nursing staff in a health care setting, the reasons cited are not far from the truth. Nurses are hired out of habit, because licensing agencies require it, because they are practical and useful, not because of an ideological commitment to our diagnostic contribution. The fact that a professional nurse can evaluate a person who is experiencing an illness, responding to being infected, injured, immobilized, unwell, in unusual surroundings, that the nurse can accurately label the problem states being experienced by the patient and can offer treatment to alleviate or correct that state, is overlooked by both the institution and the patient. It is unfortunately also overlooked by the nurse a good part of the time. On the average, nursing diagnoses are being made explicit when needed for documentation or as an overlay to a more reactive and habitual manner of providing "routine" care to "typical" patients. If nurses are not in the institution to diagnose, there is no reason to base payment on diagnosing.

Even in those situations in which the form of nursing diagnosis has become institutionalized in charting or documenting the patient's care plan, I remain skeptical that it has been internalized. Nursing as a profession has a regrettable history in which form has taken a priority over substance. I recall days when more attention was paid to my ability to print clearly in the appropriate color ink than to the content of my charting (other than the portions related to provision of prescribed medical treatments, or portions which could be misread as "judgments" about the patient), a fascinating message about nurses as doers rather than thinkers. A growing number of scholars have explored the limitations placed on nursing by its history as a religious or quasi-military profession of women trained by apprenticeship. In such a system, looking proper can loom far larger than doing the correct thing. In my years of practice, I have seen jumps from functional nursing to team nursing to primary nursing with little grasp of the real behavioral change each implies. Each time, the nurses involved were sure they would be both up-to-date and efficient. It can be far too easy to pick up the superficial jargon of nursing diagnosis without letting the diagnostic process shape our thinking and our practices. If this process of window dressing with new jargon is true, it further makes a reimbursement system based on diagnosis irrelevant, because "paying" for "diagnosing" won't buy anything different than has been purchased for years.

WHY IS DIAGNOSIS-BASED REIMBURSEMENT SOUGHT?

The more I have reflected on the title to which I committed many months ago, the more uncomfortable I have become with it. I think hidden in the title is one of the potentially more destructive problems haunting nursing today; we keep trying to come out looking like "the big boys" instead of pursuing our own ends and valuing ourselves for what we offer. "Fee-based reimbursement" implies, I think, some form of a fee-for-service, a so-many-dollars-for-each-diagnosis system, similar to that in use by medicine. It is as if we will "get there," wherever that is, when we are paid just like "them." That is not to say that as a nurse providing care to patients one should not be paid for one's ability to diagnose and treat patients. But payment can come in the form of a professional salary, a profit-sharing system, or a per-diagnosis, per-treatment or per-visit fee. The fundamental issue is the content for which pay is given. Is it merely for being present within four walls for a specific number of hours per day or per week, or is it for something accomplished on behalf of identified patients?

Another insidious implication of looking for a payment system like that used by medicine is that nurses equate such an achievement with achieving the power and independence we ascribe to the dominant health care profession. Put tersely, we spend so much time checking on how we're doing compared to physicians that we don't complete the tasks that only we can and should accomplish. Chief among those tasks, I believe, is incorporating an individual and professional responsibility for advancing the content of our practice, regardless of the basis on which we are paid for its provision. We could be paid daily based on the number of times we pick up pencils or annually based on height. Power and independence are based on client perception of value and authority, not on the content of the bill. Advancing the use of diagnostic terminology is part of the base for developing research into improved practice, and a tool for use in documenting our contribution to the well-being of society.

It is also important to remember that the form in which the dollars come may be altered without any increase. A third variation on my answer to why we seek payment based on diagnoses is that we believe that such payments will be greater than the dollars we now receive. Nurses are very much aware of tightening budgets in hospitals and other health agencies. It is a fantasy that changing from an hourly salary based on being there to fees for diagnosing will yield more money. It could simply redivide the same or a shrinking pot. If you doubt that, take a closer look at what is happening to the diagnosis-based fee reimbursement systems in medical practice. The amount of money going into illness care and health care is no longer growing rapidly as a proportion of the economy. Today adjustments to the manner in which it is distributed within the system are occurring, such as less going to hospitals, more to long-term care or to home care. We may want a shift in how funds are apportioned to nurses, say, more going to nurses who demonstrate competence in diagnosis and treatment. Or we might increase the portion of the total available for the practice of nursing by demonstrating a decrease in the administrative overhead needed to connect us with patients needing our care. It is of course possible that we could be successful in increasing dollars available for nursing by either increasing the nursing share of the current funds or by bringing in new dollars. Neither is very likely, given the current intense competition. If either occurs in the near future, nursing diagnosis is unlikely to be the reason: it is not sufficiently developed to supply the rationale.

It would be an error for me to proceed without acknowledging that dollars are, in our culture, one of the means of validating worth. It is not surprising then, that we who value nursing diagnosis strive to see our "baby," our contribution to the world of nursing, valued by others in a tangible way. That could happen in one of several arenas, the two most likely being research and practice. Nursing diagnosis research has not been distinguished by a flood of dollars from public or private sources any more than has diagnosis-based practice. One of the critical features of a nomenclature and taxomony for a discipline is that they must be useful to all members of the discipline. Those of us who have closely followed the development of nursing diagnoses know the tension that has existed between those who need clarity at a high level of conceptual abstraction (for research and theoretical development) and those who need conceptual clarity at the level of clinical utility (for describing and studying patient experience). Developing a diagnostic system that serves only one of those two needs might have short-term economic payoff for some nurses, but would, in the long run, serve the discipline poorly by isolating an essential segment of the profession and failing to support our collective professional and economic advancement.

POTENTIAL POLITICAL SUPPORT

From my present perspective as a state health director, I have the opportunity to watch groups struggle with seeking services from government at local, state and national levels. One phenomenon which occurs with some regularity is that of moving up the governmental hierarchy because it seems too difficult to make those closer to home understand the need for what is sought. Persons who cannot persuade a county commission that teenagers need access to family planning services lobby the state legislature to fund grants so that those seeking to provide the service can apply directly without county board approval. Fearing that not all state legislatures will be so open-minded, the same advocates seek to have a national program enacted so that a clinic in a conservative state can bypass both lower levels of government. Current tensions and struggles in many communities would indicate that the failure to successfully persuade local leaders, elected and other, of the need for contraceptive services can lead to the limitation and closure of clinics even when the dollars come from elsewhere. I see nurses in a similar manner proposing to meet their needs for independence, power and recognition by identifying national schemes for reimbursement for nursing activities. There was a bill in Congress to create nursing clinics which received much discussion a year or more ago. In my state, as I suspect in many others, there was nothing in the federal bill that could not have been implemented then, or today, under existing state law. But it is easier to write letters to federal representatives and to imagine a single big solution, than to picture explaining and demonstrating practice to colleagues from other disciplines who are doubtful or hostile, and local decision makers who know you as "the nurse next door." The discipline of day-to-day demonstration and articulation of the fundamentally different practice which is truly diagnosis-based can lead to reimbursement on the basis of ability to diagnose and treat. In reimbursement, law generally follows rather than leads practice, so the demonstration must come first.

Having watched the introduction of mandated benefits, I am also wary of the imposition of a mandate such as "you will pay those nurses for their diagnosing" when the service in question is not widely offered and valued. Insurers can be ordered, by state law, to assure that all subscribers have access to certain benefits, or, if services are provided by multiple providers, that all are reimbursed. Despite its inherent value, and the clear missionary zeal with which it was pursued by recipients, providers and families, the first years of hospice care have seen a payment system dedicated to controlling the costs of and access to services rather than opening the door to all in need. It almost becomes a challenge to the payer, backed into a corner by the mandate, to see how little can be gotten away with, rather than how to fully accomplish the intended goal. Slow evolution, based on a demand by satisfied customers, can yield far more in the long run. That means two things, by the way: that customers are satisfied and that they know what it was that made them feel that way.

WHAT WILL HAVE TO HAPPEN FIRST?

That last sentence leads directly to the first critical variable in moving the reimbursement for nurses to a system in which one's income is directly related to one's ability to diagnose and treat patients: patient awareness and support. Hospice happened not because nurses decided to offer what is in fact one of the best models of appropriate care available in this country (though why it should be limited to the dying is beyond me). It happened because patients and their families demanded something. Patients who have experienced relief from the discomfort of limitations of the problems we describe as nursing diagnoses must become aware that it was the professionally prescribed nursing care which provided or facilitated the relief. If our activities are seen merely as by-products of medical treatment and never made explicit, patients will continue to rally around the physicians, who make both diagnoses and treatment explicit. This is an old cause of mine, but one which I feel even more strongly about today than I did ten years ago. Aside from the marketing potential of becoming more open with our patients about our efforts, it is a violation of the ethical relationship between any professional and any client to presume to intervene in a patient's life experience without defining the reason for the interference, the intended direction of movement with its accompanying risks, and gaining consent for the treatment. Yet, nurses do just that every hour of every day in institutions all across the country. Deciding to engage in diagnosis-based practice makes the deception more difficult to hide from oneself, if not from one's patients.

Implicit in the idea that patient awareness will promote reimbursement based on diagnosis is the assumption that the awareness will be widespread. A critical mass of nurses providing diagnosis-based care may allow institutionalization of diagnostic terminology on a specific unit or in one hospital. Patient support will have to be expressed on behalf of a substantial percentage of the profession in any one geopolitical unit before it has an effect on reimbursement. That unit may be state, because many decisions about scope of practice and health and illness care reimbursement are made there. The unit could be national, but that will take a long time. Medicare and Medicaid are under too many constraints and attacks to be interested. Further, the variety of solutions possible in each of the fifty states would yield much more flexibility. Some large systems, such as the Veterans Administration, and some large prepaid services or health maintenance organizations have the capacity to change methods of paying nurses, if it were desired by the constituency. What is the percentage of nurses in a system who must be recognized by their clients directly for contributions to wellbeing to support a change? It is only a guess, but I would put it at over 45% and probably more in the vicinity of 65 or 70%.

There is a final necessity if we are to be reimbursed somehow for diagnosing. Our contribution must be documented. I am not a researcher, but I know the power that research findings carry when they are allowed to shape thinking and practice. I know the

effect it has on my decisions to develop or redirect resources when I am deciding in my own agency between two attractive options, one that merely sounds appealing, and another that is backed up by documented evidence of a reduction in morbidity or mortality. It is not enough that the care givers feel better about one program than the other. It must make a difference in the lives of the recipients. Nursing as a discipline has not grasped the necessity of testing what we do and documenting those tests. Use of diagnostic terminology can strengthen that documentation. Mere use of the words as cover for old practices will not.

If you came today to take extensive notes on how to modify your charts, time cards and billing system to incorporate nursing diagnosis and make a fortune, you have been sorely disappointed. I think I know my colleagues well enough to say that few of you are naive enough to have really expected such a simplistic answer to the question of properly compensating nurses for their efforts. Because I have spent more time on the negatives, what is getting in the way, or what may be some of the wrong reasons for changing the way we are paid, I will close with an affirmative statement regarding the relationship between nursing diagnosis and reimbursement.

Use of nursing diagnoses to describe and document practice can clarify the contribution of nursing to reduced morbidity and mortality. In order to do so, we must continue to strive for a balance between conceptual clarity which can support our theoretical development and utility in the day-to-day practice setting.

Openness with our patients about nursing's contributions can enable our clients to become advocates for our services in the complex world in which third and fourth parties have a major part in financing health and illness care.

Basing the distribution on nursing's share of the reimbursement pie on effective diagnosis and treatment can mean that better nurses are better paid, by the hour, the day or the diagnosis.

Paying better nurses more is a validation which can encourage more nurses to document more clearly nursing's overall contribution to the health of the citizenry, and over time, can increase the share of the total pie which comes to nursing. That is the unexpressed goal of many concerned with reimbursement, and a goal which is achievable only after the careful taking of many well-documented small steps. In taking those steps, nursing diagnosis can be a powerful tool, and a helpful guide.

CHAPTER 5

Approaches to the development of a nursing diagnosis taxonomy

MYRA E. LEVINE, M.S.N., R.N., F.A.A.N.

Taxonomy is often regarded as the dullest of subjects. If systems of classification were neutral hat racks for hanging the facts of the world, this disdain might be justified. But classifications both reflect and direct our thinking. The way we order represents the way we think
GOULD, *1983, p. 72*

Taxomony is the science of classification. If classification were no more than alphabetizing a list of accepted entities, then ordering "the facts of the world" would be simple indeed. But creating a taxonomy is a demanding research endeavor. It requires philosophical conviction, a structured and disciplined methodology and a clearly conceptualized purpose. There is more than one way to establish the matrix upon which a taxonomy is built, but the matrix itself must be carefully constructed.

Gould (1980) continues, "Classifications ... represent structures of thought that largely determine the status and content of a subject. ... Classification can constrain or liberate a subject." To liberate nursing means to seek its very essence and to order it in a fashion that provides a haven for all who enter its ranks. The rules that guide construction of a taxonomy must not be ignored.

The expectation that the world is orderly is the powerful stimulus that directs efforts to classify knowledge of it. Aristotle was the quintessential classifier. He observed the artifacts, catalogued and categorized them, and celebrated in this way the harmony that described the world. But is was Darwin's theory of common descent that turned classification into a scientific enterprise. In the centuries before Darwin, the *scala naturae*, the ladder of nature, was the step-by-step description of living forms from the simplest to the final, perfect form, the human being, cast in God's image. Nature's ladder restated the first taxonomy, Chapter I of the book of *Genesis*. But Darwin's theory demonstrated that there is a scientific explanation that traces the ancestry of complex forms of life back to their precursors. Many resemblances were lost, but the thread that bound living things together could be discovered if it were painstakingly sought (Mayr, 1982).

This sense of the past living on and of a future that is created in the present justifies classification as a form of organization, of formulating the structures of knowledge. In classification there are instruments to construct new knowledge, and while we draw maps of where we have been, the exercise also tells us where we are and where we might choose to go.

We think of taxonomy as classifications of living things, the ordering of relationships between species, but many systems of classification exist. Those that describe the discipline in mathematics, physics, chemistry are so elegant that we ignore the generations of searching that produced them. A taxonomy well known to nurses, nosology, the classification of disease, represents the advantage of observation and a precision of terms to describe what is seen.

Creation of a taxonomy requires the ability to identify clusters of characteristics that define a class of phenomena. Categories must be invented containing members that are similar to each other, but each category must be distinctly different from all the others. Categories of this kind are called *taxa* (the singular form is *taxon*). The decisions that finally result in taxa are complex.

1. ". . . different characters have different information content" (Mayr, 1982, p. 223). Thus, how shall the characteristics be weighted? Are some differences more significant than others? What rules for ranking will be used for all characteristics that are significant?
2. How many taxa will be necessary so that all of the entities essential to the classification are included? Will the taxon's size be justified by sufficient definition of included characteristics?
3. Is there a symmetry of relationships apparent that are useful in establishing the levels in which the taxa are placed (that is, is the hierarchy evident)?
4. What sequence of ordering provides the closest fit to the data and the way it will be used (Mayr, 1982, p. 242)?

Rank, size, symmetry and sequence successfully achieved suggest the hierarchy that is the structure or matrix of the classification. Hierarchies are not merely lists. They must display an internal "fit," so that every "higher taxon contains the taxa of the lower, subordinate rank" (Mayr, 1982, p. 206).

Every classification reflects the philosophical bias of the classifier, and often that influences the method chosen to achieve the classification. The prescientific, pre-Darwinian choice was a process of deduction. Mayr called this process "Downward classification by logical analysis" (Mayr, 1982, p. 158). Fortified by their certainty of the harmony and orderliness of the world, the classifiers adopted broad generalizations from which they deduced the step-by-step downward array of many thousands of living things. The large categories were created by identifying similarities, and subsequent levels were assigned as differences could be ascertained. It was strictly a "thought" process, never contaminated by actual examination of the specimens. (It was, however, rumored that Linneaus, the father of taxonomy, had surreptitiously examined actual specimens from time to time, Mayr, 1982, p. 190.) Classification by deduction was a method fraught with difficulty. The similarities were obvious enough, but the placing of subjects into subcategories by logic alone depended upon the differentiating characteristics (they were called *differentia*), and they tended to focus on single differences. As the explorers of the eighteenth and nineteenth centuries brought countless new species of plants and animals to light, the difficulty of classifying by logical analysis and deduction became impossible. Ever since Darwin, the evolutionary taxonomists have classified by "upward classification by empirical groups"

(Mayr, 1982, p. 190), placement being the result of careful observation, the empiric evidence, carefully gathered and weighed. Methods of observation were enhanced by the technological advances, such as the microscope, and there was exponential progress in the contributing sciences, such as physiology, biochemistry and genetics.

The importance of the inductive method and the collection of empirical evidence brought renewed vigor to classification. There was a harmony in the world vastly more wondrous than had been suspected, and vastly more complex.

The issue of weighting characteristics was well stated by Darwin himself. He wrote in *Origin of Species*, "The importance of classification of trifling characteristics mainly depends on being correlated with several other characters of more or less importance" (Mayr, 1982, p. 224). The deductive process placed emphasis on the larger taxa, the phyla, kingdoms, and classes. But the improved observation of specimens made the selection of species designation increasingly more difficult. Mayr calls modern taxonomy *microtaxonomy* because of the wealth of detail necessary for placement in the most discrete taxon, the species.

Classification is not a precise science. However carefully the characteristics are gathered, weighed, ranked and the subject placed, the entire process is dependent upon the knowledge and skill of the taxonomist. There are efforts to increase the objectivity of the process, but they have stimulated a sometimes acrimonious debate. One such school is devoted to "numerical phenetics" (from the Greek word *phaínein* to appear). The pheneticists ignore the ancestral lines that are the mainstay of evolutionary taxonomy and instead arbitrarily assign a numerical value to the characteristics of the subject. The same value is given to all characteristics without considering their relative importance, and a summarized value is reached which places the entity in a category. The pheneticists have developed valuable multivariate methods that aid in classification but their taxonomy is not widely accepted (Mayr, 1982).

Another modern school are the cladists (from the Greek word, *kládos*, meaning *twig*). They place primary importance on the branching of the ancestral tree, but they are interested only in the genealogy. The cladists believe that the branching produces a dichotomy, each branch forming two daughter branches, and when that occurs the ancestral form ceases to exist. New placement of individuals is on one or the other of the daughter branches (Mayr, 1982). By abandoning evolutionary history, the cladists place individuals on the basis of their similarities even though that sometimes results in very strange categories. For example, man, striped bass and sharks belong to a group called *Gnathostomata*, or *mouth with jaw*. But one branch is shared by man and the fish because they have fifty common characteristics including a bony skeleton. The shark is in a daughter branch because its skeleton is cartilage. The cladists would classify a Down's syndrome child with other Down's children rather than with his own parents (Webster, 1982).

The splitting into dichotomies is not a modern idea. It was the structure of the Porphyrian tree in the third century A.D. This ancient taxonomy was the work of the neoplatonist philosopher, Porphyrius, who in turn was reconstructing the positive-negative dichotomies familiarized by Aristotle. It would hardly be worth mentioning if it were not for a twentieth-century version. Decision trees are based on exactly the same premise—either-or—with the added feature of an arbitrary numerical value. It is a strange marriage of cladistics and phenetics, but it *is* a classification scheme that has been proposed to prepare nursing decisions (one might read *diagnosis* here) for computer programs.

The various philosophical schools of approach to taxonomy teach us that there are many difficulties attendant on the task of classification. Consider the dilemma facing the North American Nursing Diagnosis Association (NANDA). The 1973 charge proposed the gathering of a group of nurses who would bring empiric data from their clinical practice and from it identify the necessary categories for classifying nursing diagnosis. It was a perfectly sound inductive idea. It still is. But there was then imposed upon this activity still another, the belief that a group of theorists could come to a consensus that would create a theoretical framework out of which a diagnostic classification could be deduced. At least two nurses long involved in this enterprise have written into its proceedings the hope that the inductive approach of one group and the deductive approach of the other would somehow be reconciled and integrated (Gebbie, 1982, pp. 8–12; Kim, pp. 130–131). The situation is like that of two separate cohorts who decide to dig a tunnel through a mountain, beginning on opposite sides and hoping that somehow, the two tunnels will finally meet. First, it is essential that they dig into the same mountain.

Not only are nurses puzzled by the difficulties of describing the interactions between the caregiver and the patient. For several years physicians have recorded the conflicts that cannot be resolved over clinical issues because there is no diagnostic language available with which to do so. Feinstein writes:

. . . clinical data have no taxonomy at all. There currently exists no standard method, logic, order, system, structure, or rational procedure for classifying the clinical data of human illness (Feinstein, 1967, p. 124).

Indeed, he says, all clinical data must be converted "into the diagnostic categories of the nomenclature of pathology" (Feinstein, 1967, p. 125). Engel had much the same idea as early as 1951, and in 1960 wrote:

In the course of study of a patient, a great deal of . . . information is revealed; some may and some may not bear on the decision about diagnostic categories, but much does not lend itself to any such categorization. Yet, this unclassifiable information is essential to the physician's understanding (Engel, 1960, pp. 463–64).

Engel calls medical diagnosis "statistical and predictive," but the label "rarely, if ever, fully defines the illness" (Engel, 1960, p. 463). Feinstein demonstrates how the *nosology*, the classification of disease, is definitive only for the morbid anatomist. The clinician depends upon the evidence of his five senses and reaches conclusions based not on "evidence" but on "inferences." Inferences, he says, are "conclusions, exclusions and probability decisions" (Feinstein, 1967, p. 83). He adds:

When the endpoint of the taxonomic classification is reached after not one inference, but after a sequence of inferences, the problems of establishing reliable criteria and reproducible designations are enormous (Feinstein, 1967, p. 83).

Fabrega, describing ethnomedicine, has pointed out, ". . . occurrences of disease are significant at the point when they interfere with the social behavior of the individual. "What is relevant," he adds, "is the time-related changes in which the form of social functioning is altered or interfered with and/or the changes in the way the person uses social symbols" (Fabrega, 1975, 970). Citing these physicians places me in the dangerous area of the "regressive adaptation to a medical paradigm" (Kritek, 1985, p. 5), but it certainly is clear that they reject the notion of "cellular" diagnosis emphatically. The appeal of Weeds problem-oriented program is undoubtedly related to this strong conviction.

There may be little comfort in the discovery that physicians are as lacking in necessary clinical diagnostic language as nurses are, since it has always been assumed that the language of diagnosis of disease gave precision to medical diagnosis. Only physicians had the right to use the nosology as diagnostic labels. Nurses were required to understand and interpret it, but were forbidden to use it on patient's charts. But then, nurses were not permitted to be certain about anything; observations only "seemed" to be apparent and events only "appeared" to be unfolding. A profuse hemorrhage was described by nurses as "bright, red drainage" because only physicians could call blood *blood*. Nursing observations were recorded on short form check-lists, which reinforced the conviction that nurses had nothing important to say anyway. Nursing care was guided by pencilled notes, easily erased, on disposable Kardex cards. And for years the nurses notes were discarded when Medical Records filed a patient's chart. There is no tradition in nursing of nursing knowledge transmitted through clinical records; no sense that patient records could communicate useful information to other nurses, the recording of solutions to nursing problems, or the accumulation of useful data for nursing research. Instead, nurses struggled with a vague feeling of guilt and apology in response to criticism of the time they spent "writing" on charts; time that was alleged to be stolen from patient care.

Even if nurses themselves are now convinced that they do have essential judgments to make about patient care, the institutions in which nurses function retain their skepticism and even reluctance to permit autonomous and informed practice. This adds another imperative to the creation of a taxonomy of nursing. The classification must be unambiguous, clearly stated and definitive about nursing care. That is going to require some realism—and some straight talk.

Much ambiguity has been introduced into nursing's professional mission by the emphasis on such terms as *health care.* It is not necessary to deny the role of the nurse in health maintenance and disease prevention to acknowledge that the nurse is vital—an absolute necessity—in the care of the sick, the injured, the disabled. A diagnostic classification that does not recognize that fact fails the large population of nurses who work with the sick, and the people who desperately need their skill and expertise.

The taxonomy will fail if it is encumbered with jargon and meaningless platitudes. Why, for example, have we been so involved with the term *human responses?* First of all, what other kinds would nurses be concerned about? We are told that the human responses are the focus of nursing (Barnard, 1984, p. 5). Then there is a list of ten such human responses. The first three are mildly "physiological," dealing with self-care, and impaired rest, sleep, nutrition, elimination, and so forth, and then "pain and discomfort." The seven remaining human responses are psychosocial even psychiatric in their intent: anxiety, distortion of symbolic functions, deficiencies in decision making, self-image changes, dysfunctional perception, problematic affiliative relationships.

The confusion, however, is still manifest because the same author writes, "The patient has the health problem, the responses are the nursing problem." Confusion or not, the "diagnosed human response to actual or potential health problems are the core of nursing practice" (Barnard, 1984, p. 7).

There is a serious philosophical issue hidden in this jargon. The word *response* means *an answer, a reply.* To categorize all behavior (we will assume it is human) as a reaction to an external stimulus requires a view of the individual as a target. (Indeed, Barnard discusses "the nursing practice target area.") The kind of interventions planned for that target are very different from those that would be required by a person who, fortified with self-respect, retained control of his own life and never forfeited completely his sense of independence, choice, and strength of purpose. Allowed only to "respond," the individual assumes a role of dependency. Patients are not clinical problems; they are individuals with strengths and individuality, certain of their selfhood, unique, proud, and more than just a target that will respond.

Repeatedly there have been lamentations that diagnoses are not possible without precise terminology. But how is the issue served by adding terminology that fails not only to fill a precise role in nursing diagnosis, but is so esoteric as to confound what Gebbie once called the ordinary nurse, who must, finally, make this project succeed or fail. The effort to fit all of nursing into a list of nouns demonstrates how much more difficult the task can be when precision is lacking. The words describe a melange of behavioral possibilities, but they ask more questions than they answer. When does *communicating* exclude *relating*? How does *choosing* succeed in the absence of *valuing*? What clear lines separate *knowing* and *perceiving*? How is *feeling* separated from all the others? And how can nurses, educated in the basic sciences, lump all physiological functioning under *exchanging*?

The language choices on the approved list are little better. The wonderful ambition to build diagnoses by the gathering of empirical clinical experience seems not to have been realized. The methodology is described as *first* choosing a diagnostic category and *then* ascribing to it some justifications under the rubrics of *etiology* and *defining character-*

istics. If the process was, in fact, an inductive one as the original group visualized, the diagnostic statement would be the result of arranging the defining characteristics rather than the reverse. The methodology being used is deductive, pure and simple.

The abstracts from the Sixth Conference listed over twenty research presentations, but only five of them were clinical studies that focused on the usefulness of an accepted diagnosis. The others were studies of how various nurse populations were using the approved list. The procedure of stating the diagnosis and then finding ways to justify it is reminiscent of the traditional pattern in nursing; first the procedure was written, and then, *a posteriori*, the scientific *principles* were applied. That may account for the inconsistency in language use in the approved list. While a language as precise as that of the nosology will never be found, the substitute must be consistency in usage of the language, including its grammatical form in the diagnostic labels. Using the 1982 list (Kim and Moritz, 1982), there are several issues that would make it difficult to approach these labels for placement in a taxonomy.

There is, first of all, an overwhelmingly negative tone to the list. The labels contain words like: intolerance, impaired, ineffective, distress, isolation, dysfunctional, all descriptives of suffering. There is a difference in the way alternatives are listed. Bowel elimination, coping, fluid volume, nutrition and skin integrity are listed in separate lines for each variation covered. But injury, self-care deficit, sensory-perceptual alteration, and tissue perfusion list several possible variations in a single line. Many of the distinctions are matters of degree; some things are more or less, and many are actual or potential. There are some that are frankly pathological, for instance, rape trauma syndrome and perhaps anxiety or fear; some that unabashedly make reference to body organs (the heart, oral mucosa, skin integrity) and two euphemistic (and inaccurate) references to body functions: "bowel elimination, alteration in" and "urinary elimination, alteration in patterns." The latter two labels, perhaps in a wish to be genteel, simply mistate their intention. It is not the bowel nor the urinary (sic) that is eliminated. Constipation, diarrhea and incontinence are symptoms, and they are the only labels of so specific a category included. Pain does not rate a category of its own, but is listed under comfort so that the physiological impact of pain is lost. Meanwhile, comfort that is related to ambient light, noise, temperature and physical surroundings—the comfort that is provided by hands-on nursing care—is not included.

If the structures of thought are truly expressed in the classification system of a discipline, as Gould suggests, then the nursing structure requires some revision. It is not too late to declare a moratorium on the acceptance of diagnostic labels and begin to develop a true taxonomy of nursing.

1. Nurses everywhere, no matter where they work, should be invited to local meetings (maybe only in their own institutions) to talk about their real life experiences in nursing. A vast data base is sitting there untapped. Nurses know what they do and why they do it, and they could be encouraged to talk about it with each other. This clinical information should be gathered in a central clearing house and the defining characteristics of the clinical report teased out. Then, we can begin the essential task of creating meaningful categories, but the defining characteristics come *first*.

2. The importance of interdependent diagnostic statements that will help nurses plan intelligently for the care of the very sick, acutely ill, and severely traumatized patients who now occupy our intensive care units and acute care hospitals must be a high priority. Nurses who chose health maintenance and disease prevention as areas of practice lose nothing if a taxonomy also provides guidance for nurses who work with sick patients. Accurate, accepted terminology for normal, healthy functions such as *micturition* and *defecation* should be used.

3. We have evidence that the nosology has limited value for physicians. It also has limited value for nurses. Why shouldn't nurses identify the nursing implications in the nosology? The expressed difficulty of some physicians in finding appropriate clinical language is a problem we share. Rather than build fences that separate us from our medical colleagues, let us instead join forces to explore the clinical issues we must confront together.

4. Theory building for nursing diagnosis is premature. Now there are two processes running parallel to each other, but never quite meeting. Opportunities for contention will increase as each of the interested groups becomes more entrenched in their private designs.

   The public declarations of the association (NANDA) should be stated in clear language that will be understood by practicing nurses, no matter what their area of specialization may be. The diagnoses must make sense to them, because unless they can use the taxonomy, there is no purpose in creating one.

The search for a nursing taxonomy is not merely an exercise in semantics. The search for substantive nursing knowledge must go on in as broad a context as possible. Nursing must not be constrained, but liberated by this process. This is an opportunity to learn from each other, and to make our profession stronger and better as we do so. Let us be full partners in health care, and willingly take our place in the vanguard of those who translate the gifts of their minds into compassionate patterns of patient care.

REFERENCES

Barnard, K.: The ANA's social policy statement on nursing- implications for the conference group's work on classification of nursing diagnosis. In Kim, M.J., McFarland, G.K. and McLane, A.M., editors: Classification of nursing diagnosis: proceedings of the fifth national conference, St. Louis, 1984, The C.V. Mosby Co.

Douglas, D.J., and Murphy, E.K.: Nursing process, nursing diagnosis and emerging taxonomies. In McCloskey, J., and Grace, H., editors: Current trends in nursing, ed. 2, Boston, 1985, Blackwell Scientific Publications.

Engel, G.L.: A unified concept of health and disease, Perspectives Biol. Med. 3:459, 1960.

Fabrega, H., Jr.: The need for an ethnomedical science, Science 189:969, 1975.

Feinstein, A.R.: Clinical judgement, Huntington, N.Y., 1967, Robert E. Kreiger Publ.

Gebbie, K.M. Toward the theory development for nursing diagnosis classification. In Kim, M.J., and Moritz, D.A., editors: Classification of nursing diagnoses: proceedings of the third and fourth national conferences, New York, 1982, McGraw Hill.

Gould, S.J.: Understanding science past and present, New York Times Book Review p. 72, May 18, 1980.

Gould, S.J.: Hens' teeth and horses' toes, New York, 1983, W.W. Norton.

Kim, M.J., and Moritz, D.A.: Classification of nursing diagnosis: proceedings of the third and fourth conferences, St. Louis, 1982, The C.V. Mosby Co.

Kim, M.J.: Issues related to research on the classification of nursing diagnosis. In Kim, M.J. and Moritz, D.A. editors: Classification of nursing diagnosis: proceedings of the third and fourth conferences, St. Louis, 1982, The C.V. Mosby Co.

Kritek, P.B.: Nursing diagnosis in perspective: response to a critique, Image 17:3, 1980.

Lash, A.A.: A re-examination of nursing diagnosis, Nurs. Forum 17:332, 1978.

Mayr, E.: The growth of biological thought, Cambridge, MA, 1982, Harvard University Press.

Webster, B.: Classification is more than a matter of fish or fowl, In The New York Times, p. 8E, Feb. 14, 1982.

CHAPTER 6

Nursing's emerging paradigm: the diagnosis of pattern

MARGARET A. NEWMAN, Ph.D., R.N.

In the days of Copernicus, about 500 years ago, everyone thought the earth was the center of the universe and that the sun and all the other planets revolved around the earth. From our perspective today that was a very limited view of things. Based on his observations and mathematical calculations, Copernicus said (and people thought he was crazy), That's not the way it is. The sun is the center of things, and the earth and all the other planets revolve around the sun. What a revolutionary idea! Actually, though, it did not change what was there; it just changed the way things were viewed. For one thing, it identified the earth and its inhabitants as simply one aspect of a much larger whole.

We have been involved in a similar revolution. For a long time we thought that disease was the center of our world of nursing. We have a long history of aligning ourselves with medicine in the prevention, treatment and rehabilitation of persons, families and communities in relation to disease. Then, after a century or so of observing that this approach was not working too well, some people began to say disease is not the center of things, with everything viewed in relation to disease. The whole person, whose nature is indivisible, is the center of things. Disease is simply one aspect of the way a person manifests her- or himself.

Nursing has known this on some level all along, perhaps from the very beginning of our modern history. We have become very familiar with Florence Nightingale's emphasis on health and minimization of the information afforded by disease. She pointed out that pathology teaches us merely the disruptive characteristic of disease, and that understanding of health comes about through observation and experience. Based on observation and experience, she said, nursing can "put the patient in the best condition for nature to act upon him [sic]" (Nightingale, 1859). These words, *observation* and *experience*, have relevance to what we are trying to do today in the development of the concept of nursing diagnosis.

The generating motivations of the founders of this conference on nursing diagnosis, I submit, stem from an intuitive conviction that what nurses were observing and experiencing was different from what medicine was observing and acting upon, and so the movement to identify and elaborate the nursing perspective began in a formal way.

In 1978 the nurse-theorist group invited by NANDA to participate in the development of a classification system for nursing diagnosis met and produced a new way of viewing the phenomena of our practice. Hundreds of observations submitted by the membership of this organization were examined and were clustered into categories according to apparent similarity. At the same time, the group deliberated beliefs about nursing that provided the world view, which in my terms is the paradigm, that structures the perspective from which nursing diagnoses emerge. As in the Copernican revolution, the elements did not change, simply (though it is not simple to accomplish) the way of viewing the elements. The disease and the problems associated with disease were still there, but they were viewed not as entities within themselves but as information about the essential pattern of the person, the human being that is the center of nursing's concern and purpose.

In 1980 Marilyn Ferguson, a recognized spokesperson for new-paradigm thinking, outlined the shift that has taken place in the paradigm of health as we have moved from a paradigm in which disease is the center to a paradigm in which the person is the center. We no longer view disease as totally negative or as an entity unto itself but rather as information about the whole, as a manifestation of pattern. We seek then not to simply eliminate the symptoms of disease but to identify and understand the pattern of which the symptoms are a part. In the old paradigm based on etiology and treatment of disease, the professional is the authority and as such prescribes what the client should do. In the new paradigm based on pattern recognition, the professional is a therapeutic partner and joins with the client in the search for pattern, with its concomitant understanding and impetus for growth.

I think we can have a sense of inner satisfaction that nursing has been at the forefront of knowledge development within the paradigm of pattern. Martha Rogers (1970) emphasized from the outset, in her theory of the unitary nature of human beings, that pattern is the identifying characteristic of a person's wholeness and that the need in nursing practice is to identify *sequential patterns of man's evolving interaction with the environment.*

The point of identifying *sequential* patterns is crucial. The pattern evolves over time. The pattern of relationships that characterized one's childhood, while retaining some essential enduring characteristics, is different from the pattern of the present situation. Each pattern of person-environment interaction is time specific but at the same time contains information enfolded from the past. It is possible to discern the total pattern from the present without reference to the past, therefore, and in a crisis situation, that is probably where one starts. An example related by another nurse (A. Kelly, personal communication, April 20, 1984) illustrates this point:

The client, K., was a young divorced woman who had limited contact with her ex-husband and was not close to her family of origin, even though her mother and her brother lived in the vicinity. She reported feeling bored with her life. She supported herself and her two children, aged two and five, by providing day care for an infant and three other preschool children.

The incident that brought the client to the attention of the nurse was the sudden death of the infant while being cared for at K.'s home. K. responded appropriately, administering CPR and calling the police, but afterward felt guilty and disorganized and overwhelmed by the fighting and turmoil of the children, who had witnessed the event.

Shortly after the infant's death, the nurse telephoned the client offering information about Sudden Infant Death Syndrome (SIDS), and the client asked for help in relating to the children. The nurse visited the home, which was in disarray, and the children were fighting with each other and with the mother. K. was tearful, felt fatigued and wanted to be alone. She had lost interest in her children and was suffering from insomnia. The nurse offered some suggestions regarding the children and invited K. to attend a support group, which she later attended.

The nurse maintained periodic contact with K., and fifteen weeks later, although still sad about the experience of the infant's death, K. had gained considerable comfort from being active in the support group. She took steps to obtain an instructor's license in CPR and had begun teaching a class in it. She helped to present a program about SIDS for day-care providers, arranged to have information about SIDS supplied to each licensed day-care provider and contacted other babysitters who had had similar experiences with SIDS. She volunteered to serve on a local health service board in response to an ad in the newspaper.

At the point when the nurse entered the situation, the client's pattern of interaction was one of disorganization, feelings of sadness and guilt and frustration with child care responsibilities. When the nurse was asked what she saw as her contribution to the situation, she said she thought she provided an organizing force through which the client was able to seek assistance from her mother-in-law for the child care and move out of the home to focus on more outgoing relationships with others in the community. K. developed a close relationship with her mother-in-law for the first time and maintained a friendship with the parents of the infant who died. She was able to allow the children to discuss the experience of the infant's death and to ask questions freely. K. felt as though she had become more outgoing and caring in her relationships with other people.

A diagram of three sequential patterns from K.'s life (see Fig. 1) illustrates first a relatively closed, low-energy system in which K. existed pretty much alone with her children and the children she took care of during the day. Then the next pattern is one of disruption and disorganization, as K. dealt

with the infant's death and subsequently with her feelings and the children's behaviors. The third pattern reflects her reaching out to others to give and receive help. She establishes more intimate relationships with other adults and feels more caring. In comparison, this pattern is characterized by higher energy exchange between K. and her environment and a better quality of relationships.

The identification of the patterns of interaction at these three points in time is simply a reflection of *what is*. It requires very little or no inference or interpretation. It does not imply causality. It is not necessary to know why the client was living a relatively isolated, boring life or why or how it changed in the period following the crisis. From my point of view, this sequence reveals a pattern of expanding consciousness, i.e., a pattern of increased quality and diversity of interaction with the environment. The nurse acted as a source of power, as a pure reference beam which helped the client focus and move beyond herself to relate to others in more caring, meaningful ways.

The role of the nurse within a paradigm of pattern is to help clients recognize their own patterns. A question I have been asked many times is, "But what do you *do about* pattern even if you are able to identify it?" Nursing diagnosis, in any form, portrays the presenting phenomenon. It pinpoints what you are dealing with. It is a guide to action only insofar as we are knowledgeable about the phenomenon. The isolated phenomena of a problem-oriented paradigm are more familiar to us than the dynamic interactions of a pattern paradigm; so we think we know what to do about them. In this way we delude ourselves into thinking the diagnosis is a guide to specific action.

If diagnosis is not a guide to action, what is it? To focus again on the new paradigm, it is *pattern recognition*. It is the burst of insight that occurs when, suddenly, every-

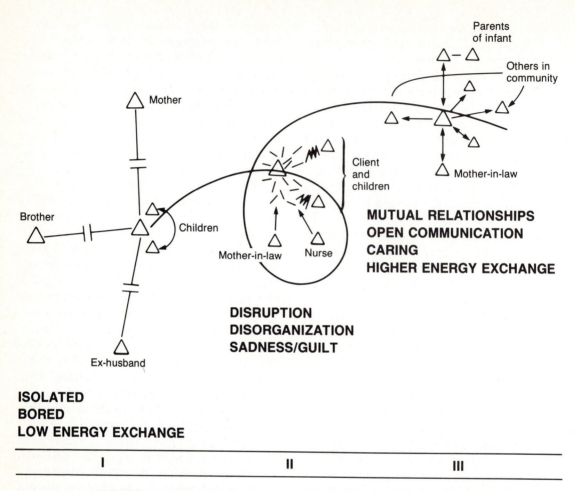

Mother

Brother

Children

Mother-in-law

Nurse

Ex-husband

Client and children

Parents of infant

Others in community

Mother-in-law

**MUTUAL RELATIONSHIPS
OPEN COMMUNICATION
CARING
HIGHER ENERGY EXCHANGE**

**DISRUPTION
DISORGANIZATION
SADNESS/GUILT**

**ISOLATED
BORED
LOW ENERGY EXCHANGE**

I   II   III

FIGURE 1   Sequential patterns of person-environment relationships.

thing fits together; everything makes sense. And when that happens, the pathway of action opens up. It is like throwing light on a situation. Then one can see clearly and take action. It is different for every situation and therefore cannot be prescribed in advance. It is facilitated by another person's involvement in the interactive process, and that's where nursing comes in.

As I've said before, I think the NANDA health assessment framework based on unitary person-environment patterns of interaction is a step in the direction of helping nurses facilitate patients' pattern recognition (Newman, 1984). I have emphasized

that this framework is not a classification system for diagnosis but a guide for assessment, a way of viewing person-environment interaction that focuses on the whole. After seeing the work of the NANDA Taxonomy Committee (March 9–10, 1986), I would propose that the nine patterns of interaction represent one step below the diagnosis level. The diagnosis level would consist of descriptions of the total pattern of the person, a pattern that would reflect the unity of the nine dimensions. This level has not been adequately explicated at this time.

From the previous cast study example, Pattern I might be characterized as one of low energy exchange and relative isolation of the person from meaningful adult relationships; Pattern II is one of disorganization, intense, conflictual feelings about herself and her children, and the beginning of an ability to receive support from other adults. Pattern III reveals an increasing number of meaningful mutual adult relationships and more open and caring relationships, which could be considered a modulated, higher exchange of energy. Exploration and elaboration of the nature of the patterns of person-environment interaction have not been undertaken systematically on a large scale; therefore at this time there is little that can be shared with certainty and specificity. I am convinced, however, on the basis of my work with graduate students' explorations and my own pilot work in this area that this unified pattern of the whole is the level at which we function in nursing and is the basis for nursing diagnosis.

As this approach to pattern identification is adopted by nursing practitioners, the skill of sensing into the whole becomes integral to practice. Sensing into the whole is the action component crucial to a paradigm of pattern, and this activity is more one of sensing into oneself than of observing another.

The holographic model of intervention explains this process. A hologram is a form of photography in which the image on the film is formed indirectly by the interaction of light waves being projected from two sources: one from the subject being photographed and one from a pure reference beam such as a laser. The interaction of waves from these two sources forms an interference pattern that reflects the visual image of the subject being photographed. The intriguing aspect of this phenomenon is that every portion of the resulting holographic film contains information about the whole! If a small corner of the film is torn off and a light is projected through that segment, the image portrayed will be the entire image originally photographed, not an arm or a leg as would have been the case if one had torn a segment from the film of a conventional photograph.

This model for the way things work has been used to explain the way the brain works (Pribram, 1971) and even the way the universe works (Bohm, 1980). And more to the point in terms of our present concern, it has been used to explain the process of therapeutic interaction.

It helps to imagine the phenomenon of interference patterns to visualize a rock being thrown into a lake. As it hits the water, a series of circular waves emanate from the point of impact and spread outward. Then imagine another rock being thrown into the water nearby with its own pattern of expanding waves. Within seconds the two wavefronts will reach each other and interact, forming a new pattern, an interference pattern (see Fig. 2). Eventually the interference pattern expands to replace the original two patterns, which have become *one pattern containing information about the whole of both.*

Now imagine two persons interacting in place of the two rocks (see Fig. 3). The waves that emanate from each person interact with the waves of the other person, forming an interference pattern that contains information from each pattern and eventually becomes the whole. One's own pattern (being) contains information about the whole. *The way to get in touch with the pattern of the other person is to sense into one's own pattern.*

Just as in holography a pure reference beam is used to depict the picture of the subject, in therapeutic relationships it is helpful to try to clear one's field to act as a mirror of the client's pattern and thereby facilitate that client's own pattern recognition.

The goal of this type of intervention (which is really nonintervention) is not so

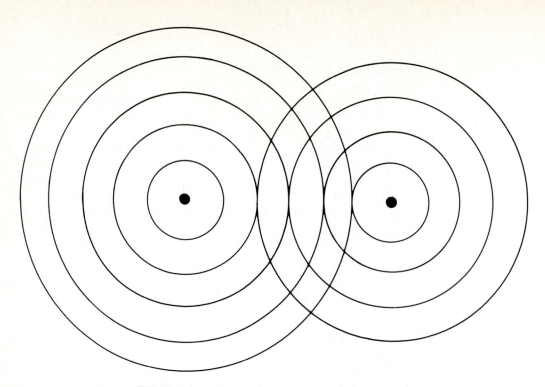

FIGURE 2   Formation of an interference pattern.

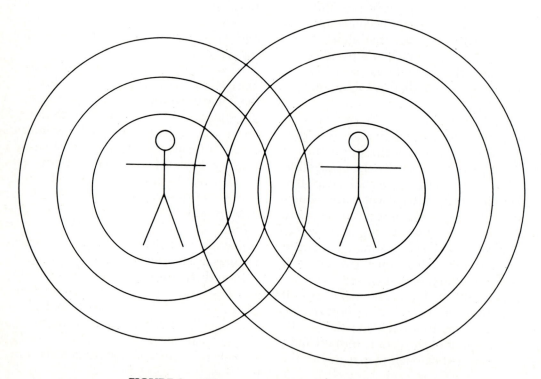

FIGURE 3   Person-to-person interference pattern.

much that we as professionals identify the pattern of the client but that clients have the experience of recognizing their own patterns of interacting with the environment. It is characteristic of the process, however, that the professional will have a similar experience. This kind of insight occurs suddenly, as when a picture comes into focus and one sees clearly, or knows thoroughly, the meaning of diagnosis.* Through this heightened understanding the pathway of action unfolds.

So what does this mean for the work of this conference? I think it means that the key to nursing diagnosis lies not so much in information outside ourselves (i.e., data *about* the client) as it does in information that is continuously available to us within our pattern of interaction with the client. This insight can occur instantly and is just as readily available to a nurse in the rapid pace of an acute care setting as it is for someone who has time for more deliberate contemplation.

For some, this approach appears to be rejecting the information that we have collected thus far. For others, it is totally subjective, not objective, and therefore not valid from their perspective.

To these charges I say first that it does include the information of the old paradigm but from a different perspective, the perspective of what that information means in terms of the total pattern of energy exchange. I agree that it is not objective, because in a paradigm of pattern things are no longer separated into subject and object. There are no separating boundaries between what is outside (objective) and what is inside (subjective), and so neither is it subjective.

A paradigm of pattern eliminates dichotomies. In a holographic model, we have access to the total information of our world through ourselves. By offering ourselves as windows of the world we can facilitate this insight, "knowing thoroughly," in others.

In the past decade, a rapidly increasing number of nurses have endorsed the concept of pattern as central to nursing diagnosis and action (Benner and Wrubel, 1982; Bramwell, 1984; Crawford, 1982; Fitzpatrick, 1983; Newman, 1979, 1983; Parse, 1981). The need now is to get on with it! When the uncertainties and doubts arise as we are faced with letting go of the safety of the old and taking the leap to the new, it's tempting to want to hold back. But as Marilyn Ferguson (1983) has said, "If you keep acting like you've always acted, you're going to get what you've always got." I am convinced that we in nursing want more for ourselves and for the patients we serve. We want the authenticity and meaning and satisfaction that comes when our relationships with patients have made a difference. Each of us has experienced the coherence of such moments from time to time and we want to be able to explicate that knowledge of the whole to others. As we are able to do this, we can have confidence that our practice derives from a nursing paradigm.

REFERENCES

Benner, P., and Wrubel, J.: Skilled clinical knowledge: the value of perceptual awareness, I and II, J. Nurs. Admin. **5:**42, and **6:**28, 1982.

Bohm, D.: Wholeness and the implicate order, London, 1980, Routledge & Kegan Paul.

Bramwell, L.: Use of the life history in pattern identification and health promotion, Advances Nurs. Sci. **7:**37, 1984.

Crawford, G.: The concept of pattern in nursing: conceptual development and measurement, Advances Nurs. Sci. **5:**1, 1982.

Ferguson, M.: The aquarian conspiracy: personal and social transformation in the 1980s, Los Angeles, 1980, J.P. Tarcher.

Ferguson, M.: Conference: power of knowing, Minneapolis, 1983.

Fitzpatrick, J.J.: A life perspective rhythm model. In

---

*The word diagnosis comes from the Greek words for *knowing* and for *through* or *thoroughly* and literally means *knowing thoroughly*.

Fitzpatrick, J.J., and Whall, A.L., editors: Conceptual models of nursing, Bowie, M.D., 1983, Brady.

Newman, M.A.: Theory development in nursing, Philadelphia, 1979, F.A. Davis.

Newman, M.A.: Editorial, Advances Nurs. Sci. **5:**x, 1983.

Newman, M.A.: Nursing diagnosis: Looking at the whole, Am. J. Nurs. **84:**1496, 1984.

Nightingale, F.: Notes on nursing: what it is, and what it is not, Philadelphia, 1900, J.B. Lippincott. (Originally published in 1859, by Harrison and Sons.)

Parse, R.P.: Man-living-health, a theory of nursing, New York, 1981, John Wiley.

Pribram, K.: Languages of the brain, Belmont, CA, 1971, Brooks, Cole.

Rogers, M.E.: An introduction to the theoretical basis of nursing, Philadelphia, 1970, F.A. Davis.

CHAPTER 7

Etiology: conceptual concerns

JOYCE J. FITZPATRICK, Ph.D., R.N., F.A.A.N.

I am pleased to be here this morning for, in my opinion, the nursing diagnosis movement, formalized through NANDA, has the potential for uniting us through our clinical practice. It is an important mission and an important goal for our discipline. While we should continue to celebrate the great strides we have made since 1973, we should also focus deliberately on major issues that remain.

The etiology, or identification of causes, of nursing diagnoses, continues to be a conceptual and practical issue in our disciplinary discussions. Our focus today, on the conceptual concerns related to etiology, may best be understood as an effort to describe the etiology of the etiological dilemmas related to nursing diagnosis. For, in fact, the issues that are to be addressed in this paper center around the basic question: Why is the etiology of a nursing diagnosis of concern? We are searching for reasons to explain an occurrence, or at least a state of mind, regarding the etiological dimensions of nursing diagnosis. And, in particular, we are asking ourselves to consider the question from alternate viewpoints, i.e., the conceptual and the practical.

This paper, focused on conceptual concerns, is organized according to three broad areas. First, I will address the question of etiology from the general perspective of the development of the discipline. Second, the question will be viewed from an analysis of the nature of etiology per se. Third, and importantly, the specific issues related to etiology of nursing diagnosis will be addressed.

The issues that confront us are not unique, but arise from the nature of our professional discipline. As a new science and an old profession (though perhaps not the oldest) nursing is presently struggling to bridge the gaps. We continue to search for links between science and professional practice, education and service, researchers and clinicians. The research-practice issue most relevant to clinical judgment as reflected in nursing diagnosis may be the distinction between statistical and clinical inference. It is important that we acknowledge that they are different *and* that we need both to carry on our work. It will continue to be important to ask ourselves how the rules of science are related to our clinical practice. Further, we must identify which rules govern our practice and articulate these clearly for the profession. The roles of scientist and clinician are complementary. It is important that we build our research and practice models for nursing diagnosis together.

Before proceeding I am compelled to alert you that I share Popper's belief that our knowledge must forever remain tentative, that the only absolute certainty resides in our belief systems, and that our goal ought to be to discover even deeper and more meaningful problems. What I will share with you are some tentative thoughts, an enthusiasm for the quest, and a readiness to explore and question. Importantly, I wish to share a hope that we will succeed, and that by discovering new knowledge about humans and their health, that we will improve the lives of many who request and seek our services, and thus influence the health of all persons.

Nurses, as practitioners and as scientists, concern themselves with persons, their environments, and their health. The conceptual agreement on the basic concepts of person, environment, health, and nursing, upon which the discipline is based, is well documented in the nursing theory literature (Fawcett, 1981; Flaskared and Halloran, 1981; Fitzpatrick and Whall, 1982; Meleis, 1985). There is general agreement that these concepts are central to a nursing perspective. Such an emphasis has been traced from Nightingale through present day nurse-theorists such as Roy, Orem, and Rogers.

There have been consistent attempts to explicate theoretically the relationships among these concepts. The conceptualization proposed by the NANDA Nurse Theorist group is one example of such an effort. Another familiar effort is the work of Donaldson and Crowley (1979) in which they identified themes central to the professional discipline.

Within the professional practice domain recently agreement has been demonstrated through the widespread acceptance of the American Nurses' Association Social Policy Statement. All of us are cognizant of the definition of nursing as focused on the diagnosis and treatment of human responses to actual or potential health problems.

In specific reference to etiology, then, what understandings are inherent in our perspective on nursing? We have consistently proclaimed the uniqueness of our perspective to be our holistic focus on persons and their health. The precise definitions of this holism have ranged from the additive or comprehensive approach to the nonadditive approach. There continues to be a basic value in the concept of holism. To be logically consistent, such a disciplinary perspective requires attention to multiple influencing factors in descriptions of diagnostic etiology. While most of us might reflexively reject the concept of single casuality, in both our professional roles of research and clinical practice and our day-to-day lives we often struggle to reduce our experiences to such simplistic understandings.

It may be helpful to discuss an example to illustrate these points. You are undoubtedly familiar with terms such as *learning-disabled, hyperactive,* and *hyperkinetic,* terms often used interchangeably. Various causes for the child's behavior have been advanced, including birth defects, perceptual deficiencies, and vitamin deficiencies. Methods of intervention flow from the basic causative factors identified. More recently, as our understanding has advanced, multiple methods of intervention have been initiated. In defining the etiology of nursing diagnosis we need to consider the direct relationships such stated causes will have on determining our interventions. In fact, etiology may be directly linked to interventions.

To return then to the more general level of discussion, several broad conceptual concerns can be identified. These include:

1. A need to delineate the processes for discipline development, and, to the extent necessary, to prioritize our focus on these processes.

Basic questions that we continue to raise here include: To what extent should our current practice determine our future? Should nursing science be developed inductively from the clinical practice perspective? Are our nursing diagnoses situation-specific or clinical-specialty-specific?

In describing and synthesizing our domain we must integrate the focus on what we do in practice with our theories and our research. Such an integrative effort is presently lacking to a large degree. It would seem imperative that we place major emphasis and energy on the movement toward conceptual integration.

2. A need to specify the norms for the discipline.

As a discipline we need to make clear and direct the conceptual and practical statements about autonomy of nursing practice in relation to nursing diagnosis. Further, in developing our research related to nursing diagnosis we should state strongly the direct value of large-scale, multisite projects. It is imperative that our efforts be directed toward complex analysis of the multifactor relationships inherent in the basic phenomena of concern to nursing. And importantly, we should evaluate nursing diagnosis as the dynamic multilevel process that in fact reflects the reality of nursing practice.

3. A need to determine the primary unit or units of analysis for the discipline.

While the assumption can be made that to a large extent our focus here is on human patterns as a basic unit of analysis, it is necessary to more fully and consistently develop this theme. For example, questions should be raised about the conceptual consistency among observations, methods of assessment, intervention plans, and patient outcomes in relation to nursing diagnosis specifically, and human patterns more generally.

Besides the more general conceptual concerns identified above, several factors related more directly to the diagnostic process will be considered. These include: the concept of causality, the process of diagnosis, the nature of clinical inferences, and the relationship of etiology to interventions.

The *concept of causality* has been debated by philosophers in general and by philosophers of science in particular since early recorded philosophic discourse. While we may wish to continue our scholarly debates regarding the validity of causality, there are more relevant questions of immediate concern within the area of nursing diagnosis. The significant issues include:

1. Relevance of singular, predominant, or multicausal models compared to multiple interaction models
2. Determination of relative weights to be placed on various etiological factors, e.g., predisposing factors, precipitating factors, etc.
3. Linearity of the etiological process and its basic relevance if determined to be primarily linear or multidimensional
4. The tentative nature of probable influencing factors and the related influences on choices of interventions

In relation to these identified issues it would seem most appropriate to our conceptual underpinnings if we chose to replace the label *etiology* with *influencing factors*. Also, it is significant that our clinical inferences are related to the processing of multiple sets of observations, facts, and other information sources. Our models for research will necessarily include a focus on complex probabilistic approaches.

The *process of diagnosis* in nursing involves a knowledge base related to a nursing perspective, an ability to collect data gathered through the observation and assessment processes, the organization of complex and multiple sets of information, and the making of clinical inferences based on the nature and organization of the data.

Based on the complexity of the phenomena of concern to nursing, *clinical inference in nursing* necessarily requires tentative hypotheses. Our knowledge about the complex human condition will continue to be somewhat imprecise. Yet it is possible to identify key related variables.

In the diagnostic model that has been tentatively adopted here, etiology must be linked directly to interventions. Therefore, it follows that the etiological factors related to nursing diagnosis must be aspects of the person's health that are amenable to nursing intervention. Perhaps if we were to concern ourselves totally with excellence in nursing practice, rather than assuming any and all functions that are presented by the situation or by other disciplines, we would more quickly and effectively advance our discipline.

Let me summarize the conceptual concerns related to the etiology of nursing diagnoses with a more general analysis of where we are and where we should go. What is reflected in the NANDA work is not so different from the profession at large. Nonetheless, it is a conceptual smorgasbord. We have so encouraged individuality and diversity in our nursing science and practice that we often fail to recognize, individually and collectively, that the product is nursing. It is time to assume professional responsibility for our discipline, and to make a clear conceptual statement about nursing. Such a conceptualization must be evaluated both by its internal logical consistency and its external validity. For example, we must recognize that the understanding of "human responses" is logically inconsistent with the conceptualization underlying the nine patterns identified by the Nurse Theorist group. Importantly, as one reads through the maze of material on nursing diagnosis published

in the past decade what is striking is both the consistency of diagnostic terms used (i.e., those approved by NANDA) and the inconsistency in conceptualization. Someone must assume leadership for clarifying the conceptual ambiguities.

My final plea, then, has direct relevance to the criterion of external validity. In a 1985 *Annual Review of Nursing Research* chapter on nursing diagnosis research, Gordon (1985) identified only eight studies on the topic. We must translate all of our clinical work on nursing diagnosis into projects that have a research dimension. The most productive mode would be a concerted movement toward large-scale investigations, across institutional settings, with large data bases and multimethod approaches. Such research is necessary not only for the validation of nursing diagnoses, but more generally, for the concerted enhancement of all aspects of our science and practice.

REFERENCES

American Nurses Association: Nursing: a social policy statement, Kansas City, Mo., 1980,

Donaldson. S.K., and Crowley, D.: The discipline of nursing, Nurs. Outlook **26**:113, 1978.

Fawcett, J.: Analysis and evaluation of conceptual models of nursing, Philadelphia, 1984, F.A. Davis.

Fitzpatrick, J.J., and Whall, A.L.: Conceptual models of nursing: analysis and application, Bowie, MD, 1983, Brady.

Flaskerud, J.H., and Halloran, E.J.: Areas of agreement in nursing theory development. Advances Nurs. Sci. **3**:1, 1980.

Gordon, M.: Nursing diagnosis. In Werley, H.H. and Fitzpatrick, J.J., editors: Annual review of nursing research, vol. 3, New York, 1985, Springer Verlag.

Meleis, A.I.: Theoretical nursing: development and progress, Philadelphia, 1985, J.B. Lippincott.

CHAPTER 8

Etiology: practical relevance

ANAYIS DERDIARIAN, M.P.H., D.N.Sc.

The topic I have been asked to examine for this conference implies two assumptions: first, that factors which cause nursing problems exist and, second, that the study of such factors and their relationships to nursing problems is important to nursing. Therefore, the purpose of this paper is to provide a conceptual framework within which to examine and to specify the central relationship of etiology to nursing practice, method, and research.

ETIOLOGY

First, it is fitting to examine the generic and practical meaning of the concept of etiology. *Webster's New World Encyclopedia* (1981) defines etiology as: "the assignment of cause; the science of causes; and, the science or theory of causes or origins of disease." *Taber's Cyclopedic Medical Dictionary* (1983) defines etiology as "the study of causes of disease which result from an abnormal state producing pathological conditions." As can be seen, these definitions concur that etiology pertains to the study of causes, diseased conditions, and the relationships between the two, i.e., that certain factors are causally related to certain diseases or disease conditions.

The practical references of etiology to health-related fields that are better established than nursing has been demonstrated in the history of their respective scientific developments. The origins of *etiology* as a concept are deeply rooted in epidemiology and medicine, based on their shared quest to understand causes of human diseases. In these disciplines, the ultimate scientific pursuit of etiology emanated from their common desire to control and prevent disease. The primary focus of epidemiology is the study of causes of disease in order to intervene in these causes and thus control disease through prevention. The primary focus of medicine, on the other hand, is the study of diseases or disease conditions in order to intervene in them as well as in their causes and, thus, to minimize harm or eradicate disease. The symbiotic relationship between epidemiology and medicine explains the advances they together have achieved in the science of factors and their causal relationships with diseases. The most recent literature reveals the multiple factors that cause human disease or contribute to it, such as behavioral, cultural, and environmental factors. Such findings imply that developments in the etiology of diseases should be pursued in the behavioral, cultural, and environmental sciences as well. Thus, medical clinicians and scientists must also collaborate in practice and research with scientists in those respective fields.

Having examined the origins of *etiology* in the epidemiologic and medical literature, it would be useful to examine the meaning of

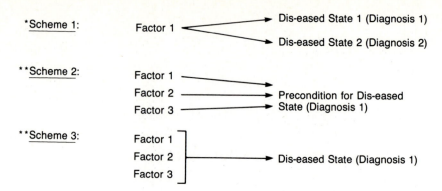

FIGURE 1   Three schemes representing possible relationships between causal factors and diseased states or nursing diagnoses.

Scheme 1 adapted from Mausner, J.S., and Bahn, A.K.: Epidemiology, Philadelphia, 1974, W.B. Saunders Co.; Schemes 2 and 3 adapted from Lilienfeld, A.M., et al.: Cancer epidemiology: methods of study, Baltimore, 1967, Johns Hopkins University Press.

cause or *causal relationships* between factors and diseases. In the epidemiologic literature, *cause* is determined if change in one variable leads to change in the other (Mausner, and Bahn, 1974, p. 100). Causal relationships between variables can be determined when, through observation and experimentation, four conditions are met. Those conditions are: (1) appropriate temporal orientation of the factors of cause and factors of diseases (or effects); (2) consistency of the relationship; (3) specificity of the cause and the effect; and (4) compatibility of the relationship with existing knowledge pertaining to it.

The first condition, correct temporal orientation, implies a sequential relationship or association between the variables. That is, causal variables preexist the conditions they cause, thus, change in them would cause change in the conditions caused as well. The next condition, consistency, requires that the same relationship persist under other similar circumstances. As a result, the more diverse circumstances under which consistency of association is observed, the stronger the relationship would be. The third condition, specificity, pertains to the extent to which the occurrence of one variable can be used to predict the occurrence of another. In the ideal specific rela-

tionship, only one variable is necessary and sufficient to cause only one condition (Susser, 1973). This is often difficult to attain for two reasons. First, a single factor may cause more than one condition (Fig. 1, Scheme 1) and second, many factors may cause the same condition (Fig. 1, Schemes 2 and 3). Lilienfeld and Pedersen (1973) demonstrated these relationships. As Figure 1, schemes 2 and 3 show, none of the factors alone would be sufficient to cause disease conditions. In the second scheme, it is implied that several factors may cause the predisease state. In the third scheme, it is implied that all three factors are needed to cause a disease state or condition.

The fourth condition requires that the strength of the relationship be congruent with existing scientific knowledge. This condition, of course, depends upon the scientific information available at a given time. The above conditions cannot be fulfilled through experimental research to determine causal relationships between variables unless the effects, or disease conditions, are induced in humans by introducing harmful factors in them first.

Since classical experimentation in research on humans cannot examine the ill effects of causal factors, systematic observation using ex-post-facto experimental and cohort designs have enabled etiology to develop, particularly following "natural experiments" though they are few and infrequent. In a limited sense, illness was considered a natural experiment as well. However, the growth of understanding of etiology of human diseases depended primarily upon systematic observation, documentation, and analysis of the coexistence of suspicious factors and diseased conditions. Such retrospective as well as prospective observations provided epidemiologists and physicians with data upon which hypotheses regarding relationships between factors and diseases could be formulated and tested. Thus, systematic search for and observations of causal factors and their relationships with disease conditions explain the development of etiology as a science.

Another explanation for the growth of epidemiology that emerged from the close collaboration between epidemiology and medicine was the defined and specific focus on human diseases and their causes. Medical science sought to determine the nature of human diseases and their signs and symptoms, to find methods to diagnose and cure them. Epidemiologists, and recently other basic scientists, sought to identify factors that cause diseases in humans. Thus, as those disciplines promoted etiology, its growth as a science was simultaneous and synergistic. Such developments explain the pivotal role etiology continues to play in determining not only diagnoses of human diseases but their control, eradication and, prevention as well. Furthermore, such historical developments point to the pivotal role etiology plays in determining medical practice. This role warrants wider understanding.

Upon closer examination, it can be seen that etiology provides the basis upon which the physician can accurately diagnose a disease. In order to make a definitive diagnosis, the physician must, whenever possible, seek and provide evidence not only of the disease's signs and symptoms but more so of its causes. Therefore, data pertaining to signs, symptoms, as well as to causes must be sought and found before a diagnosis is stated. These data are used to determine the specific interventions that are most effective and efficient. Such interventions are intended to manipulate simultaneously the disease conditions and their causes. Furthermore, changes in the evidence of causes are often used to determine the effectiveness of the interventions. Two observations in reference to the focus of interventions must be made. First, causes, when known, provide a specific target for interventions, if such intervention is possible. Second, causes for which known interventions do not exist, may direct the clinician to choose interventions that might alleviate disease or disease conditions. To the extent that causal relationships between factors and diseases or disease conditions are known, etiology has practical relevance for the diagnosis and intervention components of medical practice.

The broader effects of etiology on the control of disease are in the knowledge it provides for prevention of disease. To the extent that causal relationships between factors and diseases are established, etiology would also have a practical relevance to the preventive practices of epidemiologists and physicians. As pointed out earlier, the establishment of causal relationships between factors or causes and diseases or disease conditions depends upon systematic observation, documentation, analysis, testing, and retesting.

ETIOLOGY IN NURSING

It would be useful to examine the roots of etiology in the historical and current perspectives of nursing. This would be particularly useful, in light of the scientific development of etiology of human diseases and the practical relevance it has had on the advancement of medical practice and knowledge. It is in such a comparative examination that nursing's current state-of-the-art in etiology can be evaluated and new directions and strategies to develop etiology in nursing can be contemplated.

It is evident from the writings of Florence Nightingale (*Notes on Nursing*, 1859) that nursing had two main missions, "the nursing of the sick; and, to keep people well." The first mission refers to the art and science of diagnosing and intervening in diseased conditions of concern to nursing; the second refers to the art and science of preventing such dis-ease conditions. Disease or disease conditions are defined here as states of dis-ease, disruption of comfort, balance, healthy patterns (*Webster's New World Encyclopedia*, 1981). Nursing has done relatively well in its endeavor to fulfill the first mission. Largely owing to the efforts of NANDA, work related to the identification, definition, and progressive refinement of nursing diagnoses indicates strides toward fulfilling the mission "to nurse the sick." Nursing has not done as well in producing work related to prevention. This is so primarily because prevention depends on etiology or knowledge of causes, of which nursing possesses little. Reflecting on the discussion of etiology and medical practice earlier, it is most propitious that nursing considers etiology as the knowledge most needed to achieve its mission of early detection and prevention of the disease conditions.

In our more recent history, attention to the existing need for etiology has increased. In examining the several definitions of etiology in nursing, it becomes clear that nursing authors disagree on its meaning and practical value to nursing practice. The following provide representative examples of these definitions. Etiological factors have been defined as "those causing or maintaining a health problem that could be behavioral, environmental, or the interaction between the two" (Gordon, 1976, p. 1298). Another author refers to etiologic factors as "those physiological, situational, and maturational factors that cause a problem or influence its development" (Carpenito, 1985, p. 10). Other authors define etiologic factors as "those most likely contributing to a negative health behavior" (Leddy and Pepper, 1985, p. 216). Still another author refers to etiologic factors as stimuli causally related to patient problems (Kelly, 1985). Some authors agree that etiology has a place in the statement of nursing diagnoses, that the statement of nursing diagnoses should explicate the nature of problems as well as the etiological factors that cause or contribute to such problems (Leddy, et al., 1985; Gordon, 1976).

In analyzing the above definitions, it is evident that there is conceptual diffusion about the nature of etiological factors, nature of the problems, and the nature of the relationships between the etiologic factors and the problems. For example, as seen above, the etiologic factors could be behavioral, environmental, an interaction between these two, physiological, situational, maturational, and stimuli of some other sort. Likewise, the problems could be health problems, negative health behavior or a patient problem. Similarly, the nature of relationship of etiologic factors could be causal or contributory. Clearly, it is essential that clarity of meaning and consensus among authors on the nature of etiologic factors, problems, and the relationships between them be achieved. The most immediate challenge nursing faces in relation to this diffusion is to produce definitions of *etiologic factors*, *problems*, and the relationship between the two, explicating the distinctive characteristics of each. Rudimentary, ill-defined, and speculative as such definitions may be, they should be made explicit. Based on such definitions, work related to each of the three elements can grow and further refine each definition as such work progresses. It would be necessary to ponder each element individually and propose directions for developing meanings and definitions for each.

Causal factors

For the purposes of this paper, causal factors are those physical, physiological, psychological, social, or environmental variables that exist as a direct result of illness assumed to cause problems or disease conditions of concern to nurses. Causal factors possess certain characteristics. Their cause-and-effect relationship with nursing problems or disease conditions is compatible with existing knowledge in nursing and in disciplines allied to nursing. So, these relationships could be verifiable through scientific, theoretical, or clinical knowledge. Their assumed causal relationship with such problems can be explained by the appropriate temporal relationship with the problems they cause. They differ from contributory factors in that their relationship to problems is assumed to be causal and not intervening.

An example will be useful to illustrate. Dependence is a common problem that nurses often face. Theories of dependence indicate that it is a behavioral state brought about by unusually stressful or threatening events that impair the patient's physical, cognitive, emotional, and social resources and that act as causes of dependency on other individuals or things to compensate for diminished self-sustenance. After surgery, for instance, dependence for physical care is caused by physical disability, weakness, or pain. Physical dependence can be caused by diminished psychological self-reliance of the patient as well, such as fear of overexertion in the cardiac patient.

Nursing problems or disease conditions

Nursing problems are disease conditions that require nursing intervention. In this paper, the terms *problems* and *disease states* or *conditions* will be used inter-changeably. The nature of a nursing problem reflects a disease state. The nature of nursing problems is compatible with a corresponding item or category found in a universe of nursing problems generally known or accepted by the community of nurses. Examples of such universes are the taxonomy developed by NANDA or the universe of problems implied by known nursing models for practice. In their explications in nursing diagnoses, nursing problems reflect the nature of the disease condition as well as the likely causal factors, as supported by knowledge, theories, or clinical experience. The existence and extent of such problems are indicated by subjective and objective data also verifiable by such existing knowledge. Nursing problems could be physical, physiological, psychological, behavioral, social, or environmental in nature. In the example given above, the diagnosis of the problem based on a first-level assessment could be situational physical dependence related to physical weakness, pain, and fear of overexertion. This problem statement is compatible with theories of dependence, medical science, and clinical knowledge and it could be verifiable in the subjective and objective data potentially available. For example, Derdiarian and Clough (1976), Clough and Derdiarian (1980), and Derdiarian (1983) described the subjective and objective indicators of dependence and independence and changes in them according to the effects of the events of hospitalization, pre- and post-surgery, pre- and postdischarge.

Relationship between causal factors and disease conditions

The nature of the relationship between causal factors and disease conditions could be distinguished in some of the attributes or characteristics of causal factors enumerated above. Their distinction could be better understood if some clarification is made about the nature and characteristics of the factors contributing to nursing problems. In its generic definition, *contributing factors* are those that are not sufficient of themselves to bring about a state or condition. They contribute to the development or existence of a state or condition *(Webster's World Encyclopedia, 1981)*. It is plausible that contributing factors are those that act as intervening or extraneous variables and as such enhance or facilitate the development of the problem, or add to it, but do not cause it. They may or may not be manipulable by nursing (Derdiarian, 1981).

Again, in the example of the dependence problem, personal, cultural, and historical variables may enhance, facilitate, or complicate this problem. For instance, according to theories of dependence, personal traits of dependence (Derdiarian, 1975), cultural beliefs about patiency-behavior or, type of illness (Derdiarian, 1983), and differences in age and gender can act as contributing factors to the problem of dependence. These factors do not cause dependence. As proposed earlier, physical weakness, pain, physical disability, diminished psychological self-reliance, could all be direct results of surgical intrevention which in turn cause the problem of dependence.

As demonstrated above, definitions of the three elements of etiology should reflect their conceptual distinctions, because the practical relevance of etiology to nursing can be contemplated only on the basis of such distinctions. It is through making such distinctions that data pertinent to causal and contributing factors and nursing problems can be sought or that existing data can be distinguished and organized. Eventually, data so accumulated will reveal recurrences of factors that cause or contribute to types of problems. Data so organized can be produced from the daily practice of nursing which will provide substance to the nurse-etiologist and the nurse-clinician from which to develop research questions and hypotheses for testing. Thus, knowledge pertinent to the nature of nursing problems and their causes will develop. Such knowledge will enable nurses to provide predictable and deliberate care which is the basis for effective and efficient practice. Furthermore, such knowledge will enable nurses to anticipate and prevent problems or detect early their existence and thus check their progress.

PRACTICAL RELEVANCE OF ETIOLOGY TO NURSING

The practical relevance of etiology to nursing can be understood in terms of its relationship to nursing practice, methods and research. As etiology enabled research to improve medical practice, it is suggested here that etiology holds the potential to contribute in similar ways to the improvement of nursing practice.

Etiology and nursing practice

As used here, nursing practice is operationalized in the nursing process which consists of four component processes: assessment; diagnosis; intervention; and evaluation. Etiology is related to each of these processes and, therefore, has practical relevance to all.

Etiology and assessment

The main goal of the assessment process is to produce data in relation to the existence of a problem that should be substantiated and stated in a diagnostic statement. As was discussed earlier, the determination of a problem as expressed in its diagnostic statement should include the factor(s) suspected of causing the problem. It follows, then that the data base should include subjective and objective data substantiating not only a problem's existence but also its causes. The need for such data prompts the nurse to seek sufficient data to determine that a problem exists and to describe the causal factor(s) fully in the diagnosis. This search has a few functions. First, it prevents the nurse from making an ill-conceived decision about a problem based on incomplete data. Second, it cues the nurse to tap complete data from the appropriate sources—patient, family, colleagues, the chart, or the pertinent literature. Third, to obtain such data, the nurse either would know *a priori* (based on theory or knowledge) what type of data is needed to substantiate causality or would be able to distinguish and analyze such data when they exist. Finally, data obtained, including those pertaining to causal factors, serve as a basis to evaluate the effectiveness of nursing interventions.

Thus, the acquisition of data or analysis of existing data cue the nurse to be analytical in achieving the goal of assessment, namely, to provide sufficient appropriate data to facilitate the formulation of a nursing diagnosis. Therefore, etiologic considerations certainly determine the nurse's behavior, the quality and quantity of data obtained, and potentially, the quality of the diagnostic statements. In turn, such data obtained and carefully documented could serve as a valuable natural data base for future analysis and research.

Etiology and diagnosis

The primary goal of formulating and stating a diagnosis is to describe the problem at hand as accurately and validly as possible. As mentioned earlier, such a statement should include the nature, extent (if possible), and the causal factors of a problem. To formulate such a statement, the clinician examines all of the data obtained in terms of the problem they indicate. The clinician further evaluates the indications of the problem in light of the contributing factors (or intervening factors), which usually are demographic, situational, and environmental in nature. Taken together, the data then are analyzed in terms of the nature of the problem and its causal factor(s). The statement of the diagnosis is made. Thus, considerations for etiologic factors cue the nurse to distinguish between the data relevant to causal factors and those pertaining to contributing factors. The statement of the diagnosis serves the clinician in two ways. First, it implies the acquisition of specific interventive modes that should include plans and means to manipulate the causal factor(s) as well as the disease conditions. Second, the diagnosis implies the order of interventive manipulation, i.e., whether causal factors that are manipulated first will alleviate, minimize, or eradicate .the disease conditions, or whether the causal factors and disease conditions should be manipulated simultaneously, or whether either of the two cannot be manipulated.

Etiology and intervention

The main goal of intervention is to alleviate, minimize, or eradicate problems or disease conditions. The effectiveness of an interventive plan depends upon the degree to which it is compatible with the problem and specific to the nature and extent of the disease condition. In light of the causal factor(s) identified in the diagnostic statement, the compatibility should also include the specificity of interventions aimed at the causal factors. Based on the diagnosis, the clinician must decide to plan individual, simultaneous, sequenced, or single (a causal factor *vs.* causing a diseased condition) interventive modes. Thus, consideration of etiologic factors determines the behavior of the clinician, the health care team, and the patient and family. Such considerations furthermore determine the quality of care received as well as its cost-effectiveness. If the interventive plan is incomplete because causal factor(s) are excluded, considerations would be wanting and thus adversely affect patient care, quality of practice, and cost.

Etiology and evaluation

The primary goal of evaluation processes is to determine whether and to what extent interventions are effective in alleviating, minimizing, or eradicating a problem. An added goal of evaluation that is not often recognized in nursing practice literature is to evaluate the entire nursing process. The attainment of both evaluation goals depends upon the presence of data indicating reduction or elimination of subjective and objective evidence of the problem. It follows, then, that if assessment data were incomplete or inaccurate, they may have defined the problem poorly and thus provide an erroneous or weak basis for interventions. Likewise, interventions so ill-designed in relation to problems would impede the clinician's attempt to provide care and possibly harm the recipient of that care. Considering etiologic factors during the assessment, diagnosis, and intervention processes therefore, can serve to verify the clinician's behavior; as a result, such factors can provide criteria on which to evaluate the effectiveness of both the nursing process and the clinician's performance. The particular value of evaluating the outcomes of nursing interventions is in learning whether the factors and problems were causally related, based on theoretical understanding or clinical knowledge of the problem at hand.

Etiology and methods

Methods here can be defined as the ways, means, or instruments through which data are gathered in some organized way in relation to variables of interest. Methods are of particular importance to nursing assessment and research. To the extent that they are valid, reliable, and comprehensive, they serve the clinician well by yielding needed data. These attributes of instruments in turn can be determined by the extent of their compatibility with their underlying theories and the comprehensiveness of these theories. Therefore, it can be extrapolated that if the theories of nursing problems do not include theories about causal factors related to such problems, then the instruments derived from them will not be suitable to gather data about such factors and their rela-

tionships with the nursing problem. Such instruments are needed to gather data pertaining to factor(s) assumed to be causing problems and to the description of the problems to be assessed. Over time, it is with such documentation of data pertaining to the causal factors and the problems, that clinicians can discern whether relationships between factors and problems exist and whether these relationships are temporally sequenced, consistent, or compatible with existing theoretical or clinical knowledge. Based on such data generation and examination, the *specific* relationships between these factors and problems could be identified and studied.

Ideally, instruments as described above should be developed for daily practice. However, under less ideal situations, components to gather data pertaining to causal factors should be built in to existing clinical nursing instruments. Such data can be obtained from subjective accounts of the patient, family, other nurses or team-members as well as from objective data found in the chart, literature, and clinical knowledge. Such efforts will increase with clinicians' growing awareness of the central role etiologic considerations play in rendering practice more precise, predictable, and cost-effective.

An instrument, the Derdiarian Behavioral Systems Model (DBSM), has been developed based on the theoretical development of the Johnson Behavioral Systems model and its operational definition for nursing practice on the cancer patient.* The instrument and data have been published as a demonstration of the conceptualization presented here in relation to nursing practice and as a demonstration of pertinent data essential to its implementation. The DBSM consists of 121

---

*This work, "Comprehensive Nursing Care of the Cancer Patient" was entirely supported by the Nursing Division of U.S.P.H.S. (#R01 NU00702, 1978-1981) items that would generate subjective data in relation to changes resulting from illness with cancer. These changes cluster around 21 categories distributed throughout the eight components of the Johnson model. The changes are described by the patient in terms of direction (increase/decrease), quality (positive/negative), importance (1 to 100), and items identified as causally related with the changes from a pool of physical/physiological, cognitive/psycho- logical, emotional/affective, and environ- mental items. Changes described as nega- tive and important (above 30%) indicated problems for further exploration. One hun- dred and sixty-three patients participated in the study. They were able to indicate items they perceived as causally related to the changed. Tables 1 through 8 present the number of patients who identified factors perceived as causally related to the negative changes.

Table 1: Number of cancer patients indicating changes in achievement behavior and categories of effects perceived as causally associated with changes (n = 163)

Categories of changes	Number of patients indicating categories of effects			
	Physical/ physiological Weakness Fatigue Discomfort	Psychological/ cognitive Loss of control Thoughts about death	Emotional/ affective Sadness Depression Hopelessness	Time constraints Time needed for treatment
Ability to achieve goals	n = 40	n = 39	n = 33	n = 42
Importance of achieving goals	n = 18	n = 33	n = 16	n = 9

Table 2: Number of cancer patients indicating changes in affiliative behavior and categories of effects perceived as causally associated with changes (n = 163)

Categories of changes	Number of patients indicating categories of effects			
	Physical/ physiological Lack of content Weakness Fatigue Discomfort	Psychological/ cognitive Thoughts about death Tension	Emotional/ affective Sadness Depression Hopelessness	Time constraints Lack of time
Closeness with imme- diate family	n = 33	n = 69	n = 16	n = 11
Closeness with close friends or relatives	n = 18	n = 47	n = 31	n = 14
Closeness with friends or acquaintances at work, social groups	n = 12	n = 34	n = 17	n = 0

Table 3: Number of cancer patients indicating changes in aggressive/protective behavior and categories of effects perceived as causally associated with changes (n = 163)

Categories of changes	Number of patients indicating categories of effects		
	Physical/ physiological Pain/discomfort Fatigue Weakness Side effects of treatments	Psychological/ cognitive Lack of control over own affairs Fear of the unknown Mental fatigue	Emotional/ affective Anxiety Depression
Physical ability to protect self and loved ones	n = 57	n = 28	n = 13
Mental ability to protect interests, rights of self and loved ones	n = 34	n = 59	n = 21
Ability to maintain control over one's social affairs	n = 34	n = 43	n = 24

Table 4: Number of cancer patients indicating changes in dependence behavior and categories of effects perceived as causally associated with changes (n = 163)

Categories of changes	Number of patients indicating categories of effects			
	Physical/ physiological Pain/discomfort Infection Weakness Fatigue Side effects of treatments	Psychological/ cognitive Lack of control over situation Lack of knowledge Lack of self-sufficiency	Emotional/ affective Sadness Depression Anxiety Loneliness	Time constraints Longer time needed to do tasks
Physical reliance on others or other things	n = 60	n = 34	n = 28	n = 21
Psychological reliance on others or other things	n = 18	n = 74	n = 37	n = 13

Although perceived causal relationship between factors "effects of illness" and problematic changes in patients' lives is a weak indicator of causal relationships, it does indicate, the patient's perceptions of the reality of the experience of illness. It also provides a starting point from which objective and subjective data could be sought from scientific, theoretical, and clinical literature that may indicate the degree of causality of the relationship between the causal factors and the problematic changes. At the present time, objective indicators have been developed from literature review to substantiate the changes and the causal factors. This instrument is being tested for its usefulness

Table 5: Number of cancer patients indicating changes in ingestive behavior and categories of effects perceived as causally associated with changes (n = 163)

Categories of changes	Number of patients indicating categories of effects			
	Physical/ physiological Infection of mouth Difficulty in swallowing Lack of appetite Nausea	**Psychological/ cognitive** Nervousness Worry Aversion to foods	**Emotional/ affective** Depression Loneliness "Why eat?"	**Time constraints** Takes long to eat Change in eating times
Ability to ingest food and fluids	n = 48	n = 21	n = 38	n = 19
Ability to retain, digest and assimilate food and fluids	n = 51	n = 28	n = 11	n = 13
Enjoyment in eating	n = 66	n = 23	n = 37	n = 17

Table 6: Number of cancer patients indicating changes in eliminative behavior and categories of effects perceived as causally associated with changes (n = 163)

Categories of changes	Number of patients indicating categories of effects		
	Physical/ physiological Pain/discomfort Infections (anal) Side effects of treatments	**Psychological/ cognitive** Worry about pain Nervousness	**Time** Changes in times (pattern)
Inadequate elimination of body wastes from intestinal tract	n = 32	n = 13	n = 19
Excessive elimination of body wastes from intestinal tract	n = 23	n = 19	n = 16
Elimination of body wastes through urinary system	n = 41	n = 11	n = 0
Elimination of body wastes through skin, lungs, glands	n = 45	n = 71	n = 0

for clinical practice at UCLA School of Nursing.

Etiology and research

Research will be the ultimate means to investigate and determine causal relationships between suspected factors and problems. Research in this area can grow using inductive or deductive approaches and formal or natural means. Both are needed. The more fruitful means to generate needed data would be the natural means, which would generate

Table 7: Number of cancer patients indicating changes in sexual behavior and categories of effects perceived as causally associated with changes (n = 163)

Categories of changes	Number of patients indicating categories of effects		
	Physical/ physiological Fatigue Weakness Weight loss Changes in appearance Pain	Psychological/ cognitive Feelings of being different Feelings of being inferior Feelings of rejection	Emotional/ affective Depression Sadness
Gender identity in identity and social role	n = 74	n = 43	n = 20
Performance in and enjoyment of sexual activities	n = 33	n = 27	n = 17

Table 8: Number of cancer patients indicating changes in restorative behavior and categories of effects perceived as causally associated with changes (n = 163)

Categories of changes	Number of patients indicating categories of effects			
	Physical/ physiological Pain/discomfort Perspiration Sluggishness Side effects of treatments	Psychological/ cognitive Worry Tension	Emotional/ affective Fear Anxiety Depression	Time constraints Not enough time
Quality and quantity of sleep and satisfaction from sleep	n = 56	n = 49	n = 17	n = 7
Ability to relax through leisure activities	n = 44	n = 38	n = 19	n = 29
Other restorative mechanisms of body	n = 37	n = 19	n = 15	n = 4

data through daily practice and documentation. Both require careful observation and documentation. Such data are needed to facilitate the collaboration of the nurse-etiologists and the nurse-clinician. Apparent causal relationships between recurrent co-existence between factors and problems that occur should be tested and verified according to criteria presented earlier which quali-

fies the causality of such relationships. Such verifications, in time, will generate the study of causes, or etiology, in nursing.

The science of causes in nursing has both immediate and long-term implications. The more immediate ones pertain to the challenges nursing faces to deliver predictable (goal-oriented), accountable, rational, and cost-effective care. These qualities can largely be introduced in nursing care, if causal factors are also considered and treated. The more distant implications pertain to the challenge nursing faces to deliver predictable, accountable, cost-effective care through prevention. As discussed earlier, prevention depends largely on the knowledge of causes of problems. As health care policies so often demand, prevention of nursing problems will soon be demanded of nursing. Finally, one other distant implication etiology will have for nursing, and particularly for NANDA, is providing another conceptual reference on which classification of nursing diagnoses can be based.

In summary, it is hoped that the framework presented has specified, the central position etiology holds in relation to nursing practice, methods, and research development. Furthermore, it is earnestly hoped that the practical relevance of etiology as applied to nursing practice in this paper will be realized so that such practice can be improved and its documentation will yield more fruitful nursing research.

REFERENCES

Carpenito, L.J.: Nursing Diagnosis, Philadelphia, 1985, J.B. Lippincott.

Clough, D., and Derdiarian, A.K.: A behavioral checklist to measure dependence and independence, Nurs. Res. **29**:55, 1980.

Derdiarian, A.K.: An analysis of dependence-independence behavior variables in surgical patients with emphasis directed to trait and state dependence. In Batey, M.V. editor: Communicating nursing research, volume 8, Nursing research priorities: choice or chance, Boulder, 1977, WICHE.

Derdiarian, A.K.: Nursing in prevention of cancer. In Vredevoe, D.L., Derdiarian, A.K., Sarna, L.P., and others: Concepts of oncology nursing, Englewood, N.J., 1981, Prentice Hall.

Derdiarian, A.K.: Psychosocial variables in cancer management: considerations for nursing practice. In Vredevoe, D.L., Derdiarian, A.K., Sarna, L.P., and others: Concepts of oncology nursing, Englewood, N.J., 1981, Prentice Hall.

Derdiarian, A.: Dependence-independence behavior variables in surgical patients, Cancer Nurs. **6**:453, 1983.

Derdiarian, A.K., and Clough, D.: Patients' dependence-independence levels on the prehospitalization—postdischarge continuum, Nurs. Res. **25**:27, 1976.

Derdiarian, A.K. and Forsythe, A.W.: An instrument for theory and research development using the behavioral systems model for nursing: the cancer patient, Part II. Nurs. Res. **32**:260, 1983.

Gordon, M.: Nursing diagnosis and the diagnostic process, Am. J. Nurs. **76**:1298, 1976.

Kelly, M.A.: Nursing diagnosis source book, Norwalk, CT., 1985, Appleton-Century Croft.

Leddy, S., and Pepper, J.M.: Conceptual bases of professional nursing, Philadelphia, 1985, Lippincott.

Lilienfield, A.N., and Pedersen, E.: Cancer epidemiology, Baltimore, 1967, Johns Hopkins University Press.

Mausner, T.S., and Bahn, A.K.: Epidemiology, Philadelphia, 1974, W.B. Saunders.

Nightingale, F.: Notes on nursing, Philadelphia, 1946, J.B. Lippincott. (Originally published in 1859, by Harrison and Sons.)

Susser, M.: Causal thinking in the health sciences: concepts and strategies. In Epidemiology, New York, 1973, Oxford University Press.

Taber's Cyclopedic Medical Dictionary (1984). (28th ed.) Philadelphia, Davis.

Webster's New World Dictionary, college edition, New York, 1981, World Publishers.

CHAPTER 9

Strategies of research applicable to on-line clinical intervention

STEVEN C. HAYES, Ph.D.

My purposes in this paper are to discuss the need for research in the on-line clinical environment, to analyze the nature of the intervention questions we need answered, to identify the types of research methodologies appropriate to the task, and, finally, to relate this to assessment research. My main point will be that we have the tools available to build a scientific foundation from within the clinical environment itself.

Many of the clinical disciplines have built their practices primarily upon the experience of clinicians rather than on scientific data and theory developed by the profession. In the past, this approach was understandable. Needs had to be met. By experience, ways were developed of meeting these needs, and these ways were passed on directly to new members of the profession. Today, the lack of a strong, home-grown scientific base for professional diagnosis and intervention is costing the clinical disciplines dearly.

The need for scientific research affects both patients and professionals. The patient has a right to expect that diagnosis and intervention are based on high scientific stan-dards. Science has proven its value in health fields unquestionably over the last century. Yet many of the approaches used in the clinical disciplines have not been subjected to scientific scrutiny. History teaches us that where the scientific foundation is weak, services will often ultimately be shown to be defective.

The effects on the professional are diverse. The lack of a strong scientific base reduces the independence, standing, and funding of clinical disciplines. The independent professional status of a health field is not firmly established merely by tradition or by claims of unique professional competence. It is best established on the basis of a distinct knowledge base, and today that can only be credibly accomplished through scientific theory and research. Medicine has free rein to dominate allied health professions that do not have an independent scientific foundation. The standing and prestige of professions are also based on their scientific credibility. This is reflected in many ways, but none more directly than the salaries earned by members and the willingness of third party payers to reimburse for services. The existence of scientific demonstrations of the value of the services in question is probably one of the most powerful forms of argument for independent and adequate compensation.

Portions of this paper have been drawn from earlier writings of mine on the same topic. Correspondence should be addressed to Steven C. Hayes, Department of Psychology, University of Nevada Reno, Reno, NV, 89557-0062.

Thus, there are many reasons for the clinical disciplines to want to develop an independent scientific base. There are two major and interconnected problems. First, the great majority of the members of the profession do not see themselves as researchers. The modal number of publications by members of almost every clinical discipline is zero. Not only do practitioners not produce research, they do not consume it. Most practitioners do not read the research literature, and when they do, they do not find it very useful. Unless practitioners can become producers of research, the person power available to build a scientific foundation is greatly limited. Unless they consume research, the whole clinical research effort is wasted.

Second, even if these problems were solved, the kinds of research strategies we have traditionally been taught often do not apply well to the clinical disciplines, especially in intervention research. Indeed, this is one reason practitioners do not conduct and consume research. There are reasons why group comparison research conducted with real patients is not, for example, often seen in nursing journals, and when it is, it is rarely conducted by a practicing nurse without academic affiliation. Much of mainstream research methodology is simply not applicable in the real world of on-line clinical practice.

As a result, clinical research all too often is non-experimental (e.g., descriptive or correlational). Non-experimental research, while at times valuable, cannot ask and answer most of the critical questions in the clinical disciplines. Assessment research may seem to be an exception, but I will argue later that it is not. Another result of the poor fit of traditional group comparison research methods with clinical research is that the research that is done is often targeted towards tangential but accessible populations and questions. For example, a great deal of nursing research is directed at an understanding of nurses, rather than of patients. Research on the knowledge, attitudes and behavior of nurses is fine so far as it goes, but it does not go very far. The proper focus of research in the clinical disciplines is diagnosis and intervention with their target populations. Students are driven to avoid such research topics because group comparison experimental research with patients is extraordinarily difficult. Fortunately, there is an alternative.

CONSUMING CLINICAL RESEARCH: EXTERNAL VALIDITY AS A MATTER OF MATHEMATICAL NECESSITY

The critical question in clinical research was identified by Paul (1969) nearly twenty years ago: What treatment, delivered in what manner, is most likely to be successful for this particular patient with this specific set of problems. This is what clinicians want from research. When research can guide the actions of clinicians in this way it has a degree of external validity (Campbell and Stanley, 1963). I believe that the dominant research model is poorly designed to maximize external validity. This is one reason clinicians often ignore research. Thus, I am going to start my argument from an odd place: the consumption of research. If I can establish that the dominant research model is not only impractical but also answers the wrong kinds of questions, I hope to gain more receptivity to the alternative. This alternative fits remarkably well with the research needs of the clinical disciplines because it addresses external validity by making the production of research data possible for the practicing clinician.

The dominant model of external validity draws from sampling theory and probability theory and is closely related to theories of the internal integrity of research. Every beginning researcher learns the model, typically as a theory of proper research method. Some students even confuse it with the scientific method itself. According to the model, we must randomly select from a known population and randomly assign to groups or conditions. If variability between subjects is low relative to differences between groups, we conclude we have an effect. The effect then should also apply to other random samples from the same population as a matter of mathematical necessity.

This mathematical necessity model of external validity has a long history and powerful intellectual support. Unfortunately, no one can implement the model in the real world of clinical practice.

Problems with the mathematical necessity model

We can break down the preliminary issues into four areas: known populations, random selection, random assignment, and application to additional samples. Each presents major obstacles to clinical research. Since the model requires all its elements to maintain its mathematical integrity, a weakness in even one area seriously limits its integrity.

Known populations. Clinical researchers can easily name the populations they seek to study: stroke victims, alcoholics, patients with cardiovascular disease, and so on. These populations definitely exist, and we can often describe their defining characteristics in detail. A "known population," of course, is not simply these conceptually known populations. Some individuals may have a problem that is undetected. Others may know they have a problem but fail to seek treatment. Still others may seek treatment in a manner prohibiting their identification. In the real world, populations are detected by their contact with certain cooperative individuals or institutions. The events producing either the contact or the cooperativeness of the institution can distinguish this population from the conceptual population in important ways. For example, we may have access to

poor people entering a county hospital, but not to middle class people treated by a private practitioner.

Random selection. Even if it were possible to specify a known population matching a conceptual population, we still would have the problem of random selection. Random selection occurs when the probability of a single selection is $1/N$ for each member of the population, where N equals the total known population. In the real world, subjects are selected for practical reasons in treatment research. A given hospital may allow access to a researcher, while another may not. Any factor that leads people to use that particular hospital now also distorts the sample. For example, the hospital may draw its patients from a particular region, may enjoy a good reputation among particular religious or ethnic groups, or may be known to use treatment modalities that are attractive to certain kinds of people. It is possible to redefine the known population as all persons in a given hospital. Rarely would anyone want to generalize the results of their research to such a population, however. Thus, this maneuver seemingly meets the letter of the mathematical necessity model but does not increase its usefulness.

Even with the population of a given hospital random selection is rarely possible. Agreeing to participate in research is a significant act. Patients willing to be subjects surely differ from patients unwilling to be subjects. Researchers sometimes make mighty efforts to show that the demographic characteristics of the two groups are similar. To draw the implication that the two groups are thus functionally similar is not justified by sampling theory, however. We do not know whether other unmeasured characteristics distinguish the groups, and we do not know if these characteristics alter the applicability of research from one to the other. Demographic characteristics are far too crude for this purpose. We do know the groups are different. We do not know if the difference is important. Thus, based on mathematical necessity we can only generalize to the population of persons with this disorder, in this institution who are willing to participate in research of exactly this kind. No one is interested in generalizing to such an odd population.

Random assignment. When we have selected a sample, we then randomly assign subjects to groups. This part of the model is more feasible than its other parts, but even here trouble arises. Subjects decline assignment to particular conditions. Subjects may drop out of the study more in one condition than in another. These problems are well known, of course, and attempted solutions are common. For instance, researchers will often conduct a statistical test to see if drop-out rates differed. Even without a difference in drop-out rates, drop outs can bias a sample. Suppose we are comparing two treatments. One treatment works differently with cooperative and uncooperative people. Cooperative people respond very nicely to the treatment, but the treatment is absolutely iatrogenic for uncooperative persons. The second treatment is moderately effective for both cooperative and uncooperative people. Imagine all uncooperative people drop out of the study and the drop-out rates are thus likely to be equal in both groups. The first treatment may now look better with this sample, but not with the original sample.

Applicability to non-random samples. When you put together these three problems—known populations, random selection, and random assignment—it becomes clear that the mathematical necessity model of external validity does not exist in the world of clinical research. I am not attacking sampling theory or probability theory. If the model could be implemented, studies would indeed possess a kind of external validity. Ironically, even then the kind of external validity such studies would possess is not

the kind that would be of use to practitioners and most consumers of treatment research.

If the model were followed, research results would necessarily apply only to *other random samples from the same population.* The model can promise no more. The model does not promise that every subgroup in the sample will respond in the same manner as the entire group. A given treatment can work very nicely with the population overall and have negative effects on a subpopulation. The effects of the treatment on non-random samples are unknown. Clinicians never randomly sample from treatment populations. How an individual patient ends up being treated by a given clinician is definitely non-random. Patients seek out particular clinicians for all kinds of non-random reasons: reputation, location, sex, race, fees, availability, hours. How are we to know whether the non-random characteristics that cause an individual to be treated by someone do not also cause them to be in a sub-group for whom the overall results will not apply?

Alternatives to the mathematical necessity model

The mathematical necessity model is the only one to promise external validity as an inherent possession of a well-designed study. Every other approach to external validity relies on logical generalization (Hersen & Barlow, 1976). The principle of logical generalization is this: if a given treatment is shown to be successful with a given patient, it is more likely to be successful with another to the extent that the two are similar. This principle makes no mathematical claims. It is not based on sampling theory or probability theory. It is simply logical, based on our experience with the world. It implies that in the real world, no amount of care in experimental design will insure that the findings will be relevant, because studies do not possess external validity as a matter of mathematical necessity (Birnbauer, 1981).

Correlational analyses of factors related to outcome

There are several group comparison strategies that approach external validity based on logical generalization. It is possible in very large group studies to correlate various subject characteristics post hoc with improvement. Even if the original sample is not a random sample from a known population, it is logical to believe that if improvement is correlated with certain subject characteristics then patients who share those characteristics are likely to respond similarly. Correlational strategies occur in two forms. In one, particular characteristics are used to block subjects into various groups, arranged along a continuum. For example, high and low SES subjects might be compared. In a second type of strategy, no groups are formed but the various characteristics are examined for linear or other relationships with outcome.

The difficulties with correlational strategies are that if we include more than a few subject characteristics we quickly require either absolutely enormous groups, or we will often be basing our correlations on very small numbers of similar subjects. Correlations based on small sets are notoriously unreliable, and, indeed, correlational research of this sort is known for the variability in the results obtained across studies. In addition, we must decide before hand exactly what subject characteristics will be measured for all subjects. This is troublesome, because some of the most important variables are probably not the obvious demographic variables or universal measures usually examined in research of this kind.

Research of this sort has often failed to find consistent or strong correlations between assessment measures and outcome. It is not uncommon to see such studies reporting correlations that account for 5 to 10% of the variance in outcome. The larger correlations sometimes seen are rarely cross-validated in subsequent research. Despite the number of studies being reported of this type, there is little evidence that they are leading to greater external validity for the output of treatment research. Why are they not leading to increasingly sophisticated rules of generalization?

Probably the most difficult problem is a failure to determine individual successes and failures. There are three kinds of variability in any treatment research study. Some variability is due to inconsistent measurement. This is false variability because it exists only in the data, not in the phenomenon being measured. Other variability is caused by extraneous factors. Extraneous factors are those that are not manipulated systematically and are allowed to vary. Variability due to extraneous factors, such as maturation, or coincidental experiences, is real variability in the phenomena. Finally, there are various kinds of treatment-related variability.

All treatment research seeks to distinguish variability due to treatment from the other kinds. In group comparison research, these distinctions are made at the level of the group. Consider a typical group comparison study in which an experimental and a control group are measured before and after. We can distinguish treatment-related variability from other kinds by using the variability between subjects in the two groups as a kind of rubber rule against which treatment differences can be measured. We assume that inconsistent measurement and extraneous factors are operating, but are influencing both groups equally and that differences between the groups reflect possible treatment-related variability. If variability within the groups is large, these non-treatment sources of variability are also large and only large mean difference between the groups is unlikely. If the variability within the groups is very small, even small differences between the groups is probably due to treatment-related variability.

This is an eminently logical model, and I have no quarrel with it. Note, however, that correlational studies correlate improvement of individuals with characteristics of these same individuals. This is troublesome because in the great majority of group comparison studies all three sources of variability are *confounded at the level of the individual*. If a given person improves, we cannot say, for that individual, that improvement is due to inconsistent measurement, extraneous factors, or treatment-related variability of various kinds. It is only at the level of the group that the three types of variability are distinguished. Thus, correlational strategies of this kind correlate subject characteristics with improvement due to all three sources of variability. If we could distinguish these three sources at the level of the individual, a version of the correlational strategy would make sense. That is the model I will shortly propose.

Homogeneous groups

Another group comparison strategy is the use of homogeneous groups. Subjects are selected according to a particular set of well defined characteristics. If a given treatment works with this homogeneous group, then it seems more likely to work with others who have the same set of characteristics. Note that the principle involved here is again that of logical generalization. It is not necessary to pretend that the homogeneous group is a random sample from a known population.

The homogeneous group strategy is reasonable and deserves greater use, but is difficult to implement in the clinical environment and has certain inherent limitations. The difficulty in implementation arises because even simple group comparison research can require large numbers of subjects, and even a small set of carefully defined sub-

ject characteristics can quickly make a large group impossible to collect. The typical compromise is to limit the subject selection criteria to a few gross characteristics. Unfortunately, this undermines the principle of logical generalization supporting the strategy in the first place. If the group is not very homogeneous, how can I have confidence that my patients are like those in the group?

Other problems with group comparison research

Even if all of the above were not true, group comparison research strategies would still be out of reach of the practicing clinician. What clinician can put real patients into untreated control groups? How can a practitioner gather together large numbers of patients with the same disorders? How can a practitioner remain blind to a patients progress? Fortunately, there is an alternative that addresses both these practical problems and the limitations of group-comparison research in the area of external validity.

SINGLE-CASE DESIGNS

You can see that one solution to this problem is to relate individual subject characteristics to treatment-related improvement identified at the level of the individual and to do so many, many times. Based on the principle of logical generalization, Paul's question may then begin to be answered.

The method that promises to do this is "single-case" experimental designs (Barlow and Hersen, 1985; Barlow, Hayes, and Nelson, 1984). It is a method that opens up the possibility of contributions to the research literature by a large series of small-*n* designs, not just through a small series of large-*n* designs. It is this that makes a contribution to the scientific base of the discipline possible for the on-line practitioner. Indeed, for the single-case strategy to work, it requires their participation. If multitudes of intensive analyses of the individual are required for external validity, who will produce them? Who has access to these cases, other than practitioners? Thus, the term *single-case* is a bit of a misnomer. The issue is one of level of analysis and not one of number. A single-case approach will often require just as many subjects as the previous approach, but since individual assessment results will now be correlated with individually identified treatment effects, stronger external validity for these correlations seems likely.

In the past decade, an explosion of interest has occurred in methodological tools that are built on single-case analysis (e.g., Barlow, Hayes, and Nelson, 1984; Barlow and Hersen, 1985; Chassan, 1979; Hayes, 1981; Jayaratne and Levy, 1979; Kazdin, 1978, 1982; Kratochwill, 1978). These tools are not only scientifically defensible, they are fully applicable to the clinical environment. The fundamental idea behind single-case designs is that variability seen within an individual across time can, if examined properly, be divided into treatment-related variability, extraneous variability, and measurement error. Thus, our actual clinical cases can be used to form a strong scientific base for the clinical disciplines.

Fundamentals of single-case analysis

The fit between clinical work and the logic of single-case analysis is remarkably good. The following essentials of the analysis of treatment in the individual case closely parallel the essentials of good clinical practice.

Accurate and systematic assessment. All valid clinical knowledge is based upon systematic observation. For example, if what is observed is a function of the needs, biases, or wants of the clinician and not patient characteristics, the information gleaned from the case will necessarily be faulty. This is just good clinical practice.

Repeated measurement. Repeated measurement also parallels rules of clinical practice. Practical clinical guides often exhort clinicians to "examine regularly and consis-

tently whether therapy is being helpful" (Zaro, Barach, Nedelmann, Dreiblatt, 1977).

In clinical practice, repeated measurement should start early, using several measures if possible. Often when normal assessment ends the clinician will have a systematically collected baseline. The use of repeated measurement, more than any other single factor, allows knowledge to be drawn from the individual case, because it eliminates or restricts the plausibility of several alternative explanations for the effects seen (e.g., measurement error).

Specification of conditions. Careful specification of the treatment plan and patient characteristics allows any effects identified to be "given away." Without a clear understanding of what the clinician actually did, what the patient was actually like, and so on, we may know that something worked for someone, but not what worked for whom.

Replication. All valid knowledge should be replicable. In on-line clinical research, this requirement is increased due to the many threats to validity. All single-case designs include ways of replicating effects.

Establishment of the degree of variability. We cannot know if we have had an effect unless we have an idea of where we were headed. Measures should be taken long enough and be stable enough to know where the problem is going and to see treatment effects, should they occur. These are not absolute qualities—they depend upon what we know about the problem and its treatment. If treatment effects are expected to be large, considerable variability can be tolerated. If the problem is so variable that no effects could be seen, why proceed anyway?

If the measures are too variable, three clinically defensible options are open. First, you could wait to see if a clearer picture emerges. Second, you can search for the events that are causing improvement and deterioration. It may be sloppy measurement, or it could be real and a clue to the actual events influencing the problem. Third, the temporal unit of analysis may be too small. Perhaps the overall pattern will be clear if the specific measures are being examined in terms of days, when weeks make more clinical sense; hours if days make more sense, and so on.

Creative use of single case logic. The investigation of the individual case should be a dynamic enterprise, produced by the interaction of continuously collected clinical information and ongoing therapeutic attempts. When unanticipated effects are seen, the clinician must be ready to abandon previous decisions and to let the patient's data be the guide. This is also good clinical practice. Clinicians should "be prepared to alter your style of dealing with a client in response to new information" and "be prepared to have many of your hypotheses disproved" (Zaro et al., 1977, p. 28). This is the single biggest difference between group comparison approaches and single-case designs. Single-case designs allow design elements to be used interactively with data collected from the case. The deliberate use of these elements can increase the precision of clinical decision making.

In summary, then, a methodology for the production of clinical knowledge based on the individual case must accord itself with fundamental values of good clinical practice: accurate and repeated assessment, establishment of clinical need, specification of treatment, continuous sensitivity to the needs of patients, and establishment of the role of treatment in patient improvement. Whether the knowledge developed is valid will depend upon the degree to which these recommendations are followed. Only the last recommendation is somewhat foreign to trained clinicians, although it is implicit in clinical decision making. It is to these logical decision tools that we now turn.

The design elements in single-subject analysis

Following the format described in Hayes (1981), this paper describes single-case ex-

perimental designs in terms of a few core units, organized by the nature of stability estimates and the logic of the data comparisons. These core elements are put together as the needs of the case analysis dictate. The elements can be organized into three types: between, within, and combined series.

Within-series elements. The *within-series elements* draw their estimates of stability, level, and trend within a series of data points across time, taken under similar conditions. Changes are made in the conditions impinging upon the patient, and concomitant changes are examined in the stability, level, or trend in a series of data points taken under the new conditions. Thus, changes seen within a series of data points across time are the main source of clinical information.

There are two classes of within-series elements. In the *simple phase change* the within-series comparison is made one or more times between two conditions (for example, baseline and treatment). In the *complex phase change* there is an overall coordinating strategy which dictates a particular sequence of three or more conditions. In either case, there is one condition per phase.

Perhaps the most common example is the A/B design. (By tradition, A always stands for baseline, B, for the first treatment element, C, for the second, and so on). The A/B represents a simple case study (but with repeated measurement and careful specification of treatment) in which a period of assessment is followed by a single treatment strategy. If the stability, level, or trend of the data taken in the baseline phase changes when treatment is implemented, our confidence increases that treatment is responsible, especially if the change is marked or sudden.

Often we can think of other reasons for the change, such as the effect of extraneous events or the effects of assessment itself (see Campbell and Stanley, 1963; Barlow et al., 1984; Kazdin, 1982), so we need to replicate the effect. A simple way is then to repeat the phase change in reverse order (an A/B/A) and then perhaps to repeat it again (an A/B/A/B). Each time changes in the data coincide with phase changes, our confidence in the effect increases. For example, suppose we are interested in the effects of massage on back pain in a particular patient. After a baseline recording of the degree of back pain experienced for several days, regular massage might be implemented. If improvement in pain ratings occurs, massage can be withdrawn for a period of time and then reintroduced. If pain ratings track the relevant phases, we can conclude that massage is helpful for this patient. We would not yet know why, of course (e.g., it could be a placebo effect) but other, more complex single-case designs could tease that apart.

The alternation of phase changes can continue indefinitely, each sequence constituting a type of completed design. The two conditions could be two treatments (e.g., B/C/B/C), or elements of a treatment package (e.g., B/B+C/B). The logic of these specific types is identical; only the questions being asked and the extent of the comparisons differ owing to the specific content of the phases and the number of alternations. In a B/C/B/C design, for example, the question being asked is: Which treatment works best for this patient?

When components of a treatment package are being compared, the sequence is called an *interaction element*. It answers the question: What are the combined effects of two treatment components compared to one alone? In this element, a component of a treatment package is alternately put in and taken out, and the effects are noted. A number of specific sequences are possible (e.g., B/B+C/B/B+C, or B+C/C/B+C).

Several types of more complex phase-change elements exist. An example is an A/B/A/C/A sequence. A simple phase change comparing two treatments does not show that either work relative to baseline. If this is not already known, and if the clinician still wants to compare the two treatments, it can be done by combining simple phase change strategies for determining the effectiveness of each treatment. The sequence A/B/C/A combines an A/B/A with an A/C/A. This allows us to ask if treatments B and C are effective, and if they are differentially effective. Because order effects are possible and noncontiguous data are being compared (B and C), it is usually best for other subjects to receive an A/C/A/B/A sequence. If the conclusions are the same, then the believability of the treatment comparison is strengthened. For example, we could compare the effects of massage and stretching exercises on back pain in this manner. Some patients would receive massage first, others would receive stretching exercises first; in each case periods of intervention would be proceeded and followed by baseline. If the two treatments consistently differed, we could conclude that one was superior.

Another complex phase change element termed a *changing criterion* is available when a criterion can be set beforehand of the type of performance that must be seen in the phase to achieve a given outcome (Hartmann & Hall, 1976). If the problem repeatedly changes to match a sequence of criterion changes, the therapeutic conditions can be said to be responsible.

Between-series elements. In the between-series elements the estimates of stability level and trend of the data are made in a series of measurements taken in a specific condition, not simply across time. Effects are assessed by looking for differences between two or more of these series. The major type is an *alternating-treatments design element* (ATD; Barlow and Hayes, 1979). The ATD is based on the rapid alternation of two or more conditions, in which there is one potential alternation of condition per meaningful unit of measurement. Because a single data point associated with one condition may be preceded and followed by measurements associated with other conditions, there are no phases. Rather, measurements associated with each condition are put into separate series. If there is a clear separation between the series, differences among conditions are inferred.

Order effects are usually minimized by random or semi-random alternation of conditions. The conditions may or may not include baseline, depending upon the question being asked. The strategy is especially useful for comparing treatments or treatment elements. The ATD is also useful when measurement is cumbersome or lengthy (e.g., an entire physiological battery). Only four data points are absolutely needed (two in each condition), though more are desirable. Depending on the phenomenon of interest, alternations may incorporate many treatment sessions, or on the other extreme, may occur several times in a single session (e.g., Hayes, Hussian, Turner, et al., 1983). *Rapid alternation* refers only to the rate of treatment alternation relative to the meaningful unit of measurement.

Combined-series elements. Several elements utilize comparisons both between and within data series to draw conclusions (see Barlow et al., 1984). One is built on several repetitions of a single simple phase change, each with a new series, in which the length of the first phase and the timing of the phase change differ in each repetition. This strategy might best be termed a multiple phase change, but it is universally known as a *multiple baseline* (whether or not baseline is one of the conditions).

The different data series might be based on different problems, different individuals, or different situations, or combinations of these. By replication across different series, the multiple baseline corrects for major deficiencies of a simple phase change, that effects could be due to coincidental extraneous events, assessment, and so on. If the effects are replicated, but with different lengths of baseline for each replication (a strategy which controls for the amount of baseline assessment or mere maturation) and with the actual time of the phase change arbitrarily altered (to reduce the possibility of correlated extraneous events), the conclusions are correspondingly strengthened.

The same first condition must yield to the same second condition, since it is alternative explanations for a specific phase change effect that are being controlled for. The logic of the comparison does not require baseline. A series of B/C phase changes could easily be arranged into a multiple baseline.

No set number of phase shift replications is required between series in a multiple baseline element, but each additional series strengthens our confidence that much more. The same is true of the differences in initial phase length. If one series has an initial phase only slightly longer or shorter than the other, this is less satisfactory than if there are large differences.

Using the design elements: within and combined series

The clinician typically begins a therapeutic relationship with a period of assessment. If repeated measures are taken, this period amounts to a baseline phase. In order to establish estimates of stability, level, and trend, at least three measurement points seem to be needed though more are desirable and may be needed in a given case to discern a trend. Shorter periods of assessment may be justified when there is other information available about the problem being measured. For example, the disorder may have a known history and course (e.g., the disease may be well understood) or archival baselines may be available (e.g., family reports, records from school). Note that this issue is a clinical one (Do I know the nature and course of the problem?) not an arbitrary addition of single-case methodology.

Sometimes even though a baseline would be useful, treatment must be begun immediately. In this case, scientifically valid information may still be gained by design elements that do not require a baseline (e.g., an ATD; a B/A/B/A), or by replication (e.g., in other cases or later in the same case).

When a baseline is taken, it may show the problem to be improving, deteriorating or staying the same. In general, if substantial improvement is occurring it is not time to change course (i.e., to shift phases and to start treatment). This advice is the same on clinical grounds (Why interfere with a good thing?) as it is on methodological grounds (How can you see if you have had an effect?).

At this point, the clinician may be ready to implement treatment. Before doing so, the clinician may want to see if there is a variable that needs to be controlled first. For example, if the patient seems susceptible to mild interventions such as family support, therapeutic expectations, social encouragement and the like (especially if the treatment is dangerous, difficult, or costly), it might be worth trying the less difficult treatment first. If it is not effective the meaningfulness of subsequent therapeutic effects may be enhanced. When starting treatment, it ideally should be implemented in a powerful way. Excessively gradual implementation will make real effects more difficult to see (Thomas, 1978).

When the second phase is implemented, only three outcomes are possible: no change, deterioration, or improvement. If there is no change, the clinician can wait and see if there is a delayed effect or try another strategy. It is typically assumed that a phase producing no change can be (with caution) considered part of the previous phase (e.g., A=B/C). There are limits to this, of course. An A=B=C=D=E/F/E/F design would not be very convincing and would need to be replicated, but this is true in normal clinical work. If we seem to find the key to a case after extensive floundering, we usually aren't sure if we really have it until we try it out with others.

If treatment produces deterioration, the clinician should withdraw treatment (creating an A/B/A). If the problem improves, an iatrogenic effect is shown, which itself may be a significant if somewhat disturbing contribution to the field.

The final possible effect is improvement. There are several courses opened up: (a) to continue to completion and (perhaps) to try it with similar cases, (b) to try the intervention in other areas of the patient's life, if appropriate, or (c) to withdraw treatment briefly, with an eye toward reimplementation. Since this (an A/B) is the most common type of clinical case evaluation, these alternatives will be discussed in some detail.

Continue. An A/B design by itself often produces useful clinical knowledge. This is particularly true if the effects are marked. It makes it unlikely that such things as assessment effects or regression to the mean are responsible (Kazdin, 1981). It is, of course, always possible that the effects are due to maturation or some extraneous environmental event. This may be more or less likely, depending upon the nature of the problem, its chronicity, past history of treatment, the identification of sudden changes in the patient's world, and rapidity and the consistency of improvement in various areas of functioning. In favorable circumstances, a single A/B can produce fairly believable demonstrations of treatment impact, because the overall pattern of results significantly undermines competing explanations.

The only way to know for sure is through replication, either in the same patient or between different patients. If the A/B can be repeated in other patients, a natural multiple baseline will almost always be formed. This is probably one of the clearest examples of natural design elements that arise in clinical practice. Nothing could be more natural to clinical work than an A/B. Individual cases will naturally have different lengths of baseline (often widely so) and sequential cases usually lead to a multiple baseline across people.

Some of the earliest applied literature on

the multiple baseline (e.g., Baer, Wolf, and Risley, 1968) said that multiple baselines across persons should always be done at the same time in the same setting with the same problem. Saving cases, with perhaps periods of months or even years separating each, violates this rule, but fortunately the logic of the strategy does not really require it (Hayes, 1985). If the time of the phase shift differs in real time from patient to patient, it is unlikely that important external events could repeatedly coincide with the phase changes. The multiple baseline controls for assessment and similar effects by varying the lengths of baseline. Multiple A/Bs retain much of this protection, as long as the reasons for changing phases at the precise moment are described, vary from case to case, seem unlikely to be related to the anticipation of sudden improvement, and (ideally) are at times somewhat arbitrary. Thus, while multiple A/Bs have been described as case studies (Kazdin, 1981) they seem to be legitimate experimental designs.

The clinicians must report all cases attempted, not just those showing the desired effect. If the effect is not seen in some, the clinicians should attempt to find out why (e.g., by adding phases to those patients showing an A=B effect). A careful examination of the variables accounting for differences between patients may lead to knowledge about mechanisms of change and boundary conditions.

The multiple baseline across cases also provides a home for those cases in which most treatment is given (B only), and in which treatment is never given (baseline-only control). As anchors in a series of cases, they can provide evidence of the effectiveness of treatment even when no baseline is taken (B only), thus controlling for an unlikely order effect due to baseline assessment or of the likelihood of change when no treatment is given (baseline-only control).

A related use of these multiple A-Bs is as multiple clinical replications (Barlow, 1980). In this use, the focus is on the numbers of cases showing effects of particular types at the A/B shift.

Conduct a multiple baseline within the case. Multiple baselines often form naturally across problems owing to the tendency for practicing clinicians to tackle subsets of problems sequentially rather than all at once (e.g., Brownell, Hayes, and Barlow, 1977). Suppose, for example, that we were using biofeedback to treat spasticity in a patient's arm and leg. We could first focus on the arm, but continue to measure the degree of spasticity seen in each. If an effect was seen in the arm, but not the still untreated leg, we could then begin treatment also with the leg. If the spasticity in the leg now also improved, a multiple baseline across problems would be formed. Other types of multiple baselines within a single case are possible as well (see Barlow et al., 1984).

Withdrawal. Withdrawal of an apparently effective treatment raises ethical issues, patient fee issues, potential patient morale problems, and possible neutralization of subsequent treatment effects. However, it often seems justified and even clinically useful. It also frequently occurs naturally.

First, a withdrawal can avoid the unnecessary use of ineffective treatment. Physicians recognize this issue in the common practice of "drug holidays" (i.e., withdrawals) to assess the continued need for treatment. Second, withdrawals often present themselves naturally in treatment in the form of vacations, holidays, sickness, temporary treatment drop outs, or in terms of clinical reassessment, attention to unrelated clinical issues, and the like. With these kinds of withdrawals, the reasons for the phase change should be described and some interpretive caution should be used, since changes seen could be due to the events causing the natural withdrawal, not to withdrawal per se. Third, withdrawals can be short and given a good rationale. If this is done well, the patient may be helped regardless of the outcome. In some of my own cases, short withdrawals, when connected with deterioration, convinced patients of the need for treatment and produced greater patient involvement. In other cases, withdrawals associated with maintenance of treatment gains led to greater confidence on the patient's part that the problem was now under better control.

If treatment is withdrawn, the problem can show no change, deterioration, or continued improvement. If it deteriorates, treatment should be reimplemented (an A/B/A/B). If it shows no change (but there is room to improve) treatment could be started again to see if improvement will now occur. If the problem continues to improve, the case can be saved and the same thing tried again later (forming a multiple baseline).

Using the design elements: between series

The possibilities to use ATD elements in clinical evaluation is great but usually requires more planning. One of the advantages of an ATD is its ability rapidly to produce information. When the clinician wants to know if condition B works better than C, there are few finer ways to find out.

This is common when there are difficult treatment-related assessment decisions. Suppose, for example, a patient presents with depression. The clinician may have a difficult time determining if the patient is more likely to respond to cognitive-therapy procedures or skills-training procedures. Rather than guess, the clinician might do both, in an alternating-treatments fashion. The better treatment may quickly be revealed and all treatment effort could then go in this direction. We have recently conducted exactly such a clinical series (McKnight, Nelson, and Hayes, 1984), and were able in just a few sessions to distinguish re-

liably "cognitive responders" from "skills responders," based on ATD data.

Combining single-case and group designs

Case analyses are an exploration into the world of an individual. This kind of exploration calls for dynamic and creative use of clinical tools: assessment, intervention, and evaluation. Designs should not be a framework into which clinical procedures are injected, rather design elements should be used to support clinical decision making. In the ebb and flow of hypotheses that emerge in clinical work, design tools should be used as needed and as quickly discarded when they are no longer useful.

There are times, however, when a more formal approach is useful. For example, single-case analyses can be built into most group comparison designs. Consider a typical two-group design with an experimental and control group. Adding the needed dimension of intensive analysis can be accomplished with a minimum of three steps: repeated measurement, establishment of intrasubject variability, and within-subject comparisons. For example, at a minimum subjects in the experimental group could be exposed to a baseline phase, while measures were repeatedly taken. If the data were relatively stable (see Hayes 1981, on this point), this could be followed by a treatment phase in which repeated measurement continued. The resulting "A/B" design is probably the lowest level single-case design, but it does begin to increase the precision of the identification of individual successes and failures. Repeated measurement gives some indication within subject of the degree of variability due to measurement inconsistency and extraneous factors. If change is noticeable after the implementation of treatment, improvement is probably either due to treatment or to a coincidental extraneous factor. The strength of the analysis can be increased by adding intrasubject replication of the apparent treatment effects (e.g., through an A/B/A/B design in this example).

By using single-case designs for individual subjects *in addition* to the usual pre/post/follow-up measurement, the researcher can: (a) still analyze in a pre/post fashion, if desired; (b) identify at the level of the individual the successes and failures that seem probably due to treatment in each group; and (c) begin to correlate subject characteristics with success and failure of individuals due to treatment. Some subjects, for example, may have improved or deteriorated significantly, but in such a way that it cannot be said with confidence that treatment was the cause. Others may have shown ambiguous results. By considering these subjects separately from subjects showing clear effects due to treatment, the relationship between individual subject characteristics and individual treatment responsivity can better be determined. Thus, single-case analyses can be incorporated within group comparison designs to increase the analytic power of the research.

TREATMENT VALIDITY

Given the purposes of this association, I want briefly to address the relevance of single-case intervention research to assessment research. I have emphasized that, for research to be generalizable to the clinical situation, we will need to know more about how patient variables interact with treatment. Patient variables are in the domain of nursing and other diagnosis.

Any approach to assessment and diagnosis must specify ways to evaluate its quality. Traditionally, the quality of assessment has been determined by its psychometric properties. Psychometrics is based on the concepts of reliability and validity. Reliability refers to the consistency of scores obtained by the same persons when re-examined with the same assessment device under systematically changing circumstances (e.g., different time, different items, or different examiners), while validity refers to what an assessment device measures and how well it does so (Anastasi, 1982). To put it another way, reliability deals with relations among scores on the same device, while validity deals with relationships among scores on different devices (Campbell and Fiske, 1959). But consistency of measurement is not the same as utility.

Good applied assessment should help us predict and control clinically significant phenomena. This metric can be systematically used to evaluate the quality of assessment. For example, one of the main goals of nursing diagnosis is to select proper treatment targets. If an appropriate target is selected for treatment, presumably patients should improve more than if an inappropriate one has been selected. That is, an "appropriate" selection should allow greater prediction and control than an "inappropriate" one. Similarly, another goal of assessment is the selection of an appropriate treatment for a patient. If an appropriate treatment has been selected, patients should presumably get better faster than if an inappropriate treatment had been selected. In other words, in meeting its goals, assessment should be able to show that it can contribute to improved treatment outcome, what has been termed *treatment validity* (Hayes, Nelson, and Jarrett, in press; Nelson and Hayes, 1979).

One major type of treatment validity research relates patient classification to treatment responsivity (Hayes et al., in press). For example, recent research in our laboratory has shown the treatment validity of distinguishing cognitive distortions from overt skills deficits in the treatment of depression (McKnight, Nelson, Hayes, and Jarrett, 1984). Three subjects each were obtained who were depressed and had (a) poor social skills but few irrational cognitions, (b) irrational beliefs but adequate social skills, and

(c) problems in both areas. After a baseline phase, all subjects received both social-skills training and cognitive therapy in randomly alternating sessions (i.e., an ATD, Barlow and Hayes, 1979). Subjects with only social-skills problems improved most following social-skills training, while the reverse was true for subjects with problems only in the cognitive area. Subjects with problems in both areas improved as rapidly in either condition. Thus, the suspected relationship between these patient types and two types of therapies was obtained. The treatment validity of the diagnostic distinction between cognitive and social skills problems was confirmed. In another illustration of the treatment validity approach, only women suffering from spasmodic dysmenorrhea improved following systematic desensitization, while women suffering from congestive dysmenorrhea did not benefit from this treatment (Chesney and Tasto, 1975).

There are a number of other examples of treatment validity research addressing the question of the value of patient classification, although they are perhaps surprisingly uncommon given their obvious importance. To give a few examples, studies have shown the treatment validity of distinctions between types of insomnia (Borkovec, Grayson, O'Brian, et al., 1979), anxiety (Altmaier, Ross, Leary, et al., 1982; Elder, Edelstein, and Fremouw, 1981; Shahan and Merbaum, 1981), and depression (Paykel, Prusoff, Klerman, Haskell, et al., 1973).

Note that in studies of this type, treatment validity is based upon a nexus of assessment devices, theoretical distinctions, and treatment approaches. It evaluates devices only in the context of what is done with the knowledge obtained from them, that is, in the context of the degree to which they allow increased control over the phenomena of interest. Thus, a theoretical distinction can originally have no treatment validity, but may acquire it when treatments which make effective use of the distinction are later developed. For example, we may suspect that there are two different types of back pain, based on two patterns of assessment data, but until we have treatments that use this distinction, it may make no difference in outcome. Similarly, a device may have no treatment validity because the theoretical distinctions used to explain the assessment results are inadequate. We may use a new device correctly to identify differences in brain wave patterns in two patient subtypes, but it does not yet have treatment validity because there are no theories to explain the meaning of these data or to give use to the distinction. Thus, the interconnections between theoretical and technological advances in both assessment and treatment are underscored in treatment validity research. Treatment validity is a fairly demanding hurdle for assessment to pass over. The point is not to reject all assessment that has not yet passed this test but rather to seek to achieve this high standard before we can assert with confidence that we have quality assessment procedures.

THE PLACE OF TREATMENT VALIDITY IN ASSESSMENT RESEARCH

The notable advantage of treatment validity questions is that they relate assessment and methodological practices to functional changes in our patients. This sets the stage for important theoretical development, because it points out which of our practices are actually functionally important and thus require theoretical explanation. Once we have identified variables with treatment validity, the natural question is to determine why and how these differences occur. For example, if a given device helps match patients to effective treatment, how does this occur, and what does it say about the nature of the disorder or of the diagnostic process? Until this kind of question is answered, practices can have treatment validity and little conceptual validity.

Treatment validity provides the potential for a science of assessment that is directly related to and is built upon evidence of successful contributions to treatment. As such, it is a fundamentally different way of examining the quality of assessment—one in which the word "quality" is directly related to the central function of assessment.

Essentially, the treatment validity approach tests our view of functionally homogeneous groups. Since it does this *a priori*, is experimental and not just correlational, and concentrates on a single dimension or small number of dimensions, it does not fall prey to the same problems of the homogeneous group and correlatonal approaches. Without a demonstration of treatment validity, many of the differences identified in assessment research are differences that do not make a difference. This does not mean that we should not keep track of such non-functional differences, but only that the highest demonstration of the value of, for example, nursing diagnosis is to be found in its demonstrated utility. Because single-case designs can readily be used to test the utility of diagnoses, their use would help distinguish functional from non-functional diagnostic distinctions.

BUILDING THE SCIENCE FROM WITHIN

Like most of the clinical disciplines, nursing's greatest resource is its practitioners. They are the ones seeing the patients, trying new approaches, and applying known theories. If there is to be a strong scientific base built for nursing practice, what better way than to build it on actual work with real patients? Both academic and practicing nurses could begin to do this through the use of single-case experimental designs. It would take a major effort on the part of training programs and treatment facilities, but it could be done. The clinical disciplines have been given the sledge hammer of group comparison methods, and then have been asked to make precision constructions with this awkward tool. Not only is this impossible, but the few products that do result are inappropriate and are largely ignored. It is time for the clinical disciplines to lay aside the sledge hammer and pick up tools that fit the task at hand.

REFERENCES

Altmaier, E.M., Ross, S.L., Leary, N.R., and others: Matching stress inoculation's treatment components to clients' anxiety mode, J. Counseling Psychol. **29**:331, 1982.

Anastasi, A.: Psychological testing, ed. 5, New York, 1982, Macmillan.

Baer, D.M., Wolf, M.M., and Risley, T.R.: Some current dimensions of applied behavior analysis, J. Appl. Behav. Anal. **1**:91, 1968.

Barlow, D.H.: Behavior therapy: the next decade, Behav. Ther. **11**:315, 1980.

Barlow, D.H., and Hayes, S.C.: Alternating treatments design: one strategy for comparing the effects of two treatments in a single subject, J. Appl. Behav. Anal. **12**:199, 1979.

Barlow, D.H., Hayes, S.C., and Nelson, R.O.: The scientist-practitioner: research and accountability in clinical and educational settings, New York, 1984, Pergamon.

Barlow, D.H., and Hersen, M.: Single-case experimental designs: strategies for studying behavior change, ed. 2, New York, 1985, Pergamon.

Birnbrauer, J.S.: External validity and experimental investigation of individual behavior, Anal. Intervent. Develop. Disabilities **1**:117, 1981.

Borkovec, T.D., Grayson, J.B., O'Brien, G.T., and others: Relaxation training of pseudoinsomnia and idiopathic insomnia: an electroencephalographic evaluation. J. Appl. Behav. Anal. **12**:37, 1979.

Brownell, K.E., Hayes, S.C., and Barlow, D.H.: Patterns of appropriate and deviant arousal: the behavioral treatment of multiple sexual deviations, J. Consult. Clin. Psychol. **45**:1144, 1977.

Campbell, D.T., and Fiske, D.W.: Convergent and discriminant validation by the multitrait-multimethod matrix, Psychol. Bull. **56**:81, 1959.

Campbell, D.T., and Stanley, J.C.: Experimental and quasi-experimental designs for research, Chicago, 1963, Rand McNally.

Chassan, J.B.: Research design in clinical psychology and psychiatry, ed. 2, New York, 1979, Irvington.

Chesney, M.A., and Tasto, D.L.: The effectiveness of behavior modification with spasmodic and congestive dysmenorrhea, Behav. Res. Ther. **13**:245, 1975.

Elder, J.P., Edelstein, B.A., and Fremouw, W.J.: Client by treatment interactions in response acquisition and cognitive restructuring approaches, Cognitive Ther. Res. **5**:203, 1981.

Hartmann, D.P., and Hall, R.V.: The changing criterion design, J. Appl. Behav. Anal. **9**:527, 1976.

Hayes, S.C.: Single-case experimental designs and empirical clinical practice, J. Consult. Clin. Psychol. **49**:193, 1981.

Hayes, S.C.: Natural multiple baselines across persons: a reply to Harris and Jenson, Behav. Assess. **7**:129, 1985.

Hayes, S.C., Hussian, R.A., Turner, A.E., and others: The effects of coping statements on progress through a desensitization hierarchy, J. Behav. Ther. Exper. Psych. **14**:117, 1983.

Hayes, S.C., Nelson, R.O., and Jarrett, R.: Treatment validity: an approach to evaluating the quality of assessment. In Nelson, R.O., and Hayes, S.C., editors: The conceptual foundations of behavioral assessment, New York, Guilford. (In press.)

Hersen, M., and Barlow, D.H.: Single-case experimental designs: strategies for studying behavior change, New York, 1976, Pergamon.

Jayaratne, S., and Levy, R.L.: Empirical clinical practice, New York, 1979, Columbia University Press.

Kazdin, A.E.: Methodological and interpretive problems of single-case experimental designs, J. Consult. Clin. Psychol. **46**:629, 1978.

Kazdin, A.E.: Drawing valid inferences from case studies. J. Consult. Clin. Psychol. **49**:183, 1981.

Kazdin, A.E.: Single-case research designs: methods for clinical and applied settings, New York, 1982, Oxford.

Kratochwill, T.F.: Single subject research: strategies for evaluating change, New York, 1978, Academic.

McKnight, D.L., Nelson, R.O., Hayes, S.C., and others: Importance of treating individually-assessed response classes in the amelioration of depression, Behav. Ther. **15**:315, 1984.

Nelson, R.O., and Hayes, S.C.: Some current dimensions of behavioral assessment, Behav. Assess. **1**:1, 1979.

Paul, G.L.: Behavior modification research: design and tactics. In Franks, C.M., editor: Behavior therapy: appraisal and status, New York, 1969, McGraw-Hill.

Paykel, E.S., Prusoff, B.A., Klerman, G.L., and others: Clinical response to amitriptyline among depressed women, J. Nerv. Mental Dis. **156**:149, 1973.

Safran, J.D., Alden, L.E., and Davidson, P.O.: Client anxiety as a moderator variable in assertion training, Cognitive Ther. Res. **4**:189, 1980.

Shahan, A., and Merbaum, M.: The interaction between subject characteristics and self-control procedures in the treatment of interpersonal anxiety, Cognitive Ther. Res. **5**:221, 1981.

Thomas, E.J.: Research and service in single-case experimentation: conflicts and choices, Social Work Res. Abstr. **14**:20, 1978.

Zaro, J.S., Barach, R., Nedelmann, D.J., and others: A guide for beginning psychotherapists, Cambridge, 1977, Cambridge University Press.

CHAPTER 10

Organizing data for nursing diagnoses using functional health patterns

LAURA ROSSI, M.S., R.N.

Much time has been spent at this and other conferences evaluating various frameworks for nursing practice. The purpose of this paper is to describe the parameters for assessment within the functional health pattern typology described by Gordon and the application of this format to clinical practice. The intent is to focus on this typology as a framework for organizing data to make a diagnosis rather than as a theoretical framework for practice.

A critical part of making nursing diagnoses is related to the data base that is used for analysis (Gordon, 1982). Each pattern reflects a sequence of behavior in an area of human life (Box 1). Health status perception and management pattern refers to a patient's perceived level of wellbeing and practices for managing health. Nutritional/metabolic pattern includes a patient's 24-hour food and fluid consumption. Patterns of excretory function are described in the elimination pattern. Sleep/rest pattern refers to sleep, rest, and relaxation practices. Exercise/activity pattern addresses daily living activities that require energy expenditure such as self care, mobility, and recreation. Sexual/reproductive includes patterns of sexual preference and satisfaction as well as reproductive history. Cognitive/perceptual pattern describes a patient's ability to comprehend and use information. Self-concept/self-perception pattern refers to one's attitudes about oneself, that is, one's sense of identity and worth. Coping/stress tolerance pattern describes one's perception of stress and methods of management. Role/relationship pattern describes a patient's role or place in the world and in the entire social network. Last, value/belief pattern addresses the cultural, philosophical and religious values that guide one's decisions about life.

These eleven functional health patterns are analogous to the organ systems that physicians use to organize their data collection. Since nurses also assess, evaluate and

---

BOX 1: Functional health patterns

Health perception/management
Nutritional/metabolic
Elimination
Sleep/rest
Exercise/activity
Sexual/reproductive
Cognitive/perceptual
Coping/stress tolerance
Self-concept/self-perception
Role/relationship
Value/belief

---

document physical findings, there is overlap between a nurse's and physician's evaluation of the same person. Physical examination findings are documented by nurses at the end of a patient's history. The extent of a physical examination varies according to the nurse's specialty area and level of expertise. Many nurses have applied the functional health pattern framework to family or community assessment, however, further discussion of this area is beyond the scope of this paper.

INDIVIDUAL PATIENT ASSESSMENT

During the interview of a patient, the nurse must screen for function and dysfunction within each pattern by evaluating certain parameters. For example, in the evaluation of exercise-activity, one screens for problems with self-care, activities of daily living, mobility, and recreation and diversion preferences. These concepts resemble those identified at the second level of abstraction under the *Moving pattern* of NANDA's Human Response Framework (Kritek, 1984). It has been suggested that the eleven functional health patterns actually represent a level of abstraction between the first and second levels of the proposed Human Response Framework. Since nurses use a variety of theoretical frameworks to guide practice, they may view dysfunctional patterns as adaptation problems (Roy, 1981), or disorganized life processes (Rogers, 1970). In either situation, the nurse's observations are documented in a consistent format.

Different levels of skill and time frames are required for nurses to carry out the process of screening which accounts for variability in documentation of an assessment. The beginning staff nurse evaluating a patient admitted for cardiac surgery may not respond to subtle cues (e.g., history of periods of decreased activity to avoid anginal symptoms and medical evaluation). On the other hand, an experienced nurse-clinician

knows that delay in seeking medical attention is common among patients with cardiovascular disease and may recognize it as an overriding theme in the patient's pattern of making all decisions.

During assessments, nurses use patients' descriptions of themselves and their problems to infer functional and dysfunctional health patterns and generate hypotheses about problems. Data collection includes a patient's explanation of problems within a pattern, actions taken to alleviate the problem, and the perceived effectiveness of the actions. Using the example of exercise/activity, consider patients who describe pain on exertion. While one patient may explain the problem as angina or coronary insufficiency, another patient may describe nonspecific chest pain. Each patient describes a variety of problem-solving strategies such as taking prophylactic nitroglycerin, avoiding activities that precipitate symptoms, pacing activities to minimize myocardial oxygen demands, joining an exercise program to promote activity tolerance, or calling a physician immediately for advice. The responses prompt the nurse to ask other questions to clarify a specific problem within the pattern and define relationships among patterns.

Consider the differences between the patient who takes nitroglycerin prophylactically and the patient who avoids activities that provoke symptoms. Each patient's choice of action is related to their health perception, (health status perception and management) their understanding of symptoms and treatment (cognitive/perceptual) and/or their level of anxiety (coping/stress tolerance). This is one example of the numerous interrelationships that exist among patterns.

History taking is followed by further data analysis. Critical defining characteristics of specific nursing diagnoses may emerge from a patient's statements during assessment of one functional pattern. On the other hand, supporting signs and symptoms may be found in the evaluation of other patterns. The latter may represent the degree of severity or progression of the patient's problem (nursing diagnosis). For example, the parameters for sleep/rest pattern include usual sleep times, effect of sleep, presleep routines, and rest and relaxation practices. One would expect to learn about difficulty in falling asleep or staying asleep in this pattern, while additional data relevant to sleep and rest emerges in the assessment of the cognitive/perceptual pattern (e.g., reduced attention span or greater number of errors). Similarly, assessment of coping/stress tolerance might reveal increased irritability; exercise/activity might reveal decreased endurance. The important point to be gleaned from these examples is that assessment of all the patterns is necessary to make a complete evaluation of a patient.

Attempts to abbreviate the process by omitting certain patterns result in major gaps in the data base. Furthermore, selective use of patterns in certain specialty areas is generally based upon an assumption that specific diagnoses occur frequently in particular patient populations. Although these associations are helpful, they are not well grounded from an epidemiologic standpoint. This leads to premature closure and invalid data clustering. Research is needed to validate the functional pattern assessment parameters and to streamline history taking without jeopardizing diagnostic accuracy.

Categorization of patient problems

The organization of data extends from an individual patient's history to the classification of problems within a patient population. Consider the following retrospective chart review of 20 patients with a medical diagnosis of malignant ventricular arrhythmia (Rossi, 1984). A total of 69 patient problems was identified (mean, 3.5 problems per patient). The most common nursing diagnoses were knowledge deficit and compro-

mised coping (documented for 70% of the patients) followed by sleep disturbances and decreased activity tolerance. Although various authors have described the concurrence of nursing and medical diagnoses, the limited number of nursing diagnoses currently approved for clinical testing makes it difficult to appreciate the scope of patient problems and the impact on lifestyles. Table 1 shows the distribution of the 69 documented patient problems according to the functional pattern area affected. Notice the most common patterns affected were cognitive/perceptual, exercise/activity, and coping/stress tolerance.

Classification of nursing literature

The functional health pattern typology also permits the classification of nursing literature. This is particularly important in facilitating research and education. In a review of the last 30 years of *Nursing Research*, the topic areas of 1532 articles and briefs were examined (Rossi, unpublished). Although the percentage of clinically focused papers has increased over the years, only 469 of the

Table 1: Distribution of problems according to functional health pattern

	# Dx	Percent
Health perception/management	0	0
Nutritional/metabolic	3	4
Elimination	3	4
Sleep/rest	9	13
Exercise/activity	16	23
Sexual/reproductive	0	0
Cognitive/perceptual	19	27
Coping/stress tolerance	14	20
Self-concept/self-perception	3	4
Role/relationship	2	2
Value/belief	0	0

articles or 31% were considered to be clinically focussed.

Table 2 shows the distribution of the 469 papers according to the functional pattern area addressed. Interestingly, the highest number of studies dealt with problems affecting the cognitive/perceptual pattern, followed by role/relationship, coping/stress tolerance and health/perception management patterns. These do not correspond to the number of diagnoses on the current NANDA list and provide a different perspective on the studies of nursing phenomena conducted to date.

Application in practice

Few questions have arisen concerning the relevance of the functional health pattern framework for collecting data in clinical practice. Although one might see certain patterns as a priority for concern in particular patients or unique populations, the patterns are consistent with nursing's commitment to society as stated in the ANA Social Policy Statement. The framework's compatibility with existing practice, which cannot be overemphasized, and its advantages further support its use as a common framework for data collection. The advantages of adopting a common data collection framework are numerous. First, time for learning new assessment skills in a clinical agency is limited since nurses are accountable not only for making diagnoses but also for treating them. A common framework would decrease the cost of orientation. Secondly, cost containment has forced a serious examination of nursing's role in health care. A considerable amount of time continues to be spent on the development and redevelopment of agency-specific admission documentation and assessment formats. When documentation is poor, forms are changed in light of organizational problems that may range from inadequate administrative support to poor time management. Early discharge reinforces the profession's need for a common framework for data collection that helps nurses determine patients' readiness for discharge and their post-discharge needs for nursing care and supervision. A third advantage of the functional pattern typology as a common framework for data collection is its compatibility with existing theoretical models for nursing practice. Gordon has skillfully shown the utility of the framework in the context of four different theoretical models (Gordon, 1982).

While the functional patterns have gained widespread attention because of their clinical relevance and applicability to all areas of nursing practice, there are unresolved issues. The absence of specific parameters within the patterns and the intermingling of patterns frequently result in variations in assessment and diagnosis of the same patient. For example, a patient's health status perception and management may be affected by learning ability (cognitive/perceptual)

Table 2: Distribution of studies according to functional health pattern

	# Studies	% Clinical studies
Health perception/management	62	13
Nutritional/metabolic	33	7
Elimination	14	3
Sleep/rest	8	2
Exercise/activity	39	8
Sexual/reproductive	4	1
Cognitive/perceptual	94	20
Self-perception/self-concept	11	2
Coping/stress tolerance	77	16
Role/relationship	86	18
Value/belief	13	3
Unrelated	28	6
Total	469	99

which may be affected by coping skills (coping/stress tolerance) and the number of support systems (role/relationship).

Future investigators must examine individual nurses' use of the functional health pattern framework and its relationship to the diagnostic process in order to refine assessment parameters for each pattern. The latter is a prerequisite to consistency and precision in making nursing diagnoses and developing standards of practice for treatment.

In summary, this presentation was designed to clarify the potential uses of the functional pattern typology for nurses who have never used it. For those more familiar with its use, my ideas and enthusiasm may serve as encouragement to implement it in more clinical areas and promote consistency of patient evaluation. A unified approach to data collection will, at the very least, provide a common format that enables nurses at all levels, in all specialties to contribute to the evolution of a taxonomy of nursing diagnoses. At the very most, it will facilitate the development of a scientific basis for comparing clinical problems across individuals, cohorts, and populations.

REFERENCES

Gordon, M.: Nursing diagnosis process and application, New York, 1982, McGraw-Hill.

Kritek, P.: Report of the group work on taxonomies. In Kim, M.J., McFarland, G.K., and McLane, A.M., editors: Classification of nursing diagnoses: proceedings of the fifth national conference, St. Louis, 1984, The C.V. Mosby Co.

Rogers, M.: An introduction to the theoretical basis of nursing, Philadelphia, 1970, F.A. Davis.

Rossi, L.: Clinical research in nursing diagnosis, Unpublished manuscript, 1984.

Rossi, L.: Nursing care for survivors of sudden cardiac death, Nurs. Clin. North Am. **19:**411, 1984.

Roy, C.: An introduction to nursing: an adaptation model, ed. 2, Englewood Cliffs, NJ, Prentice-Hall, 1984.

CHAPTER 11

Organizing data for nursing diagnoses using conservation principles

JOYCE W. TAYLOR, M.S.N., R.N.

My purpose in this paper is to describe and demonstrate how Levine's conservation model can be used to develop an approach to data collection that facilitates formulation of nursing diagnoses. Since my work is largely with patients who have neurological dysfunction, my discussion focusses on that particular patient population.

In the Social Policy Statement, the American Nurses Association defines nursing as the "diagnosis and treatment of human responses to actual or potential health problems" (ANA, 1980, p. 9). The "phenomena of concern" to nurses, according to the policy statement, include responses resulting from medical diagnoses and treatments as well as responses to unique health-related needs and concerns of an individual and family.

LEVINE'S MODEL

Levine's model postulates that each individual responds "organismically"—that is, with the whole being—to both internal and external stimuli. Patients are viewed "holistically" (Levine, 1971), maintaining the unity and integrity of their being as they interact within their environments. An individual is seen in the context of the environment; both health and illness are products of a very personal pattern of adaptation. Levine describes four levels of response, which are physiologically determined, that enable an individual to make a viable adaptation to constantly changing internal and external environments. The four levels of response are: (1) response to fear (fight or flight); (2) inflammatory response (energy directed toward removal or exclusion of an irritant or pathogen); (3) response to stress (non-specifically induced changes that allow adaptation to a variety of stressors over time); and (4) sensory response (recognizable interactions between the individual and the environment).

Nursing care, according to Levine (1971), is focused on individuals and the complexity of their relationships with the environment. The goal of nursing care is to conserve or "keep together" a patient's biological, personal and social integrity in the struggle to achieve a positive (healthy) adaptation. To keep together means to maintain a proper balance between active nursing intervention coupled with patient participation, on the one hand, and within the safe limits of the patient's ability on the other. By entering a patient's eco-system, the nurse directs, activates, and sustains an organismic response as the patient strives for renewed wellbeing. When adaptation is no longer possible, the nurse supports the individual and family until care is no longer needed.

Nursing interventions are based on the four conservation principles:

1. *Conservation of Energy.* According to Levine (1967), all of life's processes are fundamentally dependent upon the production and expenditure of energy. The ability of individuals to function is predicated upon their energy potential and the specific patterns of energy exchange available. A balance between energy production and energy expenditure is essential for all activity, but is particularly crucial for neurological function. Conservation of energy is a natural defense against a disease process. The lethargy and withdrawal observed in acutely ill patients indicate a physiological response designed to prevent further damage and promote recovery. Therefore, the commonly recurring nursing diagnoses related to energy conservation in the neurological patient reflect a threat to the continuous supply of oxygen and nutrients (particularly glucose), and/or indicate an increase or decrease in energy utilization. Nursing care of a neurological patient must include measures to conserve and mobilize energy resources to meet basic metabolic needs, promote healing, and eventually develop an energy reserve sufficient to regain physical, personal, and social integrity.

2. *Conservation of Structural Integrity.* The design or structure of the body determines how it functions. Structural changes, resulting from injury, disease, and normal developmental processes, lead to changes in function. Conservation of structural integrity requires that the "wholeness" of the body be protected and that physiological functions be maintained. For a neurological patient, the common nursing diagnoses related to structural integrity evolve from threats of permanent damage to nerve tissue, concurrent or complicating disease, procedures or therapies with benefits and risks, immobility, and the impaired nutrition and hydration that may result from the disease state. Nursing interventions for such patients are based on the need to protect them from further damage or injury; prevent iatrogenic or trophicogenic (Levine, 1966) complications; preserve basic physiological functions, such as nutrition, hydration, mobility, rest, and sleep; and initiate rehabilitative measures that return patients to a state of relative independence and wellbeing.

3. *Conservation of Personal Integrity.* Both survival and rehabilitation depend upon a patient's energy resources and on some measure of structural integrity, but the body cannot be separated from the mind, emotions, and soul. The "person" who is the patient is dependent on the structural integrity of the brain itself and on the processes of the mind: the thoughts, emotions, sensations, experiences and expressions that have accumulated over a lifetime. Individuals respond to illness on their own terms, according to Levine, and the nurse is responsible for interpreting patients' behavior and responding to needs as they develop. For neurological patients, the commonly recurring nursing diagnoses relate to the loss of critical functions such as language, emotional control, and judgment which develop from abnormalities of awareness of self and environment; sudden loss of bodily functions; dependency in self care; and socially unacceptable problems such as incontinence. These problems have a serious impact upon patients' self-concept and

self-esteem and create feelings of isolation, guilt and loneliness. Patients so often helpless and vulnerable, depend upon nurses to cherish and protect their wholeness. A nurse communicates with a patient, often using what Levine refers to as "the silent language," administering meticulous physical care with warmth and gentleness; preserving the patient's privacy and dignity; respecting possessions, beliefs and values; keeping a safe and secure environment; and in all ways helping to conserve and restore personal integrity.

4. *Conservation of Social Integrity.* The ultimate goal of all health care is to return individuals to family and community in states that facilitate re-entry into productive and satisfying lives. That goal may not be fully realized because of a patient's disease or prognosis (as often occurs with neurologically damaged patients). An alternate goal of care is to assist a patient and family to cope adaptively with an inevitable outcome. For neurological patients the commonly recurring nursing diagnoses related to the resocialization process result from the patient's communication and cognitive dysfunction, social isolation and self-care deficits, extended institutionalization, and from the need for major changes in lifestyle and role relationships. Nursing care focusses on helping a patient and family adapt to the new person a patient has become, and on fostering a realignment of roles and relationships. Teaching patients to function outside of a protected environment of an institution and to establish a modified version of a preferred lifestyle are critical to the conservation of their social integrity.

Incorporating the body of neuroscience nursing into the Levine model, my approach to assessment and management of patients is made with a view of a patient as an integrated individual, continuously interacting with the environment, reacting and responding as a whole to every stimulus (including illness); a defined purpose or goal to conserve or keep together the patient's biological, personal, and social integrity when it is threatened by illness or injury; and a focus for nursing intervention on the four principles of conservation, recognizing and supporting the four levels of organismic response as the patient struggles to maintain or regain integrity.

Using the model to assess and diagnose

A fundamental purpose of a model is to direct the collection of data, based on a view of the patient, the purpose of nursing and the focus of nursing's concern. By combining concepts from the model with knowledge of neuroanatomy, physiology, and medical and nursing science it becomes possible to select from all of the possible facts one could collect about the patient those most relevant to the purposes of nursing. What Levine calls the "provocative facts" are isolated from the collected data (in medical terminology, these might be referred to as positive findings). The provocative facts are analyzed and extrapolated, and sets of defining characteristics are identified that differentiate the appropriate nursing diagnoses. A knowledge of neuroscience enables one to arrive at etiological factors although not all diagnoses have well defined etiologies or defining characteristics. The approved list is used whenever possible, and diagnoses are modified or added to adequately describe patients' problems in terms that facilitate anticipating realistic outcomes and effective nursing interventions.

In summary, using the Levine model focusses the nursing assessment on: energy exchange, structure and function, self-identity, self-concept, self-respect, social milieu, lifestyle, and relationships. An assessment guide helps direct data collection for neurological patients (see Box 1). Not all data need to be collected on every patient. The experienced nurse can quickly focus on items that are most relevant to a particular patient situation, but all items need to be kept in mind. From the collected data a nurse can isolate the provocative facts that indicate the presence of a nursing diagnosis. The facts can then be summarized and used to develop a nursing care plan (Table 1).

BOX 1: **Assessment guide***

    I. Energy exchange (resources/expenditures)
      A. Oxygen supply
         1. Airway
         2. Respirations (rate, rhythm, volume)
         3. Arterial blood gases
      B. Nutrition
         1. Present nutritional status
         2. Nutritional intake
      C. Activity, rest, sleep
         1. Medically prescribed restrictions
         2. Physical restrictions, fatigue
         3. Effects of level of consciousness, mental status changes
         4. Effects of lifestyle, patient goals
      D. Illness-related energy expenditures
         1. Fever, infection
         2. Seizures
         3. High-stimulus environment (as ICU)
         4. High stress (physiological)
         5. Pain
         6. Metabolic abnormalities
   II. Structure and function
      A. Integument
         1. Skin condition
         2. Mucous membranes, corneas
         3. Surgical wounds, injuries, tubes, catheters
         4. Skin turgor and tone, circulation
         5. Sensations (temperature, pain, touch, pressure)

---

*Assessment data in addition to routine nursing assessment
J.W. Taylor. NANDA's 7th conference on classification of nursing diagnoses.

BOX 1:   **Assessment guide—cont'd**

    B. Musculoskeletal system
       1. Strength
       2. Tone
       3. Reflexes
       4. Abnormal movement
       5. Ability to initiate, sustain, control and terminate movement
       6. Range of motion (all joints)
       7. Mobility, weight bearing
       8. Fractures, injuries
    C. Sensation, perception
       1. Vision
       2. Hearing
       3. Smell
       4. Touch
       5. Temperature
       6. Pain
       7. Proprioception
    D. Cerebral perfusion pressure
       1. Level of consciousness
       2. Blood pressure (lying, standing, sitting)
       3. Pupil size and reactivity
       4. Other cranial nerve function
       5. Posturing
       6. Intracranial pressure (when being measured)
    E. Elimination
       1. Bowel function
         a. Bowel sounds
         b. Stool (frequency, consistency)
         c. Flatus
         d. Control
       2. Urination
         a. Amount, frequency, specific gravity
         b. Bladder emptying
         c. Evidence of infection
         d. Control
    F. Fluids and electrolytes
       1. Fluid intake and output
       2. Weight
       3. Skin turgor
       4. Serum electrolytes, osmolality
    G. Treatment-related risks
       1. Steroid therapy
       2. Radiation, chemotherapy
       3. Invasive diagnostic or treatment procedures

Continued

BOX 1:   **Assessment guide—cont'd**

III. Self-identity/self-respect/self-concept
  A. Mental status
    1. Orientation
    2. Memory
    3. Judgment
    4. Problem solving
    5. Emotional lability, catastrophic reactions
  B. Communication
    1. Language (verbal, written)
    2. Speech
    3. Gestures
    4. Facial expression
  C. Image of self
    1. Degree of independence
    2. Control of bodily functions
    3. Perceived relationships with family, others
    4. Congruence of previous and present lifestyle, activity level, goals and aspirations
  D. Adaptation
    1. Evidence of grief reaction, resolution
    2. Coping strategies
IV. Social milieu, lifestyle, relationships
  A. Family, significant others
    1. Availability of support systems
    2. Willingness, ability of family or significant others to provide care or ongoing support
    3. Coping strategies of family, significant others
  B. Social situation
    1. Financial status as affected by illness, disability
    2. Career status as effected by the illness, disability
    3. Living arrangements
    4. Role relationships, expectations

Table 1: Nursing care plan

DIAGNOSIS/RELEVANT DATA: (taken from nursing assessment data)

Mrs. G. is a 73 year old *widow, living alone,* brought to the hospital by ambulance after being found unresponsive on the floor at home. Admitting *medical diagnosis is probably left middle cerebral artery infarct* (unconfirmed by CAT). Recent *cataract surgery.* At time of admission is *awake,* but does *not respond to verbal commands. Muttering unintelligibly,* is very *restless and attempting to climb out of bed.* The *right arm and leg are flaccid* with no spontaneous movement. There is a *facial droop* and *absent gag reflex. Voided in bedpan* which was placed under her, and was then *noted to be less restless.* Patient's *daughter* is the *nearest relative* and became *distraught (crying)* upon seeing her mother. *States that "everything must be done" to make her mother well.*

DISCHARGE PLAN: Deferred. Refer to Social Service

Date/Sign.	Nursing diagnosis	Expected outcome	Intervention	Resolved Date/Sign
2/27/86	**Energy exchange**			
	1. Altered nutrition (potential for less than body needs) related to: Difficulty chewing and swallowing	1. Maintains body weight	1. Mechanical soft diet Small frequent meals with between meal supplements Feed patient from left side, placing food well back in mouth	
2/27/86	**Structural integrity**			
2/27/86	2. Potential for injury, (trauma) related to: restlessness, visual impairment, right-sided weakness	2. Sustains no injury	2. Side rails at all times Posey vest Close supervision Bedside table on left and within range of vision Glasses on during waking hours Night light Anticipate care needs, especially toileting to reduce efforts to get out of bed	
2/27/86	3. Impaired musculoskeletal integrity (potential) related to: flaccid paralyses of right extremities	3. Maintains full range of motion in all extremities. Has no pain, edema in affected extremities	3. Maintain extremities in functional position: Support affected arm/hand on pillow with fingers/wrist in extension; arm slightly elevated and abducted Support upper leg on bolster when in side-lying position Small foam pads under knees and at upper outer thighs when in supine position	

Continued

Table 1: Nursing care plan—cont'd

Date/Sign	Nursing diagnosis	Expected outcome	Intervention	Resolved Date/Sign
			Range-of-motion exercises to all joints once each shift Refer to Physical Therapy when condition is stable	
	4. Impaired skin integrity (potential) related to: restlessness (shearing) decreased muscle tone (right side) immobility	4. Skin remains intact	4. Alternating pressure mattress Heal and elbow protectors Use turning sheet Turn from side to side every 1 to 2 hours Reposition right side every hour (more often if reddened areas appear) Examine all skin surfaces each time patient is turned Keep skin dry, clean, and well lubricated Gentle massage to bony prominences each time patient is turned	
2/27/86	**Personal integrity**			
	5. Impaired communication (verbal) related to: aphasia (fluent)	5. Method of communication established. Care needs are met	5. Observe patient's behavior for clues about care needs Speak to patient in one or two-word phrases Ask questions requiring only "Yes-No" responses ("Bedpan?" "Drink?" "Blanket?") Use gestures, facial expressions, touch to facilitate communication Allow time for patient response Pause between questions, subject changes	
	6. Self-care deficit (level 4 all areas) related to: right-sided weakness inability to communicate needs or follow commands	6. Begins to participate in self care	6. Anticipate and provide care needs until condition has stabilized Give simple one-step commands as care is given ("Turn", "Lift arm", etc.) Use pantomine to communicate expectations/intentions	

Table 1: Nursing care plan—cont'd

Date/Sign	Nursing diagnosis	Expected outcome	Intervention	Resolved Date/Sign
			Provide opportunities for patient to assist with personal care tasks as readiness is demonstrated Refer to Occupational Therapist when patient able to sit in chair for at least 1 hour without visible fatigue	

	Social integrity			
2/27/86	7. Altered family process (anticipated) related to: situation transition/ crisis (sudden illness of previously independent mother)	7. Daughter (and patient when able) demonstrate realization of necessary alterations by participating in realistic plan for long term care	7. Refer to Social Worker Begin exploring with daughter (and mother) to resources for long-term care With Social Worker assist daughter (and mother) identify available resources outside the family and the available options and alternatives	
	8. Grief (daughter) related to: potential loss of mother and/or permanent disability of mother	8. Daughter able to verbalize feelings and concerns Daughter verbalizes understanding of probable outcomes of illness Daughter verbalizes realistic expectations of medical therapies and nursing care	8. Keep daughter fully informed of progress, prognosis, and care/treatment needs Explain signs, symptoms, and behavioral changes Offer opportunities for daughter to express feelings/concerns Encourage daughter to participate in mother's care to the extent that is comfortable for her Support daughter's decisions about long-term care	

REFERENCES

American Nurses Association: Nursing: a social policy statement, Kansas City, MO, 1980, American Nurses Association.

Levine, M.E.: The four conservation principles of nursing, Nurs. Forum **6**:45, 1967.

Levine, M.E.: The pursuit of wholeness, Am. J. Nurs. **69**:93, 1969.

Levine, M.E.: Trophicognosis: an alternative to nursing diagnosis, In Exploring progress in medical-surgical nursing, vol. 2, New York, 1966, American Nurses' Association.

Levine, M.E.: Holistic nursing, Nurs. Clin. North Amer. **6**:253, 1971.

PART A

Validation studies: paper presentations

Clinical validation of the diagnosis anxiety

TERESA FADDEN, M.S.N., R.N.
RICHARD J. FEHRING, D.N.Sc., R.N.
EILEEN KENKEL-ROSSI, M.S.N., R.N.

Anxiety has been and continues to be a diagnosis that nurses frequently make and treat. Florence Nightingale (1859) noted that anxiety is present in patients and spoke to the need for nursing interventions in the treatment of this problem. Peplau (1963), a leader in mental health nursing, has developed a widely accepted operational definition of anxiety. In the 1970's, the North American Nursing Diagnosis Association (NANDA) included the diagnosis of anxiety on the accepted list. In 1980 it was deleted and used as a defining characteristic for the new diagnosis, fear (Kim and Moritz, 1982). Despite this action by NANDA, anxiety continued to be a diagnosis frequently made and treated by practicing nurses (Kim et al., 1982; McKeehan and Gordan, 1982; Jones, 1982). Anxiety was returned to the list of accepted nursing diagnoses in 1982.

Anxiety has been defined as the persistent feeling of dread, apprehension or disaster (Miller and Keane, 1972). It occurs in response to a threat to some value that an individual holds essential to his personal

existence (May, 1950), and can involve either biological or emotional functions. Peplau (1963) refers to this as a response to threats against biological integrity or the self system.

Anxiety is a universal phenomenon and is experienced by everyone at some point in life. While it is a normal human response, it may vary greatly in nature and degree. Spielberger, Gorsuch, and Lushene (1971) classify anxiety in terms of state or trait. Trait anxiety describes an individual's usual way of responding to life situations, while state anxiety signifies response to a particular situation.

Various levels of anxiety have been described ranging from mild apprehension to a totally disorganized state (Peplau, 1963; Jasmine and Trygstad, 1979; Murray and Zenter, 1979). The North American Nursing Diagnosis Association used four levels for diagnostic purposes. These were mild, moderate, severe, and panic. Indicators for the different levels are similar but occur on an intensity continuum (Gebbie and Lavin, 1975; Gebbie, 1976; Kim and Moritz, 1981). These levels were no longer differentiated in the 1982 listing.

Since anxiety is subjective, it cannot be measured directly, but it can be known

This study was funded by the Wisconsin Nurses Foundation.

Special recognition to the staff nurses at St. Joseph's Hospital, Milwaukee, Wisconsin, for their assistance.

through the effects that have been communicated or observed. These subjective and objective data are referred to as defining characteristics or critical indicators. The current NANDA listing for anxiety includes seventeen subjective and twelve objective indicators. These indicators include affective, cognitive, physiologic and kinetic changes (Kim, McFarland, and McLane, 1984). Through collection of objective and subjective data, it is possible to detect the presence and severity of responses in any of the above categories.

Frequently the words fear and anxiety are used interchangeably when formulating nursing diagnoses. Several authors differentiate these terms by using anxiety to describe threats from an unknown entity and fear to explain threats which have an identifiable, specific object (Jones and Jakob, 1981; Sundeen, Stuart, Rankin and Cohen, 1981). Both terms are listed on the national classification list (Kim, McFarland, and McLane, 1984). While the two terms may differ in cause, the objective and subjective data are similar, as is treatment. Because of this, it may not be important to make the distinction in clinical practice. The terms *stress* and *anxiety* are often also confused and misused. They can be differentiated by using *anxiety* as the term to explain the organism's way of responding to stressors (Murray and Zenter, 1979). In other words, stress produces or causes anxiety.

Little work has been done on validating the nursing diagnosis of anxiety. Graham and Conley (1971) reported on an evaluation study of anxiety and fear. Seventy surgical patients were observed and interviewed during the perioperative period. The most common indications of anxiety and fear were statements made by the patients. One-half of the sample admitted they were very frightened or anxious. This group could also specifically describe their fears. Significantly higher proportions of female patients and

persons facing possible disfiguring surgery or biopsy were found to have moderate to high anxiety.

Jones and Jakob (1981) published a report on a study that attempted to differentiate fear and anxiety. Although this was not a validation study, the researchers did find some interesting results. Fifty-seven volunteer nurses generated over 2,000 nursing diagnoses on 393 clients. The nursing diagnosis of fear was the third most common diagnosis. Anxiety was the seventh most common diagnosis made by these nurses. Much of the supporting subjective and objective data for the diagnosis of anxiety implied that the diagnosis under consideration was probably fear. On the other hand, when the diagnosis of fear was made by the study participants, the investigators found that the subjective and objective indicators supported this diagnosis. This study pointed out that anxiety is often mistakenly used when fear should be the diagnosis and that fear, when it is used is generally used properly. In response to this study, Burke (1982) proposed that nurses' use of the terms fear and anxiety are probably unique and may not be consistent with the definitions set forth by other disciplines. Burke suggested that nurses continue to study the phenomena of fear and anxiety.

At the Fifth National Conference on Classification of Nursing Diagnoses the group that reintroduced the diagnosis of anxiety developed three research questions pertinent to anxiety (Kim, et al., 1984). They were as follows:

1. What are the reported indicators of anxiety from the patient's view?
2. What are the indicators observed by the nurse? and
3. What is the correlation of the findings of Questions 1 and 2?

Since there is very little validation research on the present diagnosis of anxiety, this study was an effort to validate the characteristics of anxiety and to answer the questions from the Fifth National Conference. The specific questions that were addressed in this study were as follows:

1. Are the defining characteristics of anxiety, as set forth by the Fifth National Conference on Classification of Nursing Diagnoses, clinically valid?
2. How do the individual characteristics of anxiety relate (correlate) to the State-anxiety scores obtained on the State-anxiety inventory developed by Spielberger, et al., (1970).

For this study anxiety was conceptualized following the definition and defining characteristics developed by the Fifth National Conference on Classification of Nursing Diagnoses. The definition for anxiety from the Fifth Conference is as follows: "a vague, uneasy feeling the source of which is often non-specific or unknown to the individual" (Kim, et al., 1984, p. 472). The defining characteristics can be found in the *Proceedings of the Fifth National Conference* (Kim, et al., 1984). Anxiety was also conceptualized as being either state or trait in nature (Spielberger, et al., 1970). State-anxiety refers to a transitory emotional response of the human being characterized by feelings of "tension and apprehension, and heightened autonomic-nervous-system activity" (Spielberger, et al., 1970, p. 3). These characteristics are similar to those defined by the classification conference. Trait-anxiety, on the other hand, refers to a rather stable condition of anxiety-proneness.

METHODOLOGY

This study was descriptive in nature; it was based upon the clinical validation model proposed by Gordon and Sweeney (1979) and refined by Fehring (1986). The Nurse-Validation Model developed by Gordon and Sweeney consists of familiarizing trained nurse observers with a given diagnostic label and having them tabulate the defining char-

acteristics observed in an adequate number of patients with a given diagnosis. Coexistence of the observed characteristics of the diagnosis with either clinically or retrospectively identified characteristics will establish validity.

Fehring's model, the Clinical Diagnostic Validity model (CDV), is similar to Gordon and Sweeney's but includes the ability to provide quantifiable evidence that a diagnosis exists. The steps of the model are as follows:

1. Two "expert clinicians observe and assess an adequate number of patients with a previously identified nursing diagnosis.
2. The clinicians check the frequency of the previously identified characteristics of the diagnosis with those characteristics manifested by each patient observed.
3. Calculate the weighted inter-rater reliability ratios for each identified characteristic by the following formula:

$$R = \frac{A}{A+D} \times \frac{\frac{F_1}{N} + \frac{F_2}{N}}{2}$$

Where
A = Number of agreements
D = Number of disagreements
F_1 = The frequency of the characteristics observed by the first rater
F_2 = The frequency of the characteristics observed by the second rater
N = The number of subjects observed
R = Weighted inter-rater reliability ratio

4. Discard the characteristics with ratios less or equal to .50.
5. Items with ratios greater than .75 would be critical.
6. Obtain the total CDV score by summing and averaging the ratios for each characteristic.

Subjects

The criteria for subject selection were alert adult (18 years or older) medical-surgical patients with a current diagnosis of anxiety and State-anxiety scores above 45. The score of 45 or above for State-anxiety was chosen because that is the average level of anxiety for medical-surgical patients as identified by Spielberger, et al., (1970). The subjects were initially diagnosed as "anxious" by professional staff nurses caring for those patients.

There were 91 patients who were diagnosed as anxious by staff nurses and who became subjects for this study. Of those 91, only 49 had State-anxiety scores of 45 or greater. The mean age of the 49 subjects was 64.14. There were 29 females and 20 males. Their mean State-anxiety was 53.71. The mean State-anxiety for the 91 subjects was 44.88

Seventy-five percent of the subjects with anxiety scores of 45 or greater had received anti-anxiety medications or narcotics within 48 hours of their interview. Thirty-five percent of these subjects had the medical diagnosis of cancer, 14 percent had cardiovascular disease, 13 percent had an infection and the rest (38%) were hospitalized for a variety of other medical-surgical problems.

Instruments

Anxiety was assessed by use of the defining characteristics of anxiety as developed by participants at the Fifth National Conference on the Classification of Nursing diagnoses and by use of the State Trait Anxiety Inventory (STAI) of Speilberger, et al.

The defining characteristics were used by two clinical nurse-specialists as they assessed each subject. Check marks were used to indicate the presence or absence of the defined characteristics. Inter-rater reliability was obtained on each characteristic by use of the weighted inter-rater reliability formula as developed by Fehring (1986).

Anxiety was measured by the State form (X-1) of the State Trait Anxiety Inventory (STAI) developed by Spielberger, Gorsuch, and Lushene (1970). The A-State form of the STAI was designed to measure respondent's anxiety as perceived at that moment. Alpha reliability coefficients for the A-State scale range from .83 to .92 (Spielberger, et al., 1970). Validity for the STAI has been demonstrated in a wide variety of studies.

Procedure

One day a week, two clinical specialists canvassed the patient records of eight medical-surgical units for the diagnosis of anxiety. There were 35 data-collection periods. On each data-collection day there was an average of 19 patients with the diagnosis of anxiety. Two to three subjects were randomly selected from the total number of medical-surgical patients with anxiety on a given data collection day. After a subject was selected, the staff nurse caring for the patient explained the study, obtained informed consent and administered the State-anxiety inventory. The two specialists then proceeded to assess the subject for signs of anxiety using opened-ended interview and observation techniques. The two specialists alternated their role in interviewing subjects. Each specialist, however, independently rated the subject for each defining characteristic of anxiety. After the interview was complete, one of the clinical specialists obtained a blood pressure and pulse from the subject by use of an electronic instrument.

The defining characteristic "sympathetic stimulation" was assessed by taking the subject's blood pressure in the right arm while in bed with an electronic sphygnomanometer. At the same time peripheral vasoconstriction was noted. Pupil size was also observed for but dilatation was not detected in any subject. If the subject had one or more of the signs for sympathetic stimulation (i.e., elevated blood pressure, elevated heart rate, superficial vasoconstriction, or pupil dilatation) sympathetic stimulation was checked as a defining characteristic. Elevated blood pressure and heart rate were determined if the readings taken by the specialists were equal to or greater than the highest reading previously recorded on the patient's chart.

RESULTS

Data were analyzed by quantifying and ranking the frequency of observed characteristics from each specialist and by calculating the weighted inter-rater reliability ratio for each defining characteristic. The ranked frequencies of the top nine subjective and objective indicators from the 49 observed subjects are shown in Tables 1 and 2. None of the indicators reached a CDV score of 0.50 or greater.

Table 1: Ranked frequency of subjective indicators (N = 49)

	F1	F2	CDV
Worried	27	23	0.34
(Other) nervous	19	22	0.32
(Other) sleep	18	17	0.27
Concern of change	14	15	0.24
Fearful	15	13	0.22
(Other) death	12	13	0.20
Uncertainty	14	18	0.18
Scared	14	8	0.18
(Other) GI symptoms	7	10	0.14

Table 2: Ranked frequency of objective indicators (N = 49)

	F1	F2	CDV
Extraneous movement	29	28	0.40
Voice quivering	21	19	0.32
(Other) tearful	14	18	0.30
Poor eye contact	10	12	0.20
Restlessness	9	11	0.15
Facial tension	6	10	0.14
(Other) rapid speech	6	7	0.12
Glancing about	4	8	0.10
Trembling	4	6	0.08

For interest, the ranked frequencies of the subjective and objective indicators of anxiety were also categorized according to sex and medical diagnoses (See Tables 3 and 4).

The frequency of indicators noted by the staff nurses who diagnosed the 49 subjects as anxious was also calculated. Twenty percent of the subjects had the indicator of "fearful" noted, 14 percent of them were described as "uncertain," 12 percent were reported to have "extraneous movement," 8 percent were crying and 8 percent reported sleeping difficulties.

A Pearson's correlation coefficient was calculated between State-anxiety scores and the frequency of indicators that were observed. There was a modest significant correlation between state-anxiety and the total indicators (r = 0.34, p ≤ 0.01) and a modest significant relationship between state anxiety and the objective indicators (r = 0.41, p ≤ 0.01). There was no significant relationship between the subjective indicators and the State scores. However, when all 91 subjects were included in the calculations, there was a modest significant relationship between the State-anxiety scores and the total

Table 3: Ranked frequency of objective and subjective indicators by sex

Subjective	
Male	**Female**
1. Sleep disturbance*	1. Worried
2. Nervous*	2. Nervous*
3. Worried	3. Fearful
4. Change in life events	4. Sleep disturbance*
Objective	
1. Extraneous movement	1. Extraneous movement
2. Restlessness	2. Tearful*
3. Voice quivering	3. Voice quivering
4. Poor eye contact	4. Poor eye contact

*Not included on current classification list

Table 4: Ranked frequency of indicators by medical diagnoses

	Subjective	
Cancer	**CV Disease**	**Infection**
Worried	Nervous*	Nervous*
Sleep disturbance*	Change in life events	Worried
Fearful	Worried	Scared
Scared	Sleep disturbance*	Sleep disturbance*
	Objective	
Extraneous movement	Restlessness	Tearful*
Voice quivering	Extraneous movement	Extraneous movement
Tearful*	Glancing about	Voice quivering
Poor eye contact	Voice quivering	Poor eye contact

*Not included on current classification list

indicators (r = 0.51, p ≤ 0.001), a modest significant relationship between anxiety and the subjective indicators (r = 0.40, p ≤ 0.001), and a modest significant correlation between anxiety and the objective indicators (r = 0.47, p ≤ 0.001).

DISCUSSION

Although none of the defining characteristics of anxiety as defined by the participants of the Fifth National Conference on Classification of Nursing Diagnoses reached CDV levels of 0.50, all of the characteristics were observed by the two clinical specialists except "rattled," "pupil dilation," and "hand temperature." The failure of these measures to reach higher CDV levels might be due to methods. If the clinical specialists used a direct approach and asked each subject whether he was experiencing the given characteristic, there probably would have been higher CDV scores. However, the approach would have prompted the response rather than leaving it to the clinician to observe what actually occurred or was said. The reason that "pupil dilation" was not observed was because it was difficult to observe that respose in subjects owing either to darkness in the room, medications, eye changes related to aging, or because there was no obvious pupil response. How much anxiety does a person have to experience before the pupils dilate to an observable level has not been determined. Cassem and Hackett (1977) have stated that a person might have to reach a panic state before physical responses of anxiety could be detected by observation.

The results of the study also stimulated questions about the validity of Spielberger's et al. (1972) State-anxiety inventory. Out of the 91 subjects who were chosen for the study, only 49 reached the average anxiety level of 45 for medical-surgical patients. The reason that this occurred could be because of misdiagnosis by staff nurses. The staff nurses might have been observing fear rather than anxiety as speculated by Jones and Jacob (1984). Perhaps some of the patients were denying that they had anxiety. Cassem and Hackett (1977) found that many patients with heart attacks use denial as a defense mechanism. However, the usefulness of the State anxiety tool for hospitalized patients might be in question. Past studies by several nurses (eg., Juricka, 1984, Bolwerk, 1986) have found it difficult to identify patients with high levels of anxiety using the State inventory in groups of patients that theoretically have high anxiety (eg., MI patients). The evidence that there were low correlations of the State-anxiety scores with the observed frequency of indicators also supports the speculation that the State-anxiety inventory is not a valid tool for clinical use in the hospital setting. However, it might also indicate that the characteristics that nurses observe for anxiety are not characteristics of anxiety or they are not observing anxiety.

It is interesting to note that the frequently observed characteristics of anxiety by the staff nurses were also frequently observed by the two clinical specialists (i.e., fearful, uncertainty, extraneous movement, sleep disorder, and crying). Some of these characteristics and several others frequently observed by the clinical specialists are not on the classification list. The fact that the clinical specialists observed characteristics similar to those noted by the staff nurses suggests that these characteristics are indicators of anxiety to nurses, even though what they were observing might not be anxiety but actually fear. It could also be that the anxiety of psychiatric patients is manifested differently from that of mentally healthy medical-surgical patients. Most of the nurses who developed the characteristics for anxiety came from a psychiatric or mental-health background.

It could be concluded from the results of this study that most of the characteristics of anxiety on the classification list were observed and validated by the clinical specialists. The characteristics did not reach significant CDV levels. Much of the anxiety observed by the staff nurses could have been fear. There are some doubts about the clinical validity of the Spielberger's State-anxiety inventory. There are common characteristics that nurses are observing for anxiety

that are not on the classification list. It might have been better to have used a structured interview approach to elicit responses from the subjects.

The authors of this study recommend replicating it on other types of patients in different areas of the country. In other parts of the country people may have different jargon for expressing anxiety. For example, is the term or characteristic "rattled" a common expression in the Midwest? If this study *is* replicated, researchers might try a more direct approach to interviewing the subjects and might use other anxiety-measurement tools. Finally, the study might be replicated using a content-validity approach in which experts retrospectively rate the indicators of anxiety on how characteristic they are of that diagnosis. Diagnostic Content Validity (DCV) scores could be calculated on each defining characteristic and be interpreted and compared with CDV scores (Fehring, 1986). If this study were replicated using either the CDV or DCV approach, it would be recommended to differentiate the diagnoses and characteristics of anxiety from those of fear.

REFERENCES

Burke, S.: A developmental perspective on the nursing diagnoses of fear and anxiety, Nurs. Papers, **2**:59, 1982.

Cassem, N.H., and Hackette, T.P.: Psychological aspects of myocardial infarction, Med. Clin. North Am. **61**:711, 1977.

Fehring, R.J.: Validating diagnostic labels: standard methodology. In Hurley, M.E., Editor: Classification of nursing diagnoses: proceedings of the sixth conference, St. Louis, 1986, The C.V. Mosby Co.

Gebbie, K.M., editor: Summary of the second national conference: classification of nursing diagnoses, St. Louis, 1976, Clearinghouse for Classification of Nursing Diagnoses.

Gebbie, K.M., and Lavin, M.A., editors: Classification of nursing diagnoses: proceedings of the first national conference, St. Louis, 1976, The C.V. Mosby Co.

Gordon, M.: Nursing diagnosis: process and application, New York, 1982, McGraw-Hill.

Gordon, M., and Sweeney, M.A.: Methodological problems and issues in identifying and standardizing nursing diagnoses, Advances Nurs. Sci. **2**:1, 1979.

Graham, L.E., and Conley, E.M.: Evaluation of anxiety and fear in adult surgical patients, Nurs. Res. **20**:113, 1971.

Jasmin, S., and Trygstad, L.: Behavioral concepts and the nursing process, St. Louis, 1979, The C.V. Mosby Co.

Jiricka, M.J.: The use of relaxation techniques in the acute phase of myocardial infarction, Unpublished manuscript, 1982.

Jones, P.E.: The revision of nursing diagnosis terms in classification of nursing diagnoses. In Kim, M.J., and Moritz, D.A., editors: Classification of nursing diagnoses: proceedings of third and fourth national conferences, New York, 1982, McGraw-Hill.

Jones, P., and Jacob, D.F.: Nursing diagnosis: differentiating fear and anxiety, Nurs. Papers **4**:20, 1981.

Kim, M.J., McFarland, G.K., and McLane, A.M., editors: Classification of nursing diagnoses: proceedings of the fifth national conference, St. Louis, 1984, The C.V. Mosby Co.

Kim, M.J., and Moritz, D.A., editors: Classification of nursing diagnoses: proceedings of the third and fourth national conferences, New York, 1982, McGraw-Hill.

Leuders-Bolwerk, C.A.: The effect of relaxing music on state anxiety in the myocardial infarction patient, Unpublished master's thesis, Milwaukee, WI, 1986, Marquette University.

May, R.: The meaning of anxiety, New York, 1950, Ronald Press Company.

McKeehan, K.M., and Gordon, M.: Utilization of accepted nursing diagnoses. In Kim, M.J., and Moritz, D.A., editors: Classification of nursing diagnoses: proceedings of the third and fourth national conferences, New York, 1982, McGraw-Hill.

Miller, B.F., and Keane, C.B.: Encyclopedia and dictionary of medicine and nursing, Philadelphia, 1972, W.B. Saunders.

Murray, R.B., and Zentner, J.P.: Nursing concepts for health promotion, New Jersey, 1979, Prentice-Hall.

Nightingale, F.: Notes on nursing: what it is, and what it is not, London, 1859, Harrison and Sons.

Peplau, H.: A working definition of anxiety. In Burd, S.F., and Marshall, M.A., editors: Clinical approaches to psychiatric nursing, New York, 1963, Macmillan.

Speilberger, C.D., Gorsuch, R.L., and Lushene, R.E.: STAI Manual, Palo Alto, CA, 1970, Consulting Psychologist Press.

Sundeen, S.J., Stuart, G.W., Rankin, E.D., and others: Nurse-client interaction, St. Louis, 1981, The C.V. Mosby Co.

Self-esteem disturbance: a clinical validation study

JOAN NORRIS, Ph.D., R.N.
MARY KUNES-CONNELL, M.S.N., R.N.

Several authors have addressed the need for validation studies of both newly derived and established nursing diagnoses (Gordon and Sweeney 1979, McLane and Fehring 1984). Kim (1983) has called for additional development of essentialistic concepts in nursing diagnosis (i.e., self-concept, self-image). Meleis (1985) acknowledges the value of nursing diagnosis as consistent with the stages of theory development but has criticized some of the labels currently in use as esoteric or non-representative. The investigators, as psychiatric-mental health nurses, have particular interest in the concept of self-esteem and the related nursing diagnosis of self-esteem disturbance. The concept itself is commonly applied in a variety of nursing settings and is used in both a global sense and also as a measure of response to specific events or an appraisal of specific aspects of the self. The NANDA definition reads, "Self-esteem disturbance-negative feelings or conceptions of self (social self, self-capabilities)." The etiologies currently listed are loss of significant roles and unrealistic self-expectations. Refer to Box 1 for the defining characteristics accepted at the Fifth National Conference (Gordon 1982, Kim, McFarland, and McLane 1984).

PURPOSES

The purposes of this study included:

1. Development of a tentative conceptual framework for self-esteem based on the literature and study findings
2. Contributing to the clinical validity of the label, self-esteem, disturbance through

---

BOX 1:   **Self-esteem disturbance**

PROBLEM
    Self-esteem disturbance: negative feelings or conceptions of self (social self, self-capabilities)
ETIOLOGY
    Loss of significant roles; unrealistic self-expectations
DEFINING CHARACTERISTICS
Lack of eye contact
Head flexion, shoulder flexion
Self-negating verbalizations
Expressions of shame or guilt
Evaluates self as unable to deal with situations or events
*Lack of follow through
*Non-participation in therapy
*Not taking responsibility for self-care

Diagnosis and characteristics as defined in Gordon's (1982) Manual of Nursing Diagnosis and * additional characteristics added to Kim, McFarland, and McLane (Eds.) (1984) Classification of nursing diagnoses: proceedings of the fifth national conference, St. Louis, 1984, The C.V. Mosby Co.

a. Identification of the presence or absence of the defining characteristics in clients identified with this problem
b. Determination of inter-rater reliability ratios in assignment of the defining characteristics
c. Exploring factors described by clients as associated with the etiology of the problem
3. Explore defensive self-esteem as a factor in identifying self-esteem disturbance
4. Formulation of an assessment tool useful in identification of self-esteem disturbance in clinical practice

REVIEW OF THE LITERATURE
Definitions

Self-esteem is based on one's overall appraisal of the self-concept and can be described as the affective, or feeling, component of self-evaluation. A simple definition, provided by Stanwyck, is "how I feel about how I see myself" (1983:11). He describes self-esteem as relatively stable but open to modification by situational events and notes that one tends to behave in ways that are consistent with one's overall self-concept and level of self-esteem (Stanwyck 1983). These definitions are consistent with the NANDA definition of self-esteem disturbance previously cited.

In contrast, self-concept is a broad construct which describes the overall components of self-appraisal such as those proposed by Coopersmith (1967) in his classic work. These include power, significance, competence and virtue. Power is the ability to influence people and events that are considered important to the person. Significance is the sense of being valued and accepted by others, this aspect is also referred to as social self-esteem. Competence is the ability to meet one's personal goals and expectations in various performance dimensions such as the physical, intellectual and social. Virtue

consists of engaging in behavior that is consistent with one's personal moral values and beliefs.

The Bonham-Cheney nursing model for concept of self (Cheney 1984) depicts four dimensions of personal identity and three perspectives on the self. These are: the personal identity dimensions, intellectual, physical, moral and emotional; and the self perspectives, self-image, self-in-action and self-esteem.

In summary, the nursing diagnosis of self-esteem disturbance refers to an affective state (negative feelings) based on negative self-appraisal or conceptions of the self. These negative feelings tend to be somewhat globally experienced but may reflect negative conceptions that arise in perceived defects in power and significance; in the sense of being loved and valued; in physical, intellectual, emotional, and social performance or in discrepancies between one's moral beliefs and behavior.

Defensive self-esteem

A related concept first described by Freud is that of defensive self-esteem. Various mental mechanisms have been described by which persons serve to protect themselves from awareness of information that might be threatening to self-concept and self-esteem. These defense mechanisms can help one to deny negative information, project blame or responsibility onto others, or rationalize away irrational behavior. These self-protective maneuvers ward off feelings of inferiority and shame that would threaten self-esteem. Maslow (1962) cited this description by Freud in discussing his own view of man's need for self-esteem and self-actualization.

Turkat (1978) defined defensive self-esteem as self report of high self-esteem based on denial or avoidance of negative personal information. The purpose of this avoidance is preservation of a positive sense of the self. The severity of this phenomena may vary from the person who must always be considered right in order to "save face" to the restitutional symptoms of the paranoid schizophrenic who develops grandiose or persecutory delusions to defend against painful feelings of anxiety and inadequacy (Mendel 1976). Johnson (1980) also addresses the role of psychological mechanisms such as the self-concept and defense mechanisms in the regulation of behavior in her Behavioral Systems Model of Nursing.

The current diagnosis of self-esteem disturbance does not address the issue of defensive self-esteem as a label or in the related defining characteristics. Turkat (1978) discussed defensive self-esteem as a factor which had the potential to distort research findings and described the phenomena of role faking to present a positive image. This factor may also influence the accuracy of nursing diagnosis in clinical settings when assessing a client's self-esteem.

Significance of self-esteem to nurses

Nurses who care for patients at any stage of the life cycle need to be able to assess and support client self-esteem. High self-esteem in children is believed to promote productivity, leadership and motivation. Parents and others who work with children can enhance self-esteem by promoting security and clear limit setting; providing acceptance, recognition and a sense of belonging and by encouraging realistic goal setting and faith in the child's ability to achieve these goals (Reasoner 1983). Helping relationships with adult clients who are experiencing self-esteem disturbances may require focusing on the perceived gap between expectations and accomplishments. Negative thought patterns may minimize real accomplishments, exaggerate to catastrophic proportions modest deficits or problems, overly generalize weaknesses or assume helplessness or powerlessness (Crouch 1983, Dennison, Prevet, and Affleck 1980, Murphy 1982). Relationships have been shown be-

tween self-esteem level and variables such as physical or mental health and functional impairments (Antonucci and Jackson 1983, Reasoner 1983). Older adults may feel useless or rejected if they are excluded from significant opportunities to solve problems and make decisions. The perception that they are no longer esteemed by others may diminish many elders' own sense of self-worth (Stanwyck 1983). Nurses in all practice settings need to be aware of the reciprocal effects of attitudes, functional status, general health, coping and self-esteem.

TENTATIVE CONCEPTUAL MODEL

Based on review of the literature and consistent with the clinical findings, the authors developed a tentative conceptual model of self-esteem (Fig. 1). This model is global in nature and does not address specific aspects of the self-concept that may be influencing the individual's overall self-appraisal. All components of the self-concept are pertinent

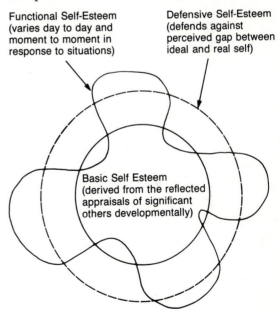

FIGURE 1 Conceptual model of the components of self-esteem.

Reprinted from Norris, J., and Kunes-Connell, M. Self-Esteem Disturbance. In C. Dougherty (Ed), *Nursing Clinics of North America*, 20(4), December, 1985, p. 748.

and they can be assessed through the use of broad questions to elicit the person's view of strengths and weaknesses, discrepancies between ideal and real self in any aspects of personal performance, and overall self-appraisal of one's coping ability. The components of the model include:

1. Basic self-esteem: a central core or relatively stable sense of self-esteem which is formed through developmental experiences and the reflected appraisals of significant others such as parents, teachers, and peers.

2. Functional self-esteem: modifications in level of self-esteem which vary somewhat above and below basic self-esteem because of day-to-day experiences or events (including rewards or reprimands, achievements or failures, gains or losses in social or functional performance).

3. Defensive self-esteem: a protective mechanism which attempts to shield the self from perceived gaps between the idealized self and real accomplishments if these gaps would pose a significant threat. It is speculated that there may be identifiable relationships between the strength of the protective defense, the intensity and nature of the threat and the relative strength of the person's basic core of self-esteem. Both Maslow (1962) and Jahoda (1959) associate higher levels of mental health and mature functioning with the ability to acknowledge one's shortcomings non-defensively.

METHODOLOGY

Fehring's (1986) clinical validation methodology was selected to provide evidence that a diagnosis occurs in clinical practice, determine the frequencies with which the defining characteristics occur in a population of diagnosed patients, and determine inter-rater reliability ratios between two clinical specialists in psychiatric-men-

tal health nursing when they identify these characteristics in patients. The weighted inter-rater reliability ratios result in an index of clinical diagnostic validity (CDV) that can be useful in differentiating indicators that occur frequently in relation to the specific diagnosis from those that occur only occasionally (see Box 2). Fehring has suggested that once adequate sample size and geographic representation are achieved in validation studies, it may be possible to drop or revise indicators with a CDV below 0.5 and to identify those with a CDV above 0.75 as key or critical indicators.

An assessment tool was developed for self-esteem disturbance based on the NANDA diagnosis characteristics and added attributes to defensive- or pseudo-self-esteem. Categories for assessment included self-description, self-report of strengths and weaknesses, self-rating of level of self-esteem, identification of influencing or etiological factors associated with self-report of low self-esteem, and observational and

---

BOX 2: Steps in developing the clinical diagnostic validity index

1. Clinicians record actual subject findings (frequencies) in relation to the defining characteristics listed.
2. Weighted inter-rater reliability ratios are calculated for each defining characteristic according to the following formula:

$$R = \frac{A}{A + D} \times \frac{\frac{F_1}{N} + \frac{F_2}{N}}{2}$$

R = **Weighted inter-rater reliability ratio**
A = **Agreements**
D = **Disagreements**
F$_1$ = **Frequency of characteristic observed by rater 1**
F$_2$ = **Frequency of characteristic observed by rater 2**
N = **Number of subjects observed**

Fehring, R.: Validating diagnostic labels: standardized methodology. In Hurley, M.E., Editor: Classification of nursing diagnoses: procedings of the sixth conference, St. Louis, 1986, The C.V. Mosby Co.

subjective data related to the NANDA indicators. An additional standardized tool was administered to obtain a self-report rating of social self-esteem. This pencil-and-paper tool was developed by Lawson, Marshall, and McGrath (1974) following literature review and critique of the available tools for measuring self-esteem. The Social Self-Esteem Inventory (SSEI) measures sense of self-worth in social situations and has a high level of reliability (r = .88) and validity. It has been used on various age groups and a normative mean of 132 was established on college-age students.

All participants in the study completed the SSEI and were observed and interviewed on separate occasions by the two nurse-investigators. Assessment tool data were recorded for future comparison.

The sample population

Four groups of patients were purposefully selected because of the likelihood that self-esteem disturbance was present. Hospitalized psychiatric patients (N=10) and chronically ill patients who were receiving home health care in the community (N=9) were prescreened by nurses. Those identified as having low self-esteem and who agreed to participate in the study were included. Residents in a domestic abuse shelter (N=6), an adolescent chemical dependency treatment center (N=11) and adult patients in chemical dependency treatment (inpatients and outpatients, N=20) who agreed to participate were also included in the study. Counselors stated that all abused and chemically dependent patients suffer from low self-esteem. Patient self-reports and the literature substantiate this (Walker 1979, Dennison et al. 1980). Fifty-six subjects agreed to participate and signed informed consent forms. Two home health care subjects were excluded by the investigators following the interviews as having only the potential for self-esteem disturbance. Males and females were equally represented in the sample. Ages ranged from 16 to 83.

RESULTS
Defining characteristics

Table 1 identifies the clinical diagnostic validity index for each defining characteristic and notes the percentage of the study population on which both investigators agreed the characteristic was present. The raters found the relatively subjective ratings of eye contact (no subjects *lacked* eye contact totally, lack was interpreted as "less than the cultural norm") and postural flexion the most difficult to rate.

Etiological influences

Subjects were asked to identify specific times and factors in their lives that contributed to feeling particularly good or bad about themselves. These responses can be categorized as follows. Half of the respondents (N=27) were unable to identify any time in their lives when they felt good about themselves. Five of the 6 abused women described consistently low self-esteem prior to the current abusive relationship. They attributed their low self-esteem to childhood abuse and/or hypercritical, unloving (emotional abuse) parental relationships. Seventeen of the 31 chemically dependent clients and three of the psychiatric patients expressed consistently low self-esteem and described similar abusive experiences in childhood. Two additional adult patients, reporting consistently low self-esteem, attributed it to lifelong experiences with prejudice (being black, being physically handicapped).

Subjects (N=12 or 22%) who described temporary disturbances in self-esteem related current experience of low self-esteem to losses. These included:

1. Not only role loss but loss of significant objects and symbolic losses such as loss of status or beliefs
2. Changes in self-concept or body image,

Table 1: Frequency of occurrence and clinical diagnostic validity (CDV) indexes for defining characteristics of self-esteem disturbance

Defining characteristics	% of all clients perceived by both investigators to manifest the characteristic	Clinical diagnostic validity CDV index
Lack of eye contact	54.5	.5
Head or shoulder flexion	12.7	.18
Self-negating verbalizations	60	.61
Expresses shame or guilt	41.8	.43
Evaluates self as unable to deal with situations	60	.58
Lack of follow-through	23.3	.26
Non-participation in therapy	1.8	.02
Self-neglect	23.6	.23
*Unrealistic verbalizations about self	16	.18

*Denial of externally validated problem/grandiosity

including dramatic changes in weight, appearance or physical capacities

3. Behavior inconsistent with held values (i.e., guilt or shame over violent behavior or thefts to maintain substance abuse supply).

A third category (N = 17 or 31%) identified themselves as having practiced massive denial of problems that were readily obvious to others or of attributing all responsibility for problems in their lives to others. One subject related being fired six times in five years but maintaining that he was always a highly valued employee who was a victim of "bad breaks." Some described long term denial of substance abuse problems leading to home and occupational problems which permitted them to maintain that "I'm OK, the rest of the world is all messed up." Others exhibited grandiosity.

Social self-esteem scores

The groups that appeared to differ by etiology were assigned to the categories derived from the model. Basic low self-esteem as a cate-gory included those subjects who were unable to describe ever feeling positive about themselves. The mean SSEI score for this group was 102. The group who described temporary low self-esteem was categorized as functional level low self-esteem. The mean SSEI score for this group was 127. The group characterized as defensive had a mean SSEI score of 123. These scores are not based on representative sampling and are merely presented for description. They do suggest variance in severity as well as duration in the group categorized as basic low self-esteem. These group means were all lower than the mean of 132 reported as the normative group score (Lawson et al. 1974).

Discussion

Based on the study, the investigators propose two or three clinical problems at a lower level of abstraction for further validation and research. The problem of low self-esteem may be categorized as two distinct basic and functional problems or as one problem on which individuals may vary in both intensity and

Table 2: Abstract of panel of experts content validation study for proposed redefinition

Clinical specialists and educators (N=300) in Psychiatric-Mental Health Nursing were surveyed nationally to provide content validity ratings of defining characteristics and to generate new indicators in a two stage process. 30% of those surveyed responded in each group resulting in usable responses from 43 educators and 46 clinical specialists. Fehring's Diagnostic Content Validity (DCV) Index was established from subjects (N=89) Lickert Scale ratings of the content validity of each indicator. DCV scores for the problems of low self-esteem (basic and functional levels) and defensive self-esteem follow below.

SELF-ESTEEM		
Low (basic)	**Low (functional)**	**Defensive**
Lack of eye contact .735	Verbalizes feelings of helplessness/uselessness .70	Denial .866
Self negating verbalization .855		Projection .88
Express shame or guilt .82		Rationalizes failures .836
Self-evaluates as unable to deal with events .855		Hypersensitive to slight or criticism .858
Rationalizes away positive, exaggerates negative feedback re: self .806		Grandiosity .795
		Superior attitude to others .76
Overly conforming or dependent on others opinions .78		Difficulty establishing and maintaining relationships .744
Hesitant to try new situations .795		
Indecisive .727		
Non-assertive/passive .769		
Seeks excessive reassurance .738		
Frequent lack of success in work, life events .718	Self-negating verbalizations .55	Hostile laugh/ridicule others .707
Head or shoulder flexion .61	Expressions of shame or guilt .56	Difficulty in reality perceptions .625
Lack of follow through .627	Self-evaluates as unable to deal with situations .63	Lack of follow through or non-participation in therapy .56
Self-neglect .67	Indecisive .565	
Self-destructive .58		

duration. The indicators of poor eye contact, self-negating verbalization, expressing shame or guilt and evaluating the self as unable to cope with situations or events appear to currently represent the most valid indicators of both problems. Further studies would be helpful in identifying and validating additional indicators. Additional work would be needed to develop the suggested alternative problem of defensive self-esteem. This seems to represent a category of behavior which is indicative of underlying self-esteem disturbance but may have manifestly different defining characteristics. It also seems likely that effective nursing approaches might vary between the problems of validated low self-esteem and that of defensive self-esteem. Table 2 presents an abstract of a panel of experts approach to generating and providing content validation for defining characteristics of these proposed new labels (Kunes-Connell, Norris 1985).

Implications for research

Further validation and correlational research needs to be done on the proposed categories to identify whether these do in fact constitute different problems with distinct major defining characteristics. Additional studies would be useful to explore possible correlations between etiological factors such as (1) abuse/neglect and basic low self-esteem consistent with Murphy's (1982) concept of learned helplessness or the related concept label of powerlessness and (2) recent losses or changes and functional low self-esteem. The new defining characteristics proposed and validated by the panel of content experts need to be validated in clinical studies. Once validation is accomplished, it will be possible to design research studies to accomplish higher levels of theory building for prescribing effective nursing interventions and predicting outcomes.

REFERENCES

Antonucci, T., and Jackson, J.: Physical health and self-esteem, Fam. Commun. Health **6:**1, 1983.

Cheney, A.: Critical indicators for the nursing diagnosis of disturbance in self-concept. In Kim, M.J., McFarland, G.K., and McLane, A.M., editors: Classification of nursing diagnoses: proceedings of the fifth national conference, St. Louis, 1984, The C.V. Mosby Co.

Coopersmith, S.: Antecedents of self-esteem, San Francisco, 1967, Freeman.

Crouch, M.A.: Future needs for self-esteem research and services, Fam. Commun. Health **6:**79, 1983.

Crouch, M.A., and Straub, V.: Enhancement of self-esteem in adults, Fam. Commun. Health **6:**65, 1983.

Dennison, D., Prevet, T., and Affleck, M.: Alcohol and behavior, St. Louis, 1980, The C.V. Mosby Co.

Fehring, R.: Validating diagnostic labels: standardized methodology. In Hurley, M.E., editor: Classification of nursing diagnoses: proceedings of the sixth conference, St. Louis, 1986, The C.V. Mosby Co.

Gordon, M.: Manual of nursing diagnoses, New York, 1984, McGraw-Hill.

Gordon, M., and Sweeney, M.: Methodological problems and issues in identifying and standardizing nursing diagnoses, Advances Nurs. Sci. **2:**1, 1979.

Jahoda, M.: Current concepts of positive mental health, New York, 1959, Basic Books.

Johnson, D.E.: The behavioral system model for nursing. In Riehl, J.P., and Roy, C., editors: Conceptual models for nursing practice, ed. 2, New York, 1980, Appleton-Century-Crofts.

Kim, H.S.: The nature of theoretical thinking in nursing, Norwalk, CT, 1983, Appleton-Century-Crofts.

Kim, M.J., McFarland, G.K., and McLane, A.M.: Classification of nursing diagnoses: proceedings of the fifth national conference, St. Louis, 1984, The C.V. Mosby Co.

Kunes-Connell, M., and Norris, J.: A panel of experts' content validation study of problems associated with self-esteem disturbance. (Unpublished manuscript.)

Lawson, J.S., Marshall, W.L., and McGrath, P.: The social self-esteem inventory, Ed. Psych. Measurement **39:**803, 1974.

Maslow, A.: Motivation and personality, New York, 1962, Harper and Row.

McLane, A.M., and Fehring, R.J.: Nursing diagnosis: a review of the literature. In Kim, M.J., McFarland, G.K., and McLane, A.M., editors: Classification of nursing diagnoses: proceedings of the fifth national conference, St. Louis, 1984, The C.V. Mosby Co.

Meleis, A.: Theoretical nursing: Development and progress, Philadelphia, 1985, J.B. Lippincott.

Mendel, W.M.: Schizophrenia: the experience and its treatment, San Francisco, 1976, Jossey-Bass.

Murphy, S.: Learned helplessness: from concept to comprehension, Perspect. Psychiat. Care **20:**27, 1982.

Reasoner, R.: Enhancement of self-esteem in children and adults, Fam. Commun. Health **6:**51, 1983.

Stansyck, D.: Self-esteem through the lifespan, Fam. Commun. Health **6:**11, 1983.

Turkat, D.: Defensiveness in self-esteem research, Psychol. Record **28:**129, 1978.

Walker, L.E.: Battered Women, New York, 1979, Harper and Row.

Impaired skin integrity

CAROL J. CATTANEO, M.N., R.N., E.T.
NANCY R. LACKEY, Ph.D., R.N.

PROBLEM

Nurses are working diligently to maintain the skin integrity of their patients to insure the body's first line of natural defense. Nevertheless, many patients experience impaired skin integrity in response to the environment, an underlying disease process, or other factors. It is very clearly a nursing function to recognize and document actual or potential impairment of skin integrity. Yet, does the approved nursing diagnosis of *impaired skin integrity* clearly define this response? And if so, how was this nursing diagnosis validated? Just how much can nurses rely on such established nursing diagnoses in clinical practice? Actually, nursing diagnoses are meaningless until their validity and clinical relevance are documented and supported by empirical studies.

PURPOSE

The purpose of this study was to operationally define the nursing diagnosis *impaired skin integrity*. Operationalizing the nursing diagnosis of impaired skin integrity offers defining criteria which can be supported by empirical data as a beginning validation process upon which nurses can base their assessment and care. The aim of this study was to expand the scientific base for nursing practice and also to provide a basis for future studies applicable to nursing practice.

THE RESEARCH QUESTION

Explicitly stated, the research question was, "What are the defining characteristics of the nursing diagnosis, *impaired skin integrity*, as perceived by randomly selected enterostomal therapy nurses throughout the United States?"

DEFINITION OF TERMS

Skin. The external covering of an animal body, integument, cutis (Random House 1967). More specifically, this study focussed on the skin as the external covering of the body.

Integrity. Soundness, completeness, unimpaired condition, perfect condition (Steadman 1982).

Impaired. Damaged or made worse by or diminished in some material respect (Webster 1984).

ASSUMPTION

Nurses are interested in caring for the skin of patients.

LIMITATION

The limitation of this study was that the focus was on the organ, skin, not on the whole integumentary system (hair, nails, glands, mucosa).

REVIEW OF LITERATURE

Discussions relative to impaired skin integrity have appeared regularly throughout the nursing literature and commonly in reference to the prevention, assessment, and management of decubitus ulcers, pressure sores, skin breakdown, and the like. In 1975, Berecek, via literature review, explored the problem of decubitus ulceration along with theories of etiology and pathophysiology. She attempted to determine contributing and predisposing conditions to the formation of decubitus ulcers to construe implications for the health care team. Berecek concluded that there was a crucial need for assessment tools to identify those patients susceptible to decubitus ulcer formation.

In an empirical study, Norton, McLaren, and Exton-Smith (1962) investigated factors concerned with the production of pressure sores and their prevention. Three separate investigations were carried out. In the first study of 250 patients in which an assessment tool was utilized, the development of pressure sores was associated with poor condition of the patient, old age, incontinence, and certain neurological disorders. In the second investigation of 218 patients, it was disclosed that local applications could not be relied on to prevent pressure sores. Finally, in their third investigation, it was noted after observing 100 patients that frequent turning of patients showed striking reductions in the number of pressure sores. For brevity, additional studies reviewed relating to pressure sores will not be discussed here.

In addition to studies concerning pressure sores, other studies concerning wound healing and factors that promote wound healing have been reported (Pollack 1982). In the second of a series of articles, Pollack (1982) addressed the roles of humidity, temperature, infection, and oxygen tension on wound healing. Finally, Pollack in his third report, expounded that wound healing proceeded more efficiently and quickly in well-nourished individuals who were in good general health . . . and individuals who were malnourished and chronically ill healed less well.

Impaired skin integrity was discussed and accepted as a nursing diagnosis by the National Conference on the Classification of Nursing Diagnoses in 1975, 1976, 1978, 1980, and 1984 (Gebbie and Lavin 1975, Gebbie 1976, Kim and Moritz 1982, Kim, McFarland, and McLane 1984). The categorizing and terminology changed somewhat in the first two conferences, but the third, fourth, and fifth conferences listed defining characteristics of impaired skin integrity as: disruption of skin surface, destruction of skin layers, and invasion of body structures. Gordon (1982) and Carpenito (1984) have expressed their interpretations of the nursing diagnosis in separate publications. It does not appear, however, that any empirical studies were used to validate the suggested defining criteria of the nursing diagnosis, impaired skin integrity.

METHODOLOGY AND FINDINGS
Phase I

Sample and setting. Six randomly selected enterostomal therapy (ET) nurses were chosen from each of 11 regions throughout the United States as outlined in the 1984–1985 Membership Directory of the International Association for Enterostomal Therapy (IAET), thereby attaining a sample size of 66. Criteria met by the enterostomal therapy nurses included: (1) graduation from an accredited IAET educational program, (2) current licensure as a registered nurse (RN), and (3) involvement in practice as an RN for at least 2 years.

Enterostomal therapy nurses were utilized as subjects in this study because of their intense clinical experience in caring for patients' skin in a variety of conditions: ostomy management, incontinence, pressure sore prevention and treatment, difficult ulcer or draining wound management, and a number of other situations resulting in actual or potential impairment of skin integrity.

Instrument. An adaptation of Kuhn's (1954) "Twenty-Statements Problem (Who Am I)" primarily developed by Hartley (1970) as the Objects Content Test (OCT), was the instrument used in this study. In adapting the OCT instrument to this study, respondents read the statement, "When I see the nursing diagnosis, *impaired skin integrity*, to me it means. . . ." The instrument was a single page, pencil-and-paper test that allowed for up to 20 responses. Simple instructions included: (1) answering as if you were giving the answer to yourself, not someone else, (2) writing your answers in the order they occur to you, (3) not worrying about logic or complete sentences or importance, and (4) going along fairly fast. Hartley (1970) recommended an allowance of not more than 30 minutes for a respondent to answer the questionnaire.

According to Jauernig (1984) reliability of the Twenty-Statements Problem and OCT could be based on results of numerous researchers who previously had used the instrument. Reliability has been established for both instruments. Multiple studies recording the test-retest reliability coefficients ranging from 0.38 to 0.85 have been reported by Spitzer, Couch, and Stratton (1970) over a time span from 1953 to 1967.

Phase II

Data analysis of the OTC questionnaire. Forty-two of 66 subjects (64%) responded with 665 different terms or phrases to the OCT questionnaire. Content analysis, a method for analyzing written, verbal, or visual materials in a systematic and objective fashion, was the procedure used in this phase (Polit and Hungler 1983).

A number of categories seemed to emerge: conceptual definitions, antecedents, defining criteria of skin integrity, outcome criteria or consequences, assessment factors, nursing interventions for impaired skin integrity (see Box 1), and a final category for words or phrases that had no apparent themes or relationships to other categories. For purposes of this discussion, attention is focussed only on the defining criteria of *impaired skin integrity*.

A panel of five nurse experts was chosen to establish reliability of the defining criteria. These experts were selected on the basis of their clinical expertise in skin care

BOX 1: Response to OCT: raw data from ET nurse respondents' 87 responses (from original 665) describing impaired skin integrity

Allergy
Alterations in
Bedsore
Blemishes
Blistered
Blood-filled vesicles
Broken skin can be very painful
Changes in color
Compromised
Color as compared to the rest of the body
Composition of skin
Consistency of skin
Denuded skin
Drainage
Dependent on the external environment
Depth of an open area
Dry
Dryness of the skin
Does it tear easily
Excoriation
Elasticity
Enterocutaneous fistula
Emaciated
Flaky
Fragile/looks like tissue paper
Fungal infection
Folds
Free of blisters
How does it feel to the touch
How long has problem existed
Hydration
Impaired skin integrity
Is it shiny
Is there burning experienced
Inflammatory process present
Is there stripping of the stratum corneum
Lesions
Layers of skin
Lack of sensation
Macerated
Macules
Mechanical exposure
Necrotic

Continued

BOX 1: Response to OCT—cont'd

Non-blanching
Normal flora involved
No burning sensation
Non-pruritic
No eschar
Non-contracting granulation tissue
Non-oily
Non-pink
Odor
Other existing medical conditions
Presence of an open area
Pressure sore
Poor
Peristomal skin eroded
Pink color
Presence or absence of hair follicle
Rash
Raw
Reddened
Recognize various skin diseases
Requires moisture
Sheared
Skin color
Signs/symptoms of infection
Skin characteristics
Skin status
Size of lesion
Staging of pressure sores
Surgical wound dehiscence
Size of area of problem
Scarring
Skin loose
Skin taut
Temperature
Texture
Tone
Type of contact (sharp, rough)
Ulceration/erosion
Visible impairment
Weeping
Wetness of skin
Warm to touch
Wrinkles

and their knowledge of content analysis. The nurse experts were utilized to help validate the presence or absence of responses in the category of impaired skin integrity according to a suggested definition. Using an equivalence approach, reliability was computed as a function of agreements among the nurse expert raters using the following equation:

$$\frac{\text{Number of Agreements}}{\text{Number of Agreements + Disagreements}}$$

(Polit and Hungler 1983, p. 392).

Phase III

Development of the second (final) questionnaire. From the results of the inter-rater reliability process, a final questionnaire was formulated that consisted of 31 terms or phrases (Box 2). It was believed that the response to this final questionnaire would validate further those characteristics that most closely defined the nursing diagnosis, impaired skin integrity.

Data analysis of the second (final) questionnaire. Of the 42 subjects who initially responded, 25 (60%) returned their completed questionnaires. As in Phase II, reliability which supported the presence or absence of a response in the category was computed as a function of agreement, this time agreement among the ET nurse respondents (Box 3). When 15 of 25 respondents agreed, the term or phrase became a part of defining criteria.

According to Polit and Hungler (1983), reliability coefficients computed in this manner can be used as an important indicator of the quality of an instrument. There is, however, no standard for what a reliability coefficient should be. Because this researcher was interested in comparing the agreement among the ET nurses, coefficients in the vicinity of 0.70 or even 0.60 were considered sufficient (Polit and Hungler 1983).

BOX 2:   **Content of the second (final) questionnaire**

Terms/Phrases

___ Inflammatory process present

___ Surgical wound dehiscence

___ Changes in color

___ Raw

___ Presence of an open area

___ Depth of open area

___ Lesions

___ Blood-filled vesicle

___ Macules

___ Pressure sore

___ Necrotic

___ Visible impairment

___ Bedsore

___ Odor

___ Skin color

___ Denuded skin

___ Flaky

___ Blemishes

___ Macerated

___ Excoriation

___ Texture

___ Sheared

___ Fungal infection

___ Drainage

___ Non-blanching

___ Ulceration/erosion

___ Size of lesion

___ Rash

___ Weeping

___ Reddened

___ Blistered

BOX 3:   **Operational definition of impaired skin integrity**

Terms/Phrases

✔ 17 Inflammatory process present

✔ 18 Surgical wound dehiscence

✔ 17 Changes in color

✔ 19 Raw

✔ 23 Presence of an open area

✔ 21 Depth of open area

✔ 18 Lesions

✔ 17 Blood-filled vesicle

✔ 18 Macules

✔ 20 Pressure sore

✔ 20 Necrotic

   13 Visible impairment

✔ 18 Bedsore

✔ 19 Odor

✔ 19 Skin color

✔ 21 Denuded skin

✔ 15 Flaky

   8 Blemishes

✔ 21 Macerated

✔ 22 Excoriation

   10 Texture

✔ 22 Sheared

✔ 18 Fungal infection

✔ 19 Drainage

✔ 14 Non-blanching

✔ 20 Ulceration/erosion

✔ 19 Size of lesion

✔ 20 Rash

✔ 22 Weeping

✔ 21 Reddened

✔ 22 Blistered

✔Agreement with Raters: 28/31 = 90%

DISCUSSION

There was a high percentage (90%) of agreement between the nurse experts and the ET respondents on the terms and phrases defining *impaired skin integrity*. An operational definition of the nursing diagnosis, impaired skin integrity, was suggested as a result (Box 3). Thereby, a beginning validation of this nursing diagnosis was under way.

RECOMMENDATIONS FOR FUTURE STUDY

Recommendations for future study are as follows:

1. Further validation should be obtained in determining that the selected defining criteria are representative of the nursing diagnosis, impaired skin integrity. Further, the terms and phrases characterized within the category need to be defined operationally for this definition to be useful in the practice of nursing.
2. Replication of this study should be done using staff nurses from across the United States to survey their thoughts on what skin integrity is and, thus, comparing results with those from the ET nurses.

IMPLICATIONS FOR NURSING

The entire human organism is vulnerable once something goes wrong with the skin. If skin integrity is maintained, contribution is made to the individual in appearance, self-esteem, and maintenance of bodily functions. Caring for patients' skin is very definitely the nurse's domain. Especially with hospitalized patients, there are many occasions for nurses to promote and maintain skin integrity.

Operationally defining skin integrity establishes criteria by which nurses can actually measure this phenomenon, thus enabling them to make decisions based on empirical data. Nurses have a basis upon which they can institute care and evaluate and justify their nursing actions. Furthermore, defining impaired skin integrity in operational terms provided a basis for future studies applicable to nursing practice.

Conceptually organizing the concept, impaired skin integrity, in a broader sense, through the development of the refined proposed conceptual model, provides flexibility and generalization of nursing knowledge. It can be used systematically in the nursing process, thereby enhancing accuracy. According to Hart, Reese, and Fearing (1981),

A conceptual organization of the body of nursing knowledge systematizes the phenomena for which nurses have primary responsibility . . . such an organization of knowledge conveniently articulates with the scientific problem-solving nursing process, and the systematic use of this type of categorization will facilitate the delineation of the foci of nursing care and suggest a logical scientific rationale for intervention approaches (p. 3).

Development of the conceptual model is a way of moving toward the development of a theoretical base for nursing practice. Upon examination and analysis of the concept, impaired skin integrity, related terms/phrases emerged, thus formulating and validating a conceptual model the first stage of theory development!

REFERENCES

Berecek, K.H.: Etiology of decubitus ulcers, Nurs. Clin. North Amer. **10:**157, 1975.

Carpenito, L.J.: Impairment of skin integrity, Handbook of nursing diagnoses, Philadelphia, 1984, J.B. Lippincott.

Gebbie, K.M., editor: Summary of the second national conference: classification of nursing diagnoses, St. Louis, 1976, Clearinghouse: National Group for Classification of Nursing Diagnoses.

Gebbie, K.M., and Lavin, M.A., editors: Skin integrity, impairment of. In Classification of nursing diagnoses: proceedings of the first national conference, St. Louis, 1975, C.V. Mosby Co.

Gordon, M.: Manual of nursing diagnoses, New York, 1982, McGraw-Hill.

Hart, L.K., Reese, J.L., and Fearing, M.D., editors: Concepts common to acute illness, St. Louis, 1981, C.V. Mosby Co.

Hartley, W.S.: Manual for the twenty-statements problem (who am I), Kansas City, KS, 1970, Dept. of Human Ecology and Community Health, University of Kansas Medical Center.

Jauernig, P.R.: Jauernig's framework for the concept force fluids. (Unpublished master's thesis.)

Kim, M.J., and Moritz, editors: Skin integrity, impairment of: actual/potential. In Classification of nursing diagnoses: proceedings of the third and fourth national conferences, New York, 1984, McGraw-Hill.

Kim, M.J., McFarland, G.K., and McLane, A.M., editors: Skin integrity, impairment of: actual/potential. In Classification of nursing diagnoses: proceedings of the fifth national conference, St. Louis, 1984, The C.V. Mosby Co.

Norton, D., McLaren, R., and Exton-Smith, A.N.: Pressure sores. An investigation of geriatric nursing problems in hospitals, London, 1962, The National Corporation for the Care of Old People.

Polit, D. and Hungler, B.: Nursing research principles and methods, ed. 2, Philadelphia, 1983, J.B. Lippincott.

Pollack, S.V.: Wound healing: a review—the biology of wound healing, J. Enterostom. Ther. **8:**16, 1981.

Pollack, S.V.: Wound healing: a review—environmental factors affecting wound healing, J. Enterostom. Ther. **9:**14, 1981.

Pollack, S.V.: Wound healing: a review—nutritional factors affecting wound healing. J. Enterostom. Ther. **9:**28, 1982.

The Random house dictionary of the English language, New York, 1967, Random House.

Spitzer, S., Couch, C. and Stratton, J.: The assessment of self, Iowa City, IA, 1970, Sernol, Inc.

Steadman's illustrated medical dictionary, ed. 24, New York, 1982, Williams and Wilkins.

Webster's 9th new collegiate dictionary, Springfield, MA, 1984, G. & C. Merriam Co.

Identifying patients with the potential for falling

JANICE K. JANKEN, Ph.D., R.N.
BETTY ANN REYNOLDS, M.S., R.N.

The nursing diagnosis *potential for injury,* and more specifically its subcomponent *potential for trauma* addresses nurses' accountability for identifying patients at risk for falls. Admittedly, this nursing diagnosis was designed to be more encompassing than just patient falls. However, it is readily apparent that many of its defining characteristics are patient attributes typically named in the fall literature as being risk factors: confusion, sensory deficits, impaired mobility, weakness, history of falls, struggling in bed restraints, balancing difficulties, alcohol abuse, and taking medications that interfere with psychomotor functioning. In practice, nurses assume that patients with these characteristics are those with the potential for falling. Yet, do these characteristics serve to differentiate between patients likely to fall from those who are not?

Overall, the research base to support that these characteristics are indeed fall risk factors has been weak. A serious limitation affecting the majority of studies aimed toward identifying risk factors has been the use of a one-group design, with investigators who conduct incident-report reviews or retrospective chart audits looking solely at patients who fell (e.g., Coyle 1979, Duran 1979, Innes and Turman 1983, Kostopoulos 1985, Kulikowski 1979, Lee and Pash 1983, Swartzbeck and Milligan 1982, Walshe and Rosen 1979). The lack of a comparison group of patients who did not fall has rendered it impossible to determine from these studies whether the characteristics observed in the patients who fell were merely characteristics of the hospital population-at-large or characteristics relatively unique to those who fell.

Also, without a comparison group it has been impossible to estimate the extent to which the so-called risk factors actually serve to differentiate between patients who fall and those who don't. Thus, despite the common assumption that fall-prone patients can be identified, there is a dearth of research to support this premise. In turn, this raises question about the utility of the diagnosis *potential for injury,* at least as it pertains to patient falls.

This study was developed to identify patient characteristics associated with falls in the acute care setting and to examine the extent to which the characteristics explained whether or not falls occurred. More specifically, the study examined the extent to which the defining characteristics of potential for injury served to distinguish between patients who did and did not fall during hospitalization and explored whether defining characteristics of other nursing diagnoses might better aid in identifying fall-prone patients. The five questions addressed in the study were:

1. Which patient characteristics extant upon admission to the hospital are significantly related to falling?
2. Which patient characteristics extant on the day of fall are significantly related to falling?
3. To what extent do the significant admission-day characteristics explain fall status?
4. To what extent do the significant fall-day characteristics explain fall status?
5. To what extent do the defining characteristics of *potential for injury* explain fall status?

136

METHOD

Design: The study design was a retrospective comparative chart audit.

Sample: The data came from the charts of 631 patients aged 60 and older, 331 of whom fell during their hospital stay. Since it is well documented that being elderly is a risk factor, only the charts of patients aged 60 and older were used in an effort to control for age and determine which qualities of the elderly predispose them to falls. The charts were from one hospital, a 719-bed tertiary care medical center. Incident reports were used to identify the patients who fell. The charts of all patients aged 60 and older who fell between the dates of 7/1/82 and 3/31/84 made up the fall-group sample. A simple random sample was drawn from the charts of patients aged 60 and older who were hospitalized during the same time period but did not fall.

In each chart, two days of documentation on patient characteristics were sampled. Since it is desirable to make an early assessment of which patients are predisposed to falls, data recorded during the first 24 hours of hospitalization were collected from the charts of both the fall and no-fall groups. Given that patient status is not constant throughout hospital stay, for the fall group, data recorded on the chart for the 24 hours preceding the fall were collected. For purposes of comparison, one day of hospital stay was randomly selected for audit in each chart of the no-fall group.

Instrumentation: A coding manual for interpreting chart data was developed for use in this project. The selection of independent variables was based on the Nursing Diagnosis framework. Although it was recognized that the work of the National Conference Group for Classification of Nursing Diagnosis is by no means complete, for the purposes of the study it was assumed that the defining characteristics for all accepted nursing diagnoses cited in Kim and Moritz (1982) represent the universe of signs and symptoms that nurses look for in working with patients.

Beginning with entire list of defining characteristics for all accepted nursing diagnoses, those that were non-patient characteristics (i.e., family and environmental factors) were deleted. Then, fifty charts not in the sample were examined to determine the remaining defining characteristics: (1) the types of chart documentation that were indicative of their presence, (2) those that were not mutually exclusive and needed to be combined in one category, and (3) those that either were not reliably documented or occured so infrequently that they could not be included in the study. This process resulted in 24 dicotomous independent variables. With the exception of fall history which was assessed only on admission, data were sought on these patient characteristic variables from each of the sampled two days of chart documentation.

In addition, data were collected on what will herein be referred to as *sample characteristics*. The sample characteristic variables were: age, sex, service (medical, general surgical, or surgical specialty), living arrangement (home alone, home with someone, or nursing home), employment status, room type (private or nonprivate), and nursing unit. The last variable was later recoded to *building* when results showed that all nine units in one building of the hospital consistently had a greater proportion of patients in the fall group and the reverse was true on 10 of the 13 units in the other building. For the fall group only, data were collected on the time and site of the fall.

A coding manual was written with explicit descriptions of the chart documentation needed to infer a variable's presence. Three registered nurses served as coders. Intercoder reliability assessed on the initial 75 charts coded was 88.1%. Intercoder reliability assessed on a 5% random sample of charts throughout the coding period was 90.3%. Assessment of the intercoder discrepancies revealed that the variable categories were clear but that coders had overlooked applicable chart documentation.

Data analyses: To answer the first two questions posed in this study, chi-square analyses were used. Since the large sample size increased the likelihood of attaining statistical significance on relatively small differences, the alpha level was set at .01.

Stepwise multiple regression analyses were computed to answer the remaining three study questions. The regression analyses were terminated when the increase in R^2 attributed to a variable ceased to be significant at the $p \leq .05$ level.

RESULTS

Chi-square analyses revealed significant associations between fall status and 10 of the 24 patient characteristic variables examined on admission and 11 of the 23 patient characteristic variables examined on the fall/random day. Table 1 shows the percent of patients demonstrating the statistically significant characteristics by fall status on both data collection days.

As can be seen, seven variables were significantly related to fall status on both admission and the fall/random day: general weakness, decreased mobility of the lower extremities, sleeplessness, incontinence, confusion, depression, and alcohol abuse. In all instances, the direction of the relationship was that a greater proportion of fall patients demonstrated the characteristic. Of these variables, weakness, decreased mobility of the lower extremities, confusion, and alcohol abuse are defining characteristics of *potential for injury*, while sleeplessness, incontinence, and depression are not.

Table 1: Percent of patients demonstrating significant* characteristics by fall status on admission and fall/random days

Characteristic	Admission		Fall/random	
	Fall (n=331)	No fall (n=300)	Fall (n=331)	No fall (n=300)
General weakness	63.3	37.3	53.8	26.0
Sleeplessness	60.1	36.3	64.6	32.7
Decreased mobility lo extremities	61.3	38.7	63.4	36.0
Incontinence	40.8	23.0	48.6	20.0
Confusion	28.7	13.3	42.3	11.3
Depression	8.2	2.3	12.7	3.3
Alcohol abuse	14.2	7.7	14.8	6.3
Narcotic taken	24.2	36.3	NS	NS
Impaired speech	21.4	13.3	NS	NS
Imposed restriction of movement	69.8	79.0	NS	NS
Assessed for posey	NS	NS	19.6	6.3
Agitation	NS	NS	31.4	11.0
Decreased mobility up extremities	NS	NS	33.5	20.7
Vertigo	NS	NS	24.5	12.3

*$p \leq .01$

Sleeplessness, a variable not previously reported in the literature as being related to falls was examined to determine its relationship to time of fall; interestingly, the falls experienced by patients with sleeplessness were evenly distributed throughout the 24-hour period and not limited to the nighttime hours.

Narcotic taken, impaired speech, and imposed restriction of movement, although significant on admission, were not significantly related to fall status on the fall/random day. In contrast to other significant patient characteristic variables, narcotic taken and imposed restriction of movement were inversely associated with fall status, being more common to patients in the no-fall group. Assessed for posey, impaired mobility of the upper extremities, agitation, and vertigo, while not significant on admission, were significantly related to fall status later in the hospital stay.

Nine variables were not significantly related to fall status on either data collection day: hypoxia, hypnotic taken, impaired hearing, arrhythmia, hypertension, complete bed rest, non-extremity pain, obesity, and impaired vision. Fall history, measured only on admission, was not significant. Of particular interest is the finding that impaired vision and hearing, hypnotic taken, and fall history were not significantly related to falling even though they are defining characteristics of potential for injury.

Of the seven sample characteristic variables, only sex ($X^2 = 4.73$, df = 1, p = .030) and living arrangement ($X^2 = 4.33$, df = 2, p = .288) were not significantly related to fall status. Despite the attempt to control on age by limiting the sample to the charts of patients aged 60 and older, the fall-group mean age of 74.4 years was significantly older than the no-fall-group mean age of 71.8 years (t = 6.13, df = 629, p<.001). Significantly more (67.7%) of the 56 employed patients were in the no fall group, an inverse relationship with fall-

ing ($X^2 = 10.34$, df = 1, p<.01). Service was significant with 57.4% of the 380 medical patients, 50.4% of the 127 general surgical patients, and 38.8% of the 121 surgical specialty patients in the fall group ($X^2 = 12.88$, df = 2, p<.001).

Of the 334 patients in private rooms, 60.2% fell, contrasted with 43.8% of the 297 patients in non-private rooms ($X^2 = 17.05$, df = 1, p<.000). And as noted earlier, falls were significantly more prevalent in one of the two hospital buildings ($X^2 = 43.13$, df = 1, p<.001). To determine whether patients with different characteristics were concentrated in private rooms or in one building, chi-square analyses were computed on all study variables both by room and by building; no significant differences were found. Building is a perplexing variable because it is not generalizable to other settings. Thus, it is important to note that a moderately significant association existed between building and room (r = .50, p<.000), with the majority of private rooms in the building with the majority of falls.

These initial analyses supported the idea that differences exist between patients who do and do not fall. An unexpected finding further supported the idea that patients who fall are different from those who do not; at the same time, the finding confounded interpretation of the study results. A significant difference was found between the mean day of hospital stay on which falls occurred and the mean day of hospital stay randomly selected for the no-fall group (t = 6.13, df = 629, p<.001). The mean day of fall was 14.2 (SD = 14.6). The mean random day of patient stay for eliciting information on the no fall group was 8.3 (SD = 8.7). This finding suggests that a substantial proportion of patients who fell were destined for a longer hospital stay prior to any injuries that might have resulted from the fall and extended the need for medical care. While an interesting finding, at the same time, it raises questions about the scientific soundness of comparing the fall and random-day data, since the increased length of stay increased the probability of falling in the hospital just by virtue of spending more time there, regardless of patient characteristics.

Having found significant differences between patients who did and did not fall on numerous variables, the next analyses were directed toward identifying which variables were most important in distinguishing fall from no fall patients and getting an overall picture of how well these variables did in predicting whether or not a patient fell. For these purposes, stepwise multiple regression analysis were used.

First, using the admission day data, the 10 patient characteristics significant upon admission and the five significant sample characteristics were used as potential predictor variables for fall status. As shown in Table 2,

Table 2: Stepwise regression analysis: admission day patient and sample characteristics as independent variables

Variable	Beta
General weakness	.224***
Building	.207***
Decreased mobility of lower extremities	.163***
Sleeplessness	.160***
Imposed restriction of movement	−.136***
Room type	.101*
Employment status	−.094**
Impaired speech	.094**
Incontinence	.093**
Confusion	.091*
Narcotic taken	−.088*
Alcohol abuse	.076*

$R^2 = .307$

***$p \leq .001$
** $p \leq .01$
* $p \leq .05$

of the 15 potential explanatory variables, 12 entered the regression equation as significantly adding to the explained variance of fall status. The R^2 for this equation was .307; in other words, knowing whether or not a patient had these characteristics over knowing nothing at all reduced the error in predicting whether or not a patient fell by 30.7%.

The beta gives the relative weight of each variable in predicting fall status. Thus, general weakness was the most important variable in predicting fall status, followed in descending order by building, decreased mobility of the lower extremities, sleeplessness, imposed restriction of movement, room type, employment, impaired speech, incontinence, confusion, narcotic taken, and substance abuse.

To assess the extent to which the fall/random-day data explained fall status, the 11 significant fall/random-day patient characteristics and the five significant sample characteristics were used as potential predictor variables. Of the 16 potential predictors for fall status, 10 entered the equation as significantly adding to the explained variance of 34.5%. Table 3 summarizes the results of this analysis. Although the ordering of their relative weights varied, seven of these variables also entered the admission-day equation: confusion, building, sleeplessness, decreased mobility of the lower extremities, incontinence, general weakness, and employment status. Further, the explained variances of the two analyses were relatively similar, suggesting that the ability to identify patients with the potential for falling may not improve greatly as time goes on during hospitalization.

The final analysis used the defining characteristics for the nursing diagnosis potential for injury as independent variables. Theoretically, these are the predictors staff nurses use to identify patients at risk for falls. The 12 variables that were regressed on fall status as being indicators of the defining characteristics were: general weakness, decreased mobility of the lower extremities, decreased mobility of the upper extremities, posey, fall history, impaired hearing, impaired vision, vertigo, alcohol abuse, confusion, hypnotic taken, and narcotic taken. Variables from fall/random-day data were used, since they had the stronger relationship with fall status. Table 4 summarizes the results of this regression. As can be seen, five of the 12 variables entered the equation, achieving an R^2 of .219. This was the weakest model obtained.

DISCUSSION AND SUMMARY OF FINDINGS

The findings of this study must be interpreted in the context of the methodology used. Although this study examined the ability to predict falls, the design was retrospective. Consequently, the data coders were aware of the outcome variable of interest, fall status, as they audited charts, introducing a potential source of bias. Also, reliance on incident reports for identifying the fall group sample was a methodological weakness, since it is possible that falls were reported at the discretion of the nursing staff.

The study relied upon chart documentation, and it is generally acknowledged that a number of the examined variables are underreported, such as alcohol abuse and history of falls. Thus, the relative importance of the variables in explaining fall status may very well be different than that shown in this study.

Many of the variables that this study sought to examine occurred so infrequently that it was impossible with a reasonable sample size to obtain a sufficient number of cases with the trait. Consequently, conditions that conceptually made sense together were collapsed into one variable. For example, the variable "incontinence" included fecal and urinary incontinence, frequency, and diarrhea. Thus, the variable definitions were broad and the degree to which subcategories contributed to the overall category is unknown.

And as discussed previously, the significant difference between the mean fall and random days raises question about the comparability of their data. It seems likely that if

Table 3: Stepwise regression analysis: fall/random day patient and sample characteristics as independent variables

Variable	Beta
Confusion	.217***
Building	.209***
Sleeplessness	.181***
Decreased mobility lower extremities	.174***
Incontinence	.129***
General weakness	.093**
Depression	.082*
Vertigo	.079*
Employment status	−.072*
Surgical specialty	−.067*
R^2=.345	

***p≤.001
**p≤.01
*p≤.05

Table 4: Stepwise regression analysis: potential for injury defining characteristics as independent variables

Variable	Beta
Confusion	.265***
Decreased mobility lower extremities	.189***
General weakness	.168***
Vertigo	.116**
Alcohol abuse	.077*
R^2=.219	

***p≤.001
**p≤.01
*p≤.05

matching had been done between fall days and the sampled day of hospital stay for the no-fall group, the results would have been different, with a different sample of non-fallers being required to find those who had a lengthier hospital stay.

With the above limitations in mind, this study has produced a number of suggestive findings. The findings lend support to having a nursing diagnosis *poential for injury* with falls being one aspect of the diagnosis. Data that nurses routinely collect in their work with patients differentiate, to a significant degree, between those who do and do not fall. Further, it is possible to identify a substantial proportion of patients who will fall during hospitalization from data available to nurses within the first 24 hours of hospitalization even though the falls often do not occur until much later in the hospital stay.

While the findings give credence to the diagnosis potential for injury, they also suggest a re-evaluation of its defining characteristics and particularly those of potential for trauma. Other combinations of variables may provide a stronger prediction model. Admittedly, replication studies are needed to determine whether certain variables such as depression, private room, and sleeplessness warrant inclusion. However, since this project was undertaken, several other studies with comparison groups of no-fall patients have become available (Lund and Sheafor 1985, Morse, Tylko, and Dixon 1985, Shepherd and Clapsadle 1981). In viewing the findings of these studies together, specific recommendations concerning defining characteristics of potential for trauma can be made. Specifically:

1. Confusion, impaired mobility of the lower extremities, and alcohol abuse repeatedly have been shown to be related to falling, suggesting these are appropriate defining characteristics.

2. Being elderly is well documented as a fall risk factor. Although physiological age is a defining characteristic of potential for injury, it is not included among those of potential for trauma. It should be included.

3. As in this study, incontinence was found to be related to falling by Morse et al. (1985). Thus, consideration should be given to including it as a defining characteristic.

4. Finally, although commonly viewed as risk factors, there is increasing evidence that taking narcotics and hypnotics do not predispose patients to falls. Other investigators have observed that such medications play little, if any, role in contributing to falls (Lund and Sheafor 1985, Rubenstein, Miller, Postel, and Evans 1983, Sehested and Severin-Nielson 1977, Shepherd and Clapsadle 1981, Tinker 1979), lending support to the notion that, at least in relationship to falls, these are not valid defining characteristics for potential for trauma.

REFERENCES

Coyle, N.: A problem-focused approach to nursing audit: falls, Cancer Nurs. **10**:389, 1979.

Duran, G.: Positive use of incident reports, Hospitals **53**:60, 64, 68, 1979.

Gordon, M.: Nursing diagnosis: process and application, New York, 1982, McGraw-Hill.

Innes, E.M., and Turman, W.G.: Evaluation of patient falls, Quart. Rev. Bull. **9**:30, 1983.

Janken, J.K., Reynolds, B.A., and Swiech, K.: Patient falls in the acute care setting: identifying risk factors through comparative and multivariate analyses, Nurs. Res. (In press.)

Kim, M.S., and Moritz, D.A., editors: Classification of nursing diagnoses: proceedings of the Third and Fourth national conferences, New York, 1982, McGraw-Hill.

Kostopoulos, M.R.: Reducing patient falls, Orthop. Nurs. **4**:14, 1985.

Kulikowski, E.S.: A study of accidents in hospitals, Supervisor Nurs. **10**:44, 1979.

Lee, P.S., and Pash, B.J.: Preventing patient falls, Nurs. 83 **13:**119, 1983.

Lund, C. & Sheafor, M.L.: Is your patient about to fall? J. Geront. Nurs. **11:**37, 1985.

Morse, J.M., Tylko, S.J., and Dixon, H.A.: Examination of patient falls final report, Edmonton, Alberta, 1985, University of Alberta Hospitals.

Nickens, H.: Intrinsic factors in falling among the elderly, Arch. Intern. Med. **145:**1089, 1985.

Perry, B.C.: Falls among the elderly—a review of the methods and conclusions of epidemiologic studies, J. Amer. Geriat. Soc. **30:**367, 1982.

Radebaugh, T.S., Hadley, E., and Suzman, R., editors: Falls in the elderly: biologic and behavioral aspects, Clin. Geriat. Med. **1:**497, 1985.

Rubenstein, H.S., Miller, G.H., Postel, S., and others: Standards of medical care based on consensus rather than evidence: the case of routine bedrail use for the elderly, Law, Med. Health Care **11:**271, 1983.

Shepherd, R., and Clapsadle, N.: A study of inpatient falls at Presbyterian Hospital during 1979. (Unpublished manuscript.)

Sehested, P., and Severin-Nielsen, T.: Falls by hospitalized elderly patients, causes and prevention, Geriatrics **32:**101, 1977.

Swartzbeck, E.M.: The problems of falls in the elderly, Nurs. Management **14:**34, 1983.

Swartzbeck, E.M., and Milligan, W.L.: A comparative study of hospital incidents, Nurs. Management **13:**39, 1982.

Tinker, G.M.: Accidents in a geriatric department. Age Aging **8:**196, 1979.

Venglarik, J.M., and Adams, M.: Which client is a high risk? J. Geront. Nurs. **11:**28, 1985.

Walshe, A., and Rosen, H.: A study of patient falls from bed, J. Nurs. Admin. **18:**31, 1979.

Diagnostic content validation of ten frequently reported nursing diagnoses

KAREN L. METZGER, M.S., R.N.
ELIZABETH F. HILTUNEN, M.S., R.N.

Nursing diagnosis has increasingly gained recognition and acceptance within the nursing community. Proponents of this concept generally agree that nursing diagnoses permit professional nurses to articulate the independent domain of nursing practice, enhance quality patient care and contribute to research and theory generation. However, experts (Fehring 1986, Gordon 1982) have also noted that nursing diagnoses may be poorly defined and lack validity and thus lead to lack of confidence in diagnostic judgment. Accuracy in the diagnostic process is affected by the use of valid defining characteristics for a given diagnosis. These characteristics (i.e., signs and symptoms, cues) provide criteria for the existence of the diagnosis, permit discrimination among health problems, and enhance confidence in diagnostic judgment.

The paucity of diagnostic validity studies and the lack of practical validation models have been noted by Fehring (1986). Until more nurses contribute to this research effort, nursing diagnoses will have limited value as valid nomenclature in nursing (Kim, McFarland and McLane 1984). Therefore, the purpose of this study was to contribute to the validation of 10 frequently reported nursing diagnoses by retrospective nurse identification.

Factors contributing to concept identification that were considered in this study were: presence of relevant and irrelevant cues, number of cues, and control of memory strain. The concept in this case is represented by a nursing diagnosis.

Bourne and Dominowski (1972) demonstrated that the presence of relevant and irrelevant attributes (cues) of a concept have been shown to influence concept identification. Although relevancy of a cue is an essential criterion for the accurate identification of a concept, they determined difficulty increases linearly with the number of cues present. Cianfrani (1984) found there was a decrease in accuracy in nurse's identification of health problems with increased amounts of data and the presence of low-relevance data.

Both the quality of information and the processing of information influence diagnostic concept identification. Use of memory stores is inherent in the process of concept identification. Whereas memory has several stages and processes (Bourne and Dominowski 1972, Bourne, Dominowski, and Loftus 1979), it is the short-term memory that processes both information received from the environment and past information retrieved from long-term memory stores. The limited capacity for short-term memory provides an argument for controlling the number of relevant cues to be processed (Carnevali, Mitchell, Woods and Tanner 1984 Gordon 1984). Miller (1956) postulates that the human mind can hold only five to nine units of information in short-term memory store. Hence, when amounts of data are minimized, memory strain, recall time, and the risk of error are substantially reduced.

The strategies suggested for concept identification are applicable to the processes necessary in the formulation of a nursing diagnosis. The basis for formulating nursing diagnoses depends upon identifying and evaluating the discriminating cues for each diagnosis (Gordon 1982, Matthews and Gaul 1979). Nevertheless, in the current list of diagnoses, 47 of the 62 diagnoses have no critical defining characteristics specified (Gordon 1986).

Gordon and Sweeney (1979) described three models for the quantification and validation of nursing diagnoses: a retrospective identification model, a clinical model, and a nurse-validation model. Studies have employed the retrospective identfication model (Riordan 1984, Vincent 1985). In fact, it was used as the method for identifying nursing diagnoses at the first four national conferences. The clinical model has been implemented in studies that have examined frequency and patterns of nursing diagnoses in selected populations (Gould 1983) and in a variety of practice settings (Jones and Jakob 1982). The nurse-validation model has been applied to the clinical testing of identified diagnoses (Kim et al. 1982, McFarland and Naschinski 1985, Ryan and Falco 1985). These methods have contributed to the validation of critical diagnostic criteria (Cheney 1984, Miller 1984). Fehring (1986) has proposed practical models to validate nursing diagnoses based on methods proposed by Gordon and Sweeney. Norris and Kunes-Connell (1985) utilized Fehring's model in identifying the clinical diagnostic validity (CDV) of self-esteem disturbance.

RESEARCH QUESTIONS

The specific research questions for this study were:

1. What is the diagnostic content validity (total DCV score) of 10 frequently reported, NANDA accepted nursing diagnoses?
2. What are the critical and supporting defining characteristics of 10 frequently reported, NANDA accepted nursing diagnoses when utilizing the DCV scoring model?
3. What NANDA accepted critical defin-

ing characteristics are supported when utilizing the DCV scoring model?

METHODOLOGY

This descriptive study utilized a structured survey to collect data that were analyzed for diagnostic content validity using a validation model described by Fehring (1986).

SAMPLE

Nurses with knowledge and experience in nursing diagnosis were the target population. Two groups of nurses in the Northeast were sampled, members of a regional nursing diagnosis interest group that held regular meetings with emphasis on diagnostic categories and diagnostic process, and graduate nursing students who had completed a graduate course in theory and process which emphasized diagnostic categories and cue perception.

A convenience sample of 76 registered nurses was obtained. It consisted of 57 members of the nursing diagnosis interest group and 19 medical-surgical graduate nursing students. Of those surveyed, 67.9% responded. The majority (78.9%) of the subjects were between 26 and 45 years of age. A baccalaureate degree was held by all of the subjects, 60.5% held a master's degree, and 6.6% a doctoral degree. The majority (69.7%) practiced in a medical-surgical area. Functional roles most frequently reported were clinical practitioner (38.2%) and educator (32.9%). Self-ratings of experience with nursing diagnosis (four categories) ranged from novice to expert. The majority (97.4%) rated themselves as at least competent. Of these, 51.3% considered themselves proficient or expert. Seventy-three (97.3%) reported basing their nursing interventions on nursing diagnosis.

INSTRUMENT AND DATA ANALYSIS

The instrument used for data collection, *Diagnostic Content Validity Tool*, was a graphic rating scale which listed 10 nursing diagnoses, their definitions and accompanying defining characteristics (Gordon 1985a, Kim and Moritz 1982, Kim, McFarland and McLane 1984). These diagnoses were the ten most frequently reported NANDA accepted nursing diagnoses in a nursing literature review, 1980–1984 (Gordon 1985b). Diagnoses that met study criteria were identified after ranking categories or subcategories by number of cases. The diagnoses represented those common to a variety of nursing settings. A pretest of the instrument was conducted among a panel of four experts in nursing diagnosis for clarity, research adequacy, and freedom from bias. Changes were made in the tool based on the responses of the panel. Content validity of this tool was supported. The ten diagnoses selected have been officially accepted for clinical testing by NANDA.

Subjects were requested to recall a representative sample of clients from their most recent clinical experience who had each of the nursing diagnoses. They then were requested to rate, on a 5-point scale with 5 indicating very characteristic and 1 indicating not characteristic, those defining characteristics that best represented each diagnostic category. Based on the diagnostic content validation (DCV) method proposed by Fehring (1986), a weighted ratio was calculated for each characteristic. The ratio was obtained by summing the weights assigned to each response and then dividing by the total number of responses. Those cues with ratios greater than or equal to .75 were considered critical. Those with a ratio greater than .50 but less than .75 were considered supporting characteristics. (The term *supporting* was selected by the researchers.) Those with a ratio less than or equal to .50 were discarded. A total DCV score for each diagnosis was obtained by summing ratings of all cues and averaging the results. The maximum score possible was 1.0.

PROCEDURE

The self-administered questionnaires were distributed to the graduate students, and a mailing was sent to all the members of the nursing diagnosis interest group. Subjects were informed that completion and return of the questionnaire was considered informed consent to participate in the study.

RESULTS

The total DCV scores were calculated for each of the ten nursing diagnoses from combined group scores (see Box 1). The two diagnoses with the highest content validity ranking were *alteration in urinary elimination pattern* and *impaired physical mobility*.

Following total DCV scoring, critical cues (Table 1) and supporting cues (Table 2) were ranked. The cue with the highest DCV score (.962) was inability to wash body or body parts for the diagnostic category *self-care deficit: bathing/hygiene*.

The average number of cues for the diagnostic categories prior to DCV scoring was 13.5 (see Table 3). With DCV scoring, the

---

BOX 1: Total DCV scores for ten frequently reported nursing diagnoses

Alteration in urinary elimination pattern	.848
Impaired physical mobility	.782
Alteration in comfort: pain	.779
Self-care deficit: bathing/hygiene	.745
Impairment of skin integrity: actual	.735
Anxiety	.667
Disturbance in self-concept: body image	.652
Sleep pattern disturbance	.618
Impairment of skin integrity: potential	.609
Alteration in nutrition: less than body requirements	.536

Table 1: Critical cues for ten frequently reported nursing diagnoses

Diagnostic category	Critical cue	DCV score
Self-care deficit: bathing/hygiene	*Inability to wash body or body parts	.962
Impaired physical mobility	Inability to purposefully move within the physical environment, including bed mobility, transfer, and ambulation	.961
	Decreased muscle strength, control, and/or mass	.830
	Limited range of motion	.802
	Imposed restrictions of movement, including mechanical, medical protocol	.792
Alteration in comfort: pain	Communication of pain descriptors	.946
	Guarding behavior, protective	.855
	Facial mask of pain	.834
	Distraction behavior	.787
	Autonomic responses not seen in chronic stable pain	.777
Sleep pattern disturbance	*Verbal complaints of difficulty falling asleep	.940
	*Verbal complaints of not feeling rested	.933
	*Awakening earlier or later than desired	.853
	*Interrupted sleep	.830
Impairment of skin integrity: actual	Disruption of skin surface	.932
	Destruction of skin layers	.800
Alteration in urinary elimination pattern	Incontinence	.909
	Frequency	.890
	Urgency	.863
	Retention	.854
	Nocturia	.824
	Dysuria	.821
	Hesitancy	.777
Anxiety	Anxious	.909
	Apprehension	.854
	Increased tension	.834
	Worried	.774
	Fear of specific consequences	.764
	Distressed	.750
Impairment of skin integrity: potential	Mechanical factor: pressure	.907
	Physical immobilization	.885

*Cue identified by NANDA as critical defining characteristic (Kim and Moritz 1982)

Continued

Table 1: Critical cues for ten frequently reported nursing diagnoses—cont'd

Diagnostic category	Critical cue	DCV score
	Mechanical factor: shearing forces	.861
	Altered circulation	.861
	Alteration in nutrition state (obesity, emaciation)	.830
	Excretion/secretion	.787
	Altered sensation	.763
	Skeletal prominence	.750
Alteration in nutrition: less than body requirements	20% or more under ideal body weight	.865
	Reported inadequate food intake less than RDA	.830
Disturbance in self-concept: body image	*Verbal response to actual or perceived change in structure and/or function	.861
	Negative feelings about body	.850
	Verbalization of: fear of rejection or of reaction by others	.757
	Preoccupation with change or loss	.753
	*Nonverbal response to actual or perceived change in structure and/or function	.753

*Cue identified by NANDA as critical defining characteristic (Kim and Moritz 1982)

average number of cues was 10.5 (4.4 critical and 6.1 supporting).

Of those diagnostic categories with eight or fewer cues listed by NANDA, all but one retained the cues as supporting or critical. The least reduction (one cue) occurred in *anxiety,* the diagnostic category with the largest number of cues (29).

The number of critical cues after DCV scoring ranged from one to eight, with *impairment of skin integrity: potential* assigned the highest number. All of the original cues (seven) for *alteration in urinary elimination pattern* were rated as critical. *Alteration in comfort: pain, impaired physical mobility,* and *self-care deficit: bathing/hygiene* also retained all cues as critical or supporting.

Three diagnostic categories with critical cues identified by NANDA were used in this study *(self-care deficit: bathing/hygiene, sleep pattern disturbance, disturbance in self-concept: body image).* At least 73.7% of the respondents supported these cues as critical. The lowest DCV score (.753) was obtained for the cue "nonverbal response to actual or perceived change in structure and/or function" for the diagnosis *disturbance in self-concept: body image.*

DISCUSSION

The ranking of the diagnoses by total DCV score revealed that the most highly valid contained the majority of cues in the biophysical domain. The physical cues of these diagnoses seemed to have a higher information value for the respondents. This lends support to a reliability factor for the cues utilized in diagnostic identification as discussed by Gordon (1982). Gordon post-

Table 2: Supporting cues for ten frequently reported nursing diagnoses

Diagnostic category[a]	Supporting cue	DCV score
Anxiety	Restlessness	.747
	Uncertainty	.740
	Sympathetic stimulation	.722
	Fearful	.712
	Painful and persistent increased helplessness	.693
	Scared	.692
	Jittery	.685
	Insomnia	.685
	Facial tension	.670
	Focus "self"	.656
	Extraneous movements	.632
	Increased wariness	.625
	Voice quivering	.620
	Glancing about	.618
	Trembling/hand tremors	.609
	Shakiness	.603
	Poor eye contact	.589
	Rattled	.568
	Increased perspiration	.568
	Expressed concerns re: change in life events	.555
	Overexcited	.545
	Inadequacy feelings	.527
Disturbance in self-concept: body image	Not touching body part	.747
	Not looking at body part	.737
	Actual change in structure and/or function	.726
	Feelings of helplessness, hopelessness or powerlessness	.703
	Verbalization of refusal to verify actual change	.696
	Hiding or overexposing body part	.692
	Verbalization of focus on past strength, function or appearance	.679
	Change in social involvement	.655
	Missing body part	.636

[a]Supporting cues in eight categories met criteria.

Continued

Table 2: Supporting cues for ten frequently reported nursing diagnoses—cont'd

Diagnostic category[a]	Supporting cue	DCV score
	Verbalization of change in lifestyle	.633
	Depersonalization of part or loss by impersonal pronouns	.611
	Change in ability to estimate spatial relationship of body to environment	.521
Sleep pattern disturbance	Frequent yawning	.747
	Dark circles under eyes	.697
	Increasing irritability	.697
	Lethargy	.670
	Restlessness	.642
	Listlessness	.640
	Disorientation	.537
Impairment of skin integrity: potential	Mechanical factor: restraint	.743
	Altered metabolic state	.649
	Alterations in skin turgor	.593
	Radiation	.593
Alteration in nutrition: less than body requirements	Lack of interest in food	.716
	Loss of weight with adequate food intake	.710
	Aversion to eating	.647
	Reported or evidence of lack of food	.632
	Perceived inability to ingest food	.623
	Sore, inflamed buccal cavity	.547
	Reported altered taste sensation	.530
	Weakness of muscles required for swallowing or mastication	.524
	Diarrhea and/or steatorrhea	.510
Self-care deficit: bathing/hygiene	Inability to obtain or get to water source	.712
	Inability to regulate temperature or flow	.562
Impaired physical mobility	Impaired coordination	.698
	Reluctance to attempt movement	.608
Alteration in comfort: pain	Self-focusing	.683
	Narrowed focus	.677
	Alteration in muscle tone	.675

[a]Supporting cues in eight categories met criteria.

Table 3: Number of cues for diagnostic categories before and after DCV scoring

Diagnostic category	Total cues NANDA	Total cues after DCV scoring	Critical cues NANDA	Critical cues after DCV scoring	Supporting cues NANDA	Supporting cues after DCV scoring
Anxiety	29	28	0	6	29	22
Disturbance in self-concept: body image	21	17	2	5	19	12
Alteration in nutrition: less than body requirements	21	11	0	2	21	9
Impairment of skin integrity: potential	20	12	0	8	20	4
Sleep pattern disturbance	17	11	4	4	13	7
Alteration in comfort: pain	8	8	0	5	8	3
Alteration in urinary elimination pattern	7	7	0	7	7	0
Impaired physical mobility	6	6	0	4	6	2
Impairment of skin integrity: actual	3	2	0	2	3	0
Self-care deficit: bathing/ hygiene	3	3	1	1	2	2
Total cues	135	105	7[a]	44	128	61
Mean	13.5	10.5	.7	4.4	12.8	6.1

[a]From 3 diagnostic categories only.

ulates that practitioners generally consider observable physical cues to be more reliable and valid indicators of a diagnosis than subjective feeling states because they are observable and thus may have greater agreement between diagnosticians. Without verbal reports of subjective feelings and perceptions, the clinician may be required to make inferences. These inferences are interpretations and thus may be associated with less agreement.

Number of cues seemed to have an influence as well. Those diagnostic categories with eight or fewer cues prior to scoring were in the upper half of the ranking. Many of the cues were interpreted as critical indicators when the initial number of cues was low. The lower half of the ranking represented categories with 17 to 29 cues prior to scoring. These retained a range of 11 to 28 cues following DCV scoring. The majority attained DCV scores of less than .75. These findings supported the arguments of Bourne and Dominowski (1972) that number of cues and relevant and irrelevant cues are factors in concept identification.

Alteration in nutrition: less than body requirements, ranked tenth and received a total DCV score of .536. Fehring (1986) has suggested that those diagnoses with total scores below .60 be further evaluated. This diagnosis had the greatest decrease in cues after scoring. Although respondents identified relevant and irrelevant cues, the diagnosis did not meet Fehring's recommended criteria for content validity.

Analysis indicated a substantial reduction in the average number of cues after DCV scoring. The average number of *critical cues* (4.4) fell below the limits suggested by Miller (1956) for information processing. However, when supporting cues are included this limit is exceeded. This finding suggests a need to evaluate the DCV scoring criteria and the use of critical and supporting cues. Since the clinician may be testing multiple diagnostic possibilities, strategies to control memory strain, such as limiting the number of highly valid cues, should be employed. Analysis also demonstrated quantifiable evidence for the support of the critical cues identified by NANDA for three diagnoses used in this study. These seven critical cues seem to be highly valid indicators of the diagnoses and should enhance accuracy and confidence in diagnostic judgment.

Limitations of this study included the lack of random and geographical sampling of nurse-subjects. The type and amount of diagnostic training of subjects as well as experience with a given diagnosis may have influenced reliability of their ratings and thus the DCV scores obtained. Furthermore, use of this model required that nurses retrospectively rate characteristics based on their memory of clients' manifestations, which may have decreased reliability.

Implications for nursing resulting from this study include quantifiable evidence for establishing validity and increasing confidence in nursing diagnoses. If nurses are to be held accountable for the diagnosis-based care they provide, confidence and accuracy in the diagnostic process guiding that care is critical.

Further analysis of the data in this study is proposed. Statistical analysis is under way to examine the data for cue clustering and to identify discrete categories. Analysis of differences in cue selection between the two subgroups in the sample and relationships of cues and sample demographic characteristics is planned. The relationship between education and clinical experience and cue selection may assist in describing factors affecting judgment about diagnostic cues.

Further studies utilizing this model are recommended in testing these and other accepted nursing diagnoses. Randomly selected samples that are geographically representative should be utilized to estimate content validity of diagnoses. With additional studies contributing to the pool of data on diagnostic categories, evaluation of the criteria for acceptable scores for diagnostic categories as well as critical and supporting cues is recommended. Data from these studies also could be employed by diagnostic review committees on a regional and national level.

The purpose of this study was to obtain validity estimates on selected nursing diagnoses. Findings reflected the immaturity of some diagnoses in the present classification system and identified a need for further refinement studies. Utilization of this validation model is encouraged as a means to contribute to research needed for standardization of nursing diagnoses.

REFERENCES

Bourne, L.E., and Dominowski, R.L.: Thinking, Ann. Rev. Psychol. **24**:105, 1972; Bourne, L.E., Dominowski, R.L., and Luftus, E.P.: Cognitive processes, Englewood Cliffs, N.J., 1979, Prentice-Hall, Inc.

Carnevali, D.L., Mitchell, P., Woods, N. and others: Diagnostic reasoning in nursing, Philadelphia, 1984, J.B. Lippincott.

Cheney, A.M.: Critical indicators for the nursing diagnosis of disturbance in self concept. In Kim, M.J., McFarland, G., and McLane, A., editors: Classification of nursing diagnoses: proceedings of the fifth national conference, St. Louis, 1984, The C.V. Mosby Co.

Cianfrani, K.L.: The influence of amounts and relevance of data on identifying health problems. In Kim, M.J., McFarland, G.K., and McLane, A., editors, Classification of nursing diagnoses: proceedings of the fifth national conference, St. Louis, 1984, The C.V. Mosby Co.

Fehring, R.: Validating diagnostic labels: standardized methodology. In Hurley, M. E., editor: Classification of nursing diagnoses: proceedings of the sixth conference, St. Louis, 1986, The C.V. Mosby Co.

Gordon, M.: Nursing diagnosis: process and application, New York, 1982, McGraw-Hill.

Gordon, M.: Manual of nursing diagnosis, New York, McGraw-Hill, 1985a.

Gordon, M.: Practice based data set for a nursing information system, J. Med. Systems **9**:43, 1985b.

Gordon, M.: Structure of diagnostic categories. In Hurley, M.E., editor: Classification of nursing diagnosis: proceedings of the sixth conference, St. Louis, 1986, The C.V. Mosby Co.

Gordon, M., and Sweeney, M.: Methodological problems and issues in identifying and standardizing nursing diagnosis, Advances Nurs. Sci. **2**:1, 1979.

Gould, M.: Nursing diagnoses concurrent with multiple sclerosis, J. Neurosurg. Nurs. **15**:339, 1983.

Jones, P.E., and Jakob, D.F.: The definitions of nursing diagnoses: phase 3 and final report, Toronto, 1982, University of, Toronto, Faculty of Nursing.

Kim, M., Ambroso, R., Gulanick, M., and others: Clinical use of nursing diagnosis in cardiovascular nursing. In Kim, M.J., and Moritz, D., editors: Classification of nursing diagnoses: proceedings of the third and fourth national conferences, New York, 1982, McGraw-Hill.

Kim, M.J., McFarland, G.K., and McLane, A.M., editors: Classification of nursing diagnoses: proceedings of the fifth national conference. St. Louis, 1984, The C.V. Mosby Co.

Kim, M.J., and Moritz, D.A., editors: Classification of nursing diagnoses: proceedings of the third and fourth national conferences, New York, 1982, McGraw-Hill.

Kim, M.J., Seritella, R., Gulanick, M., and others: Clinical validation of cardiovascular nursing diagnoses. In Kim, M.J., McFarland, G., and McLane, A., editors: Classification of nursing diagnoses: proceedings of the fifth national conference, St. Louis, 1984, The C.V. Mosby Co.

Matthews, C., and Gaul, A.: Nursing diagnosis from the perspective of concept attainment and critical thinking, Advances Nurs. Sci. **2**:17, 1979.

McFarland, G.K., and Naschinski, C.E.: Impaired communication: a descriptive study, Nurs. Clin. North Amer. **20**:775, 1985.

Miller, G.: The magical number seven, plus or minus two: Some comments on our capacity for processing information. Psychol. Rev. **63**:81, 1956.

Miller, J.: Development and validation of a diagnostic label: Powerlessness, In Kim, M.J., McFarland, G.K., and McLane, A.M., editors: Classification of nursing diagnoses: proceedings of the fifth national conference, St. Louis, 1984, The C.V. Mosby Co.

Norris, J., and Kunes-Connell, M.: Self-esteem disturbance. Nurs. Clin. North Amer. **20**:745, 1985.

Riordan, M.: Validation of the defining characteristics of the nursing diagnosis: alteration in comfort: pain, (Unpublished manuscript.)

Ryan, P., and Falco, S.M.: A pilot study to validate the etiologies and defining characteristics of the nursing diagnosis of noncompliance, Nurs. Clin. North Amer. **20**:685, 1985.

Vincent, K.G.: The validation of a nursing diagnosis: a nurse consensus survery. Nurs. Clin. North Amer. **20**:631, 1985.

Delphi survey to gain consensus on wellness and health promotion nursing diagnoses

MARILYN D. FRENN, M.S.N., R.N.
CAROL A. JACOBS, M.S.N., R.N.
HELENA A. LEE, M.S.N., R.N.
MONICA T. SANGER, M.S.N., R.N.
KATHLEEN A. STRONG, M.S., R.N.

Within the health care system there has been a steady shift in emphasis from illness to health and a reorientation of both providers and consumers to the importance of health promotion. However, the current list of nursing diagnoses is based on illness care and is, therefore, incomplete in describing nurses' health promotion focus.

The significance of health promotion as a part of nursing practice has been identified (Brubaker 1983, Gleit and Tatro 1981, Keller 1981, Pender 1982). As health-promoting nursing interventions continue to be studied and tested, clustering of phenomena relevant to these activities helps nurses to describe the domain of their practice. The taxonomy of nursing diagnoses is an organizing framework of nursing phenomena and assists nurses in explicating their health-promotion roles.

Members of the wellness special interest group who attended the Sixth Conference of the North American Nursing Diagnosis Association (NANDA) expressed concern about the limited applicability of the current nursing diagnosis taxonomy and the absence of labels reflecting wellness and health-promotion nursing practice. Although nurses use nursing diagnoses in wellness and health promotion nursing practice areas, there is a paucity of research identifying these diagnostic labels. The purpose of this study was to use the delphi survey technique to develop and gain consensus on a list of health-promotion nursing diagnoses. The research question guiding the study was "What are clinically useful nursing diagnoses in a wellness and health-promotion framework?"

REVIEW OF THE LITERATURE

The definition of health used by health professionals influences practice, education, and research. If the definition is vague, a clear direction is not provided. If it is disease-oriented, it will be reflected in the focus of care (Nowakowski 1979). Health is defined in the American Nurses Association (ANA) *Nursing: A social policy statement* as "a dynamic state of being in which the developmental and behavioral potential of an individual is realized to the fullest possible extent" (ANA 1980).

The core of nursing practice has centered around the health promotion role of nursing. The concept of health has been explicated throughout the history of nursing by such leaders as Nightingale (1946), Goodrich (1932), Frost (1939), Henderson (1964), and others.

Nurses have a primary responsibility to understand health processes and help clients develop positive health practices (Pender 1982). Pender has designed and tested a health promotion model appropriate to a variety of clinical settings; this model facilitates the organization of client data into

The cooperation of participating NANDA nurses is gratefully acknowledged. This study was funded, in part, by a grant from Sigma Theta Tau, Delta Gamma Chapter, Marquette University, and from the Center for Nursing Research, University of Wisconsin-Milwaukee.

meaningful patterns (1982). Siegel (1973) stated, however, that health professionals were not well-equipped conceptually to study health. There had not been a vocabulary or classification system of healthy functional capacities. Gordon (1982) subsequently outlined functional patterns of living to serve as a guide in assessment and diagnostic formulation.

The absence of a vocabulary of health with conceptual clarity may derive from a medical or pathological orientation in the health care system and from the difficulty of quantifying the phenomenon of health. Lamb and Richmond (1975) have identified the deficiency of the usual coding of medical diagnoses with its neglect of health maintenance and ambulatory practice categories. Similarly, because the focus of the accepted list of nursing diagnoses has been on problem identification, actual or potential, its usefulness to nurses in health promotion and wellness nursing practice has been limited.

In a survey of studies published in major nursing journals, Brown, Tanner, and Padrick (1984) found a significant shift during the 1970's and 1980's from acute illness to wellness and health promotion. Current as well as projected health-care trends indicate a need for research on nursing effectiveness in facilitating clients' health-promoting behaviors (Andreoli and Musser 1983).

The centrality of the concepts of health, person, environment, and nursing has been demonstrated by Fawcett (1984) in her description of a metaparadigm of nursing. Presently, nurse scientists have examined the concept of health philosophically (Smith 1981), through the use of ethnographic methods (Tripp-Reimer 1984), as well as through the use of quantitative measures (Brown, Muhlenkamp, Fox, and Osborn 1983, Fontes 1983). Thus, examination of a vocabulary and taxonomy for health promotion is central to further development of the body of nursing knowledge.

The delphi technique was the method used for this study, experts in the areas of nursing diagnosis and health promotion generated the data that formed the basis of the findings. These data originated from subjects' nursing practice experience; no definitions or guidelines were used in order that the diagnostic labels might better reflect nursing practice phenomena.

ASSUMPTIONS

There are a few assumptions basic to this study. Nurses who have expertise in the areas of nursing diagnosis and health promotion are able to identify and rate nursing diagnoses clinically relevant to wellness and health promotion. Nursing diagnoses generated by a group of nurses who practice in a variety of settings reflect the range of health promotion needs that are treated in nursing practice. It is finally assumed that the delphi technique is a valid method to gain consensus on issues in nursing practice.

SUBJECTS

Questionnaires were mailed to 495 nurses who attended the Sixth Conference of NANDA. Subjects for the study were the 104 registered nurses (21% response rate) who completed the three rounds of the survey. The majority of the subjects (72%) were prepared at the master's or doctoral level. (Seventy-five percent of the over 1200 NANDA members are master's of doctoral-prepared nurses.) Mean years active in nursing was 18 years with a range of 3 to 37 years. Subjects identified the percentage of their time spent in various professional nursing activities. Mean of time collectively spent in administration was 22%; in education, 46%; in practice, 24%; in research, 7%; and in other (e.g., graduate school), 1%. By comparison with NANDA members in general, 18% are clinicians, 54% are educators, and 18% are administrators.

Using a Likert-type scale of one (minimal)

to seven (extensive), the majority of subjects indicated a knowledge level of four to five (mean = 4.4) in wellness and health promotion and a knowledge level of five to six (mean = 5.7) in nursing diagnosis. Thus, the subjects were qualified as experts in the areas of health promotion and nursing diagnosis to participate in the delphi survey.

METHOD

The delphi technique is a survey method that originated in the field of business and was developed to determine experts' opinions on projected trends. Its use as a research technique in nursing has been documented. Lindeman (1975) used the delphi technique to identify research priorities for clinical nursing. Other researchers who have used the delphi method include Oberst, Ventura, and Frederickson (1978) to determine priorities for cancer nursing and Shoemaker (1984) who examined essential characteristics of nursing diagnoses.

There are three aspects of the delphi technique that distinguish it from other survey methods: anonymity of group members, controlled feedback during successive survey rounds, and statistical group response (Couper, 1984). Advantages of the technique are that individuals who have expertise in the area of study generate the data and respond to each others' ideas in an anonymous and equal manner. Repeated rounds of the survey are conducted to help respondents gain consensus as they consider responses and comments.

For this study a three-round delphi technique was used. Based on results of a pilot study (N = 10), the initial questionnaire was designed as an open questionnaire for the generation of diagnostic labels appropriate to nursing practice in a wellness and health-promotion framework; demographic information was also requested. Researchers examined the data resulting from Round I, grouped similar diagnoses, and removed from the list any previously accepted nursing diag-

noses. In subsequent rounds, subjects used a Likert-type scale of one (low) to six (high) to rate the labels according to relevance for use in practice within a wellness and health-promotion framework. Data analysis for Rounds II and III consisted of calculation of means and rank ordering of the diagnoses according to means. Comments of subjects were included to provide rationale for other subjects to consider.

FINDINGS

The 104 nurse respondents in this study generated a total of over 800 nursing diagnoses, of which 76 labels appropriate to the domain of nursing practice in a wellness and health-promotion framework were rated in Rounds II and III. Nursing diagnoses that are already on the accepted list were not included in subsequent rounds unless the respondents changed the diagnosis to include a positive qualifier. From the total of 76 diagnoses that were developed, the final means ranged from a high of 4.95 (sleep/rest pattern, effective/ineffective) to a low of 1.77 (growth/relapse, potential for).

Table 1 includes a listing of the 76 nursing diagnoses and their rankings from Rounds II and III. The rankings of the highest and lowest diagnoses indicate consistency among the subjects in their responses to the items.

The final question of the survey requested the subjects to rank on the scale of one to six the clinical usefulness of "positive" nursing diagnoses (e.g., effective, intact, potential for). The mean for this item was 3.74 indicating favorable but not complete support for the idea of using positive diagnoses in practice. Some respondents who favored the use of positive diagnoses stated that positive nursing diagnoses:

- Direct reinforcing and supporting interventions
- Are needed with a healthy population not at risk

Table 1: Rank order of Round II and Round III delphi generated diagnoses

Round III	Round II	
1.	(2)	Sleep/rest pattern, effective/ineffective
2.	(6)	Activity/exercise pattern, effective/ineffective
3.	(1)	Stress management, effective/ineffective
4.	(5)	Communication patterns, effective/ineffective
5.	(10)	Developmental tasks, age-appropriate/delay
6.	(4)	Health maintenance, effective/ineffective
7.	(11)	Pain management, effective/ineffective
8.	(7)	Coping strategies, effective/potential for growth
9.	(8)	Grieving, functional
10.	(3)	Support system, effective/ineffective
11.	(22)	Activity tolerance/deficit
12.	(16)	Parenting skills, potential for growth
13.	(18)	Infection, potential for
14.	(9)	Decision making, effective/ineffective
15.	(61)	Crisis management, adequate/inadequate
16.	(36)	Self-perception/self-concept, positive
17.	(71)	Problem-solving skills, inadequate
18.	(21)	Role changes, awareness of potential, accepted/impaired
19.	(29)	Change in family dynamics (specify)
20.	(23)	Physical disability, adaptation to
21.	(15)	Community resource use, effective/ineffective
22.	(42)	Motivation, intact/decreased
23.	(26)	Risk factor management, effective/ineffective
24.	(13)	Substance misuse/abuse (specify)
25.	(62)	Cultural adaptation, potential for growth
26.	(69)	Maternal/infant attachment, healthy/problematic
27.	(20)	Bonding, effective/ineffective
28.	(30)	Environmental hazards, potential for injury
29.	(14)	Relaxation management, effective, ineffective
30.	(68)	Leisure management: effective/ineffective
31.	(32)	Assertiveness, effective/ineffective
32.	(25)	Nutritional patterns, adequate
33.	(74)	Role conflict
34.	(12)	Health practices, knowledge of (specify)
35.	(75)	Social skills, inadequate
36.	(31)	Conflict resolution skills, impaired
37.	(67)	Fatigue
38.	(60)	Anticipatory role transition (specify), desire for future growth
39.	(28)	Independence/dependence, accepted/unresolved
40.	(24)	Lifestyle modification (specify), potential for
41.	(19)	Home maintenance management, effective
42.	(34)	Dentition, intact/impaired
43.	(63)	Decisional conflict
44.	(73)	Role ambiguity
45.	(17)	Health perception, realistic/unrealistic
46.	(35)	Spiritual integrity: faith, hope, love intact
47.	(65)	Dietary insufficiency (specify)
48.	(66)	Emotional self-care deficit
49.	(27)	Immunological protection, adequate/inadequate
50.	(76)	Vulnerability to peer pressure

Continued

Table 1: Rank order of Round II and Round III delphi generated diagnoses—cont'd

Round III	Round II	
51.	(33)	Environmental health management, effective/ineffective
52.	(38)	Self-care wellness behavior (specify)
53.	(41)	Resource deficit (specify)
54.	(39)	Physical mobility, adequate
55.	(37)	Relationship building, potential for growth
56.	(43)	Self-actualization potential, maintained/impaired
57.	(45)	Values-actions dissonance
58.	(47)	Motivation for wellness
59.	(40)	Increased health promotion, potential for
60.	(51)	Well child (specify age group)
61.	(72)	Regression
62.	(46)	Spiritual rituals impairment
63.	(44)	Thought patterns/attitudes, positive
64.	(70)	Overcommitment
65.	(49)	Losses, awareness of potential
66.	(48)	Sexual integrity
67.	(52)	Well family
68.	(54)	Self-awareness, diminished
69.	(55)	Depression
70.	(59)	Anticipatory guidance
71.	(50)	Sexual reproductive pattern, effective (specify)
72.	(64)	Desire for increased harmonious functioning (specify)
73.	(53)	Enhancement of well-being, potential for
74.	(58)	Altered states, awareness of potential for
75.	(56)	Maintenance of normotension
76.	(57)	Growth relapse, potential for

- Are a part of health care (not illness care), health promotion, and the prevention aspect of nursing
- Show that nursing is concerned with areas even though client/family/community is well
- Direct nursing interventions that must be enacted to ensure continued effectiveness in maintaining a healthy state, encouragement to continue the present course, validation and recognition of and agreement with clients' present actions.

Other respondents indicated concern for the use of positive nursing diagnoses. These subjects made comments about the lack of a problem focus to clarify the need for nursing:

- Of little value except as assessment data

- If effective, where is the need for nursing?

Although there was considerable feedback about the use of positive qualifiers for nursing diagnoses, subjects identified the clinical usefulness in a wellness and health-promotion nursing practice.

LIMITATIONS

About 20% of the nurses present at the Sixth Conference on the Classification of Nursing Diagnoses participated in this study. Although health promotion is integral to all nursing practice, only a select group of nurses participated in the study. Health promotion, wellness, and nursing diagnosis were not operationally defined for the subjects. While the absence of definitions enabled participants to use their knowledge and experience to interpret the questionnaire, it may have also contributed to a lack of consistency in their responses.

DISCUSSION

Through the delphi technique process this study examined the identification of nursing diagnoses in the areas of wellness and health promotion as consensus by the subjects was reached. Clinical testing and validation of nursing diagnoses that received the highest rankings will be the next steps in the development of the nursing diagnosis taxonomy. Further research to identify and define critical indicators of the wellness and health promotion nursing diagnoses would facilitate the description of the domain of health-promotion nursing practice.

Additional study with clinical testing of the generated nursing diagnostic labels is indicated to add to the knowledge of wellness and health-promotion nursing practice. Identification of nursing diagnoses already in use by clinicians could be compared with the listing of labels from this study. Also, diagnoses could be studied in terms of Pender's (1982) concepts of stabilizing (health protection focus) and actualizing (health-promotion focus) health behaviors.

Finally, analysis of the delphi technique as a method to gain consensus among nurse experts requires further study to determine the validity and usefulness of this method.

REFERENCES

American Nurses Association: Nursing: a social policy statement, Kansas City, MO, 1980, American Nurses Association.

Andreoli, K.G., and Musser, L.A.: Trends that may affect nursing's future, Nurs. and Health Care **5**:47, 1984.

Brown, N.J., Muhlenkamp, A.F., Fox, L.M., and Osborn, M.: The relationship among health beliefs, health values, and health promotion activity, Western J. Nurs. Res. **5**:155, 1983.

Brown, N.J., Tanner, C., and Padrick, K.P.: Nursing's search for scientific knowledge, Nurs. Res. **33**:26, 1984.

Brubaker, B.H.: Health promotion: a linguistic analysis, Adv. Nurs. Sci. **5**:1, 1983.

Couper, M.R.: The delphi technique: characteristics and sequence model, Adv. Nurs. Sci. **7**:72, 1984.

Fawcett, J.: The metaparadigm of nursing: present status and future refinements, Image. **16**:84, 1984.

Fontes, H.: An exploration of the relationships between cognitive style, interpersonal needs, and the eudaimonistic model of health, Nurs. Res. **32**:92, 1983.

Frost, H.: Nursing in sickness and health, New York, 1939, Macmillan.

Gleit, C., and Tatro, S.: Nursing diagnoses for healthy individuals, Nurs. Health Care. **2**:456, 1981.

Goodrich, A.W.: The social and ethical significance of nursing, New York, 1932, Macmillan.

Gordon, M.: Nursing diagnosis: process and application, New York, 1982, McGraw Hill.

Henderson, V.: The nature of nursing, Amer. J. Nurs. **64**:62, 1964.

Keller, M.: Toward a definition of health, Adv. Nurs. Sci. **4**:43, 1981.

Lamb, G.A., and Richmond, J.B.: Putting health in health administration. In Education for health administration, vol. 2, Ann Arbor, 1975, Health Administration Press.

Lindeman, C.A.: Delphi survey of priorities in clinical nursing research, Nurs. Res. **24**:434, 1975.

Nightingale, F.: Notes on nursing, Philadelphia, 1946, J.B. Lippincott.

Nowakowski, L.: Examination of assumptions: a necessary prelude to the development of health services, Paper presented at the Nursing Practice with Self-Care Focus Conference, Georgetown University, Feb. 1979.

Oberst, M.T., Ventura, M., and Frederickson, K.: Priorities in cancer nursing research, Cancer Res. **1**:280, 1978.

Pender, N.J.: Health promotion in nursing practice, Norwalk, 1982, Appleton-Century-Crofts.

Shoemaker, J.: Essential features of a nursing diagnosis. In Kim, M.J., McFarland, G.K., and McLane, A.M., editors: Classification of nursing diagnoses: proceedings of the fifth national conference St. Louis, 1984, The C.V. Mosby Co.

Siegel, H.: To your health—whatever that may mean. Nurs. Forum. **12**:280, 1973.

Smith, J.A.: The idea of health: a philosophical inquiry, Adv. Nurs. Sci. **3**:43, 1981.

Tripp-Reimer, T.: Reconceptualizing the construct of health: integrating the emic and etic perspectives, Res. Nurs. Health, **7**:101, 1984.

Developing a method for validating the output of computerized expert systems in nursing

JOAN NORRIS, Ph.D., R.N.
JANET CUDDIGAN, M.S.N., R.N.
SHEILA RYAN, Ph.D., R.N.

Artificial intelligence applications of computer technology have generated expert systems that can support decision making in education and clinical practice for various health professionals. These systems simulate behavior or provide decision making support cues which, if initiated by humans, can be said to be intelligent. These expert systems are developed by combining expertise in applying knowledge engineering to expertise in the content domain. Some examples of these computerized expert consultants in nursing have been achieved by the Creighton Online Multiple Modular Expert System (COMMES; Ryan 1985). These include:

1. *Education consultant* which selects and organizes educational goals and key media references in response to a nurse's requests for information on a given topic. This consultant designs a mini-curriculum for self-study based on individualized needs that may arise in response to either clinical problems or a desire to obtain continuing education updating and credit.

2. *Evaluation consultant* which generates brief essay questions as a mechanism for obtaining CEU credits. The nurse-user demonstrates knowledge acquired following use of the education consultant. Responses to the test items can be mailed to Creighton Nursing faculty to evaluate and award CEU credits.

3. *Protocol consultant* which systematically provides specific guidelines or cues to guide the nurse in developing a plan of care or in creating standards of care appropriate to particular patient problems. This clinical decision support consultant will be the focus of the validation study for which the methodology being presented was developed.

These three consultants described are based on the COMMES generalist nursing knowledge base. Additional consultants have been developed based on specialized knowledge bases. These include a gerontology consultant, an oncology risk assessment consultant and a nursing diagnosis consultant who assists the novice in identifying a nursing diagnosis based on consideration of the presenting signs and symptoms. This knowledge base consists of the NANDA diagnoses, etiologies and defining characteristics based on Gordon's (1984) *Manual of Nursing Diagnosis*.

EARLY DEVELOPMENT AND VALIDATION EFFORTS

The COMMES project was initiated as an interdisciplinary effort by the Health Sciences Schools at Creighton University and was originally funded through a grant by the W.K. Kellogg Foundation of Battle Creek. A common taxonomy was developed and implemented by the various schools in writing their curricular goals and objectives. This common format, the total systems design taxonomy, assured consistency in communicating the educational goals and resources of each program in the development of the knowledge bases.

The functional components of the COMMES system incorporate (1) an expert knowledge base, (2) a semantic network and

(3) a reasoning system. The knowledge base we refer to in this discussion is a definition of the clinical capabilities of the generalist nurse derived from the educational goals and media resources developed by the nursing faculty for its BSN program (see Fig. 1 for the steps in developing the nursing consultants in the COMMES system). The semantic network is developed by selected nurse faculty who "teach the system" that certain terms are associated. This capture of nursing's cognitive expertise is a key characteristic of expert systems in the artificial intelligence area. Using deductions and inference rules from the reasoning program, information can then be retrieved in various intelligent ways, not merely by major topic. The nurse can describe complex, multifaceted clinical situations for which information is needed. For instance, pulmonary edema can

be associated with several nursing diagnoses, with trauma and pregnancy. By using one or more key words joined by "and" or "in the context of," the nurse can request various aspects of information pertinent to the immediate need, such as nursing care and pulmonary edema in the context of pregnancy.

These decision support services permit nurses in off-campus settings to seek consultation about necessary components of care or to update their nursing knowledge at any hour of the day or night. The nurse who wishes to plan care or write policies or standards of care for a patient problem can seek guidelines or cues for all aspects to be considered by consulting the nurse protocol consultant (NPC).

Development and initial testing of the system proceeded over a 7-year period. Early efforts at knowledge base validation and evaluation were focused on the quality and specificity of the goals and objectives, the relevance and currency of information in the learning resources provided (i.e., text books, journal articles, audiovisual materials) and the overall completeness of the information provided. The primary mechanism was the peer review process via the curriculum committee. There was considerable confidence in the consensual validation which was provided by comparing the textbook and media resources to the faculty member's goal definition and development of the objectives for instruction. On-site evaluation was provided by staff nurses who used the services in test settings. The computer printed out nurse inquiries and the system's responses. Inadequate responses were analyzed to determine whether the problems were rooted in semantic access to the knowledge base or to deficiencies in the knowledge base itself.

Major strengths inherent in the COMMES system are: (1) the reliability of the computerized consultant which consistently provides reliable information in response to

BSN PROGRAM CURRICULUM

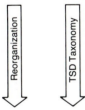

GENERALIST KNOWLEDGEBASE

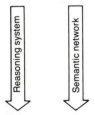

COMMES EXPERT CONSULTANTS IN NURSING

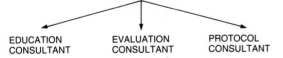

EDUCATION CONSULTANT   EVALUATION CONSULTANT   PROTOCOL CONSULTANT

FIGURE 1   Steps in developing the COMMES expert consultants in nursing.

questions and (2) the ability to continue to provide an updated knowledge base. The computerized consultant never sleeps, does not take sick days or vacations, and does not lower the quantity or quality of its output because of fatigue, illness or mood swings. It continues to produce reliable, regularly updated information.

The systematic procedure used by the computer expert provides a comprehensive cueing system that reviews pertinent factors for consideration and provides support to the human expert who must make the clinical decisions, often in less than optimal conditions. It is important to emphasize that the computer expert does not make the decisions or attempt to duplicate the experience, judgment, empathy or intuition of the professional nurse. It can however provide decision support through cueing the reader as to specific components of nursing care planning for consideration. See Box 1 for a protocol concerning the patient problem of insulin reactions.

PURPOSE

In order to evaluate the validity and usefulness of the output of a computerized expert consultant in nursing, approaches had to be devised which addressed the special com-

---

BOX 1: **Sample protocol for nursing care of the patient problem of insulin reactions**

Insulin reactions: describe manifestations of insulin reaction, time of occurrence, kind of insulin, and means used to treat insulin reaction and complications of insulin therapy

---

Clinical practice should incorporate or integrate the following:

1. The various kinds of insulin, indication for each, action onset, action peak and duration, and usual time and method of administration

Specific aspects of insulin might include:

protamine zinc insulin	globin zinc insulin	ultra lente insulin	nph insulin
semilente insulin	human insulin	regular insulin	lente insulin
isophane insulin			

Specific aspects of indication for insulin might include:

hypoinsulinism	hyposecretion of insulin	hyperglycemia

Specific aspects of insulin administration might include:

IV administration	injection	subcutaneous	subcutaneous
subcutaneous		injection	ous
injection			injection

Specific aspects of action might include:

action onset	action peak	action duration

2. Manifestations of insulin reaction, time of occurrence, kind of insulin, and means used to treat insulin reaction and complications of insulin therapy

Specific aspects of assessment of insulin reaction might include:

pallor	staggering gait	delirium	yawning
weakness	drowsiness	cold perspiration	headache
speech difficulty	oral paresthesia	tachycardia	coma
brain damage	seizure	confusion	tremor

plexities of a comprehensive nursing knowledge base while incorporating methods which have some established credibility. The methodology that follows was derived from the literature and consultation with experts in computer systems in nursing. The research question is: Does the NPC provide valid and useful information for planning nursing care and writing standards of care?

DEVELOPMENT OF CONCEPTS, DEFINITIONS, AND APPROACHES

Two key terms in testing and measurements for education, research and evaluation are reliability and validity. Sax (1980) describes re-

liability as the extent to which information (generally derived from tests or measurements) is consistent and dependable, not subject to random conditions or chance. As previously noted, computerized experts are highly reliable, consistently producing the appropriate information in response to the same question. For the purposes of this particular evaluation project, validity becomes the primary issue. The American Heritage Dictionary (1971) defines *validate* as "to substantiate or verify" and uses terms such as *well-grounded, sound* and *producing desired results*. Major types of validity pertinent to demonstrating the accuracy and usefulness

---

hyperkalemia	blurred vision	hypoglycemia	slurred speech
hunger	irritability	vasodilation	shock
bradycardia	paralysis	hypothermia	

Specific aspects of nursing diagnosis of insulin reaction might include:
nutritional deficit   impaired thought process   potential for injury

Specific aspects of desired outcome of insulin reaction might include:
normal blood sugar   alert and oriented   return to previous problem-solving
free from injury   free from seizure   ability

Specific aspects of intervention for insulin reaction might include:

half cup orange juice	1 tsp sugar	glucose paste	IV glucose
candy	50% dextrose IV	avoid excess exercise	solution
discuss cause	avoid alcohol	carry rapid-acting	IV or subcu-
high-protein and low-carbohydrate diet		carbohydrate	taneous gly-
		instruct for signs of	cogen
		hypolgycemia	

Specific aspects of intervention for insulin reaction might include:
discuss conditions that decrease insulin   check sleeping patient for diaphoresis
need   assess insulin administration tech-
diabetic identification tag   nique
assess compliance with therapy plan   administer glucocorticoid
treat shock

Specific aspects of complication of insulin therapy might include:

tissue hypertrophy	hypoglycemia	hyperglycemia	lipodystrophy
insulin allergy	insulin resistance	erratic insulin action	Somogyi effect

Specific aspects of insulin reaction might include:

hypoglycemia	insulin allergy	insulin shock	local reaction

of products of an expert computer system include content validity, face validity, and external validity. The internal validity of the research study itself is also of key concern.

Problems in developing accurate and complete knowledge in AI systems have been addressed by Suwa, Scott and Shortliffe (1982). The content expert may provide incomplete or erroneous information, or the information may be inadequately transferred to the computer representation. Spelling and syntax errors are also common.

CONTENT VALIDITY

Content validity refers to the ability of a measure or item of information to effectively relate to its goal or purpose. In testing, this refers to the extent to which items reflect the skills and competencies required by the stated objectives (Sax 1980). In nursing diagnosis, content validity can be established by determining whether the defining characteristics identified for a particular diagnosis actually occur and are representative of that condition as an entity in actual clinical practice (Fehring 1984, 1986). Content validity is commonly established through review of the literature and the use of a panel of experts (Fehring 1984, Miller, Pople and Myers 1982, Gordon and Sweeney 1979, Borg and Gall 1979).

For the purposes of this methodology, content validity is defined as the extent to which nurses with expertise in specific clinical practice domains find the output of the computerized expert system in nursing comparable to that of qualified human experts in that domain.

INTERNAL AND EXTERNAL VALIDITY

Internal validity pertains to the study design and conditions that control for potential sources of bias. *External validity* refers to the ability to generalize findings to the larger population (Borg and Gall 1979). Issues particularly pertinent to conditions in this study

include selection bias, testing effects and population validity.

Aspects of internal validity include: (1) selecting the patient problems to be used in the study on a random basis to assure a representative sample of the system's output, and (2) random presentation of the various protocol sets to the panel of evaluators. It is important to control for sources of bias such as evaluator fatigue based on consistent final placement of one set of items..

In order to promote external validity, the panel of experts selected to compare the output of the computer and human experts needs to be geographically dispersed and knowledgeable about the content domain to be evaluated. For the purposes of population validity, the panel of experts consists of geographically selected nurse educators (M.S.N. or higher degree) and clinicians (B.S.N. or M.S.N.) who are experienced in the domain of clinical patient care problems to be evaluated.

FACE VALIDITY

Face validity is described by Sax (1980) as the extent to which items appear relevant, important and interesting to the reviewer. In testing and measurement this is considered to be a secondary form of validity, since the importance or interest of items which are also lacking in accuracy, relevance or reliability does not increase their value. Conversely, items perceived to be trivial, unclear or irrelevant to the reviewer will not likely be taken seriously despite their empirical validity and reliability. Face validity is also pertinent to expressions of doubt as to whether the output of a machine can really be a valuable adjunct to human decision making.

The panel of quality assurance nurses provides a sample most similar to the nurse-consumer of the protocol consultant services. They are generalists rather than specialists in a specific content area and will look at the various protocols in all domains from the standpoint of their value in planning patient care and developing standards of care. This is face validity.

THE TURING TEST

A.M. Turing, an English mathematician, proposed that the output of a computer system be considered expert or intelligent if it could not be distinguished from the work of a competent human expert. The Turing Test has come to be considered an ideal criterion for acceptance of artificial intelligence expert systems. To apply this test, the output of both the computer and human experts will be typed so that the form of presentation does not indicate which is human and which machine generated. This protects against biases for or against computer systems in the panel of evaluators (Turing 1950, Chandrasekaran 1983). Both groups of nurse-evaluators, content experts and quality-assurance nurses, will compare the output of the human experts and the computer expert on ratings of usefulness, importance and relevance (face validity) as well as items related to content validity. These ratings will be compared for evidence of comparability or indistinguishability between the computer and human output in the study.

METHODS AND PROCEDURES

The study design involves:

1. *Content validity*—a geographically dispersed panel of nursing experts to compare sets of nursing protocols generated by the computer (NPC) with protocols written by educators (EDC) and clinical specialists (CSC) in selected content domains.
2. *Face validity*—a geographically dispersed panel of quality-assurance nurses will compare all sets of protocols written by the computer (NPC) and the educational (EDC) and the clinical (CSC) content experts.
3. *The Turing Test*—mean ratings of all

evaluators for each of the experts (NPC, EDC, and CSC) will be compared for indistinguishability.

PRELIMINARY PROCEDURES

The investigators selected three domains of patient problems for their breadth and common occurrence in practice: (1) gastrointestinal, (2) cardiovascular and (3) endocrine conditions. Chandrasekaran (1983) notes the importance of representational selection from the practice domain. Within each of these domains, three patient problems were selected for inclusion in the study. Random selection was employed to avoid biased sampling since the quantity and quality of a particular protocol may vary somewhat according to the skills and expertise of the faculty members who developed that section of the knowledge base.

An educator and a clinical specialist in each of the three content domains were selected on the basis of their expertise and geographic diversity. These human experts, who agreed to write protocols, were provided with format guidelines and examples to assist in developing the educator (EDC) and clinical-specialist (CSC) sets of protocols. Upon completion of these protocol sets there were three separate sets of expert protocols generated in each of the three content domains for three patient problems:

1. Gastrointestinal—pyloric stenosis, pancreatitis and cirrhosis
2. Cardiovascular—angina/arteriosclerotic heart disease, pericarditis and bacterial endocarditis
3. Endocrine—diabetes mellitus, hyperthyroidism and syndrome of inappropriate ADH secretion.

The investigators developed and piloted a Lickert Scale evaluation tool that asked respondents to compare each set of protocols on (1) specific items related to accuracy, comprehensiveness, relevance to practice and currency of information and (2) general items including usefulness, importance and relative preference ranking of the three experts in each category.

SAMPLE

The total panel for evaluation (N=105) is purposefully selected to meet criteria for geographic diversity, educational preparation and experience in a selected content domain or quality assurance. Nurse-educators (45) with a minimum of a master's degree in nursing and nurse-clinicians (45) with a minimum of a bachelor's degree in nursing will be selected on the basis of 2 years or more of experience focused on one of the three specific content domains (15 educators and 15 clinicians in the gastrointestinal, endocrine or cardiovascular domain). An additional group of quality-assurance nurses (N=15) with BSN preparation and 2 years experience will evaluate all three complete sets of protocols.

The sample was selected by contacting directors of over 200 NLN-accredited schools of nursing and 300 JCAH-accredited hospitals according to geographic region. The directors were acquainted with the criteria for selection of panel members and were asked to contact qualified nurses who would agree to be contacted to participate in the study. The final study population was drawn from these qualified volunteers.

ANALYSIS AND SIGNIFICANCE

An assessment of the return rate and a power analysis will be used to assure adequate sample size and estimate the probability of Type II error. Analysis of variance will be used to determine whether significant ($p. < .05$) differences exist in the panel of experts' ratings of the NPC and human-generated protocols. If significant differences in ratings are found in any categories, the category's summary preference ratings will indicate whether the NPC was preferred by the evaluators over the human experts.

Following statistical analysis of the study results, consultation will be obtained from a nursing expert in quality assurance and a computer systems expert (with extensive experience in nursing computer systems) to obtain recommendations for improving the content (nursing knowledge base) or process (computer system) of this expert computerized consultant in nursing. Miller, Pople and Myers (1982) note that once validation and system improvement of decision support experts have been accomplished, evaluation of actual system performance in clinical settings is appropriate.

If validity and usefulness can be demonstrated, there are significant implications for implementation and further research. Potential consumers could be given assurance of the system's accuracy and value. Further research could be developed to test cost effectiveness, time savings and quality of care issues related to actual use of the system in hospitals and other agencies. This would be of particular importance in the current health care milieu in which cost effectiveness and quality of care issues are pervasive concerns.

ACKNOWLEDGEMENTS

1. The authors wish to acknowledge the efforts of Steve Evans and the Office of Instructional Science Research in the development and ongoing implementation of the COMMES system.
2. The authors wish to also acknowledge the participation of Dr. Sam Schultz and Dr. Judy Ozbolt as consultants in the preliminary planning stages for this project. Their assistance was very helpful in defining issues and potential approaches.
3. A study using this methodology was funded by grant #1 R01 NU011279-01 by the Division of Nursing of the Department of Health and Human Services.

REFERENCES

American Heritage Dictionary New York, 1971, American Heritage Publishing.

Borg, W., and Gall, M.: Educational research, ed. 3, New York, 1979, Longman.

Chandrasekaran, B.: On evaluating AI systems for medical diagnosis, The AI Magazine, Summer: 34-37, 1983.

Fehring, R.: Validating diagnostic labels: standardized methodology. In Hurley, M.E. editor: Classification of nursing diagnoses: proceedings of the sixth national conference, St. Louis, 1984, The C.V. Mosby Co.

Gordon, M., and Sweeney, M.A.: Methodological problems and issues in identifying and standardizing nursing diagnoses, Adv. Nurs. Sci. **2:**1-15, 1979.

Miller, R., Pople, H., and Myers, J.: Internist I—an experimental computer-based diagnostic consultant for general internal medicine, New Engl. J. Med. **307:**468-476, 1982.

Ryan, S.: An expert system for nursing practice: clinical decision support. Comput. Nurs. **3:**77-84, 1985.

Sax, G.: Principles of evaluation and psychological measurement and evaluation, ed. 2, Belmont, Ca., 1980, Wadsworth.

Suwa, M., Scott, A., and Shortliffe, E.: An approach to verifying completeness and consistency in a rule-based expert system, AI Magazine **3:**16-21, 1982.

Turing, A.M.: Computing machinery and intelligence, Mind **59:**433-468, 1950.

Validation studies: poster presentations

Proportion of specific agreement as a measure of intrarater reliability in the diagnostic process

CATHY RODGERS WARD, M.S., R.N., C.C.R.N.

Reporting reliability is an important component in research often neglected in nursing studies (Goodwin and Prescott 1981). The reliability of a measurement such as identifying a nursing diagnosis concerns the extent to which the measuring procedure yields the same diagnosis on repeated trials. In nursing diagnosis research the most frequently reported method of calculating reliability is by interrater percentage of agreement (Kim, McFarland, and McLane, 1984). Interrater reliability for identifying nursing diagnoses ranges from zero to 100% (Castles 1982), however precise methods of calculating these figures are not often cited.

Intrarater reliability is another form of reliability in diagnostic methods not frequently utilized in nursing diagnosis research. Intrarater agreement measures the consistency with which a single rater classifies data using a specified measuring tool after rating the data on two separate occasions.

PURPOSE

The purpose of this study was to determine the reliability of identifying nursing diagnoses, or the extent to which one rater formulating nursing diagnoses from assessment data will formulate the same diagnoses from the same data at another time.

METHOD

Ten second-year graduate nursing students assessed a total of 50 adult patients with a known cardiovascular medical diagnosis. All participants had completed the same courses in nursing theory, clinical decision making, and clinical content. Participation in the study was voluntary and informed consent was obtained from each student.

Participants were instructed to utilize the Functional Health Pattern Assessment Tool (Gordon 1982) in collecting the data and to identify nursing diagnoses for each patient according to the North American Nursing Diagnosis Association (NANDA) accepted list of diagnoses (Kim, McFarland, and McLane 1984) and to note other diagnoses as appropriate. NANDA definitions, etiologies, and defining characteristics also served as guides for the identification of the diagnosis.

This study was conducted in two phases. At time one (T_1) each student assessed five patients for a total of 48 patient assessments (two patient assessments were rejected due to incomplete data). Diagnoses were listed on a separate sheet from the subjective and objective assessment data and the assessments were coded and numbered 1 through 5. Five months later at time two (T_2), the written assessment data (without the diagnoses) were returned to each student. The participants were then asked to review the written assessments performed at T_1 and identify diagnoses according to the NANDA list with the same approach utilized at T_1.

One potential concern with intrarater reliability has been that the first rating may affect the second rating (Waltz, Strickland, and Lanz 1981). Efforts to decrease the memory effect in this study included maximizing the length of time between T_1 and T_2 to 5 months and altering the order in which the patient assessments were reviewed at the second rating. A table of random numbers was used to place the five assessments in a random order and students reviewed the assessments in that sequence.

Diagnoses identified at T_1 and T_2 were compiled and compared to determine reliability. *Reliable* in this study meant agreement between the first and second assessment. Agreement could have referred to each nursing diagnosis, summing over the students, or to each student, summing over the diagnoses. The former method seems more relevant to determine the reliability of individual NANDA diagnoses.

METHODS OF DETERMINING AGREEMENT

Numerous methods of calculating agreement are available, but not all are applicable to all types of research. For example, one method of determining agreement would have been to compare the number of diagnoses identified at T_1 to the number of diagnoses identified at T_2 and report an overall percentage of agreement. While this approach may be accurate for certain observa-

tional research of repetitive behavior, it is not appropriate in this study, because the accuracy of interest is the identification of specific diagnoses. A student may have formulated five diagnoses at both T_1 and T_2 but the five diagnoses may not be identical, therefore this method is not specific to each diagnosis, could produce an inaccurate, high percentage of agreement, and is therefore not acceptable.

Another frequently used index of agreement divides the number of agreements by the number of agreements plus the number of disagreements. Figure 1 demonstrates diagnoses present or absent at T_1 and T_2. Figure 2 provides an example of this method for the diagnosis of Alteration of Tissue Perfusion. In this example there are two agreements that the diagnosis was present at both ratings and 42 agreements that the diagnosis was absent in both ratings. Using the following formula a 92% agreement was determined for this diagnosis:

$$\frac{\text{number of agreements}}{\text{number of agreements} + \text{number of disagreements}} = \frac{(a+d)}{(a+d) + (b+c)}$$

$$= \frac{2 + 42}{(2+42) + (1+3)} = \frac{44}{48} = .92 \text{ agreement}$$

In this study cell d, (the number of agreements that the diagnosis was absent) was likely to be large and therefore tended to inflate agreement. This method of calculating overall agreement is dependent upon the total number of observations made and has been utilized in other nursing diagnostic studies and found to overestimate reliability (Halloran 1985). It was therefore rejected as an approach to determining agreement in this study.

Fleiss (1981) proposed another approach which eliminates the inflationary trends connected to cell d. This method, termed the *proportion of specific agreement* (p_s) calculates reliability using only cells a, b, and c. It is not dependent on the total number of assessments made, but rather focuses on the probability of the diagnosis recurring at T_2. The formula for this method is:

$$p_s = \frac{2a}{2a + b + c} \text{ or } \frac{\text{reuse of the diagnosis}}{\substack{\text{average use} \\ \text{of the diagnosis}}}$$

T_2

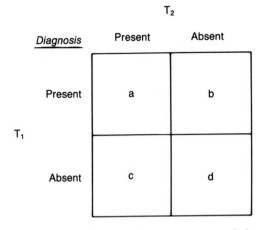

FIGURE 1 Determining agreement of diagnoses between ratings. a = diagnosis present in both assessments (T_1 and T_2); b = diagnosis present at T_1, absent at T_2; c = diagnosis absent at T_1, present at T_2; d = diagnosis absent in both assessments (T_1 and T_2).

T_2

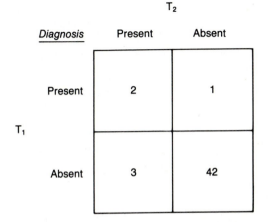

FIGURE 2 Agreement for the diagnosis of alteration in tissue perfusion

This method was selected to compute reliability in this study. Determining specific agreement for the diagnosis of Alteration in Tissue Perfusion (see Figure 2) with this approach would yield:

$$\frac{2 \times 2}{(2 \times 2) + 1 + 3} = \frac{4}{8} = .50 \text{ agreement}$$

An agreement of .50 for this diagnosis was determined using the proportion of specific agreement method as compared to .92 using the overall proportion of agreement frequently reported in nursing diagnosis research. Thus, the proportion of specific agreement method subjects the data to more rigorous tests of reliability than previously reported methods.

Diagnoses with agreements of .80 or better were considered to be "reliable." Agreements of .61 to .79 were considered marginal and diagnoses with agreements of .60 or less were considered unsatisfactory or unreliable.

RESULTS

Of the 51 NANDA diagnoses accepted for testing, 35 were found in this sample. Students identified a mean number of 4.81 ± 2.24 nursing diagnoses per patient at the first rating and 5.29 ± 2.02 diagnoses per patient at the second rating.

Table 1 lists the results of specific agreement computations for the 35 diagnoses. Seven diagnoses were found to be reliable, 11 diagnoses were marginal, and the remaining 17 diagnoses were unsatisfactory or unreliable in this study.

DISCUSSION

This study addressed the question of whether a nurse assessing the same patient at two different intervals will formulate consistent diagnoses while utilizing the NANDA defining characteristics and definitions. Findings demonstrate that certain diagnoses are more likely to be consistent than others, and therefore reliability indices

Table 1: Reliability of NANDA diagnoses identified

Reliable diagnoses		Unreliable diagnoses	
P_s	Diagnosis	.60	Sleep pattern disturbance
1.00	Powerlessness	.60	Health maintenance, alteration in
.90	Nutrition, alterations in: less than body requirements	.50	Self-concept, disturbance in
		.50	Social isolation
.86	Ineffective airway clearance	.50	Tissue perfusion, alteration in
.83	Knowledge deficit	.40	Skin integrity, impairment of: actual
.83	Nutrition, alterations in: more than body requirements	.40	Grieving, anticipatory
		.40	Coping, ineffective individual
.81	Activity intolerance	.40	Fear
.80	Urinary elimination, alteration in	.29	Self-care deficit
Marginal diagnoses		.29	Impaired mobility
.75	Impaired gas exchange	.29	Fluid volume excess
.75	Diversional activity deficit	.25	Coping, ineffective family: compromised
.73	Comfort, alteration in: pain	.20	Cardiac output, alteration in: decreased
.67	Injury, potential for	.00	Ineffective breathing pattern
.67	Non-compliance	.00	Spiritual distress
.67	Bowel elimination, alterations in: constipation	.00	Sensory perceptual alterations
.67	Family processes, alterations in		
.67	Sexual dysfunction		
.67	Thought processes, alterations in		
.67	Grieving, dysfunctional		
.63	Anxiety		

are variable for each diagnosis. The proportion of specific agreement method provided a stringent test for determining reliability. The problem of overestimated agreement commonly seen with traditional methods was avoided by eliminating the high number of agreements on absent diagnoses at both ratings.

Reliability is a necessary but not sufficient condition of validity. Consistency of a diagnosis over time contributes to its validity and can be interpreted to mean that those NANDA diagnoses found to be reliable are those most clearly delineated or understood by the nurse. Although the nurse used the same definitions and defining characteristics as guidelines for both ratings, agreement on

the presence of the diagnoses was low on 17 of the 35 diagnoses. This would indicate that some defining characteristics and definitions are not explicit to provide specific criteria for deciding if the diagnosis is present or absent. The diagnoses of fear and anxiety for example have many of the same defining characteristics which can confuse the diagnostician if the definitions are not distinctly stipulated.

It is interesting to note that the diagnostic label with the highest reliability (powerlessness) in this study does have a clearly delineated definition and specific defining characteristics. This diagnosis is a product of concept development by Miller (1984) from a theoretical perspective. Findings of this study support the need for further concept explication work on the nursing diagnostic labels currently proposed for clinical testing.

REFERENCES

Castles, M.: Interrater agreement in the use of nursing diagnosis. In Kim, M., and Mortiz, D., editors: Classification of nursing diagnoses: proceedings of the third and fourth national conferences. New York, 1982, McGraw Hill.

Fleiss, J.L.: Statistical methods for rates and proportions, New York, 1981, John Wiley & Sons.

Goodwin, L., and Prescott, P.: Issues and approaches to estimating interrater reliability in nursing research, Res. Nurs. Health, **4**:323-337, 1981.

Gordon, M.: Nursing diagnosis: process and application, New York, 1982, McGraw-Hill.

Halloran, E.J.: Nursing workload, medical diagnosis related groups, and nursing diagnoses, Res. Nurs. Health, **8**:421-433, 1985.

Kim, M., McFarland, G., and McLane, A.: Classification of nursing diagnoses: proceedings of the fifth national conference, St. Louis, 1984, The C.V. Mosby Co.

Kim, M., McFarland, G., and McLane, A.: Pocket guide to nursing diagnoses, St. Louis, 1984, The C.V. Mosby Co.

Miller, J.F.: Development and validation of a diagnostic label: powerlessness, In Kim, M.J., McFarland, G.K., and McLane, A.M., editors: Classification of nursing diagnoses: proceedings of the fifth national conference, St. Louis, 1984, The C.V. Mosby Co.

Waltz, C., Strickland, O., and Lenz, E.: Measurement in nursing research, Philadelphia, 1984, F.A. Davis.

Validation and identification of nursing diagnoses labels for psychiatric mental health nursing practice

GERTRUDE K. McFARLAND, D.N.Sc., R.N.
CHARLOTTE E. NASCHINSKI, M.S., R.N.

During the last decade, nursing diagnosis has become an increasingly significant step of the nursing process. The American Nurses' Association Congress for Nursing Practice included diagnosis in their definition of nursing: "Nursing is the diagnosis and treatment of human responses to actual or potential health problems" (1980 p. 9). The North American Diagnosis Association (NANDA) was formed to develop a taxonomy of nursing diagnoses for use by professional nurses. Since its inception in 1973, NANDA has promoted the development and refinement of this taxonomy through nursing research, education and practice. However, development of the nursing diagnosis statement continues to be identified as a problematic area in nursing practice. This is especially true for certain clinical specialty areas such as psychiatric mental health nursing practice.

Although in the holistic practice of nursing, any one or a combination of nursing diagnosis labels may have relevance for psychiatric mental health nursing practice, psychosocially oriented nursing diagnostic labels are more frequently used in this clinical specialty area. Psychiatric nurse experts are pointing out that the phenomena of concern for psychiatric nursing practice have not been identified completely.

STATEMENT OF PROBLEM AND PURPOSE

Between the First and the Sixth National Conferences on the Classification of Nursing Diagnoses, the identification and classification of the phenomena of concern for nursing practice has undergone significant revision. Nursing diagnosis labels have been altered deleted, or added. Psychiatric nurse experts are expressing concern that there are "gaps" in the currently developed NANDA list of nursing diagnostic labels. That is, the phenomena of concern for psychiatric mental health nursing practice have not been identified completely. In addition, psychiatric nurse experts have expressed concern about the clarity and usefulness of some of the nursing diagnoses currently identified by NANDA.

The purposes of this study are to:

1. Determine the degree of usefulness and clarity of meaning of selected nursing diagnostic labels currently accepted by NANDA for psychiatric nursing practice.
2. Identify alternate labels for those selected nursing diagnostic labels currently accepted by NANDA but found unclear or low in usefulness for psychiatric nursing practice.
3. Determine the degree of usefulness and clarity of selected nursing diagnostic labels proposed as, "to be developed," by NANDA or identified by psychiatric nurse experts in nursing literature.
4. Identify alternate labels for selected nursing diagnostic labels proposed to be developed by NANDA or identified by psychiatric nurse experts in nursing literature but found unclear or low in usefulness for psychiatric nursing practice.
5. Identify additional nursing diagnostic labels that are useful for psychiatric nursing practice.

METHODOLOGY

A descriptive study was conducted to determine professional judgments regarding the clarity of meaning and degree of usefulness of selected nursing-diagnosis labels for psychiatric and mental health nursing. The population consisted of 66 master's or doctorally prepared psychiatric nurses with 2 or more years of experience in psychiatric-mental health nursing. The response rate was 68% (N=45). Of the 45 respondents, 17.8% (N=8) were prepared at the doctoral level and 82.2% (N=37) were prepared at the master's level. All had in excess of 2 years of psychiatric-mental health nursing experience. All subjects were currently employed at the same large, federal, mental hospital and were involved in providing a wide range of treatment modalities and services to a variety of psychiatric clients. A survey tool was developed on which were listed selected nursing diagnostic labels relevant to psychiatric-mental health nursing practice that are accepted or proposed for further development by NANDA, as well as diagnostic labels identified in the literature and through research by the authors and other psychiatric nurse experts. The survey tool was piloted among members of a psychiatric nursing faculty in order to ensure its clarity. Using a 5-point Likert scale, respondents were asked to indicate the degree of usefulness of selected diagnostic labels. Respondents were also asked to indicate the clarity of each diagnostic label by checking "yes" or "no." In addition, the respondents were asked to identify alternate diagnostic labels and suggestions for improvement for any labels rated unclear or low in usefulness. The data generated from the survey tool were tabulated and reported in both raw numbers and percentages. Written suggestions for modifications, improvements or new labels were content analyzed and the data was summarized for each diagnostic label.

MAJOR FINDINGS AND IMPLICATIONS

The findings of the survey related to the clarity of meaning of the diagnostic labels are reported in Tables 1 and 2. Table 1 documents the number and percentage of respondents agreeing or disagreeing with the clarity of meaning of each nursing-diagnosis label. The NANDA accepted nursing diagnoses (see Table 2, *Column 1*) and the nursing-diagnosis labels identified by the Authors and other psychiatric nurse experts (Table 2—*Column 2*) are rank ordered in Table 2. Ninety percent or more of the respondents agreed that the meanings of five of the 12 nursing-diagnosis labels identified by psychiatric nurse experts (depressive mood; suicide, threatened or attempted; suspiciousness; hyperactive behavior; regressive behavior) were clear in meaning. None of the nursing-diagnosis labels accepted by NANDA were viewed as clear in meaning by 90% or more of the respondents. Between 80 and 89% of the respondents agreed that the meaning was clear for 15 out of 19 NANDA accepted nursing-diagnosis labels and six of the 12 nursing-diagnosis labels identified by psychiatric nurse experts. Four NANDA accepted labels and one label identified by psychiatric nurse experts fell below 80%.

The findings of the survey related to the degree of usefulness of the nursing diagnoses labels for psychiatric-mental health nursing practice are reported in Tables 3 and 4. Ninety percent or more of the respondents rated three of the 12 labels identified by psychiatric nurse experts to be moderately to very useful for psychiatric-mental health nursing (Table 4). None of the nursing-diagnosis labels identified by NANDA were rated as moderately to very useful for psychiatric-mental health nursing by 90 percent or more of the respondents. Between 80 and 89% of the respondents rated eight of the 12 labels identified by psychiatric nurse experts to be moderately to very useful for psychi-

Table 1: Clarity of meaning

		Is this diagnosis clear in meaning?				
	Yes		No		No response	
Nursing diagnosis label	N	%	N	%	N	%
Aggressive behavior	38	84.4	6	13.3	1	2.2
*Anxiety	38	84.4	7	15.6	0	0
Communication, impaired	38	84.4	6	13.3	1	2.2
*Coping, ineffective individual	39	86.7	5	11.1	1	2.2
Crisis: maturational, situational	35	77.8	10	22.2	0	0
Denial, ineffective	38	84.4	7	15.6	0	0
Depressive mood	42	93.3	2	4.4	1	2.2
*Diversional activity, deficit	40	88.9	4	8.9	1	2.2
*Family process, alteration in	29	64.4	15	33.3	1	2.2
*Fear	37	82.2	6	13.3	2	4.4
*Grieving, anticipatory	40	88.9	5	11.1	0	0
*Grieving, dysfunctional	38	84.4	7	15.6	0	0
*Health maintenance, alteration in	32	71.1	12	26.7	1	2.2
Hyperactive behavior	41	91.1	3	6.7	1	2.2
*Knowledge deficit	38	84.4	7	15.6	0	0
Manipulation	36	80	8	17.8	1	2.2
*Non-compliance	35	77.8	7	15.6	3	6.7
*Parenting, alteration in: actual or potential	37	82.2	7	15.6	1	2.2
*Powerlessness	39	86.7	5	11.1	1	2.2
*Rape trauma syndrome	40	88.9	3	6.7	2	4.4
Regressive behavior	41	91.1	3	6.7	1	2.2
Ritualistic behavior	37	82.2	8	17.8	0	0
*Self-concept, disturbance in: body image, self-esteem, role performance personal identity	39	86.7	5	11.1	1	2.2
*Sensory-perceptual alteration: visual, auditory, kinesthetic, gustatory, tactile, olfactory	39	86.7	5	11.1	1	2.2
*Sexual dysfunction	36	80	7	15.6	2	4.4
*Social isolation	34	75.6	9	20	2	4.4
Substance misuse (drug or alcohol)	40	88.9	4	8.9	1	2.2
Suicide, threatened or attempted	42	93.3	2	4.4	1	2.2
Suspiciousness	42	93.3	2	4.4	1	2.2
*Thought processes, alteration in	38	84.4	6	13.3	1	2.2
*Violence, potential for: self-directed or directed at others	36	80	8	17.8	1	2.2

*Nursing-diagnosis labels accepted as of the sixth national conference.

Table 2: Degree of clarity by rank order

Column 1 NANDA accepted nursing-diagnosis labels	Column 2 Nursing-diagnosis labels identified by psychiatric nurse experts
Diversional activity, deficit (88.9%);	Depressive mood (93.3%);
Grieving, anticipatory (88.9%);	Suicide, threatened or attempted (93.3%);
Rape trauma syndrome (88.9%);	Suspiciousness (93.3%):
Coping, ineffective individual (86.7%):	Hyperactive behavior (91.1%);
Powerlessness (86.7%):	Regressive behavior (91.1%);
Self-concept, disturbance in (86.7%);	Substance misuse (89.9%);
Sensory perceptual alteration in (86.9%);	Aggressive behavior (84.4%);
Anxiety (84.4%):	Communication, impaired (84.4%):
Grieving, dysfunctional (84.4%):	Denial, ineffective (84.4%)
Knowledge deficit (84.4%);	Ritualistic behavior (82.2%);
Thought processes, alteration in (84.4%):	Manipulation (80%);
Fear (82.2%):	Crisis: maturational, situational (77.8%).
Parenting, alteration in (82.2%);	
Sexual dysfunction (80%);	
Violence, potential for (80%);	
Non-compliance (77.8%):	
Social isolation (75.6%):	
Health maintenance, alteration in (71.1%);	
Family process, alteration in (64.4%).	

atric nursing practice (Table 4). Fourteen out of 19 nursing diagnostic labels identified by NANDA were rated as moderately to very useful for psychiatric mental health nursing by 80 to 89% of the respondents (Table 4).

Seventy to 79% of the respondents rated one out of 12 labels identified by psychiatric nurse experts to be moderately to very useful for psychiatric-mental health nursing (See Table 4). Five of the 19 nursing-diagnosis labels identified by NANDA were rated as moderately to very useful for psychiatric-mental health nursing by 70 to 79% of the respondents (Table 4).

The four NANDA labels found to be most unclear in meaning (supported by 79% or less of the respondents) were: non-compliance; social isolation; health main-

tenance, alteration in; family process, alteration in. No alternative labels were identified by the respondents for non-compliance.

Several respondents considered non-compliance to be a negative labeling of patient behavior which may result from not listening to the patient or identifying what the patient is capable of accomplishing. Non-compliance may also imply that the patient is deviant if he or she makes a decision that differs from the nurse's expectation.

An alternate label suggested for family process, alteration in is "family process, alteration in coping." Respondents suggested that alteration in family process does not necessarily imply alteration in effective functioning.

Table 3: Degree of usefulness

	No response		0 Of no use		1		2 Moderately useful		3		4 Very useful		5	
Nursing-diagnosis label	N	%	N	%	N	%	N	%	N	%	N	%	N	%
Aggressive behavior	2	4.4	0	0	0	0	3	6.7	9	20	15	33.3	16	35.6
*Anxiety	2	4.4	0	0	1	2.2	4	8.9	7	15.6	14	31.1	17	37.8
Communication, impaired	3	6.7	0	0	0	0	1	2.2	13	28.9	15	33.3	13	28.9
*Coping, ineffective individual	4	8.9	0	0	2	4.4	1	2.2	7	15.6	18	40	13	28.9
Crisis maturational, situational	4	8.9	0	0	3	6.7	4	8.9	4	8.9	14	31.1	16	35.6
Denial, ineffective	4	8.9	2	4.4	0	0	3	6.7	7	15.6	11	24.4	18	40
Depressive mood	2	4.4	0	0	1	2.2	0	0	3	6.7	15	33.3	24	53.3
*Diversional activity, deficit	1	2.2	3	6.7	2	4.4	0	0	10	22.2	10	22.2	19	42.2
*Family process, alteration in	5	11.1	1	2.2	1	2.2	3	6.7	9	20	9	20	17	37.8
*Fear	3	6.7	1	2.2	1	2.2	2	4.4	7	15.6	13	28.9	18	40
*Grieving, anticipatory	2	4.4	1	2.2	1	2.2	3	6.7	5	11.1	9	20	24	53.3
*Grieving, dysfunctional	2	4.4	0	0	1	2.2	4	8.9	7	15.6	12	26.7	19	42.2
*Health maintenance, alteration in	2	4.4	1	2.2	4	8.9	4	8.9	12	26.7	7	15.6	15	33.3
Hyperactive behavior	2	4.4	0	0	1	2.2	0	0	3	6.7	16	35.6	23	51.1
*Knowledge deficit	2	4.4	0	0	0	0	4	8.9	8	17.8	12	26.7	19	42.2
Manipulation	3	6.7	0	0	3	6.7	2	4.4	9	20	9	20	19	42.2
*Non-compliance	7	15.6	0	0	2	4.4	3	6.7	8	17.8	12	26.7	13	28.9
*Parenting, alteration in: actual or potential	4	8.9	1	2.2	1	2.2	3	6.7	15	33.3	7	15.6	14	31.1
*Powerlessness	5	11.1	1	2.2	0	0	2	4.4	8	17.8	12	26.7	17	37.8
*Rape trauma syndrome	5	11.1	0	0	0	0	2	4.4	3	11.1	14	31.1	19	42.2
Regressive behavior	6	13.3	0	0	1	2.2	0	0	4	8.9	10	22.2	24	53.3
Ritualistic behavior	3	6.7	1	2.2	2	4.4	2	4.4	4	8.9	10	22.2	23	51.1

*Nursing-diagnosis labels accepted at the sixth national conference.

Table 3: Degree of usefulness—cont'd

Nursing-diagnosis label	What is the degree of usefulness of the nursing-diagnosis label for psychiatric nursing?												
	No response		0 Of no use		1		2 Moderately useful		3		4 Very useful		5
	N	%	N	%	N	%	N	%	N	%	N	%	N	%
*Self-concept, disturbance in: body image, self-esteem, role performance, personal identity	4	8.9	2	4.4	0	0	1	2.2	8	17.8	13	28.9	17	37.8
*Sensory-perceptual alternation: visual, auditory, kinesthetic, gustatory, tactile, olfactory	4	8.9	2	4.4	0	0	0	0	13	28.9	9	20	17	37.8
*Sexual dysfunction	5	11.1	2	4.4	1	2.2	2	4.4	9	20	8	17.8	18	40
*Social isolation	6	13.3	2	4.4	2	4.4	1	2.2	3	6.7	16	35.6	15	33.3
Substance misuse, drug or alcohol	6	13.3	0	0	0	0	2	4.4	6	13.3	8	17.8	23	51.1
Suicide, threatened or attempted	4	8.9	0	0	0	0	1	2.2	5	11.1	7	15.6	28	62.2
Suspiciousness	5	11.1	1	2.2	0	0	1	2.2	2	4.4	11	24.4	25	55.6
*Thought processes, alteration in	4	8.9	1	2.2	1	2.2	2	4.4	6	13.3	9	20	22	48.9
*Violence potential for: self-directed, or directed at others	6	13.3	0	0	1	2.2	2	4.4	4	8.9	9	20	23	51.1

*Nursing-diagnosis labels accepted at the sixth national conference.

An alternate label suggested for social isolation is withdrawal. The current definition of social isolation is, "condition of aloneness experienced by the individual and perceived as imposed by others and as a negative state" (Kim, McFarland, and McLane 1984, p. 56). Several respondents commented on the fact that at times social isolation is self-imposed and not necessarily perceived as negative.

An alternate label suggested for health maintenance, alteration in is "health maintenance, dysfunctional." Several respondents commented that "alteration" suggests change that can be either positive or negative. More specificity is needed in this label.

The five NANDA labels found to be least useful (supported by 79% or less of the respondents) were family process, alteration

Table 4: Degree of usefulness by clusters

Percentage of respondents	NANDA accepted nursing-diagnosis labels	Nursing-diagnosis labels identified by psychiatric nurse experts
90–100%		Communication, impaired
		Depressive mood
		Hyperactive behavior
80–89%	Anxiety	Aggressive behavior
	Coping, ineffective individual	Denial, ineffective
	Diversional activity, deficit	Manipulation
	Fear	Regressive behavior
	Grieving, anticipatory	Ritualistic behavior
	Grieving, dysfunctional	Substance misuse
	Knowledge deficit	Suicide, threatened or attempted
	Parenting, alteration in: actual or potential	Suspiciousness
	Powerlessness	
	Rape trauma syndrome	
	Self-concept, disturbance in	
	Sensory perceptual alteration	
	Thought processes, alteration in	
	Violence, potential for	
70–79%	Family process, alteration in	Crisis: maturational, situational
	Health maintenance, alteration in	
	Non-compliance	
	Sexual dysfunction	
	Social isolation	

in; health maintenance, alteration in; non-compliance; sexual dysfunction; social isolation. Except for sexual dysfunction, these labels are the same as those found most unclear in meaning by the respondents.

Several respondents commented that the label, "sexual dysfunction," is too broad in scope. It was suggested that this diagnosis label needs subdiagnoses; one such suggested subdiagnosis is, "sexual identity disturbance."

The one label identified by psychiatric nurse experts found to be most unclear (supported by 79% or less of the respondents) was crisis: maturational, situational. No alternate label was offered. However, respondents suggested the separation of maturational from situational crisis with separate definitions for both. In addition, the label "crisis: maturational, situational" was the only label that was supported by 79% or less in relation to its usefulness.

Additional nursing diagnostic labels suggested by the respondents as useful for psychiatric nursing practice were:
• Withdrawn behavior
• Impulsiveness
• Institutionalization

- Dependency
- Passivity
- Euphoric mood
- Underactive behavior
- Interpersonal relationship, inability to establish
- Bizarre behavior
- Guilt, exaggerated
- Control, ineffective individual
- Affect, inappropriate
- Trust dysfunctions
- Judgment, impaired

RECOMMENDATIONS

After consideration of the findings of this study, the following recommendations are made:

1. That the study be replicated utilizing a national sample of psychiatric nurse experts.
2. That studies be designed to identify the etiologies and defining characteristics of the newly identified nursing-diagnosis labels for psychiatric-mental health nursing.

REFERENCES

American Nurses' Association: Nursing: a social policy statement, Kansas City, MO, 1980, American Nurses' Association.

Balistrieri, T., and Jiricka, M.: Validation of a nursing diagnosis: role disturbance. In Kim, M.J., McFarland, G.K., and McLane, A.M., editors: Classification of nursing diagnoses: proceedings of the fifth national conference, St. Louis, 1984, The C.V. Mosby Co.

Jones, P., and Jakob, D.: Anxiety revisited—from a practice perspective. In Kim, M.J., McFarland, G.K., and McLane, A.M., editors: Classification of nursing diagnoses: proceedings of the fifth national conference, St. Louis, 1984, The C.V. Mosby Co.

Luetje, V., and McSweeney, M.: Nursing diagnoses of abusive patients. In Kim, M.J., McFarland, G.K., and McLane, A.M., editors: Classification of nursing diagnoses: proceedings of the fifth national conference, St. Louis, 1984, The C.V. Mosby Co.

McFarland, G.K., and Naschinski, C.: Impaired communication: a descriptive study, Nurs. Clin. North Amer. **20:**775-785, 1985.

McFarland, G.K., and Naschinski, C.: Communication pattern. In Thompson, J., McFarland, G.K., Hirsch, J., and others, editors: Clinical nursing, St. Louis, 1986, The C.V. Mosby Co.

McFarland, G.K., and Naschinski, C.: Inappropriate aggression, dysfunctional grieving, and anticipatory grieving: a descriptive study. In Hurley, M.E., editor: Classification of nursing diagnoses: proceedings of the sixth conference, St. Louis, 1986, The C.V. Mosby Co.

McFarland, G.K., and Wasli, E.: Psychiatric nursing. In Brunner, L., and Suddarth, D.: The Lippincott manual of nursing practice, Philadelphia, 1982, J.B. Lippincott.

McFarland, G.K., and Wasli, E.: Nursing diagnosis and process in psychiatric mental health nursing. Philadelphia, J.B. Lippincott. (In press.)

Mills, W.: Alienation: a basic concept underlying social isolation. In Kim, M.J., McFarland, G.K., and McLane, A.M., editors: Classification of nursing diagnoses: proceedings of the fifth national conference, St. Louis, 1984, The C.V. Mosby Co.

Validation of the nursing diagnosis, spiritual distress

JUDI WEATHERALL, M.S., R.N.
NANCY S. CREASON, Ph.D., R.N.

Illness, suffering, and death affect a person's biological, psychosocial, and spiritual selves. To understand and identify the spiritual manifestations of such crises on clients, nurses must have knowledge about the spirit of a person and what are valid cues to spiritual distress.

PURPOSE

The purpose of this study was to begin to validate the defining characteristics of the diagnosis *spiritual distress*, as accepted by NANDA, through a content analysis of nursing literature and patient data.

REVIEW OF LITERATURE

Stallwood and Stoll (1975) proposed that man has a spiritual core that strives to establish and maintain a relationship with a god that the individual defines. As man experiences positive and negative life events, his spirit emits psychosocial and biological cues about the impact of these events on his relationship with his deity. Frankl (1975) described the human spirit as a core surrounded by the psychological and physical aspects of man that seeks purpose and meaning in life. Dickinson (1975) defined the spirit as "animating," "intangible," and giving "liveliness to the physical organism as well as the literal breath of life" (p. 1790).

Stallwood and Stoll (1975) defined spiritual needs as "any factors necessary to establish and maintain a person's dynamic personal relationship with God (as defined by that individual)" (p. 1088). Frankl (1963) noted that "a man's concern, even his despair, over the worthwhileness of his life is a spiritual distress" (p. 104). NANDA defined spiritual distress as "a disruption in the life principle that pervades a person's entire being and that integrates and transcends one's biologic and psychosocial nature" (Kim, McFarland, and McLane 1984b, p. 57).

METHODOLOGY

Articles on spirituality, spiritual needs or care and religious needs or care were identified in the *Cumulative Index to Nursing and Allied Health Literature* and in a bibliography on spiritual distress (Kim, McFarland, and McLane 1984a, pp. 509-510). Each article retained for the project was written by a professional nurse or a student in a professional nursing program, published in a nursing publication and contained cues to spiritual distress. Thirty-four articles met these criteria and appeared in print from 1959 to 1984.

Data on 13 patients came from assessments in which registered nurses diagnosed a patient as being in spiritual distress. Appropriate permission to use the data was obtained. The patients were hospitalized in two different hospitals in the Midwestern United States and included seven women and six men. Women ranged in age from 24 to 92 years and men ranged from 22 to 80 years with a mean age of 46.8 years.

Content analysis was used on the nursing literature and patient data. The articles were reviewed for cues to indicate that a patient had spiritual needs or required spiritual care, since none of the articles used the term *spiritual distress*, but described conditions similar to spiritual distress. Cues from the articles and patients were compared to 24 NANDA defining characteristics. The seven descriptors of "alteration in behavior and mood" were counted as individual characteristics and there were 17 other NANDA characteristics. Frequencies and percentages were calculated on the cues, articles, and patients that supported each characteristic or suggested other characteristics of spiritual distress.

RESULTS

The nursing literature yielded 379 cues, of which 228 cues (60%) supported 22 NANDA defining characteristics with a range of one (0.3%) to 39 cues (10%) per characteristic. The 22 characteristics were supported by one (3%) to 18 articles (53%). No cues supported the NANDA characteristics of "preoccupation" and "denies responsibilities for problems." The remaining 151 cues (40%) suggested other defining characteristics.

Patient data yielded 85 cues. Fifty-three cues (62%) supported 18 NANDA characteristics with a range of 1 (1%) to 12 cues (14%). From one (8%) to five patients (38%) experienced these characteristics. No cues supported the NANDA characteristics of "seeks spiritual assistance," "questions moral and ethical implications of therapeutic regimen," "anxiety," "apathy," "does not experience that God is forgiving," and "description of somatic complaints." The remaining 32 cues (38%) suggested other defining characteristics.

The data supported a large number of characteristics. It was decided that the literature suggested validity when a characteristic was supported by 5% or more of the cues and/or 25% or more of the articles. Patient data suggested validity when a characteristic was supported by 5% or more of the cues and/or 25% or more of the patients. Characteristics supported by both the literature and patient data in the manner described above were considered the most valid. Three NANDA characteristics and two others met these latter criteria and can be seen in Table 1.

The literature supported four additional NANDA characteristics and two others, while support from patient data for these characteristics was minimal. See Table 2.

Patient data supported two additional NANDA characteristics and one other. These were mildly supported by the literature and can be seen in Table 3.

In addition, the seven characteristics most strongly supported by the patient data were analyzed to see whether there were differences in each characteristic related to sex or age. Table 4 shows these differences in the experience of spiritual distress.

Table 1: Defining characteristics supported by the nursing literature and patient data

Characteristic	% of literature cues	% of articles	% of patient cues	% of patients
Questions meaning of suffering*	7	53	14	38
Verbalizes concern about relationship with deity*	10	47	6	38
Verbalizes inner conflict about beliefs*	7	35	6	23
Hopelessness	5	32	11	46
Cues having to do with relationships with others	5	35	7	31

*NANDA defining characteristics

Table 2: Defining characteristics supported by nursing literature with minimal support from patient data

Characteristic	% of literature cues	% of articles	% of patient cues	% of patients
Seeks spiritual assistance*	5	35	0	0
Questions meaning for own existence*	5	35	4.7	15
Expresses concern with meaning of life and death and/or belief systems*	4	32	1	8
Anxiety*	4	27	0	0
Guilt feelings	5	38	0	0
Fear	5	29	0	0

*NANDA defining characteristics

Table 3: Defining characteristics supported by patient data with mild support from the nursing literature

Characteristic	% of patient cues	% of patients	% of literature cues	% of articles
Crying*	7	38	1	12
Unable to choose or chooses not to participate in usual religious practices*	7	31	2	12
Inadequate coping	11	8	0	0

*NANDA defining characteristics

Table 4: Sex- and age-related differences in spiritual distress demonstrated by patient data

Characteristic	Patients experiencing characteristic		Ages or age range
Questions meaning of suffering*	Men:	1	58 yrs.
	Women:	4	28 to 34 yrs.
Verbalizes concern about relationship with deity*	Men:	1	35 yrs.
	Women:	4	28 to 58 yrs.
Verbalizes inner conflict about beliefs*	Men:	0	0
	Women:	3	28 to 34 yrs.
Crying*	Men:	3	58 to 80 yrs.
	Women:	2	24 & 29 yrs.
Unable to choose or chooses not to participate in usual religious practices*	Men:	2	56 & 62 yrs.
	Women:	2	58 & 92 yrs.
Hopelessness	Men:	4	28 to 80 yrs.
	Women:	2	28 & 58 yrs.
Cues have to do with relationships with others	Men:	3	22 to 80 yrs.
	Women:	1	58 yrs.

*NANDA defining characteristics

DISCUSSION

Study limitations include the non-randomness and small size of the patient sample, and that the data analysis was a secondary analysis. The content analysis was a subjective process, which may affect reliability.

The data suggest that five characteristics are the most valid and clinically useful, (Table 1). Three of these are NANDA characteristics, but "hopelessness" and "cues having to do with relationships with others" are not presently listed as defining characteristics of spiritual distress.

A framework of spiritual distress is needed to link these five characteristics. It is proposed that suffering be added as a major etiology to spiritual distress. When suffering is intense or prolonged, the client's spirit seeks purpose, meaning, and hope in his experience. The person may find spiritual strength or hope in relationships with a diety, self, or with others. If spiritual strength cannot be found through these relationships, the person experiences spiritual distress or even hopelessness, the ultimate spiritual distress.

The study highlights several issues. One is why the literature supports characteristics of spiritual distress that were not seen in the patient data. Does this reflect the particular patients in the sample and their cues to spiritual distress, or can nurses describe the cues but not connect them with spiritual distress in clinical practice? Another issue is what to do with the observed differences in spiritual distress between men and women in various ages. Will nursing need defining characteristics for each sex in different adult developmental stages? These issues need to be explored with further research.

REFERENCES

Dickinson, C.: The search for spiritual meaning, Amer. J. Nurs. **75:**1789-1793, 1975.

Frankl, V.E.: Man's search for meaning: an introduction to logotherapy, New York, 1963, Washington Square Press.

Frankl, V.E.: The unconscious god: psychotherapy and theology, New York, 1975, Simon and Schuster.

Kim, M.J., McFarland, G.K., and McLane, A.M., editors: Classification of nursing diagnoses: proceedings of the fifth national conference, St. Louis, 1984, The C.V. Mosby Company.

Kim, M.J., McFarland, G.K., and McLane, A.M.: editors: Pocket guide to nursing diagnoses, St. Louis, 1984, The C.V. Mosby Co.

Stallwood, J., and Stoll, R.: Spiritual dimensions of nursing practice. In Beland, I.L., Passos, J.Y., editors: Clinical nursing: pathophysiological and psychosocial approaches, New York, 1975, McMillan.

Hopelessness and its defining characteristics

SUZANNE C. BEYEA, M.S.N., R.N.
DEBORAH D. PETERS, M.S.N., R.N.

The development of a nursing taxonomy is an attempt to describe those phenomena observed by nurses on a daily basis. One such phenomenon is hopelessness. To date the term seems to represent a wide variety of interpretations, but among nurses it lacks precision. The purposes of this research were to define the term *hopelessness,* and to identify those defining characteristics most frequently used when using the category in clinical practice.

REVIEW OF LITERATURE

Hopelessness, the loss of hope, is an elusive concept often best understood when the entity of hope is explored. "Hope is in essence a psychic commitment to life and growth" (Skolny and Riew 1974, p. 208-209). An individual with hope possesses the knowledge and feeling that life's stressful events can be dealt with and will have an optimistic conclusion (Lynch 1965). Hope is a powerful coping mechanism which is used to ward off despair (Korner 1970). In a healthy person, hope facilitates self-restorative activities and has a soothing effect on a person, creating in him or her a sense of power and control in dealing with life's stressors.

Korner (1970) describes three components of hope, the purpose of hope, the emotional commitment to hope, and the dynamic rationalizing chain of hope. The purpose of hope is to hypothesize future gratification so as to ward off hopelessness. The affective component of hope or the emotional commitment to hope is often captured in the conceptualization of a person "clinging to hope".

The last component of hope is represented by a dynamic rationalizing chain of events consisting of reality, hope, logic and reasoning. This process permits the individual to continuously receive input from the environment, interpret it in an organized, self-protective manner, and respond appropriately to the stimulus.

Hopelessness, on the other hand, is based on a conviction that there is nothing to hope for and that the future is bleak (Korner 1970). The individual becomes trapped in the present and loses sight of the future if the future considered is too fraught with impossibility and dread (Schneider 1980; Lynch 1965).

The concept of hopelessness is thought to be "rooted in a structure of thought, feeling, and action that is rigid and inflexible" (Lynch 1965, p. 31). A sense of hope is thought to develop in early childhood as a result of successful resolution between parental trust and mistrust (Erikson 1964). When a lack of trust is present in early childhood experiences, the child's coping strategies become less effective, rendering the individual vulnerable to hopelessness.

According to the literature, individuals displaying hopeless behavior exhibit various characteristics. Lange (1978) and Fromm (1968) have outlined these responses (Table 1), while Gottschalk (1974) and Engel (1968) have developed themes that they feel are exhibited by persons displaying hopelessness (Table 2).

Although hopelessness is discussed in the literature, it has not yet been described in terms of a diagnostic category. This research is an attempt to contribute to the growing body of knowledge so that the phenomenon can be used more effectively in clinical practice.

METHODOLOGY

Subjects for the study consisted of a convenience sample of 100 nursing diagnosis experts, who were master's prepared and had studied nursing theory and process within the diagnostic framework as presented by Marjorie Gordon. Each subject was asked to complete a questionnaire in which each defining characteristic was rated according to its degree of reliability in formulating the diagnosis of hopelessness. The defining characteristics used were found in the literature and were thought to best describe the concept. Hopelessness was defined as an emotional state displaying the sense of impossibility, the feeling that life is too much to handle, apathy, when one is resigned to fate.

DATA ANALYSIS

Descriptive statistics were used to analyze the data. Fifteen defining characteristics were rated on a Likert scale of one through five (with one being "very characteristic" and five being "not at all characteristic"). Only three defining characteristics were rated as either very or quite characteristic of the diagnosis by 85% or more of the sample. These defining characteristics included feelings of emptiness, pessimism, and the expression of feeling overwhelmed.

Four additional defining characteristics were rated as very or quite characteristic by 75% to 84% of the sample. These are included in Table 3.

Defining characteristics that were rated as very or quite characteristic by 65% to 74% of the sample were social withdrawal, expression of vulnerability, sense of entrapment, and a sense of incompetence. While lack of gratification from roles and relationships and feelings of irritability and tension were rated by 65% or less of the population as very or quite characteristic.

DISCUSSION

Through data analysis it is apparent that there is a group of defining characteristics that have high face and content reliability for the nursing diagnosis of hopelessness. However, within the context of this study there is

Table 1: Responses to the loss of hope

Investigator	Response indicating hopelessness
Lange	Hypoactivation: "empty, drained" General psychological discomfort: "loss, deprivation" Social withdrawal: emotional distress Sense of incompetence: vulnerability, helplessness
Fromm	Resignation to fate Social isolation, withdrawal Destructiveness

Table 2: Consistent themes of individuals displaying hopelessness

Researcher	Theme
Gottschalk	Not being a recipient of good fortune Not receiving help or esteem from others Pessimism Lack of ambition or interest
Engel	Feeling at the end of one's rope Loss of gratification in roles and relationships Sense of discontinuity between past, present and future Recalling past helplessness

Table 3: Defining characteristics rated very or quite characteristic by 75% to 84% of the sample

Defining characteristic	% very or quite characteristic
Sense of loss, deprivation	76
Lack of interest or ambition	78
Sense of impossibility	82
Expression of helplessness	80

also a group of defining characteristics that do not reliably and consistently predict this diagnosis.

One consideration of these findings must be that the concept of hopelessness may indeed be so abstract that it is, in fact, a conceptual category within which lie several additional diagnoses. These diagnoses have yet to be described, but may more accurately be the descriptors of phenomena, or be defining characteristics or etiologies for other phenomena yet to be defined.

Another explanation of the results may in fact be that hopelessness is a term often used in the literature, but less frequently described by nurses in practice. Increased sophistication with the use of the diagnostic process in addition to defining and looking at etiologies for hopelessness may help refine the category.

IMPLICATIONS

This study explored the concept of hopelessness and its defining characteristics. The results indicated a specific group of defining characteristics felt to be exhibited by persons displaying hopelessness.

Further research is needed to explore and refine both the category and defining characteristics of hopelessness, as well as the investigation of both the concepts of hope and hopelessness. Nurses have been cited as providers of realistic hope to patients and clients, however there are only a few studies addressing this concept. Despite this very limited study, it is apparent to the researchers that hopelessness is a condition seen and treated by nurses and one that needs recognition and more effective interventions.

REFERENCES

Engel, G.L.: A life setting conducive to illness: the giving up—given up complex, Ann. Intern. Med. **69:** 293-300, 1968.

Erikson, E.: Childhood and society, ed. 2, New York, 1964, W.W. Norton and Co.

Fromm, E.: The revolution of hope, New York, 1968, Harper and Row.

Gottschalk, L.A.: A hope scale applicable to verbal samples, Arch. Gen. Psych. **30:**779-785, 1974.

Korner, I.N.: Hope as a method of coping, J. Consult. Clin. Psychol. **34:**134-139, 1970.

Lange, S.: Hope. In C.E., Carlson, and B., Blackwell, editors: Behavioral Concepts and Nursing Intervention, Philadelphia, 1978, J.B. Lippincott.

Lynch, W.F.: Images of hope, Baltimore, 1965, Helicon Press.

Miller, J.F.: Inspiring hope, Amer. J. Nurs. **85:**22-25, 1985.

Rothlis, J.: The effect of self group on feeling of hopelessness and helplessness, West. J. Nurs. Res. **6:**157-167, 1984.

Schneider, J.S.: Hopelessness and helplessness. J. Psych. Nurs. Mental Health Serv. **3:**12-21, 1980.

Skolny, M.A., Riew, J.P.: Hope: solving patient and family problems by using a theoretical framework. In Riehl, J.P., and Roy, S.C., editors: Conceptual models of nursing practice, New York, 1974, Appleton-Century-Crofts.

Powerlessness in a nursing home population

REBECCA J. SHAW, M.S., R.N.

Nursing home residents have typically suffered several losses, such as loss of spouse, friends, home, occupation and sensorimotor capability. Inherent in these losses is the assumption that they have also lost some degree of power or control over their lives. A beginning step in determining the application of the nursing process to clients with the nursing diagnosis of "powerlessness" is to validate its commonly held defining characteristics.

Powerlessness has been defined as "the perception of the individual that one's own action will not significantly affect an outcome (or) a perceived lack of control over a current situation or immediate happening" (Kim et al, 1984a, p. 118; Miller 1983, p. 3). Lambert and Lambert (1981) found that hospitalized patients in their study defined powerlessness as lack of control, immobility, dependence, and uncertainty. While powerlessness seems to be similar to locus of control, Miller points out that powerlessness is situational and locus of control is innate (1983).

Older persons are among those who are especially at risk for powerlessness. They have experienced role loss, sensory loss, and an increasingly restrictive environment, all of which decrease their options (Miller and Oertel 1983). Lipman and Slater (1977) state that the physical restrictions of the nursing home environment automatically place the resident in a position of powerlessness.

METHODOLOGY

This was an exploratory, qualitative study focusing on nursing home residents' sense of control over space and situation. Lofland's (1971) suggested methodology for conducting qualitative research was followed. Specifically, subjects were interviewed, using a semi-structured interview guide focusing on residents' feelings about their control over space and situations.

Contents of transcripts of the interviews were then analyzed for statements indicating feelings of powerlessness, based on the subjective defining characteristics listed in nursing diagnosis handbooks (Carpenito 1984, Gordon 1985, and Kim, et al. 1984b), the proceedings of the Fifth NANDA Conference (Kim, et al. 1984a) and Miller's paper from that conference (Miller 1984). These defining characteristics are listed in Table 1.

SAMPLE

The setting for this study was a non-proprietary, church-sponsored nursing home in the Midwest. A convenience sample of 20 residents agreed to be interviewed. Only two subjects were male. The mean age of subjects was 81.7 years. The average occupancy time in the facility was 20.5 months. Six subjects were fully mobile; 13 were wheelchair mobile but could walk with help; and one was wheelchair bound. Two subjects described themselves as blind, nine wore glasses and nine had good eyesight. Ten subjects were hard of hearing. Intellectual functioning was measured by the Pfeiffer (1975) Short Portable Mental Status Questionnaire, which showed that seven subjects had intact intellectual functioning, three had mildly impaired intellectual functioning and ten had moderately impaired intellectual functioning. The latter were retained as subjects since they were nevertheless able to express their feelings.

Table 1: Defining characteristics identified in the literature

Defining characteristics	Expressions of powerlessness*
Expresses lack of control over situation	
Feelings of unrelieved boredom	— 1
Need to follow agency rules	— 1
Poor eyesight	— 2
Poor hearing	— 1
Invasions of privacy	— 1
Staff rearranges belongings	— 5
Placement in the nursing home	— 8
Designated bath day	— 4
Loss of home	— 1
Disagreements with roommates	— 2
Dependence on grown child	— 1
Expresses lack of control over outcome	
Unable to mobilize in the nursing home	— 1
Expresses lack of control over self-care	
Blindness	— 1
Disability	— 1
Verbalizes depression over physical deterioration that occurs despite compliance with regimens	— 0
Verbalizations of apathy, e.g., "I don't care."	— 0
Expresses dissatisfaction or frustration over inability to do ADL's	— 1
Expresses doubt over role performance	— 0
Expresses doubt that self-care measures can affect outcome	— 0
Displays reluctance to express true feelings or expresses fear of alienation from caregivers	— 0
Expresses uncertainty about fluctuating energy levels	— 0
Expresses resignation	— 15
Expresses giving up	— 0
Expresses fatalism	— 0
Expresses uneasiness	— 0
Seeks staff interventions in disagreements over control over space	— 12

*Any one subject may have more than one expression of powerlessness

RESULTS

Eighty-five percent of the subjects verbalized at least one of the defining characteristics of powerlessness (Table 1). Seventy-five percent of the subjects expressed lack of control over their situations. The majority of situations in which subjects verbalized this defining characteristic were as follows: placement in the nursing home (n=8), staff invasions into personal belongings (n=5), designation of a certain bath day (n=4). Other situations over which one or two subjects expressed lack of control were feelings of unrelieved boredom, need to follow agency rules, poor eyesight, deafness, invasions of privacy, loss of home, disagreements with roommates, and dependence on children.

Only one subject verbalized lack of con-

Table 2: Defining characteristics showing power

Defining characteristics	Expressions of power[*]
Expresses control over situation	
Roommate is bedridden and demands little space or control in the room	– 10
Could handle invasions of dining room seat if needed	– 3
Able to choose whether to participate in activities	– 3
Made the decision to enter the nursing home	– 3
Able to refuse bath on assigned bath day	– 2
Able to get away for privacy in own room	– 2
Able to negotiate sharing of hall spaces	– 2
Completely able to do own activities of daily living	– 2
Will return to own home when able to do own activities of daily living	– 1

[*]Any one subject may have more than one expression of power

trol over outcome, her inability to be freely mobile ("I'd rather go where I want to"). Two subjects verbalized lack of control over self-care, one owing to blindness, the other resulting in admission to the nursing home.

Seventy percent of the subjects expressed resignation, with statements such as, "This is just where I have to be;" "I've just had to put up with it;" "It can't be helped;" "It (placement in the facility) had to be;" and "There is nothing else I can do."

No subjects displayed apathy, doubt over role performance, doubt that self-care measures would affect outcome, reluctance to express feelings, uncertainty about fluctuating energy levels, giving up, fatalism, or uneasiness.

Sixty percent of the subjects stated that they asked for help from the staff in dealing with difficult interactions with other residents, such as disputes over closet or hallway spaces. This is another possible indication of powerlessness, but further research is needed to determine whether this may more accurately be described as learned helplessness.

An unexpected outcome of this study is the finding that 60% of the subjects expressed some degree of power over certain situations (Table 2). Notably, ten subjects stated that their roommates were bedridden and demanded little space or control over their rooms. Subjects saw this as positive, because they then could control room spaces, placement of items on window ledges, programs which were dialed on the television, etc. Despite the fact that dining room seats were assigned by the facility, three subjects felt that they could get another seat if needed or that they could defend that space successfully. The agency allows all residents control over whether to attend activities; three subjects verbalized control over choosing to go to activities. Three subjects stated they had control over the decision to enter the nursing home, two felt that they could refuse a bath on their assigned bath day, two felt they could control their room spaces, and one stated that she had a favorite sitting space which was rarely challenged by other residents. Two stated that they had kept active to facilitate the adjustment to the restrictive nature of the nursing home environment. One subject stated she would be able to return to her own home as soon as she was able to do her own activities of daily living.

DISCUSSION

This study validates several of the common defining characteristics for powerlessness. It also suggests the need to explore this nursing diagnosis in positive as well as negative terms, that is, as power as well as powerlessness.

Another possible defining characteristic for powerlessness, asking for staff intervention in disputes, was identified. Further concept development and research is needed to distinguish whether this behavior is related to learned helplessness rather than powerlessness or whether learned helplessness is a contributing factor in powerlessness. Research relating powerlessness to locus of control would further refine the definitions of these terms.

Additional validation of powerlessness in other nursing homes, in retirement homes, and in subjects' family homes, as well as in other age groups, would lead to more accurate assessment of those most at risk for powerlessness. Nursing interventions could then be developed to increase or maintain the nursing client's sense of power over a situation.

REFERENCES

Carpenito, L.J.: Handbook of nursing diagnosis, Philadelphia, 1984, J.B. Lippincott.

Gordon, M.: Manual of nursing diagnosis, New York, 1985, McGraw-Hill.

Kim, M.J., McFarland, G.K., and McLane, A.M., editors: Classification of nursing diagnoses: Proceedings of the fifth national conference, St. Louis, 1984, The C.V. Mosby Co.

Kim, M.J., McFarland, G.K., and McLane, A.M.: Pocket guide to nursing diagnosis, St. Louis, 1984, The C.V. Mosby Co.

Lambert, V.A., and Lambert, C.E.: Role theory and the concept of powerlessness, J. Psych. Nurs. Mental Health Serv. **19**:11-14, 1981.

Lipman, A. and Slater, R.: Homes for old people—toward a positive environment, Gerontologist **17**:146-156, 1977.

Lofland, J.: Analyzing social settings, Belmont, CA, 1971, Wadsworth.

Miller, J.F.: Concept development of powerlessness: a nursing diagnosis. In Miller, J.F., editor: Coping with chronic illness: overcoming powerlessness, Philadelphia, 1983, F.A. Davis.

Miller, J.F.: Development and validation of a diagnostic label: powerlessness. In Kim, M.J., McFarland, G.K., and McLane, A.M., editors: Classification of nursing diagnoses: proceedings of the fifth national conference, St. Louis, 1984, The C.V. Mosby Co.

Miller, J.F., and Oertel, C.B.: Powerlessness in the elderly: preventing hopelessness. In J.F. Miller: Coping with chronic illness: overcoming powerlessness, Philadelphia, 1983, F.A. Davis.

Pfeiffer, E.: A short portable mental status questionnaire for the assessment of organic brain deficit in elderly patients, J. Amer. Geriat. Soc. **23**:433-441, 1975.

Etiologies of sleep pattern disturbance in hospitalized patients

KATHLEEN BEYERMAN, M.S.N., R.N.

Sleep is a requisite for health, yet many hospitalized patients have sleep pattern disturbances. What are the causes of these disturbance? Nurses list many—pain, noise, anxiety, daytime sleeping, and interruptions for treatments are a few. But what does the patient identify as the cause of his sleep difficulty?

The importance of eliciting the patient's belief regarding the cause of his sleep pattern disturbance was illustrated by Gillis in 1976. In a study of nine medical-surgical patients with a control group of ten, it was found that when the meaning of the patient's sleep problem was not determined by the nurse, the patient did not experience relief from sleeplessness even when medication was administered. In the experimental group, the nurse deliberately tried to determine the specific meaning of the patient's difficulty in sleeping. Seven of these nine patients did not need medication and were able to sleep.

This supports Gordon's contention that "Etiological factors identified in the diagnosis are the focus of the intervention. If these can be changed, the problem should begin to resolve" (Gordon, 1982, p. 244). Establishing the etiology of sleep pattern disturbance is necessary before effective nursing interventions can be implemented.

STATEMENT OF THE PURPOSE

The purpose of this study is to determine what hospitalized adult medical patients perceive as the causes of their sleep pattern disturbance. Hospitalization-induced sleep pattern disturbance is distinguished from preadmission sleep pattern disturbance in order to identify those etiologies specific to hospitalization.

DEFINITION OF SLEEP PATTERN DISTURBANCE

Sleep pattern disturbance is a nursing diagnosis, defined as a "disruption of sleep time which causes the patient discomfort or interferes with the patient's desired lifestyle" (Kim and Moritz 1982, p. 313). Sleep pattern disturbance was operationally defined by its critical defining characteristics (Kim and Moritz 1982, p. 313):

- Difficulty falling asleep (sleep latency)
- Interrupted sleep
- Awakening earlier or later than desired
- Not feeling well rested

REVIEW OF THE LITERATURE

In previous studies, subjective reports of sleep patterns have been obtained by questionnaire and interview. Questions have been either closed- or open-ended and usually fell into categories of sleep latency, duration of sleep, quality of sleep and the nature of dreams (Johns, 1971). Information about sleep patterns has been gathered from both patient and non-patient populations. Standardized tests such as the Sleep Behavior Self-Rating Scale (Kazarian, Howe, Nerskey, and Deinum 1978) and the Stanford Sleep Inventory (SSI) (Price, Coates, Thorensen & Grinstead 1978) have been used by some researchers.

Causes of sleep pattern disturbance identified by subjects using the SSI were tension and worry; personal, social, and family problems; school problems; lack of sufficient exercise; and alcohol or drug use (Price, et al. 1978). Although the findings of studies using the SSI were similar to other studies of hospitalized patients, the drawback to the SSI is that it was developed specifically for the purpose of understanding how to help adolescent students.

Researcher-designed questionnaires and interviews have been developed to examine patient-ascribed etiologies of sleep pattern disturbances. Hilton (1976) studied nine patients in a respiratory intensive care unit (ICU). During their interviews the patients listed noise, oxygen administration, conversation, other patients, uncomfortable position, tension, procedures, pain, lighting, frustration, and fear and anxiety related to the nurses' competence as interferences with sleep.

These same deterrents to sleep were found in a study in another ICU. The sleep disturbers noted by patients, in order of importance, were activity and noise, pain and physical condition, nursing procedure, vapor tents, and hypothermia (Dlin, Rosen, Dickstein, Lyons, and Fischer 1971).

A study of 16 ward patients revealed a total of 96 sleep disturbers. They were categorized into five areas of decreasing frequency: health problems, environmental interferences, uncoordinated daily activities, psychological factors, and changed personal habits. Pain was the most frequently expressed health problem. Restricted position and dyspnea were listed as the second and third most influential factors in sleep disturbance. Almost all patients complained about the noise and all commented on the poor ward organization, complaining about the many interruptions that interfered with sleep. Most of the psychological factors were related to anxiety, such as thinking about the illness, financial worries, and concern about family members (Choi-Lao 1976).

In another study 70% of 40 ward patients stated that they had problems sleeping and identified discomfort, noise, other patients, daytime sleeping, and middle-of-the-night nursing care as some of the causes (Grant and Dlell 1974).

Fass (1971) interviewed 60 presurgical and convalescing cardiac surgical patients to identify specific sleep disturbers. They listed nightmares, cardiac monitor wires, noise in the corridor, pain, room temperature, equipment noises, worry, other patients in pain, the nurses' station telephone, and other patients receiving care as reasons for having trouble sleeping. Many of these patients complained of loud conversation and laughing by the doctors and nurses at the nurses' station.

To summarize, etiologies of sleep disturbances have been elicited from subjects through the use of standardized instruments and researcher-designed questionnaires and interview schedules. A weakness in all of the studies has been that the patient with sleep pattern disturbance induced by hospitalization has not been distinguished from the patient who had sleep pattern disturbance before admission. Therefore, the etiologies of hospitalization-induced sleep pattern disturbance have not been isolated.

CONCEPTUAL FRAMEWORK

Since there are so many factors disturbing sleep, a categorization system is helpful in understanding them. Walker (1972) groups the etiologies of sleep pattern disturbance into two categories, physiological and psychological. However, this system does not allow for environmental factors, which researchers and patients alike list as major sleep disturbers (Choi-Lao 1976, Dlin et al. 1971, Fass 1971, Grant and Dlell 1974, Hilton 1976, Walker 1972).

The Roy Adaptation Model for Nursing offers a framework which allows the findings of research on etiologies of sleep pattern disturbance to be organized in a useful way. Roy describes man as an open, adaptive system that receives input from both internal and external stimuli (Roy and Roberts 1981). Sleep disturbers may be categorized as internal and external stimuli.

The Fourth National Conference on

Nursing Diagnoses used the concept of internal and external stimuli in grouping the etiologies of sleep pattern disturbance. Internal factors included illness and psychological stress. External factors included environmental changes and social cues (Kim and Moritz 1982).

Since sleep is an adaptive function (Ellis and Dudley 1969, Kramer, Hlasny, Jacobs, and Roth 1976), the investigation of its disturbers may be more appropriately undertaken within the framework of the Roy Adaptation Model than by simply categorizing them as physiological or psychological.

METHODOLOGY

The purpose of this descriptive study was to identify patient-perceived etiologies of sleep pattern disturbance. Hospitalization-induced sleep pattern disturbance was distinguished from preadmission sleep pattern disturbance in order to identify etiologies which were specific to hospitalization.

The sample was an accidental one drawn from two medical units in an urban teaching hospital. One hundred patients were interviewed. To be eligible, patients must have spent three nights in the hospital; this was to avoid the first-night effect, a mild insomnia associated with sleeping in a strange place (Hartman and Elion 1977).

Volunteer subjects were used and were guaranteed confidentially (see Box 1). Patients who did not speak English and patients who were judged by the staff nurse as unable to answer questions were not interviewed.

The questions on the interview schedule assessed the presence of the critical defining characteristics of sleep pattern disturbance (see Box 1). Content validity was verified by three practicing clinical nurse specialists.

BOX 1   **Sleep pattern disturbance interview**

Introduction

I am speaking with patients about their sleeping patterns to try to determine the causes of hospitalization-induced sleep disturbances. I am asking all the patients on the unit who have spent at least 3 nights in the hospital to participate in this study. The results of this study will be used to try to help nurses understand the causes of sleep disturbances in hospitalized patients. Your answers to these questions will be kept confidential.

Interview Schedule

1. Do you have trouble falling asleep at home?
2. Do you frequently wake up at night at home?
3. Do you wake up early at home and find it difficult to fall back asleep?
4. Do you feel well rested after a night's sleep at home?
5. Do you have trouble falling asleep in the hospital? If so, why?
6. Do you frequently wake up at night in the hospital? If so, why?
7. Do you wake up early in the hospital and find it difficult to fall back asleep? If so, why?
8. Do you feel well rested after a night's sleep in the hospital? If not, why not?

The interview schedule was then pretested by three patients and deemed ready to be used as written.

After informed consent was obtained, the patient was asked the questions in the interview schedule. All interviews took place at the bedside between 1:00 p.m. and 6:00 p.m. in an effort to avoid questioning the patient too close to rising or retiring.

Additional data, collected by chart review, included gender, age, medical diagnoses, nursing diagnoses, the sleeping medication ordered, and whether that medication was taken by the patient.

RESULTS

Of the 100 patients interviewed, 43 were men and 57 were women. Ages ranged from 27 to 96, with a mean age of 68. These patients were hospitalized for a variety of reasons. Chart reviews indicated that neither nurses nor physicians diagnosed sleep pattern disturbance or insomnia in any of these 100 patients, even though 48 patients stated during the interview that they had had at least one critical defining characteristic of sleep pattern disturbance before admission. Thus, a problem common to almost half of the patients went undocumented. When the number of patients with hospitalization-induced sleep pattern disturbance was added to the number of patients who had the problem before admission, there were a total of 80 patients out of 100 who had difficulty sleeping while in the hospital. The incidence of sleep pattern disturbance was as follows: at home, 48%; after admission, 32%; and none 20%.

Twenty patients did not have sleep pattern disturbance at home or in the hospital. Thirty-two had no disturbance at home, but did in the hospital. It was this group that was isolated for study of sleep pattern disturbance etiologies.

The problem most often identified by patients with hospitalization-induced sleep pattern disturbance was sleep latency. This

Table 1: Presence of critical cues of sleep pattern disturbance

Critical cue	Number of times the cue was reported
Sleep latency	20
Interrupted sleep	17
Early awakening	13
Not well rested	10
Total	60

was followed by interrupted sleep, then early awakening, and finally, not feeling rested (Table 1). In spite of the large percentage of patients complaining of sleep latency and frequent sleep interruptions, less than one third felt that they were not well rested. This was an unanticipated finding. The lack of feeling rested did not correlate significantly with the presence of any of the other critical defining characteristics of sleep pattern disturbance.

The 32 patients with hospitalization-induced sleep pattern disturbance identified a total of 70 causes for this problem. These causes were grouped according to the Fourth National Conference on Nursing Diagnoses classification (Kim and Moritz 1982) and their frequencies were noted (Table 2).

Seventy percent were external stimuli; 30% were internal stimuli. None of the causes were classified as social cues. The most frequently cited cause of sleep pattern disturbance was noise (24%). This was followed by seven complaints (10%) of "nurses wake me" and six each of taking medication and the strangeness of the hospital environment (9%).

These findings were consistent with the findings of previous research. All of the studies cited in the literature review of hospitalized patients identified noise as a cause of sleep pattern disturbance (Choi-Lao 1976, Dlin, et al. 1971, Fass 1971, Grant and Dlell 1974, Hilton 1976). When several of these researchers rank-ordered sleep disturbers in terms of frequency, noise was the most fre-

Table 2: Classification and frequencies of etiologies

Classification	N
External	
Environmental changes	
Noise	17
Nurses wake	7
Medication administration	6
Strangeness of the hospital	6
Lights	3
Vital signs	3
Uncomfortable bed	2
Tests	2
Others	2
Social cues	0
Internal	
Illness	
Need to void	4
Pain	2
Others	4
Psychological stress	
Bored during the day	2
Thinking about home	2
Others	7

quent disturber found (Choi-Lao 1976, Grant and Dlell, 1974).

The second most frequent cause found in this study was being awakened by the nurse. Choi-Lao (1976), Dlin, et al. (1971), Grant and Dlell (1974), and Hilton (1976) also found this to be a common factor in sleep disturbance. If this cause were to be combined with medication, vital signs and tests, it could be classified as "disturbances for therapeutic and diagnostic measures." By combining these causes in this manner, 26% of the sleep disturbers could be grouped in this one category.

DISCUSSION

With external stimuli comprising 70% of the total number of sleep disturbers identified, there is little doubt that patients could be helped significantly by decreasing the amount of stimuli in the environment.

Many external stimuli are within the nurse's control. Not all noise and activity could be eliminated in an acute care setting, but consideration could be given to the scheduling of medication, treatments, and vital signs, as well as to decreasing the amount of noise. The finding that many patients enter the hospital with sleep pattern disturbance already present leads one to speculate that there is a large group of patients whose recovery will be impeded by this problem.

It is significant that in spite of the frequency of sleep pattern disturbance, none of the nurses made the diagnosis. Possible reasons may be that nurses have not been taught about sleep pattern disturbance, that they do not believe that it is important, that they expect patients to have sleeping problems, that they do not believe that they can affect the problem, or that they are truly unaware of this problem in patients.

The results of this study also suggest that the subcategory "social cues" is not a useful one for hospitalized patients. The meaning of "social cue" is not clear. Kim and Moritz do not define it, and it does not meet the criteria for etiological subcategories which they list in their book (Kim and Moritz 1982, p. 340). The proposed subcategory "therapeutic and diagnostic measures" is very useful and does meet the criteria.

The labeling of the etiologies of sleep pattern disturbance is important not only because it gives us a better understanding of the problem and its scope, but also because it provides us with a focus for interventions.

RECOMMENDATIONS

There are many strategies that would decrease the problem of sleep pattern disturbance in hospitalized patients. Several are:

- Use of a functional health pattern assessment at admission to determine usual sleeping pattern and pre-existing sleep pattern disturbance

- Daily monitoring of patients' perception of their sleep
- Conferences for evening and night nurses focusing on diagnosing and developing interventions for sleep pattern disturbance
- Elimination of unnecessary noise
- Reduction of the number of times a patient must be awakened for nursing care activities

Recommendations for further research are:

- Identify etiologies for sleep pattern disturbance in other populations and in other settings.
- Determine nursing interventions that most effectively treat sleep pattern disturbance.

Increasing nurses' awareness of the frequency and severity of the problem of sleep pattern disturbance will lead them to develop more interventions which will not only treat the problem, but also prevent it. The development of these interventions will depend upon nurses recognizing sleep as a requisite for the maintenance and recovery of health.

REFERENCES

Choi-Lao, A.T.: The sleep assignment: a way to learn problem solving, Canad. Nurse, **72**:34-35, 1976.

Dlin, B.M., Rosen, H., Dickstein, K., and others: The problems of sleep and rest in the intensive care unit, Psychosomat **12**:155-163, 1971.

Ellis, B.W., and Dudley, H.A.: Some aspects of sleep research in surgical stress, J. Psychosomat. Res. **20**:303-308, 1969.

Fass, G.: Sleep, drugs, and dreams, Amer. J. Nurs. **71**:2316-2320, 1971.

Gillis, L.: Sleeplessness—can you help? Canad. Nurse **72**:32-34, 1976.

Gordon, M.: Nursing diagnosis: process and application, New York, 1982, McGraw-Hill.

Grant, D.A., and Dlell, C.: For goodness sake let your patients sleep, Nurs. 74 **4**:54-57, 1974.

Hartman, E., and Elion, R.: The insomnia of 'sleeping in a strange place': effects of l-tryptophane, Psychopharmacol. **53**:131-133, 1977.

Hilton, B.A.: Quantity and quality of patients' sleep and sleep-disturbing factors in a respiratory intensive care unit, J. Adv. Nurs. **1**:453-468, 1976.

Johns, M.: Methods for assessing human sleep, Arch. Intern. Med. **127**:484-491, 1971.

Kazarian, S., Howe, M., Merskey, H., and others: Insomnia: anxiety, sleep-incompatible behaviors and depression, J. Clin. Psychol. **34**:865-867, 1978.

Kim, M., and Moritz, D., editors: Classification of nursing diagnoses: proceedings of the third and fourth national conferences, New York, 1982, McGraw-Hill.

Kramer, M., Hlasny, R., Jacobs, G., and others: Do dreams have meaning? An empirical inquiry, Amer. J. Psych. **133**:778-781, 1976.

Price, V.A., Coates, T.J., Thorensen, C.E., and others: Prevalence and correlates of poor sleep among adolescents, Amer. J. Dis. Children **132**:583-586, 1978.

Roy, C., and Roberts, S.: Theory construction in nursing, Englewood Cliffs, N.J., 1981, Prentice-Hall.

Walker, B.B.: The postsurgery heart patient: amount of uninterrupted time for sleep and rest during the first, second, and third postoperative days in a teaching hospital, Nurs. Res. **21**:164-169, 1972.

Validation of the nursing diagnosis "knowledge deficit: restorative measures"

SUSAN COPELAND-OWEN, B.S.N., R.N.
THERESA DiBENEDETTO, B.S.N., R.N.
GAIL FURNEY, B.S.N., R.N.
DAVINA GOSNELL, Ph.D., R.N.
MARTHA HORST, B.S.N., R.N.
SHEILA KELLY-KNOX, B.S.N., R.N.
MARY MARCELLO, B.S.N., R.N.
MARILYN MORGENSTERN-STANOVICH, B.S.N., R.N.
CAROL PONTIUS, B.S.N., R.N.

Nursing is defined as the diagnosis and treatment of human responses to actual or potential health problems (ANA, 1980). The nursing process is used to identify the phenomena of concern to nurses, that is, the human responses to actual or potential health problems. Those responses that are amenable to nursing therapy are known as nursing diagnoses. Gordon (1976) describes three essential components of a nursing diagnosis: the health problem, the etiology, and the defining cluster of signs and symptoms, i.e., defining characteristics.

Martin and York (Kim, McFarland, and McLane 1984) report the three most prevalent nursing diagnoses accepted by the Fourth National Conferences to be (1) alteration in comfort, (2) ineffective breathing patterns, and (3) knowledge deficit. In our clinical experiences with chronic diabetics and peripheral vascular, renal, and cardiac clients we have found that the diagnosis 'knowledge deficit: restorative measures' is very common. Kim et al. (1984, p. 497) define this diagnosis as "lack of specific information regarding activities that move the individual toward an optimal level of function."

An analysis and critique of the literature related to long-term care of clients with diabetes, peripheral vascular disease, coronary artery disease and chronic renal disease revealed numerous examples of the relevance of the diagnosis "knowledge deficit: restorative measures" in these client populations. The literature clearly indicated that continued contact with health professionals may be necessary in order to maintain new behavior patterns and to provide support and encouragement for modification of behavior. Without identification of this diagnosis in these populations, however, needed nursing care beyond the usual short-term period of hospitalization is seldom recognized or provided.

Validation of a nursing diagnosis refers to how accurately the diagnostic cues and corresponding etiologies describe the client's response to actual or potential health problems. The importance of validating nursing diagnoses is a recurring theme in the literature, however, to date there only minimal work has been done. The nursing diagnosis "knowledge deficit: restorative measures" is in need of validation and testing. It is hoped that this study will contribute to the development of nursing diagnoses and stimulate other nurses to pursue this line of inquiry.

The purpose of this study was to validate the nursing diagnosis "knowledge deficit: restorative measures." Specifically, the focus of inquiry was on validation of the defining characteristics and etiologies for the diagnosis with four chronically ill populations—persons with diabetes, peripheral vascular disease, cardiac disease, and renal disease.

The specific defining characteristics addressed were:

- Inability to identify community resources
- Inability to verbalize methods to minimize sequelae of the chronic disease
- Inability to recognize the need for long-term health maintenance
- Inability to explain the relationship between therapeutic modalities and long-term health maintenance.

Corresponding etiologies were identified as:

- Previous history of low readiness for learning
- Previous history of lack of interest or motivation to learn
- Lack of access to health care personnel for ongoing instruction
- Lack of reinforcement for previous teaching
- Inability to access community resources

Delineation of the specific diagnostic cues, i.e., characteristics and etiologies, was based on an extensive literature review including the proceedings of the North American Nursing Diagnosis Association (NANDA) conferences as well as clinical expertise of the authors.

METHOD

A short questionnaire by the authors was the measurement instrument used to examine the defining characteristics and etiologies for the nursing diagnosis "knowledge deficit: restorative measures." The questionnaire was designed for use with the four chronically ill client populations: diabetic, peripheral vascular, cardiac, and renal disease patients. Objective questions were used to address the validation items. Each population was asked essentially the same questions, however there were four variations of

the questionnaire with content such as risk factors and health practices made specific to each chronic disease. For example, a question related to knowledge of community resources varied as follows: "What resources are available to you in your community for your health care of _____ [one of the four diagnoses were inserted]?" No reliability measures were established for the instrument. Face and content validity were established by literature validation and content experts review.

Demographic data such as medical diagnosis, length of illness, previous teaching and by whom were collected.

Data were collected in settings in northwestern Pennsylvania and northeastern Ohio including offices of two endocrinologists and one cardiovascular and thoracic surgeon, two cardiac rehabilitation centers, one home training dialysis center and one visiting nurse association. The time period of data collection was June through July, 1985.

A convenience sample of 69 subjects was used for this study. To participate in the study, clients needed to be associated with one of the aforementioned agencies and have one of the four designated chronic illnesses.

The questionnaires were completed by subjects at the time of one of their regularly scheduled visits to the agency. Participation was voluntary. Data collection was done by eight graduate nursing students.

FINDINGS

Frequencies and percentages were used to analyze the data. In Table 1 a summary of the frequencies (percentages) of defining characteristics is presented.

The findings indicate that the majority of subjects in the sample had had previous health teaching. Further analysis revealed, however, that there was lack of reinforcement of previous teaching, and for some sub-

Table 1: Presence of defining characteristics for knowledge deficit: restorative measures

Chronic illness groups (N=69)

Defining characteristics	Diabetes (n=15)		Peripheral vascular disease (n=7)		Cardio-vascular disease (n=27)		Renal disease (n=20)	
	YES	NO	YES	NO	YES	NO	YES	NO
Previous health teaching	87%	13%	71%	29%	44%	56%	100%	0%
Able to recognize risk factors	94%	6%	43%	57%	96%	4%	93%	7%
Able to recognize community resources	67%	33%	29%	71%	78%	22%	100%	0%

jects a considerable period of time had elapsed since any teaching had occurred.

The four chronic illness groups varied in their ability to recognize risk factors. Subjects with diabetes, cardiovascular disease or renal disease were able to identify at least some risk factors to a high degree (93—96%), however, only 43% of subjects with peripheral vascular disease were able to identify any risk factors. While most subjects could identify risk factors, their level of understanding regarding the need to engage in specific care measures for long-term health maintenance and the ability to recognize the relationship between therapeutic modalities and long-term health maintenance was quite limited. For example, nearly all diabetic subjects (93%) knew that diabetes was not curable, but only 47% could identify the normal range of blood sugar. All subjects with peripheral vascular disease felt that it was important to examine their feet on a daily basis for cuts and bruises but only 57% felt that palpating peripheral pulses was an important task to complete on a regular basis. Only 29% of the peripheral vascular disease subjects could identify the effects of a low-salt, -fat, and -cholesterol diet and 43% stated they did not know what physiological effect resulted from dietary restrictions. Thirty-three percent of the

cardiac subjects did not understand how a low-salt diet affects the heart, and 22% did not know the effect of a low-fat, low-cholesterol diet on the heart.

The ability of subjects to recognize community resources varied considerably. Sixty-seven percent of the diabetic subjects could identify at least one community resource. Most identified the American Diabetes Association and some listed the hospital diabetic classes, diabetic clinical specialist, or diabetic clinic. Renal dialysis subjects were also quite familiar with community resources. All identified the dialysis center as a resource. The American Kidney Foundation was also cited frequently. A more diverse group of community resources were identified by cardiac subjects and included malls, parks, bike clubs, racquet clubs, a blood pressure screening program, and the American Heart Association. Only 29% of the subjects with peripheral vascular disease could identify any community resource available to assist them in management of their disease.

When asked who had provided education about their disease, subjects identified the registered nurse most often, i.e., 84% to 100% of the time. Physicians and dieticians were also identified as providing education but far less frequently. As mentioned previously, the teaching tended to be somewhat limited and occurring at the time of hospitalization. The exception was renal dialysis patients who had all participated in an intense, ongoing home dialysis training program.

In general, the defining characteristics as delineated were found to be valid to support the nursing diagnosis of knowledge deficit: restorative measures in the four chronically ill groups of subjects included in this study. The corresponding etiologies of lack of access to health care personnel for ongoing instruction and a lack of reinforcement for previous teaching were also found to be present and valid. The etiologies of previous history of low readiness for learning, previous history of lack of interest or motivation to learn, and ability to access community resources were not examined in this study.

SUMMARY

Today, the number one illness is chronic illness. Knowledge deficit: restorative measures is a nursing diagnosis of major importance in the long-term care of chronic illness. Further validation of the diagnosis and development of effective nursing interven-

tion to assist the patient in assuming self-care is essential. Based upon the findings of this study the following recommendations are offered:

- The study be extended to a larger, more diverse population of chronically ill patients
- The number and variety of settings for data collection be increased
- Reliability be established for the instrument
- The instrument be revised to incorporate all etiologies and a "no response" item
- A longitudinal study be conducted to validate the existence of the defining characteristics and etiologies over time

REFERENCES

American Nurses' Association: Nursing a social policy statement, Kansas City, MO, 1980, American Nurses' Association.

Gordon, M.: Nursing diagnosis and the diagnostic process, Amer. J. Nurs. **76:**1298-1300, 1976.

Kim, M.J., McFarland, G.K., and McLane, A.M., editors: Classification of nursing diagnoses: proceedings of the fifth national conference, St. Louis, 1984, The C.V. Mosby Co.

Individual and aggregate client focus of nursing diagnosis among four clinical areas

ADELITA GONZALES, B.S.N., R.N.

In the nursing literature of the past 10 to 15 years, the concept of nursing diagnosis has been defined and investigated. However, definitions and examples of nursing diagnoses given in the literature focus on the individual. This, despite various nursing models' characterization of nursing as encompassing the individual, family, aggregate, and community (Neuman 1980, Roy 1980, and Johnson 1980).

Nursing standards also suggest nursing includes both individual and aggregate clients. In reviewing the various American Nurses' Association's Nursing Standards for Practice among clinical groups—community health, maternal-child health, psychiatric-mental health, and medical-surgical—the primary recipient of nursing care may be the family, group, or community as a whole. However, these standards provide little to guide the nurse in considering and diagnosing the community, family, or group as the primary recipient of care.

Hamilton (1983), disagreed with the assumptions made by many authors when writing about nursing diagnosis that conclusions drawn concerning ways to develop, classify, and act on nursing diagnoses will be the same whether nursing relates to individuals, families, groups, or entire communities. Despite significant work in defining and classifying nursing diagnosis (Newman 1983, Kim and Moritz 1982, Higgs and Gustafson 1985, and Muecke 1984), the formulation of nursing diagnoses, when applied to the primary recipient of care other than the individual, has been largely ignored.

A study to determine whether current nursing practice reflects conceptual nursing models and nursing standards would clarify the clients diagnosed and acted upon among clinical areas. A descriptive, comparative study on the client focus of nursing diagnoses among clinical areas would indicate whether current nursing practice reflects standards or conceptual models.

The problem of this investigation was to determine if a difference existed in the focus of clients' diagnoses among nurses of the four clinical areas of community health, maternal-child health, psychiatric-mental health, and medical-surgical. The investigator hypothesized that there is a difference in the focus of clients diagnosed among nurses in the four clinical areas. To conduct this study, the researcher assumed that the subjects were familiar with the concept of nursing process and diagnosis and that the client focus of diagnosis is reflected in the etiology component of the nursing diagnosis statement (Ziegler, Vaughan-Wrobel, and Erlen 1986).

RESEARCH DESIGN

An ex post facto, descriptive, comparative design was utilized in this study. Two investigators developed instruments and described the data for this study. A Demographic Data Sheet was utilized to describe the sample. The Client Focus Instrument (Appendix A), obtained the focus of each clinical area practice, which included a case study, describing eight client situations or problems that were amendable to nursing interventions (Appendix B). A set of four nursing diagnoses for each of the eight client situations or problems was generated. The

Table 1: Frequency and percentage distribution of client focus of diagnosis by clinical group

	Client focus of diagnosis							
	Individual		Family		Group		Community		Total
Clinical group	Frequency	Percentage	Frequency	Percentage	Frequency	Percentage	Frequency	Percentage	frequency
Medical-surgical	12	18.75	30	46.88	19	29.69	3	4.68	100%
Psychiatric-mental health	28	35.00	25	31.25	24	30.00	3	3.75	100%
Community health	28	35.00	30	37.50	16	20.00	6	7.50	100%
Maternal-child health	11	23.00	21	43.75	12	25.00	4	8.30	100%

$x^2(9) = 11.03, p > .05$.

four nursing diagnoses in each set included an individual, family, group, and community diagnostic focus. The subjects read the case study and then selected the nursing diagnosis from each set that best described their practice. Each subject received four scores, the number of diagnoses selected from each of the classifications of individual, family, group, and community.

Content validity of the classification of the diagnoses was established by a panel composed of three experts on nursing diagnosis. The members, working independently, were asked to classify each of the nursing diagnosis statements as being an individual, family, group, or community diagnosis. A consensus as to the classifications required at least two of the three members to classify the diagnosis under the same category. Reliability was improved by utilizing a second panel of graduate nursing students to evaluate the instruments for clarity of instructions and time requirement to complete.

SAMPLE

A convenience sample of American-educated registered nurses who received their baccalaureate degree within the past 10 years comprised the sample. There were eight subjects in medical-surgical group, ten in the psychiatric-mental health group, ten in the community health group, and eight in the maternal-child health group.

DESCRIPTION OF SAMPLE

The mean age of the 34 nurses (two MCH nurses were dropped as they did not fully complete the instrument) was 32.5 years, with the mean years of experience being 6.8. A one-way analysis of variance was computed to determine whether there was a difference in age and years of experience among the four clinical groups. For age, the findings were $F(3.33)=12.5, p>.05$; for years of experience, the findings were $F(3.33)=.40, p>.05$. Since no differences were found in either

case, the clinical groups were homogenous in age and years of experience.

FINDINGS

The hypothesis was tested by the chi-square statistic and was rejected. No difference in the focus of clients diagnosed among the four clinical groups was found $(x^2(9)=11.03, p>.05,$ Table 1). When the client focus of diagnosis was analyzed separately for each of the eight client problems, a significant difference among the clinical groups was found for the nursing problem labeled "grieving/death" $(x^2(9)=17.32, p<.05,$ Tables 2 and 3).

When the groups were reviewed separately, significant differences existed in their selection pattern of client focus. The medical-surgical group selected more family (47%) and group (40%) and less community diagnoses (6.25%) than was expected by chance (Table 4). The psychiatric-mental health group selected fewer community diagnoses (3.75%) and selected the individual (35%), family (31.25%), and group (50%) diagnoses approximately equally (Table 5). The community-health group selected fewer community diagnoses (7.5%) and more individual

Table 2: Summary table of results of chi-square test of focus of diagnosis by clinical group and problem

Problem	X^2 value	df	p
Unplanned teenage pregnancy	8.32	9	>.05
Low employment opportunities	13.62	9	>.05
Developmental delays	6.25	9	>.05
Inadequate transportation	5.40	9	>.05
Wife abuse	10.20	9	>.05
Nutritional imbalance	5.00	9	>.05
Long-term health care	13.10	9	>.05
Grieving/death	17.52	9	<.05*

*Statistically significant.

Table 3: Frequency and percentage distribution of grieving/death client focus nursing diagnosis by clinical group

| Clinical group | Client focus of diagnosis | | | | | | | | Total frequency |
| | Individual | | Family | | Group | | Community | | |
	Frequency	Percentage	Frequency	Percentage	Frequency	Percentage	Frequency	Percentage	
Medical-surgical	2	25.00	6	75.00	0	0.00	0	0.00	100%
Psychiatric-mental health	4	40.00	6	60.00	0	0.00	0	0.00	100%
Community health	10	100.00	0	0.00	0	0.00	0	0.00	100%
Maternal-child health	2	33.34	3	50.00	1	16.67	0	0.00	100%

$X^2(9) = 17.52, p < .05.$

Table 4: Frequency and percentage distribution of client focus of nursing diagnosis by medical-surgical nurses

Client focus of diagnosis	Observed frequency	Percentage	Expected frequency
Individual	12	18.75	16
Family	30	46.88	16
Group	19	29.69	16
Community	3	4.69	16
Total	64	100.00	64

X^2 (3) = 13.81, $p<.05$.

Table 5: Frequency and percentage distribution of client focus of nursing diagnosis by psychiatric-mental health nurses

Client focus of diagnosis	Observed frequency	Percentage	Expected frequency
Individual	28	35.00	20
Family	25	31.25	20
Group	24	30.00	20
Community	3	3.75	20
Total	80	100.00	80

X^2 (3) = 19.7, $p<.05$.

Table 6: Frequency and percentage distribution of client focus of nursing diagnosis by community health nurses

Client focus of diagnosis	Observed frequency	Percentage	Expected frequency
Individual	28	35.00	20
Family	30	37.50	20
Group	16	20.00	20
Community	6	7.50	20
Total	80	100.00	80

X^2 (3) = 18.8, $p<.05$.

Table 7: Frequency and percentage distribution of client focus of nursing diagnosis by maternal-child health nurses

Client focus of diagnosis	Observed frequency	Percentage	Expected frequency
Individual	11	23.0	12
Family	21	43.0	12
Group	12	25.0	12
Community	4	8.3	12
Total	48	99.3	48

X^2 (3) = 12.16, $p<.05$.

(35%) and family diagnoses (37.5%) than expected by chance (Table 6). The maternal-child health group selected more family (43%) and fewer community diagnoses (8.3%) than expected by chance (Table 7).

DISCUSSION OF FINDINGS

The findings of the study indicated there was no significant difference in the client focus among the four clinical groups. This may suggest that the Standards of Practice for the study's clinical subjects do not describe the client focus of the subjects' actual practice.

Analyses of the selection pattern of client focus of nursing diagnoses within each clini-

cal group revealed that two most closely reflected their Standards of Nursing Practice. The findings suggest that the nursing practice of this study's PMH and MCH subjects closely resemble their standards for practice. The PMH Standards of Nursing Practice (ANA 1973a) stated the society, the community, and those individuals and families within it can be the focuses of PMH nursing care. The PMH subjects selected equally individual, family, and group client focus nursing diagnoses. The MCH Standards of Practice (ANA 1980), stated that the family is the primary recipient of care. The MCH subjects demonstrated a congruence with their standards of practice, they primarily selected family-client focus nursing diagnoses.

However, this study provided evidence of incongruence between CH and MS subjects and their Standards of Practice (ANA 1973b and ANA 1974). According to the CH standards, the community as a whole is the focus of nursing care. In this study, the CH subjects selected individual and family-client focus nursing diagnoses, community client focus nursing diagnoses rarely. While the MS Standards of Nursing Practice stated that the primary focus of MS nurses is the individual's physiological alteration and related social and behavioral problems, this study's MS subjects selected family and group client focus more often than the individual. This may suggest that the nursing standards need to be modified or that nursing practice needs to be modified to reflect standards.

In the generation of an instrument of nursing diagnoses that were classified individual, family, group, and community, the investigator considered Mundinger and Jauron's (1975) contention that nursing diagnostic components included a client response related to its etiology. However, Smith (1984) suggested that nurses were unable to write group diagnoses and that literature was not available that described how aggregate nursing diagnoses are reflected in the etiology component (Ziegler et al. 1986). They contended that the etiology component of the nursing diagnosis directs nursing interventions. Therefore, the etiology must reflect the client focus.

CONCLUSIONS AND IMPLICATIONS

Based upon this study's findings, the following conclusions were drawn. The Standards of Practice for each of the study's clinical groups may not describe the client focus of actual practice. Secondly, the client focus of the PMH and MCH subjects closely reflected their standards, while the client focus of the MS and CH subjects differed

from their standards. Lastly, the Client Focus Instrument may be a useful tool for identifying the client focus of nursing practice.

The above conclusions imply that nursing should consider the inclusion of aggregate nursing diagnoses in their taxonomy to more accurately reflect the scope of nursing. Also implied is that standards should be investigated for purposes of revision or that practice need to be upgraded to reflect standards. Lastly, nursing educators need to develop guidelines that closely differentiate how nursing-diagnosis statements are formulated compared to actual practice.

This study's recommendations for further study would be that a similar study be done to examine the relationship between the selection pattern of nursing diagnoses of BSN and MSN nurses within a similar clinical group. Also, additional studies should be conducted to refine characteristics of the etiology component for writing aggregate nursing-diagnosis statements, and whether an educational program utilizing this study's format for classifying diagnoses would best facilitate the classification of nursing diagnoses.

REFERENCES

American Nurses' Association: Psychiatric-mental health nursing practice standards, Kansas City MO, 1973, American Nurses' Association.

American Nurses' Association: Standards for community-health nursing practice, Kansas City, MO, 1973, American Nurses' Association.

American Nurses' Association: Medical-surgical nursing practice, Kansas City MO, 1974, American Nurses' Association.

American Nurses' Association: A statement on the scope of the maternal and child health nursing practice, Kansas City MO, 1980, American Nurses' Association.

Gonzales, A.: Individual and aggregate client focus of nursing diagnosis among four clinical areas. Unpublished master's thesis, Texas Women's University, 1985.

Hamilton, P.: Community nursing diagnosis, Adv. Nurs. Sci. **5:**21-36, 1983.

Higgs, Z.R., and Gustafson, D.D.: Community as client: assessment and diagnosis, Philadelphia, 1985, F.A. Davis.

Johnson, D.E.: The behavioral system for nursing. In Riehl, J.P., and Roy, C., editors: Conceptual models for nursing practice, New York, 1980, Appleton-Century-Crofts.

Kim, M.J., and Moritz, D.A.: Classification of nursing diagnoses: proceedings of the third and fourth national conferences, New York, 1982, McGraw-Hill.

Muecke, M.A.: Community health diagnosis in nursing, Pub. Health Nurs. **1**:23-35, 1984.

Mundinger, M., and Jauron, G.: Developing a nursing diagnosis, Nurs. Outlook **23**:94-98, 1975.

Neuman, B.: The Betty Neuman health-care systems model: a total person approach to patient problems. In Riehl, J.P., and Roy, C., editors: Conceptual models for nursing practice, New York, 1980, Appleton-Century-Crofts.

Newman, M.A.: Newman's health theory. In Clements, F.W., and Robert, F.B., editors: Family health: a theoretical approach to nursing care, New York, 1983, John Wiley.

Roy, C.: The Roy adaptation model. In Riehl, J.P., and Roy, C., editors: Conceptual models for nursing practice, New York, 1980, Appleton-Century-Crofts.

Smith, P.: Group nursing diagnosis, Unpublished master's thesis, Texas Woman's University, 1984.

Ziegler, S., Vaughan-Wrobel, B., and Erlen, J.: Nursing process, nursing diagnosis, and nursing knowledge, New York, Appleton-Century-Crofts. (In press.)

APPENDIX A
Client focus instrument

1. Problem: Unplanned teenage pregnancy
— Increasing unplanned teenage pregnancy related to lack of community programs in comprehensive sexual education
— Sharon's second unplanned teenage pregnancy related to her inconsistent use of contraceptives
— Increasing unplanned teenage pregnancies related to early adolescent sexual activity without comprehensive sexual education
— Second unplanned teenage pregnancy related to the failure of marital partners to assume contraceptive responsibilities
2. Problem: Low financial status and few teenage employment opportunities
— Decreased employment opportunities among low-income teenagers related to inadequate integration for low-income teenagers of vocational preparation in high school curriculum
— Decreased teenage employment opportunities related to the community's lack of on-the-job training programs
— Sharon's decreased employment opportunities related to her lack of knowledge of available adult basic education resources
— Lack of consistent above-minimum-wage employment related to the family's inability to plan long-term for breadwinner's educational preparation
3. Problem: Developmental delays
— Brian's developmental delays related to his ineffectual muscle coordination
— Increased developmental delay in toddlers related to the lack of community awareness of the need for parental skills' training
— Brian's developmental delays related to the family's lack of sufficient parental skills in providing appropriate environmental stimuli
— Inadequate environmental stimulation in toddlers of teenage parents related to the lack of adolescent knowledge of sufficient parental skills
4. Problem: Transportation for low-income persons
— Inadequate transportaton for low-income persons related to the lack of community interest in acquisition of city, state, federal funds
— Inadequate transportation for low-income persons related to ineffectual use, by the financially disadvantaged, of the political mechanisms to acquire needed funds
— Decreased mobility related to the marital partner's lack of cooperation in seeking other modes of transportation

— Sharon's decreased mobility related to her unfamiliarity with bus routes

5. Problem: Wife abuse

— Repeated incidents of wife abuse related to inadequate stress management among marital partners

— Wife abuse related to Mexican-American cultural beliefs of sex roles and marriage

— Sharon's acceptance of physical beatings related to her feelings of helplessness regarding options in current marriage situation

— Increasing rate of wife abuse related to the community's lack of effective stress management programs and severe legal condemnation of the phenomena

6. Problem: Nutritional status

— Sharon's poor nutritional status related to the family's unhealthful dietary patterns

— Sharon's poor nutritional status related to her lack of knowledge of iron-rich foods

— Inadequate nutritional status related to the community's lack of interest in nutritional wellbeing and nutritional maintenance programs

— Inadequate nutritional status in teenage mothers related to adolescent preference for foods deficient in the Recommended Daily Requirements

7. Problem: Jonathan's acute/long-term health problems

— Infant long-term health problems related to the lack of strategically placed prenatal care community programs

— Infant long-term health problems related to the increasing teenage pregnancy rate and the accompanying high birth risk rate

— Increasing anxiety over Jonathan's continuing, acute health problem related to the disruption to the family's need for reasonable security

— Sharon's increasing anxiety over Jonathan's illness related to her lack of knowledge of Jonathan's physical anomalies

8. Problem: Grieving/death

— Incomplete grieving process among Mexican-Americans related to their cultural belief of grieving as a sign of weakness

— Sharon's preoccupation with death of child related to the marital partners' inability to seek out the need for mutual support

— Inadequate coping with death and grieving related to the lack of community-support programs for the bereaved

— Sharon's increasing fear of her preoccupation with death of child related to her lack of knowledge of the stages of grief

APPENDIX B
Case study

Sharon P. was in her 6th month of pregnancy at her first prenatal visit. A medical and psychosocial interview revealed the following:

— Sharon was a gravida II, para I, AB O.

— Sharon was 18 years old, unemployed, a high school dropout.

— Brian, Sharon's son, was 15 months old, was not walking and still taking all fluids from the bottle despite Sharon describing him as holding the bottle and having a neat pincer grasp.

— Because Sharon could not drive, she had to rely on a friend to bring her to this prenatal visit.

— Johnny, Sharon's husband, was Mexican-American, 19 years old, and worked at various construction sites, She spoke of him losing a job often due to his "temper."

— Sharon has on occasion suffered physical beatings from her husband, even during both pregnancies. She expressed a wish to separate from her husband, but was unable to manage alone financially and emotionally.

___ Sharon was found to be moderately anemic.

Sharon's second son, Jonathan, was born 4 weeks prematurely. When making a routine 2 weeks postpartum visit, the community health nurse noted that Jonathan had not gained weight, was listless, and ashen colored. Jonathan was admitted to the hospital with a diagnosis of failure to thrive. Jonathan was released after he gained 4 pounds. Despite the nurse's continued home visits, Jonathan did not gain weight and Sharon continued to speak of his feeding difficulties. At 2 months of age, Jonathan was again hospitalized with failure to thrive. Child welfare investigated for possible child neglect, but neglect could not be documented. Jonathan continued being listless, had no eye contact, and only maintained his weight. At 3½ months, the nurse recommended a change of doctors. A new pediatrician hospitalized Jonathan again, diagnosed an abnormal gastric reflex, discharged him after 4 days. At 4 months of age, Jonathan was found dead in his crib by his mother. For the next few weeks, Sharon called the nurse repeatedly with fears of going crazy, "I go to the grave every day. That's crazy, isn't it? That's what Johnny's family says."

Alteration in growth and development: a nursing diagnosis validation study

CYNTHIA PELTIER COVIAK, M.S.N., R.N.

Since the inception of the Task Force of the National Group for Classification of Nursing Diagnoses and its descendent organization, the North American Nursing Diagnosis Association (NANDA), over 40 potential and actual nursing diagnoses have been defined and are being tested. During this time, it has become evident that there is a paucity of diagnoses identified that describe health problems and responses to health problems that are unique to children and adolescents.

Several authors have suggested that developmental alterations are of concern to nursing, and that this concern should be reflected in a nursing diagnosis taxonomy (Coviak and Derhammer 1983, Lunney 1982). Others have attempted to illustrate examples of cases in which developmental alterations are evident (Aspinall, Jambruno and Phoenix 1977), and to label the alterations they had observed (Bumbalo and Siemon 1983, Oldaker 1984). Burns and Thompson (1984) reported using "developmental delay" as a diagnostic label, however, no formal definition of a diagnosis of "alteration in growth and development" or "developmental delay" was reported.

As graduate students in a course on management of the care of children, Coviak and Derhammer (1983) attempted to define a diagnosis of "alteration in growth and development," to determine possible etiologies of the diagnosis and to identify some possible defining characteristics of such a diagnosis. Through a literature review and observation and recall of child clients they had cared for, they proposed that "alteration in growth and development" described a condition in which there was "a primary or secondary failure of the client to meet expected growth and development norms of his or her age group" (Coviak and Derhammer 1983). Primary failures included cases in which the client never had met the norm, while secondary failures included cases of regression to earlier levels of growth and development.

Since validation studies are required to establish the accuracy of definitions and defining characteristics of newly described nursing diagnoses, the purpose of this investigation was to obtain validation data to support the acceptance of a nursing diagnosis of "alteration in growth and development" and to determine whether a group of defining characteristics parallel to those proposed by Coviak and Derhammer (1983) could be identified.

Several research questions and hypotheses were tested. Some questions were related to issues of agreement with the diagnosis. Those were:

- Do nurses recognize and diagnose the signs and symptoms of altered growth and development? (Will there be agreement between the diagnoses identified by nurses in this study and the primary diagnosis identified by the researcher for a client portrayed in a case study?)
- Will the signs and symptoms identified by participants in the investigation (from a case study) agree with those defining characteristics identified by previous authors? (Coviak and Derhammer 1983).
- What will be the most frequent signs and symptoms identified?
- What will be the average number of

signs and symptoms of the diagnosis that nurses who accurately identify altered growth and development indicate as being most important for making the diagnosis? (Coviak 1985, p. 16)

Other research questions and hypotheses predicted the characteristics of nurses who would identify altered growth and development:

- Do nurses with a greater degree of expertise show a higher degree of accuracy in making this diagnosis (from a case study) than those with lesser amounts of expertise?

  Hypothesis: Accuracy in making the diagnosis of altered growth and development from the case study will be significantly greater ($p<.05$) in nurses with greater amounts of expertise than in nurses with lesser amounts of expertise.

- Do nurses who identify more than 75% of the signs and symptoms of altered growth and development depicted in the case study diagnose the alteration more often than nurses who identify fewer signs and symptoms?

  Hypothesis: Nurses who identify 75% or more of the signs and symptoms of altered growth and development displayed in the case study will diagnose altered growth and development significantly more often ($p<.05$) than nurses who do not identify at least 75% of the signs and symptoms of the diagnosis presented in the case study.

- How will the number of signs and symptoms identified by nurses vary with the level of expertise of the nurse?

  Hypothesis: Nurses with greater amounts of expertise will identify 75% of the signs and symptoms of altered growth and development exhibited in the client of the case study significantly more frequently ($p<.05$) than will nurses with lesser amounts of expertise.

- How will the level of experience with

nursing diagnosis affect agreement in the diagnosis of altered growth and development?

Hypothesis: Nurses with greater amounts of experience in nursing diagnosis will identify altered growth and development as primary diagnosis for the case study client significantly more frequently than nurses with less experience in nursing diagnosis ($p<.05$). (Coviak, 1985, pp. 16-18.)

METHODOLOGY

This investigation was descriptive in nature. A case study depicting a child who displayed some of the characteristics of a developmental alteration and a professional profile questionnaire were mailed to a random sample of 200 nurses listed as members of the Maternal-Child Health Division of the Michigan Nurses Association (MNA). The nurses were asked to identify their major nursing diagnosis for the child, to list the cues in the case study which led them to this diagnosis, and to list any other diagnoses they would make for the child or family depicted. They were also asked to complete the professional profile questionnaire, which asked information about their professional background, experience with nursing diagnosis, and other descriptive data. Thus, the design was derived from the retrospective identification and the nurse-validation models of Gordon and Sweeney (1979), and utilized mailed questionnaires to obtain a larger geographic sampling of nurses which Fehring (1986) suggests is necessary for true validation.

The mailing list obtained from the MNA for sample selection held 1,774 names of members of the Division of Maternal and Child Health. The sample chosen (200) was, therefore, slightly more than 10% of the target population. Although the population and sample were not totally comprised of nurses holding at least a master's degree, the nurses were members of a professional organization and listed their area of practice or interest as that of maternal-child nursing. It was deemed likely that altered development would be familiar to this group of nurses.

The instruments were developed by the investigator. The case study was based on an actual client history. Names, family background, and other identifying circumstances were changed, but developmental alterations reflected the original client. The case study and the professional profile questionnaire were reviewed by four nurses who held at least a master's degree, for the purpose of establishing content validity. The questionnaires were modified using the experts' suggestions, and tested through a pilot study. There were minor changes in each instrument following the pilot study, which were incorporated for the formal study.

Instruments and procedures for the investigation were approved by the Human Subject Review Committee of the college. For both the pilot and formal studies, mailings included: (1) an informational cover letter, (2) the case study, (3) the respondent profile, (4) a postcard for requesting study results, and (5) a stamped, self-addressed envelope for returning the questionnaires to the investigator. As the questionnaires were returned, a code number was assigned to each set to allow matching of case studies with profiles (questionnaires remained anonymous). Two weeks following each initial mailing, a reminder postcard was sent to all of the sample, encouraging them to reply if they had not already done so. Data collection ceased 2 weeks after the second mailing. A total of 62 responses were obtained for the final study (31% of the sample). Two sets of questionnaires were discarded since the case study had not been completed. This allowed 60 questionnaires (30%) for data analysis. Descriptive statistics, the chi-square statistic, and Pearson and Spearman correlational statistics were used.

RESULTS

The respondent profile provided data on many of the characteristics of the respondents. Respondents reported their areas of practice to be child-adolescent health (40% of the sample), community health (16.7%), maternity nursing (13.3%), neonatal I.C.U. (8.3%), newborn nursery (5.0%), ambulatory care (3.3%) and other (11.7%). The respondents held the positions of staff nurse (41.7%), clinical nurse-specialist (10%), community health nurse (10%), administrator (8.3%), nursing school faculty (6.7%), and various other roles. The levels of education reported as the highest completed were diploma (15%), associate degree (18.3%), baccalaureate in nursing (28.3%), baccalaureate in other fields (5%), master's degree in nursing, (26.7%), master's degree in another field (5%) and doctorate in education (1.7%). Most respondents (63.3%) had less than 15 years experience in nursing, and practice time in maternal-child health was less than 10 years for the majority of the sample (68.3%).

Research Question One asked if there would be agreement on the primary diagnosis for the child in the case study. Primary diagnoses identified were categorized as: (1) failure to thrive (30%), (2) developmental lag or delay (21.7%), (3) altered growth and development (15%), (4) alteration in nutrition (15%), (5) altered parenting (8.3%), (6) alteration in one aspect of growth and development (e.g., motor, language, fine motor, etc.; 3.3%). Other diagnoses had a frequency of one. Alternate (secondary) diagnoses identified were categorized as: (1) developmental lag or delay (25%), (2) altered nutrition (25%), (3) altered family processes (25%), (4) altered parenting (23.3%), (5) alteration in one aspect of growth and development (11.7%), (6) altered bowel elimination (11.7%). Other diagnoses identified as secondary diagnoses had frequencies of identification less than seven.

As failure to thrive is an accepted medical

diagnosis, but does describe a child with developmental and growth lags, analyses were completed both including failure to thrive in the developmental diagnosis category, and excluding failure to thrive from this category because of its medical origins. When developmental lag or delay, alteration in growth and development, and alteration in one aspect of growth and development are grouped, the total frequency of identification of a developmental diagnosis as *primary* diagnosis was 24 (40% of the sample). When failure to thrive is added to this group, the developmental diagnosis category had a frequency of 27 (45.8% of the sample) for primary diagnosis.

In considering all diagnostic choices of the respondents, 50 of the 60 respondents (83.3%) identified a developmental diagnosis for *either* the primary or an alternate diagnosis for the child in the case study (including failure to thrive). When failure to thrive is excluded as a developmental nursing diagnosis, the frequency of identification of diagnoses in the developmental category was 42 (70%).

Research Question Two asked whether there would be agreement in the signs and symptoms identified by respondents from the case study with proposed defining characteristics of Coviak and Derhammer (1983), while *Research Question Three* asked which would be the most frequent signs and symptoms identified. Listed in order of descending frequency, specific cues from the case study that were identified by over 60% of the respondents represented the categories of (1) altered physical growth, (2) delay in performing motor skills of age, (3) delay in performing language skills of age, (4) delay in performing manipulative skills of age, and (5) inability to perform self-care activities appropriate to age (feeding). *Research Question Four* asked what the average number of signs and symptoms of the diagnosis would be indicated as most important

for making the diagnosis. This question remained unanswered, as a large number of the respondents did not mark those cues they thought most pertinent, as had been requested.

Testing of research hypotheses through use of the chi-square test revealed that expertise scores based on levels of education attained, years of experience in maternal-child health and in nursing, and experience with children were found to be significantly related to diagnosis of altered development as either a primary or alternate diagnosis (*research hypothesis for Question Five*), but not to identification of over 75% of the cues which had been validated with content validity experts (*research hypothesis for Question Seven*). It was found that when failure to thrive was excluded from the developmental nursing diagnosis group, nurses who had identified over 75% of the validated cues were significantly more likely ($p = .038$) to identify a developmental diagnosis as primary diagnosis for the child (*research hypothesis for Question Six*). Finally, in testing the *research hypothesis for Question Eight,* two printing errors (in questions asking the respondents the number of years they had used nursing diagnosis, and at what levels of education they had used it) limited the findings. A trend was found, however, when failure to thrive was excluded from the developmental nursing diagnosis category. Nurses with longer experience in nursing diagnosis appeared to be more likely to diagnose a developmental alteration than those with less experience with nursing diagnosis (this relationship approached, but did not meet significance; $p = .0595$). This hypothesis, and the others, will require further testing before conclusions can be made.

CONCLUSIONS

There were too few nurses in the sample with master's degrees and doctoral degrees to definitely validate a developmental diagnosis, but the existence of this clinical entity was supported by its recognition by a majority of the nurses in this study. Use of a wide variety of terms to describe the condition depicted in the case study illustrates a need for nurses in maternal and child health to adopt a common term for the child who displays delayed development. The investigator proposes that "alteration in growth and development" or "developmental delay" be considered for testing by the NANDA, so that more formal validation studies may be undertaken. It is further suggested that research should be conducted to determine whether inorganic failure to thrive (i.e., delayed growth and development which is *not* caused by disease, but which can be diagnosed and treated by nurses, and only requires a physician's interventions to order the tests which rule out disease) should be classified as a nursing diagnosis, collaborative problem (as described by Carpenito 1983, 1985), or medical diagnosis.

REFERENCES

Aspinall, M.J., Jambruno, N., and Phoenix, B.S.: The why and how of nursing diagnosis, MCN **2:**354-358, 1977.

Bumbalo, J.A., and Siemon, M.K.: Nursing assessment and diagnosis: mental health problems of children, Topics Clin. Nurs. **5:**41-54, 1983.

Burns, C.E., and Thompson, M.K.: Developing a nursing diagnosis classification system for PNPs, Ped. Nurs. **10:**411-414, 1984.

Carpenito, L.J.: Nursing diagnosis: application to clinical practice, Philadelphia, 1983, J.B. Lippincott.

Carpenito, L.J.: Nursing diagnosis, Conference presentation. Grand Rapids, MI, 1985.

Coviak, C.P.: Alteration in growth and development: a nursing diagnosis validation study, Unpublished master's thesis, Grand Valley State College, Allendale, MI, 1985.

Coviak, C.P., and Derhammer, J.: A proposal for a new nursing diagnosis: actual alteration in growth and development, Unpublished manuscript, Grand Valley State College, Allendale, MI, 1983.

Fehring, R.J.: Validating diagnostic labels: standardized methodology. In Hurley, M.E., editor: Classification of nursing diagnoses: proceedings of the sixth conference, St. Louis, 1986, The C.V. Mosby Co.

Gordon, M., and Sweeney, M.A.: Methodological problems and issues in identifying and standardizing nursing diagnoses, Adv. Nurs. Sci. **2:**1-15, 1979.

Lunney, M.: Nursing diagnosis: refining the system, Amer. J. Nurs. **82:**456-459, 1982.

Oldaker, S.M.: Nursing diagnosis among healthy adolescents. In Hurley, M.E., editor: Classification of nursing diagnoses: proceedings of the sixth conference, St. Louis, 1986, The C.V. Mosby Co.

Validation of a nursing diagnosis: neonatal thermal instability

NANCY MATULICH, M.S.N., R.N.C.

Although the term *nursing diagnosis* has had a relatively short history, nurses have been using the diagnostic process to identify and label health problems and nursing care needs since the founding of modern nursing. In *Notes on Nursing* Nightingale (1859) illustrates the use of the diagnostic process for patients with "no appetite" and urges the use of "sound and ready observation" in the identification of the patient's problems. More recent authors (Gordon 1982, Newman 1984) have also been clear in their call for the use of the diagnostic process and the nursing diagnostic terminology as a way to build the clinical science of nursing and identify nursing's realm of accountability. Although the call seems to be clear, the process of implementation does not seem to be. Some authors (Gordon 1979, Carpenito, 1984) call for the restriction of nursing diagnosis to those areas where a nurse can practice independently of a physician. Others (Kim et al. 1984, Jacoby 1985) feel that there is a place for nursing diagnoses that have independent and dependent elements. Others (Stolte 1986, Burke 1984) feel that patient strengths should be diagnosed. Regardless of how these questions are resolved it is clear that nursing must continue to work toward identification and validation of a nursing language and clinical science.

PURPOSE

This descriptive survey attempted to validate the need for a nursing diagnosis in the area of neonatal thermal regulation. For research purposes three subproblems were identified:

1. Is neonatal thermal instability a clinically significant problem?
2. Is neonatal thermal instability within the realm of nursing?
3. What neonatal characteristics are commonly associated with neonatal thermal instability?

REVIEW OF THE LITERATURE

As early as 1907, investigators began describing the thermal characteristics of the neonate and the neonate's response to cold stress (Budin 1907). Since then physiologists and neonatologists have gone to extensive lengths to evaluate the neonate's thermal characteristics and to describe the numerous problems that can result from abnormal body temperatures in the neonate (Blackfan and Yaglou 1933, Silverman and Blanc 1957, Abrams 1978, Adamsons 1965, Bruck 1968, Hill and Rahentullo 1965). These authors, and others, have more than adequately demonstrated that the "Maintenance of an optimal thermal environment is one of the most important aspects of effective neonatal care," (Korones 1981, pp. 81). A variety of nursing publications and textbooks also indicate that temperature regulation is an important aspect of the care of the neonate. (Korones 1981, Clark 1979, Perez 1981, Rutter (undated), Seaver 1978).

From these and other sources it is clear that the neonate has special needs in the areas of temperature control and thermal environment. What is not clear is who is, or should be, accountable for this area of neonatal care.

DEFINITIONS

Neonatal thermal instability. Neonatal thermal instability is the inability of the neonate to maintain his core or skin temperature within the normal range without external heat or increased metabolism. For the purpose of this research the neonate was determined to be thermally unstable when two or more body temperatures were outside of the normal range.

Normal neonatal temperature range. Normal neonatal axillary temperatures range between 36.3 degrees Centigrade and 37.0 degrees Centigrade.

Nursing interventions. Nursing interventions are independent actions taken by a nurse to treat or prevent an undesired patient response to a health problem.

METHODOLOGY

The sample. The sample consisted of the first 50 babies born during one month at each of four hospitals. Neonates remaining in the hospital less than 24 hours and babies born outside of a Labor and Delivery Unit were not included in the sample. As illustrated in Table 1 the gestational age

Table 1: Characteristics of the sample

Gestational age	Number	Percent
Preterm (<38 weeks)	9	6.0
Term (38–40 weeks)	122	81.3
Post-term (>40 weeks)	19	12.7

Intrauterine growth	Number	Percent
SGA (Small for gestational age)	3	2.0
AGA (Appropriate for gestational age)	116	77.3
LGA (Large for gestational age)	31	20.6

classifications and the intrauterine growth patterns of the sample were not unusual.

Data collection. Data collection procedures consisted of a retrospective review of the medical records of each study baby. The data collected included:

1. The axillary temperatures taken during the first 24 hours of life
2. The number of medical orders written during the first 24 hours of life
3. The number of temperature-related medical orders written during the first 24 hours of life
4. The number and type of temperature-related interventions or assessments (other than temperature measurements) documented during the first day of life
5. The discharge diagnosis of each baby and the related ICDM-9CM codes as assigned by the hospital's medical records personnel
6. The gestational age and intrauterine growth of each neonate, when available.

RESULTS

Abnormal body temperatures were common in a large number of the babies studied. At least one abnormal temperature was identified in 84.5% of the babies studied. One hundred thirteen babies (56.5%) had two or more abnormal temperatures and were identified as thermally unstable. Additionally, 30% of the 1487 temperatures taken were not within the normal range (Fig. 1).

To a large extent the physicians ignored the area of temperature and temperature control in the neonate. Only 342 (7.9% of the total number of orders written) orders out of a total of 4332 medical orders pertained to temperature. By comparison, 213 orders (5%) were written to discharge the baby from the hospital. A typical baby had an average of 21 medical orders written during the first 24 hours of life, and only one or two of these orders pertained to temperature. At discharge one baby had a medical diagnosis of "other hypothermia" (ICD-9CM code 778.3). However, a review of the temperatures taken on this baby failed to identify a single abnormal temperature in the baby's entire hospital stay (Table 2).

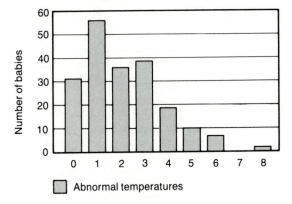

FIGURE 1 Frequency of abnormal temperatures.

Table 2: Medical diagnoses documented at discharge

	Frequency
Normal newborn	155
Hyperbilirubinemia	10
Transient tachypnea of the NB	9
Preterm	5
Cephalhematoma	5
Neonatal hypoglycemia	3
R/O Sepsis	3
Post-term	3
Meconium stained	3
Respiratory distress syndrome	2
Low birth weight	2
Meconium aspiration	2
Twin gestation	2
Hypothermia	1
All other diagnoses	6

During a baby's first 24 hours of life nurses spent a considerable amount of time assessing the baby's thermal status and intervening to correct or prevent temperature-related problems. A total of 1487 temperatures (7.4 per baby) were taken in the first 24 hours of life. A total of 2772 temperature-related nursing interventions (an average of 13.9 per baby) were documented in the first day of life (Box 1).

There was no association between the occurrence of unstable temperatures and either of the two most commonly identified characteristics of the neonate, gestational age or intrauterine growth. A one-sample chi-square test was used to determine whether the frequency of unstable temperatures differed among the three gestational age groups or among the three intrauterine growth groups. The obtained chi-squares, $\chi^2 = 0.62$ (gestational age) and $\chi^2 = 2.60$ (intrauterine growth), df = 2, were not significant.

DISCUSSION

Based on the data from this study it appears that thermal instability is a clinically significant problem and that nurses are making as-

BOX 1: Documented temperature-related nursing interventions

Extra blanket applied
Wrapped in warm blanket
Dressed in shirt and diaper
Dressed in shirt, diaper and hat
Cared for in servo controlled incubator
Cared for in non-servo controlled incubator
Transferred to incubator
Placed under radiant warmer
Cared for under radiant warmer
Transferred to radiant warmer
Transferred to incubator
Transferred to open crib
Weaned to open crib
Heat shield in use
Thermo pad in use

sessments and intervening based on an un-documented, and possibly subconscious, nursing diagnosis of neonatal thermal instability. Further, supporting the belief that this problem is within the realm of nursing is the fact that physicians generally ignored this area of newborn care when writing medical orders and documenting diagnoses.

Unfortunately, this study was not able to provide any guidelines for the practicing nurse to use to identify neonates at increased risk for neonatal thermal instability. But, given the high incidence of abnormal temperatures in the sample, it appears that all infants deserve careful assessment and preventive interventions.

One weakness in this study was its failure to identify and evaluate problems that occur secondary to thermal instability.

REFERENCES

Abrams, R.M.: Thermal physiology of the fetus. In Sinclair, J.C., editor: Temperature regulation and energy metabolism in the newborn, New York, 1978, Grune & Stratton.

Adamsons, K., Jr., Gandy, G.M., and James, L.S.: The influence of thermal factors upon oxygen consumption of the newborn human infant, J. Ped. **66**:495-502, 1965.

Blackfan, K., and Yaglou, C.: The premature infant: a study of the effects of atmospheric conditions on growth and development. Amer. J. Dis. Child. **46**:1175-1190, 1933.

Bruck, K.: Which environmental temperature does the premature infant prefer? Pediatrics **41**:10027, 1968.

Budin, P.: The nursling, London, 1907, Caxton Publishing Co.

Burke, B.: Special interest group report: nursing diagnosis and the healthy client. In Kim, M.J., McFarland, G.K., and McLane, A.M., editors: Classification of nursing diagnoses: proceedings of the fifth national conference, St. Louis, 1984, The C.V. Mosby Co.

Carpenito, L.J.: Is the problem a nursing diagnosis? Amer. J. Nurs. **84**:1418-1419, 1984.

Clark, A.L., and Affonso, D.D.: Childbearing: a nursing perspective, ed. 2, Philadelphia, 1979, F.A. Davis.

Gordon, M.: The concept of nursing diagnosis, Nurs. Clin. North Amer. **14**:487-496, 1979.

Gordon, M.: Nursing diagnosis, process and application, New York, 1982, McGraw-Hill.

Hill, J.R., and Rahentullo, K.A.: Heat balance and the metabolic rate of newborn babies in relation to environmental temperature, and the effect of age and of weight on basal metabolic rate, J. Physiol. **180**:239, 1965.

Jacoby, M.K.: The dilemma of physiological problems: eliminating the double standard, Amer. J. Nurs. **85**:281, 285, 1985.

Kim, M.J.: Without collaboration, what's left? Amer. J. Nurs. **85**:281-284, 1985.

Kim, M.J., Amoroso-Seritella, R., Gulanick, M., and others: Clinical validation of cardiovascular nursing diagnoses. In Kim, M.J., McFarland, G.K., and McLane, A.M., editors: Classification of nursing diagnoses: proceedings of the fifth national conference, St. Louis, 1984, The C.V. Mosby Co.

Korones, S.B.: High risk newborn infants: the basis for intensive nursing care, ed. 3, St. Louis, 1981, The C.V. Mosby Co.

Newman, M.A.: Nursing diagnosis: looking at the whole, Amer. J. Nurs. **84**:1496-1499, 1984.

Nightingale, F.: Notes on nursing: what it is and what it is not, London, 1859, Harrison and Sons. (Facsimile reprint by J.B. Lippincott).

Perez, R.H., editor: Protocols for perinatal nursing practice, St. Louis, 1981, The C.V. Mosby Co.

Rutter, N.: A guide to incubator care of infants, Basinstake, Hampshire (England), undated, Vickers Medical Publication.

Seaver, J., editor: Thermoregulation and temperature stress in the newborn, Hatboro, PA, 1978, Narco/Air-Shields.

Silverman, W., Agate, F., and Fertig, J.: A sequential trail of the nonthermal effect of atmospheric humidity on survival of newborn infants of low birth weight, Pediatrics, **31**:477, 1963.

Silverman, W., and Blanc, W.: The effects of humidity on survival of the newly-born premature infants, Pediatrics, **20**:477, 1957.

Stolte, K.M.: Nursing diagnosis and the childbearing woman, MCN **11**:13-15, 1986.

Wessel, S.L., and Kim, M.J.: Nursing functions related to the nursing diagnosis *decreased cardiac output.* In Kim, M.J., McFarland, G.K., and McLane, A.M., editors: Classification of nursing diagnoses: proceedings of the fifth national conference, St. Louis, 1984, The C.V. Mosby Co.

World Health Organization: International classification of diseases: clinical modification, 9th revision, Ann Arbor, MI, 1978, World Health Organization.

Validation of the defining characteristics of the nursing diagnosis, alteration in comfort: pain*

MARY P. RIORDAN, M.S., R.N.

BACKGROUND OF THE PROBLEM

The human response of pain is a complex phenomenon affected by a multitude of factors, physical, psychological, emotional and social. Pain is an individualized response that varies among people, cultures, age and sex.

Nursing is a service-oriented profession concerned with providing goal-directed care to patients, families and communities in situations where health care needs have been assessed. The Nursing Social Policy Statement has defined nursing in the following way: "Nursing is the diagnosis and treatment of human responses to actual or potential health problems" (ANA 1980, p. 9). Pain and discomfort have been identified by the ANA in The Nursing Social Policy Statement as a response to a health problem. According to the ANA Standards of Nursing Practice (1973) it is the responsibility of the nurse to assess the health status of an individual and to make a nursing diagnosis from the data which have been collected.

Nurses are the health care providers who have the closest contact with patients on a daily basis and therefore are in the optimal position to diagnose the problem of pain and help the individual, whether through relief or coping mechanisms, or both.

In order to diagnose a problematic response a nurse must gather data through communication with and observation of the patient. He or she must process the data using scientific knowledge as a background. This will lead to the generation of hypotheses and the eventual labeling of the collected cues into a nursing diagnosis.

The goal of nursing is to help patients relieve a problem or cope with and manage it. A complete and thorough assessment provides the nurse with necessary data to provide the care that leads to patient relief or improved management of the problem.

STATEMENT OF THE PROBLEM

In order to help alleviate problems and be accountable for interventions, the nurse must have a broad knowledge base upon which to base her actions. The purpose of this study was to further validate the defining characteristics of the nursing diagnosis "alteration in comfort: pain." Differentiation between the cues utilized by nurses in diagnosing acute pain versus chronic pain were also studied. Through further validation, it was the investigator's goal to contribute to the body of knowledge for nursing in order to increase nurses' levels of awareness in the area of pain assessment.

CONCEPTUAL FRAMEWORK

The framework of the self-care agency model of nursing proposed by Orem (1980) and pain as a stressor as described by Selye (1978) in stress theory were utilized in this study.

Pain can be considered a stressor on both the physical and emotional level. A person will initially adapt to pain as a stressor, but as the pain intensifies the person's resistance may become weakened and susceptible to exhaustion. It is at this point that the person may need the assistance of a nurse.

The nurse takes on the role of the dependent-care agent in Orem's theory

*This research project was funded in part by a Federal Nurse Traineeship.

221

(1980). As a dependent-care agent she provides or assists in caring for those who are unable to provide their own self-care. It is the responsibility of the nurse to actively conduct ongoing assessment of a patient experiencing the stress of pain. The nurse would determine at what point during the stages of stress adaptation the patient's ability to perform his or her own self-care may be threatened, and it would be at this point that the nurse would intervene. The nurse's role would be to assist the patient with self-care and to encourage greater independent self-care.

In order for the nurse to adequately assess the self-care capabilities, life- and health-sustaining behaviors, and to help a patient recover and cope, he or she must have a complete data base, founded on enough scientific knowledge to identify nursing diagnoses and a prescription for care.

REVIEW OF THE LITERATURE
Definition of pain

Pain is an individualized, subjective experience expressed differently by different people. It is affected by cultural, social, psychological, emotional and physical norms. As Sternbach (1968) states, "Pain is a hurt that we feel" (p. 1). One of the reasons for such an individualized response can be related to structural differences in the nervous system. The sensitivity of the nervous system varies from person to person. Experience can affect one's attitude toward pain. Varied perceptions of the situation in which pain is occurring will result in different responses.

The most comprehensive definition of pain which considers its many aspects is, "Pain is an abstract concept which refers to (1) a personal, private sensation of hurt; (2) a harmful stimulus which signals current or impending tissue damage; (3) a pattern of responses which operate to protect the organism from harm" (Sternbach 1968, p. 12).

Nursing assessment of pain

The role of the nurse in pain assessment has been discussed in the literature.

The professional nurse assumes responsibility for pain assessment for the purpose of providing information that will assist the physician in diagnosis and therapy, and that will assist the nurse in (1) making a nursing diagnosis, (2) evlauating and instituting nursing care measures or prescribed therapy for pain relief, (3) helping the individual with chronic pain achieve positive adaptive mechanisms and (4) evaluating the effectiveness of interventions by determining the degree of relief obtained (Johnson 1977, p. 139).

Patient observation by the nurse is a key component in the process of pain assessment. The importance of patient observation is brought out in a study of 102 patients with short-term, long-term, and progressive pain done by Jacox (1980). Seventy percent of the patients responded that they preferred not to discuss their pain with others and approximately two thirds said they try to keep their pain to themselves and suffer quietly.

Objective pain assessment by nurses is supported by Davitz and Davitz (1981). In a study, 81 nurses were asked to rate the degree of pain and psychological discomfort caused by certain illnesses compiled from a list of 80 illnesses. The results of the study exhibited that: (1) nurses infer greater psychological distress than physical pain in most illnesses and injury, (2) inferences on psychological distress are separate from physical pain, (3) in some illnesses, nurses do see an increased relationship between physical and psychological distress and therefore recognize increased suffering in these particular situations, (4) nurses consider trauma and cardiovascular illnesses the most painful conditions and (5) diseases which are associated with death or long-term disability cause psychological distress.

Jacox (1980) and Johnson (1977) offer assessment guidelines which are helpful to nurses and include: (1) following up verbal report of pain with evaluation of the pain, (2) assessment of physiologic signs, especially in situations where the level of consciousness is altered, (3) use other terms besides *pain* in assessing presence of pain, (4) chronic pain patients do not exhibit the usual signs and symptoms of pain and will not recognize that they are in pain, (5) obtain detailed description of the types of situations that are painful for the patient, (6) be empathetic and (7) determine how the patient deals with pain at home.

The use of these guidelines is supported by a study by Jacox (1980) of 442 nurses and nursing students. Forty-six patient behaviors were identified, and the nurses responded that the physiologic signs and behaviors were easier to assess than were verbal communication indicators.

RESEARCH QUESTIONS

The questions of interest to the investigator which were answered in this study were:

- What cues are utilized by nurses in making the diagnosis of Alteration in Comfort: Acute Pain?
- What cues are utilized by nurses in making the diagnosis of Alteration in Comfort: Chronic Pain?
- What cues are common to both categories of pain?

METHODOLOGY

This study was a descriptive study conducted for the purpose of validation of the accepted clinical cues utilized in formulating the nursing diagnosis of alteration in comfort: pain.

The subjects who were asked to participate in this study were registered professional nurses who were familiar with nursing diagnosis. The sample included: (1) colleagues of the investigator enrolled in the master's degree program for nursing at a New England college; (2) members of a conference group for the clas-

sification of nursing diagnosis; and (3) graduate nursing faculty at a New England college.

The sampling method was a convenience sample from the above-mentioned groups. Return of the completed form of the Alteration in Comfort: Pain Checklist was considered consent to participate.

The investigator obtained her data through the administration of a survey questionnaire which was adapted with permission of the author from a graphic rating scale developed by Vincent (1983) and utilized in a study for the validation of a nursing diagnosis.

The investigator modified the graphic rating scale, which had a reliability of 0.740 using Cronbach's alpha reliability coefficient (Vincent 1985, p. 637). The modified graphic rating scale utilized for the purposes of this study was called the Alteration in Comfort: Pain Checklist, which had a Chronbach's Alpha Reliability coefficient of 0.9779.

Part I of the survey was a list of 53 clinical cues taken from a review of the literature and the Fourth National Conference for Classification of Nursing Diagnoses (Kim and Moritz 1982, p. 285). All cues were listed on the checklist twice. The first listing was categorized under acute pain and the second listing was categorized under chronic pain. For each clinical cue, a percentage range was given indicating how often a cue was used in arriving at the diagnosis of alteration in comfort: pain. The participants were asked to think of a representative sample of patients from their most recent clinical practice whom they had cared for and had diagnosed as having pain. The participants were then asked to check off the applicable cues they had utilized in making the diagnosis of alteration in comfort: pain and the percentage of times they utilized those cues.

RESULTS

The sample consisted of 86 registered nurses (R.N.'s). The age of the subjects ranged from under 25 to 55 years of age with the majority (83.8%) of the sample being 26 to 45 years of age. The educational preparation of all participants was a minimum of a BS degree. A master's degree was held by 53.5%; 44.2% held a bachelors degree; and 2.3% held a doctoral degree. Of those subjects who held an advanced degree, 32.6% obtained that degree in the medical-surgical area, and 57% of the entire sample practiced in the medical-surgical specialty. The remainder of the sample represented diverse areas of nursing practice.

Seventy-two subjects (83.7%) were involved with working with patients at the time of data collection. The subjects' years of experience in nursing ranged from "under 5 years" to "over 28 years," the majority (48.8%) reporting 5 to 10 years of clinical experience in nursing. The subjects' experience with caring for patients having alteration in comfort: pain was reported as moderate to extensive by 96.5%. Experience with nursing diagnosis was evenly divided between competent and proficient, 38.4% each.

The remainder reported evidence as novice and expert, 12.8% and 10.4% respectively. Seventy-seven participants (89.5%) reported they based their nursing interventions on nursing diagnosis.

Analysis of the data was accomplished through the utilization of descriptive statistics.

The only cue reported as used in diagnosing acute pain "nearly always" (80–100%) by over 75% of the subjects was "statement regarding pain" (77.9%; see Table 1). The only other cue utilized by more than 50% of the subjects in the same "nearly always" category was "protective guarding behavior" (61.6%).

No chronic pain cue was reported as utilized by more than 75% of the respondents in the "nearly always" category. "Statements regarding pain" was utilized by over 50% of the sample in the "nearly always" category for chronic pain (see Table 1).

No cue was reported as used "nearly always" in diagnosing acute or chronic pain by 95.0% or more of the sample.

Table 1: Acute and chronic pain cues utilized "nearly always" by 50% of sample (n=86)

Category of pain	Cue	F	%
Acute	Statements regarding pain	67	77.9%
	Protective guarding behavior	53	61.6%
Chronic	Statements regarding pain	51	59.3%

Table 2: Acute and chronic pain cues utilized "sometimes" or above by 95% of sample (n=86)

Category of pain	Cue	F	%
Acute	Protective guarding behavior	84	97.6%
	Statements regarding pain	83	96.5%
	Restlessness	83	96.5%
	Moaning	82	95.3%
	Crying	82	95.3%
Chronic	Statements regarding pain	85	98.9%
	Self-focusing	82	95.3%

Cues used "sometimes" and above (40–100%) by 95% or more of the sample in diagnosing acute pain were "protective guarding behavior" (97.6%), "statements regarding pain" (96.5%), "restlessness" (96.5%), "moaning" (95.3%) and "crying" (95.3%) (see Table 2).

Chronic pain cues reported as utilized 40% or more of the time by 95% or more of the subjects included "statements regarding pain" (98.9%) and "self-focusing" (95.3%).

Cues utilized by more than 75% of the subjects 40–100% of the time in diagnosing pain were analyzed. Twenty-five cues were reported as utilized "sometimes" or above in formulating the diagnosis acute pain (see Table 3), and 17 cues were reported utilized in

arriving at the diagnosis chronic pain (see Table 4).

From the categories of "sometimes" and above (40–100%), 10 cues were reported which were the same for both acute and chronic pain (Table 5). There were 15 cues utilized in formulating the diagnosis of acute pain which were not used in formulating the diagnosis of chronic pain, and 7 cues utilized in formulating the diagnosis of chronic pain but not utilized in formulating the diagnosis of acute pain (Table 5).

DISCUSSION

As indicated by the results, the cue "statements regarding pain" was the most frequently utilized diagnostic cue for alteration in comfort: pain in both acute pain and chronic pain. This result lends further support to McCaffery (1972), who defined pain as being what that patient says it is and exists whenever the patient says it does. From the data, this cue might be considered as a critical defining characteristic of pain;

Table 3: Frequency distribution of acute pain cues utilized "sometimes" or above by 75% of sample (n=86)

Cue	F	%
Protective guarding behavior	84	97.6%
Statements regarding pain	83	96.5%
Restlessness	83	96.5%
Moaning	82	95.3%
Crying	82	95.3%
Anxiety	81	94.2%
Change in respiratory rate	80	93.0%
Grimace	80	93.0%
Change in pulse rate	79	91.8%
Whimpering	78	90.7%
Self-focusing	77	89.6%
Irritability	77	89.5%
Clenched teeth	75	87.2%
Tightened muscles of jaw	74	86.0%
Agitation	74	86.0%
Unusual posture (knees to abdomen)	72	83.7%
Writhing	71	82.6%
Change in blood pressure	69	80.2%
Change in skin color (pallor)	69	80.2%
Grunting	69	80.2%
Knotted brow	69	80.2%
Pinched features	66	76.7%
Diaphoresis	66	76.7%
Rubbing	65	75.6%
Widely open/tightly shut eyes	65	75.6%

Table 4: Frequency distribution of chronic pain cues utilized "sometimes" or above by 75% of sample (n=86)

Cue	F	%
Statements regarding pain	85	98.9%
Self-focusing	82	95.3%
Irritability	81	94.2%
Protective guarding behavior	81	94.2%
"Beaten" look	78	90.7%
Restlessness	76	88.3%
Depression	75	87.2%
Withdrawal from social contact	75	87.2%
Anxiety	74	86.1%
Agitation	69	80.2%
Sighing	68	79.0%
Regression	67	77.9%
Muscle aches/heaviness	66	76.7%
Knotted brow	66	76.7%
Eyes lack luster	65	75.6%
Crying	65	75.6%
Rubbing	65	75.6%

Table 5: Common and differential cues utilized "sometimes" or above by 75% of sample (n=86)

Category of cue	Specific cue		Rank
Common cues for acute and chronic pain	Statements *re* pain	($\bar{x}$ 97.7%)	1
	Protective guarding behavior	($\bar{x}$ 95.9%)	2
	Self-focusing	($\bar{x}$ 92.5%)	3
	Restlessness	($\bar{x}$ 92.4%)	4
	Irritability	($\bar{x}$ 91.9%)	5
	Anxiety	($\bar{x}$ 90.2%)	6
	Crying	($\bar{x}$ 85.5%)	7
	Agitation	($\bar{x}$ 83.1%)	8
	Knotted brow	($\bar{x}$ 78.4%)	9
	Rubbing	($\bar{x}$ 75.6%)	10
Cues utilized for acute pain only	Moaning	(95.3%)	1
	Change in respiratory rate	(93%)	2
	Grimace	(93%)	2
	Change in pulse rate	(91.8%)	3
	Whimpering	(90.7%)	4
	Clenched teeth	(87.2%)	5
	Tightened muscles of jaw	(86.1%)	6
	Unusual posture (knees drawn up to abdomen)	(83.7%)	7
	Writhing	(82.6%)	8
	Change in blood pressure	(80.3%)	9
	Change in skin color (pallor)	(80.3%)	9
	Grunting	(80.3%)	9
	Pinched features	(76.8%)	10
	Diaphoresis	(76.7%)	11
	Widely open/tightly shut eyes	(75.6%)	12
Cues utilized for chronic pain only	"Beaten" look	(90.7%)	1
	Depression	(87.2%)	2
	Withdrawal	(87.2%)	2
	Sighing	(79.0%)	3
	Regression	(77.9%)	4
	Muscle aches/heaviness	(76.7%)	5
	Eyes lack luster	(75.6%)	6

however, it does not meet the criteria of being reported as "nearly always" present (80–100%) by the total sample.

No cues were utilized "nearly always" (80–100%) by 95% or more of the participants. Five cues were used in diagnosing acute pain by 95% or more subjects in the "sometimes" or above category. Two cues were utilized in formulating a diagnosis of chronic pain for the mentioned criteria. This result may lend support to a reliability factor for the cues utilized in diagnosing alteration in comfort: pain as discussed by Diers (1979). Diers postulates that the more data one must consider in formulating a judgment, the less reliable that judgment may be. Hence, the fewer the cues necessary for determining the diagnosis alteration in comfort: pain, the more reliable those cues would be for this diagnosis and therefore could perhaps be considered more reliable defining characteristics.

Data obtained which indicated cues utilized by 75% of the nurses "sometimes" or above may be cues which could be considered diagnostic and may have implications for nursing practice and education in terms of refining the list of diagnostic cues for alteration in comfort: pain.

The differences indicated by the results between acute and chronic pain support Johnson's work (1977) in which she indicates that a critical aspect of chronic pain is that it imposes an emotional, physical and financial stress on the individual. It is interesting to note that the results indicated that there was a predominance of behavioral cues utilized in diagnosing chronic pain, whereas there was more of a mixture of behavioral and physiological cues utilized in diagnosing acute pain. Behavioral cues could be interpreted as indicators of the emotional and financial stress which Johnson discusses as a result of chronic pain. The physiological cues represented the changes which occur in acute pain owing to stimulation of the autonomic nervous system.

Tables 3 and 4 indicate that this sample utilized different cues in diagnosing acute and chronic pain. This finding may lend support to further refinement and definition of specific pain diagnoses, i.e., alteration in comfort: acute pain and alteration in comfort: chronic pain. Further, the data from this study would support the postulation that both the general diagnosis of alteration in comfort: pain and acute pain and chronic pain could have the critical defining characteristics of "statements regarding pain."

The data from this study lend validity to the cues designated as defining characteristics at the Third and Fourth National Conferences (Kim and Moritz 1982). The data indicated that all high-frequency cues were listed by the Conference Group also.

IMPLICATIONS FOR NURSING PRACTICE

Implications for nursing practice resulting from this study include a further refinement and validation of the multitude of diagnostic cues utilized in the nursing diagnosis of alteration in comfort: pain.

In terms of education, nurses should be made aware of the broad range of diagnostic cues, and should be alert to identify possible critical defining characteristics for this diagnosis.

Further refinement of the diagnostic cues contributes to the development of a body of highly reliable cues utilized in the formulation of this diagnosis. Nurses need a set of highly reliable cues to further delineate and support their decision to diagnose a patient with alteration in comfort: pain.

Education plays a role in increasing nurses' awareness of these highly reliable cues as well as the utilization of different cues in diagnosing alteration in comfort: acute pain and alteration in comfort: chronic pain.

RECOMMENDATIONS FOR FUTURE STUDY

The investigator suggests further research and testing of the findings. In particular, further testing of the validity and reliability of cues utilized at least sometimes (40–100%) by 75% of the nursing population in this study is recommended.

Studies that would further refine and validate the diagnostic cues for this nursing diagnosis and support the critical defining characteristics would serve to expand the knowledge base of nursing science.

Studies are needed to further refine the critical defining characteristics for alteration in comfort: pain, and to further test highly reliable defining characteristics for diagnosing acute and chronic pain. This could be the basis of studies that would test for the existence of specific diagnoses within the category of alteration in comfort: pain, i.e., acute and/or chronic pain.

Research in the area of pain has important applications in nursing practice and patient care. Pain is such a complex and subjective phenomenon that research that contributes to the expansion of the nursing knowledge base will serve to refine and improve the pain assessment process. The more specific and accurate the assessment process is, the more definitive nursing interventions will be and, therefore, the quality of patient care will improve.

REFERENCES

American Nurses' Association: Standards of nursing practice, Kansas City, 1973, American Nurses' Association.

American Nurses' Association: Nursing: a social policy statement, Kansas City, 1980, American Nurses' Association.

Copp, L.A.: The spectrum of suffering, Amer. J. Nurs. **74:**491-495, 1974.

Davitz, J.R., and Davitz, L.L.: Inferences of patients' pain and psychological distress, New York, 1981, Springer Verlag.

Diers, D.: Research in nursing practice, Philadelphia, 1979, J.B. Lippincott.

Gordon, M.: Nursing diagnosis and the diagnostic process, Amer. J. Nurs. **76:**1298-1300, 1976.

Gordon, M.: Nursing diagnosis process and application, New York, 1982, McGraw-Hill.

Gordon, M., and Sweeney, M.A.: Methodological problems and issues in identifying and standardizing nursing diagnoses, Adv. Nurs. Sci. **2:**1-15, 1979.

Jacox, A.K.: The assessment of pain. In Smith, L.W., Merskey, H., and Gross, S.C., editors: Pain: meaning and management, New York, 1980, Spectrum.

Johnson, M.: Pain: how do you know it's there and what do you do? Amer. J. Nurs. **76:**48-50, 1976.

Johnson, M.: The assessment of clinical pain. In Jacox, A.K., editor: Pain: a source book for nurses and other health professionals, Boston, 1977, Little, Brown.

Johnson, R.I.: Orem self-care model of nursing. In Fitzpatrick, J.J. and Whall, A.L., editors: Conceptual models of nursing: analysis and application, Bowie, MD, 1983, Robert J. Brady.

Kim, M.J., and Mortiz, D.A., editors: Classification of nursing diagnoses: proceedings of the third and fourth national conferences, New York, 1982, McGraw-Hill.

Mahoney, C.A.: Some implications for nursing diagnosis of pain, Nurs. Clin. North Amer. **12:**613-619, 1977.

Mallick, J.: Nursing diagnosis and the novice student. Nurs. Health Care **4:**455-459, 1983.

McCaffery, M.: Nursing management of the patient with pain, Philadelphia, 1972, J.B. Lippincott.

McCauley, K., and Polomano, R.C.: Acute pain: a nursing perspective with cardiac surgical patients, Topics Clin. Nurs. **2:**45-55, 1980.

McLachlan, C.: Recognizing pain, Amer. J. Nurs. **74:**496-497, 1974.

Melzack, R.: Phantom limbs, Psychol. Today, **4:**63-68, 1970.

Melzack, R.: The puzzle of pain, New York, 1973, Basic Books.

Merskey, H.: The nature of pain. In Smith, L.W., Merskey, H. and Gross, S.C., editors: Pain: meaning and management, New York, 1980, Spectrum.

Munley, M.J., and Keane, M.C.: Symposium on impressions of pain: a nursing diagnosis (Foreword), Nurs. Clin. North Amer. **12:**609-611, 1977.

Orem, D.: Nursing: concepts of practice, ed. 2, New York, 1980, McGraw Hill.

Polit, D., and Hungler, B.: Nursing research, Philadelphia, 1983, J.B. Lippincott.

Rankin, M.: The progressive pain of cancer, Topics Clin. Nurs. **2:**57-73, 1980.

Selye, H.: The stress of life, revised edition, New York, 1978, McGraw-Hill.

Sternbach, R.: Pain: a psychophysiological analysis, New York, 1968, Academic Press.

Vincent, K.G.: The validation of a nursing diagnosis by psychiatric clinical specialists, Boston College, Chestnut Hill, MA, Unpublished research paper.

Vincent, K.G.: The validation of a nursing diagnosis: a nurse consensus survey, Nurs. Clin. North Amer. **20:**631-640, 1985.

Wallace, K.G., and Hays, J.: Nursing management of chronic pain, J. Neurosurg. Nurs. **14:**185-191, 1982.

Wong, J., and Wong, S.: An assessment of postoperative pain (theatre nursing), Nurs. Times **76:**18-20, 1980.

Content validation of the nursing diagnosis fluid volume deficit related to active isotonic loss

GMAC-AACN RESEARCH COMMITTEE
JILL GERSHAN, M.S.N., R.N., C.C.R.N.
MARY KAY JIRICKA, M.S.N., R.N., C.C.R.N.
CAROL SMEJKAL, M.S.N., R.N., C.C.R.N.
CECILIA FREEMAN, M.S., R.N., C.C.R.N.
KAY GREENLEE, M.S.N., R.N., C.C.R.N.
GENEE BRUKWITZKI, M.S.N., R.N.
MARY ROSS, M.S.N., R.N.
DAWN L. JOHNSON, M.N., R.N., C.C.R.N.
TONI BALISTRIERI, M.S.N., R.N., C.C.R.N.

The nursing diagnosis "fluid volume deficit" and the identified etiologies and defining characteristics have not been validated. This nursing diagnosis is complex, because defining characteristics differ depending upon the etiology. For example, fluid volume deficit related to free water loss is manifested by signs and symptoms of intravascular volume depletion as well as neurologic changes. Whereas, fluid volume deficit related to isotonic loss is primarily associated with signs and symptoms of intravascular volume depletion. The purpose of this study is to validate defining characteristics of the nursing diagnosis "fluid volume deficit related to active isotonic loss."

DEFINITION OF TERMS

Operational definitions of key words in the study include:

Nursing diagnosis: A clinical judgment about an individual, family or community which is derived through a deliberate, systematic process of data collection and analysis. It provides the basis for prescriptions for definitive therapy for which the nurse is accountable. A nursing diagnosis is expressed concisely and includes the etiology of the condition when known (Shoemaker 1985).

Active isotonic loss: acute loss of both water and serum electrolytes, such that serum electrolyte values do not change.

Relevant: the amount of significance a defining characteristic has in the determination of a nursing diagnosis (Fehring 1986).

Fluid volume deficit: an imbalance in body fluids caused by deficient intake or excessive excretion.

Defining characteristics: signs and symptoms or other information that, when clustered together, identify the nursing diagnosis and have a weighted ratio greater than or equal to 0.50 according to the diagnostic content validity (DCV) methodology (Fehring 1986).

Critical indicators: defining characteristics that have a weighted ratio greater than or equal to 0.75 (Fehring 1986).

Nurse experts: registered nurses who are members of the Greater Milwaukee Area Chapter of the American Association of Critical Care Nurses (GMAC-AACN) and who voluntarily completed the Validation Tool.

THEORETICAL FRAMEWORK

Nursing diagnosis has been called a foundation for nursing theory. Some theorists believe it is the initial step in the development of nursing science (Kritek 1978).

As a theoretical framework, nursing diagnosis has several important characteristics. First, it provides common terminology for labelling or naming related concepts. This is considered to be first-level theory (Kritek

1978). Second, nursing diagnosis emerges from practice, because it describes what nurses see and do. Third, nursing diagnosis has clinical relevance as it is useful in guiding practice (McKay 1977).

Nursing diagnoses also possess the characteristics of a science as described by Jacox (1974). These characteristics are as follows: (1) science is cumulative; (2) the knowledge is incomplete and is modified by building upon previous knowledge; (3) new hypotheses can be generated; and (4) it is useful to clinical practice.

In addition, according to Bircher (1975), the natural history of a science includes three steps. These are: (1) identifying shared critical attributes, (2) grouping them into related phenomena, and (3) connecting interrelated phenomena to theoretical concepts. When nurses correlate indicators or signs and symptoms with a clinical state they are implementing the first two steps.

Nursing diagnosis as a theoretical framework and a foundation for science provides countless opportunities for research. At present, 65 diagnostic labels have been identified; however, there is little research data to validate these labels.

DESIGN AND METHODOLOGY

The diagnostic content validity (DCV) method was used to validate the nursing diagnosis "fluid volume deficit, related to active isotonic loss." The DCV model utilizes retrospective evidence obtained from experts on the characteristics of a given diagnostic label. The DCV model is an adaptation by Fehring (1984) of the content validity index (CVI) method described by Waltz and Bausell (1981).

The steps to apply the DCV method are as follows:

1. The characteristics of an identified diagnosis are rated by nurses on a scale of 1 to 5. The ratings indicate how representative each characteristic is of a given diagnosis: (1) not at all relevant, (2) very little

relevancy, (3) somewhat relevant, (4) quite relevant, and (5) very relevant.
2. The delphi technique is used to obtain consensus.
3. The responses are assigned weights: $5 = 1.0$, $4 = 0.75$, $3 = 0.50$, $2 = 0.25$, $1 = 0.0$. The weights for each characteristic are summed, and then divided by the total number of responses. The result is the weighted ratio for each characteristic.
4. The characteristics with ratios greater than or equal to 0.75 are identified as critical indicators.
5. The characteristics with ratios greater than or equal to 0.50 are identified as defining characteristics.
6. The characteristics with ratios less than 0.50 are not considered representative of the nursing diagnosis.

Procedure for collection of data

Characteristics associated with fluid volume deficit were obtained through a review of the nursing literature. A validation tool containing a list of characteristics was developed and sent to nurse experts along with an introductory letter, a demographic questionnaire, and a self-addressed stamped return envelope.

The delphi Technique was used. Three rounds of data collection were completed. After each round of data collection the validation tool was revised and sent to the participating respondents. Participation in the study was voluntary. Anonymity was maintained. The nurse experts received a coded envelope to return completed questionnaires and their names did not appear on the validation tool.

DATA ANALYSIS

Data analysis for this pilot study was divided into two parts. Nurse-expert demographic data were described, and the variables identified in the literature review were clustered according to weighted ratios.

Returns from 53 volunteer nurse experts

Table 1: Demographics of nurse-experts from round 3 (N=20)

	Frequency	%
Certified critical-care nurse (CCRN)	13	65%
Full-time employment	15	75%
BSN as basic education	16	80%
BSN as highest degree	9	45%
MSN as highest degree	8	40%
Employed in a community or private hospital	16	80%
Provide care in a variety of critical care settings	17	85%
Use nursing diagnosis in practice	19	95%

were obtained in the first round, 25 in the second round, and 21 in the final round. Demographic data for 20 of the final 21 experts were available. The majority of nurse experts (85%) were under 40 years of age and had 8.5 years of experience in critical-care units. Other characteristics of those who completed all three rounds of data collection are shown in Table 1.

The proficiency in use of nursing diagnosis is central to the issue of validation of nursing diagnosis. In this sample, 95% of the nurse experts used nursing diagnosis regularly in their practice. Hospital inservice, self-study, and continuing education offerings were the most frequent methods of learning about nursing diagnosis. In addition, 50% had taken academic courses.

The descriptive statistics generated for this analysis were calculated on a Sperry Univac mainframe computer using the Statistical Packages for the Social Sciences. Since each variable was rated on a scale of 1 to 5, a program to recode these numbers was used to provide a weighted ratio.

There were a total of 72 variables used in the survey. Of these variables, 9 were identified as critical indicators and 14 were identified as defining characteristics (see Box 1). A summary of the progress of each of the 72 variables through the three rounds is provided in Table 2.

BOX 1: Critical indicators and defining characteristics

Critical indicators

Negative intake and output balance
Postural blood pressure changes
Changes in body weight
Decreased central venous pressure
Increased hematocrit/hemoconcentration
Decrease blood pressure
Decreased urine output
Concentrated urine/increased specific gravity
Pulmonary capillary wedge pressure <6

Defining characteristics

Normal serum sodium
Decreased venous filling
Decreased pulse volume/pressure
Confusion
Dry mucous membranes
Poor skin turgor
Narrow pulse pressure
Weakness
Thready pulse
Decreased cardiac output
Increased heart rate
Moist or clammy skin
Increased thirst
Increased blood urea nitrogen

Table 2: Summary of variable results on each round

Variables	Round			Variables	Round		
	1	2	3		1	2	3
1. Neg. I & O balance	CI	CI	CI	37. ↑ Hematocrit/hemoconc.	CI	CI	CI
2. Decreased PaO₂	—	—	—	38. Rhonchi	—	—	—
3. Normal serum sodium	D	D	D	39. Decreased urine osmo.	—	—	—
4. Poor judgment	—	—	—	40. Elevated temperature	D	D	—
5. Postural BP changes	CI	CI	CI	41. Poor capillary refill	D	D	—
6. Deep respirations	—	—	—	42. Shallow respirations	D	D	—
7. Changes in body weight	CI	CI	CI	43. ↑ Serum creatinine	D	D	—
8. Resp. acidosis	—	—	—	44. Anxious	D	D	—
9. Elevate systolic BP	—	—	—	45. Decreased cardiac output	D	D	D
10. Paranoia	—	—	—	46. Dry skin	D	D	—
11. Increased urine output	—	—	—	47. Increased heart rate	CI	CI	D
12. Decreased venous filling	D	D	D	48. Agitation	D	D	—
13. Nausea	—	—	—	49. Decreased BP	CI	CI	CI
14. Muscle cramping	D	D	—	50. Moist or clammy skin	D	D	D
15. Paradoxical pulse	—	—	—	51. Decreased urine output	CI	CI	CI
16. Flaring nares	—	—	—	52. Increased thirst	CI	CI	D
17. Edema	D	—	—	53. Cool skin	D	D	—
18. ↓ Venous pulsations	D	D	—	54. Increased resp. rate	D	D	—
19. Personality changes	—	—	—	55. Increased BUN	D	D	D
20. Tracheal tugging	—	—	—	56. Coma	D	D	—
21. Metabolic acidosis	D	D	—	57. Pale skin	—	—	—
22. Seizures	—	—	—	58. Conc. urine/ ↑ sp. grav.	D	CI	CI
23. ↓ Pulse vol./pressure	CI	D	D	59. Restlessness	D	—	—
24. Confusion	D	D	D	60. Decreased temperature	—	—	—
25. Dry mucous membranes	CI	CI	D	61. Weight loss	D	—	—
26. Decreased CVP	CI	CI	CI	62. Altered sleep patterns	—	—	—
27. Lethargy	D	D	—	63. Hypoventilation	—	—	—
28. Poor skin turgor	CI	CI	D	64. Irritable	D	—	—
29. Wheezes	—	—	—	65. Use of accessory muscles	—	—	—
30. Decreased hematocrit	—	—	—	66. Dizziness	D	D	—
31. Cyanosis	—	—	—	67. Apathy	—	—	—
32. Narrow pulse pressure	D	D	D	68. Urine sodium < 15mEq/L	D	—	CI
33. Weakness	D	D	D	69. Headache	—	—	—
34. Diaphoresis	D	D	—	70. PCWP <6	CI	CI	CI
35. Thready pulse	D	D	D	71. Metabolic alkalosis	CI	D	—
36. Respiratory alkalosis	—	—	—	72. ↓ Venous saturation	—	—	—

CI = Critical indicator, variables with a weighted ratio ≥ .75
D = Defining characteristic, variables with a weighted ratio ≥ .50
— = not useful variables for this nursing diagnosis

Discussion

This study sought to validate a nursing diagnosis with a specific etiology. The etiology, active isotonic loss, may account for the differences that were found between the defining characteristics for fluid volume deficit as listed by the North American Nursing Diagnosis Association (NANDA) and the findings of this study. The defining characteristics described by NANDA included decreased urine output, concentrated urine, output greater than intake, sudden weight loss, decreased venous filling, hemoconcentration, and increased serum sodium (Kim, McFarland, and McLane 1984). Findings from this validation study also identified these characteristics, but as critical indicators. Increased serum sodium was listed as a defining characteristic of fluid volume deficit by NANDA, whereas normal serum sodium was identified as a critical indicator in this study. In addition, four characteristics that were not included on the NANDA list were identified. These additional critical indicators were postural blood pressure changes, decreased central venous pressure, decreased blood pressure, and pulmonary capillary wedge pressure less than six.

The implications of this study for nursing focus on the development of nursing as a science. Validation of diagnostic labels may enhance the development of a common language for nursing, thereby creating the foundation for theory development. In nursing education, a common language provides structure and content for curriculum design and development. It also provides a common base for nursing practice and nursing research.

Content validation of the nursing diagnosis fluid volume deficit related to active isotonic loss by nurse-experts contributed to the development of a common language as a foundation for theory development. Recommendations for further research include content validation of this diagnosis by a more diverse sample of nurse-experts as well as validation in the clinical setting.

REFERENCES

Bircher, A.U.: On the development and classification of diagnoses, Nurs. Forum, **14:**10-29, 1975.

Fehring, R.J., Validating diagnostic labels: standardized methodology. In Hurley, M.E., editor: Classification of nursing diagnosis: proceedings of the sixth conference, St. Louis, 1986, The C.V. Mosby Co.

Jacox, A.: Theory construction in nursing: an overview, Nurs. Res. **23:**4-13, 1974.

Kim, M.J., McFarland, G.K., and McLane, A.M., editors: Pocket guide to nursing diagnosis, St. Louis, 1984, The C.V. Mosby Co.

Kritek, P.B.: The generation and classification of nursing diagnosis: toward a theory of nursing, Image **10:**33-40, 1978.

McKay, R.P.: Research Q and A: what is the relationship between the development and utilization of a taxonomy and nursing theory? Nurs. Res. **26:**222-224, 1977.

Shoemaker, J.K.: Characteristics of a nursing diagnosis, Occup. Health Nurs. **33:**387-9, 1985.

Waltz, C., and Bausell, R.B.: Nursing research, design, statistics and computer analysis, Philadelphia, 1981, F.A. Davis.

Predictability of clinical indicators of infection

LINDA S. BAAS, M.S.N., R.N., C.C.R.N.
GORDON A. ALLEN, Ph.D.
MARILYN SAWYER SOMMERS, M.A., R.N., C.C.R.N.
ADELE M. BEITING, M.S.N., R.N., C.I.C.

STATEMENT OF THE PROBLEM

Potential for infection is a nursing diagnosis frequently used in clinical settings, even though it has not yet been reviewed by the North American Nursing Diagnosis Association (NANDA). Carpenito (1984, p. 38) defines the potential for infection as "the state in which an individual is at risk for being invaded by a pathogenic agent." Hospitalized patients are at high risk of developing nosocomial infections owing to the frequent use of invasive devices, a lowered immunologic response to infection as a result of medication taken for treatment of the disease, and the proliferation of strains of bacteria indigenous to the hospital that are resistant to antibiotics (Maki 1981). Among health care professionals, the nurse has the major role in identifying patients at risk for infection and planning interventions to reduce the risk of infection (Larson 1985).

Two invasive monitoring devices frequently used in critically ill patients are arterial catheters and pulmonary artery catheters. These devices are inserted by physicians, but nurses are responsible for the assembly, maintenance and replacement of the components of the system (Lewandowski and Kositsky 1983). Furthermore, the nursing protocols ensure that aseptic technique is employed to enter the line to infuse medications or remove blood samples and to cleanse and protect the catheter entry site (Hudson-Civetta and Banner 1983, Abbott, Walrath and Scanlon-Trump 1983).

Nosocomial infections related to hemodynamic monitoring have been reported in numerous studies. An early report by Stamm (1975) described an epidemic of flavobacterium species secondary to contamination of the ice bath used to chill the syringes for arterial blood specimens. The infection rate reported by Stamm was 7%. Walruth, Abbott, Caplan and Scanlan (1979) report a 13% infection rate in trauma patients with arterial and/or intravenous catheters; however, a higher rate of stopcock contamination was found. Band and Maki (1979) reported an 18% incidence of local infection with a 4% bacteremia rate in patients with hemodynamic monitoring catheters. Michel, Marsh, McMichan, and others (1981) studied 153 critically ill patients with arterial or pulmonary artery catheters and found an infection rate of 19%. A more recent study by Shinozaki, Deane, Mazuzan, and associates (1983) reported a lower infection rate of 5% in patients with arterial catheters.

The definitive evidence for the presence of

The investigators would like to thank the following for their assistance with the study: Anne Russell, R.N., data collector; Lana Weckbach, Ph.D. microbiologist; Karen Morris, R.N., Head Nurse; the nursing staff of the Medical Intensive Care Unit of University Hospital, University of Cincinnati Medical Center; Peter Frame, M.D.; Joseph Staneck, Ph.D.; Mitchell Rashkin, M.D.; Robert Toltzis, M.D.; Calvin Linnemann, M.D.; Patricia O'Conner R.N., M.S.N.; Beverly Malone, R.N., Ph.D.; Grace Lemasters, R.N. Ph.D.; Cheryl Schneider R.N., and Peter Fisher. This study was partially supported by a grant from Cobe Laboratories Inc., Lakewood, Colorado.

infection is the identification of colonies of an organism grown on culture. In most clinical situations, however, frequent cultures of the catheter tip are not practical, economical, or obtainable. Cultures of the infusate or stopcocks, which are more easily obtained, have not correlated highly with the results of cultures of catheter tips obtained upon discontinuation of the device (Walruth et al. 1979, Maki 1981). Instead, the nurse has traditionally relied on clinical indicators, such as redness, tenderness, or presence of drainage, to predict the occurrence of infection (Larson 1985).

The predictive value of particular clinical indicators has not been validated. It would be valuable to know that the presence of a specific indicator has a known probability of associated infection. Likewise, the absence of certain indicators may predict that infection is unlikely. The application of Bayes' theorem allows such decision making in nursing diagnosis.

PURPOSE

The purpose of this study is to validate the predictability of clinical indicators of infection in patients with invasive arterial and/or pulmonary artery catheters.

METHODOLOGY

The present data were collected during the course of a study designed to evaluate the efficacy of different types of hemodynamic monitoring systems and nursing protocols for maintenance. The study was conducted over 6 months, in a medical and cardiac Intensive Care Unit in a 600-bed teaching hospital. All patients requiring hemodynamic monitoring were approached for consent to participate in the study. The subjects were randomly assigned to one of four study groups. The purpose of the study was to determine whether there was a difference in infection rates owing to the frequency of tubing changes, and whether disposable or reusable sterile transducers were used. The purpose, design and result of this phase of the research are reported by Sommers, Baas and Beiting (1985).

Daily inspection of the catheter insertion site as well as a chart review was performed by a member of the research team. The clinical indicators examined were: redness at the puncture site, tenderness, presence of drainage, highest daily body temperature and white blood cell count. After examination of the catheter site, a sterile scrub was performed and an occlusive dressing was applied.

When the monitoring device was no longer required or the patient expired, the catheter was asepticly removed. The tip of the catheter and the interdermal segment were retrieved for cultures according to the procedure described by Maki (1981). The catheter segment was rolled across a 100-milliliter 5% sheep blood agar plate and incubated. A colony count of 15 or greater confirmed infection. The growth of the same bacteria on a catheter segment and on blood culture confirmed catheter-induced bacteremia.

BAYES' THEOREM

In general, there are four possible relationships between the occurrence of a clinical indicator and the presence of a problem (Sackett, Haynes and Tugwell 1985). First, the subject may have the clinical indicator and have the problem; this is called a true positive. Second, the subject may have the clinical indicator but not have the problem; this is called a false positive. Third, the subject may not have the clinical indicator or the problem; this is a true negative. Finally, the subject may not have the clinical indicator but does have the problem; this is a false negative. The schematic below illustrates the possible events.

	Problem	
	Present	**Absent**
Positive	True positive (TP)	False positive (FP)
Negative	False negative (FN)	True negative (TN)

Indicator

Three terms are frequently used in the nursing and medical literature when the information in the table is used in diagnostic decision making.

Sensitivity (SENS) is a measure of the ability to identify as positive those patients who actually have the problem; it is also known as the true positive rate.

$$\text{Sensitivity} = \frac{TP}{TP + FN}$$

Specificity (SPEC) is a measure of the ability to identify as negative those patients who do not have the problem; it is also known as the true negative rate.

$$\text{Specificity} = \frac{TN}{TN + FP}$$

Prevalence (PREV) is the likelihood of the problem occurring among all patients; it is also known as the prior probability of the problem. If there are no clinical indicators available, the likelihood of making a diagnosis should equal the prevalence rate, i.e., if the prevalence is .10, then one would expect that a patient has the problem one time in ten.

$$\text{Prevalence} = \frac{TP + FN}{TP + FN + TN + FP}$$

When the sensitivity and the specificity of an indicator have been obtained, a revised estimate of the probability that a patient has the problem is provided by Bayes' theorem.

Thomas Bayes, an English clergyman, proposed this theorem of conditional probability in 1763. The theorem states:

P(problem/positive indicator) =

$$\frac{(SENS)(PREV)}{(SENS)(PREV) + (1-SPEC)(1-PREV)}$$

Bayes' theorem provides the mechanism for modifying the diagnosis as one gains knowledge from clinical indicators. If a clinical indicator is a true indicator, then the occurrence of that indicator will increase the probability the problem actually exists. However, if a clinical indicator is not specific to the problem or is insensitive to the problem, the probability provided by Bayes' theorem will not increase above the prevalence rate of the problem.

RESULTS

Of the 90 subjects studied, 7 patients developed a local infection as evidenced by the growth of 15 or more colonies on the semiquantitative culture of the tip or interdermal segment of the catheter. Figure 1. shows the sensitivity and specificity for each clinical indicator. Using a prevalence rate of .08 (7/90) in Bayes' theorem generates the revised probability of a diagnosis of infection. It is apparent that none of the clinical indicators dramatically increase the probability that the patient has an infection. The two best indicators are a white blood cell count (WBC) of less than 4.0 (thousand/ml^3) and the joint occurrence of drainage, tenderness and redness, with revised probabilities of .20 and .17, respectively. Although neither probability is large in an absolute sense, the probability of the patient having an infection has been increased by a factor of two over the prevalence rate.

CONCLUSIONS

In conclusion, the clinical indicators of infection examined in this study provide little additional data for the nurse who assesses

Clinical Indicator	True Positive	False Positive	False Negative	True Negative	Sensitivity	Specificity	Bayes Probability
Redness	1	19	6	64	.14	.77	.05
Tenderness	3	25	4	58	.43	.69	.11
Drainage	3	24	4	59	.43	.71	.11
Temp > 101.3	0	11	7	72	0	.87	0
WBC > 12.5	0	45	7	38	0	.46	0
WBC < 4.0	1	4	6	79	.14	.95	.20
Drainage Tenderness Redness	1	5	6	7.8	.14	.94	.17

FIGURE 1   Predictive value of clinical indicators of infection.

the patient for this problem. That the clinical indicators do not add much diagnostic information is the result of a combination of factors. Not all patients who had an infection showed a positive clinical indicator (i.e., low sensitivity). And many patients who did not develop infection had a clinical indicator (i.e., low specificity).

The low predictive value of the clinical indicators of infection does not negate the use of the nursing diagnosis of potential for infection, since it remains a real threat to the health of patients. The nurse remains responsible for the care of the patient with multiple invasive devices. Nursing interventions with patients at risk require careful attention to prevent contamination and the introduction of possible pathogens. Finally, the nurse should be aware of the presence of false positive clinical indicators of infection. Reliance on clinical indicators alone may result in a false identification of infection.

RECOMMENDATIONS

Nursing diagnosis research has primarily focused on the validation of the clinical relevance of specific diagnoses. As nursing diagnoses are accepted by the North American Nursing Diagnosis Association, studies of the predictability of clinical indicators are warranted. The use of sensitivity, specificity and Bayes's theorem will enhance the clinical decision making ability of the nurse assessing patients and identifying health problems.

REFERENCES

Abbott, N., Walrath, J.M., and Scanlon-Trump, E.: Infection related to hemodynamic monitoring: venous and arterial catheters, Heart and Lung **12**:28-34, 1983.

Band, J., and Maki, D.: Infections caused by arterial catheters used for hemodynamic monitoring, Amer. J. Med. **67**:735-742, 1979.

Carpenito, L.: A handbook of nursing diagnosis, Philadelphia, 1984, J.B. Lippincott.

Hudson-Civett, J. and Banner, T.: Intravascular catheters: guidelines for care and maintenance, Heart and Lung **12**:466-476, 1983.

Larson, E.: Infection control issues in critical care: an update, Heart and Lung **14**:150, 1985.

Lewandowski, L., and Kositsky, A.: Research priorities for critical care nursing: study by the American Association of Critical-Care Nurses, Heart and Lung **12**:40, 1983.

Maki, D.: Nosocomial bacteremia: an epidemiologic overview, Amer. J. Med. **70**:719-732, 1981.

Michel, L., Marsh, H.M., McMichan, J.C., and others: Infection of pulmonary artery catheters in critically ill patients, JAMA **245**:1032-1036, 1981.

Sackett, D.L., Haynes, R.B., and Tugwell, P.: Clinical epidemiology: a basic science for clinical medicine, Boston, 1985, Little Brown.

Shinozaki, T., Deane, R., Mazuzan, J., and others: Bacterial contamination of arterial lines: prospective study, JAMA **249**:223-225, 1983.

Sommers, L., Baas, L., and Beiting, A.: Nosocomial infections related to four methods of hemodynamic monitoring, Heart and Lung **14**:286-287, 1985.

Stamm, W., Colella, J., and Anderson, R.: Indwelling arterial catheters as a source of nosocomial bacteremia, N. Engl. J. Med. **292**:1099-1103, 1975.

Walruth, J., Abbott, N., Caplan, E. and others: Stopcock: bacterial contamination in invasive monitoring systems, Heart and Lung **8**:103-108, 1979.

Alterations in protective mechanisms

KATHLEEN C. SHEPPARD, M.S.N. R.N., C.C.R.N.

Evolving is a term used to describe the science of nursing. Nursing diagnosis as a classification of the phenomena of nursing is also in a beginning state. The North American Nursing Diagnosis Association (NANDA) has emphasized that the list of diagnoses accepted for clinical testing at the Fifth National Conference for Classification of Nursing Diagnosis in 1982 is neither exhaustive nor validated (Roy 1984). In order to validate the labels already identified, nurses are encouraged to use the labels in practice. However, it is acknowledged that not all problems with which nurses may deal are on the list, and nurses are encouraged to develop appropriate diagnoses for those situations.

The Taxonomy Committee of NANDA is categorizing the existing diagnoses into "patterns of unitary persons." In the process of taxonomic development, several areas of "unidentified diagnoses" were recognized.

In theory and in practice, it is known that more diagnoses need to be developed if the list is to be complete. There are, however, areas of controversy surrounding the development of nursing diagnoses. Some authors define nursing diagnoses as those dealt with exclusively by the nurse (Gordon 1982). Other authors argue that nursing diagnoses should encompass all that nursing does independently and interdependently. If we accept that nursing is an applied science based on many sciences, then the existence of physiological diagnoses is legitimate (Kim 1985).

NANDA has encouraged identification of diagnoses. In the practice of oncology nursing, there are human responses to the diseases of cancer and their treatments that present a significant concern. The responses to the physiological phenomena of myelosuppression and immunosuppression in persons with cancer have profound implications for nursing therapy. In addition, implications for nursing are evident in persons with conditions other than cancer. There is not a specific label for these phenomena. The diagnosis "potential injury" currently includes these areas in a general way. Therefore, the need for a specific nursing diagnosis was identified.

SIGNIFICANCE OF THE PROBLEM

Infectious complications are a frequent cause of morbidity, and in many centers, they are the major cause of death in persons with cancer (Pizzo and Young 1985). The increased risk and severity of infection result from profound alteration of normal host defenses secondary to underlying malignancy and its treatment. A thorough understanding of impaired host defenses and interaction with microbes is encouraged in order to increase prompt recognition and management for prevention of complications (Pizzo and Young 1985).

The most common side effect of chemotherapy is bone marrow suppression. The results of the suppression are leukopenia, thrombocytopenia, and erythrocytopenia. The nurse has a primary role in protecting the patient from infection, bleeding, and anemia. The Oncology Nursing Society (ONS) has noted the significance of the problem by formulating the ONS Standard on protective mechanisms with the following rationale: (1) Protective mechanisms are compromised by disease and treatment. (2) Morbidity and mortality are related to altered protective mechanisms. (3) Clinical signs of compromised protective mechanisms can be absent or greatly modified (ONS 1979).

POTENTIAL FOR INJURY

The current classification for responses to myelosuppression, immunosuppression, and altered clotting factors is with the defining characteristics of the nursing diagnosis "potential for injury" (Kim, McFarland and McLane 1984). This label guides, in a general way, the formulation of the goal of providing safety. However, many of the concepts with which the nurse deals are involved in preventing injury in the broadest sense. Detecting complications of renal calculi by monitoring urinary output prevents injury to the kidney.

The diagnosis potential for injury has three subcomponents: poisoning, suffocation, and trauma. The definition of potential for poisoning is the risk of accidental exposure to or ingestion of drugs or dangerous products in doses sufficient to cause poisoning. Potential for suffocation is defined as the accentuated risk of accidental suffocation. Potential for trauma is the accentuated risk of accidental tissue injury (e.g., wound, burn, fracture; (Kim, McFarland, and McLane 1984).

The three subcomponents assist in defining injury as an external factor. They are events of trauma, a hurt, or damage (Taber 1968). The diagnosis potential for injury defined by the three subcomponents has clarity and directs practice. In the hospital situation, fall precautions and electrical safety are of utmost importance. It is in this scope of trauma that the category of "injury" is a large concept but specific enough to guide action. The potential for injury references in the Fifth National Conference proceedings are related to falls and accidents (Kim, McFarland, and McLane 1984).

However, the use of "potential for injury" is open to such broad interpretation that the concept does not elicit strategies or focus care. For example, patients' charts contain statements such as potential for injury related to infection, potential for injury related to hypokalemia, and potential for injury related to seizures. No one would argue that these are injurious states, but risk for all kinds of injury is a major issue in nursing practice. Further research is needed on the nursing diagnosis potential for injury to delineate its scope. The term becomes too broad to be useful when it includes abnormal blood and coagulation profiles.

IDENTIFICATION
Phase I

Identification of a problem sometimes begins as a felt need. In oncology practice, nurses who attempt to use diagnoses soon become discouraged. They express disappointment in the list accepted for clinical testing, because it does not meet their high-priority needs, namely, the responses of persons with cancer who have myelosuppression, immunosuppression, and coagulation disorders. This is very important in the area of oncology.

The occurrence of these responses in persons other than those with cancer had to be addressed also. Myelosuppression, typical of cancer and cancer chemotherapy, involves leukopenia, thrombocytopenia, and erythrocytopenia, and may occur in patients with other diseases. For example, leukopenia may be found in cyclic neutropenia or granulocytopenia as a side effect of antibiotics. Anemia has many categories, such as sickle cell anemia and thalassemia. Platelet disorders such as idiopathic thrombocytopenic purpura are separate from the cancer diagnosis (Reich, 1984).

Immunosuppression results from cancer and its treatment, but it also exists in acquired immune deficiency syndrome (AIDS), graft-versus-host disease (GVHD), and hypogammaglobulinemia (see Box 1). Persons receiving organ transplants, for example a renal transplant, receive immunosuppressants (Blattner and Hoover 1985). Persons

BOX 1: Persons at risk

Diseases:
Cancer (especially lymphoma, leukemia, multiple myeloma)
Immune disorders (e.g., AIDS, acute GVHD, hypogammaglobulinemia)
Autoimmune disorders (RA, chronic GVHD, SLE, CAS)
Splenic disorder (primary splenic neutropenia)
Coagulation disorders (DIC, hemophilia, von Willebrand's disease)
Anemic disorders (sickle cell, thalassemia)
Platelet disorders (idiopathic thrombocytopenic purpura)
Leukocyte disorders (cyclic neutropenia)

Treatments: Radiation
              Drugs
                  Antineoplastics
                  Corticosteroids
                  Immunosuppressants
                  Anticoagulants
                  Thrombolytic enzymes
                  Antibiotics (penicillins, cephalosporins)

Conditions: Alcohol
              Stress
              Age (elderly, newborn)
              Inadequate nutrition

with autoimmune disorders, such as rheumatoid arthritis (RA), systemic lupus erythematosus (SLE), and chronic GVHD may also have defects in the immune system (Dale, 1981). Cold agglutinin syndrome (CAS) is an autoimmune response that causes "clumping" of red blood cells and may lead to red blood cell hemolysis (Donham and Denning 1985).

Coagulation disorders occur in persons with hemophilia and von Willebrand's disease (Reich, 1984). Disseminated intravascular coagulopathy (DIC) is a coagulation disorder seen across patient populations. Cardiovascular patients as well as others, receive anticoagulants or thrombolytic en-

zymes, or both. Persons treated with corticosteroids have the side effect of immunosuppression.

Persons with cancer (especially, lymphoma, leukemia, and multiple myeloma) are a major immunosuppression population. Persons receiving cancer chemotherapy or radiation are also at risk for myelosuppression, immunosuppression, and coagulation disorders. But, conditions other than cancer and its treatment are within the nurse's area of concern. Alcohol abuse leads to abnormal blood and coagulation profiles. Stress can depress the immune system. The immune systems of newborns and elderly are more apt to be compromised. Inadequate nutrition compromises blood and coagulation profiles (Donley 1976).

Further identification was done in November 1985 at the Southern Regional Conference for Nursing Diagnosis. At the conference, the critical-care interest group discussed concerns and formulated recommendations to be forwarded to NANDA. Two of those recommendations were further research in and definition of "potential for injury" and development of the diagnosis "alterations in protective mechanisms."

In March 1983, a national conference on nursing diagnoses in critical care was cosponsored by the American Association of Critical Care and Marquette University. At that meeting critical-care nursing concerns not included in the accepted list of the Fifth National Conference were identified. The third most frequently identified concern was compromised immunologic defenses (Wake, McLane and Gotch 1985).

Therefore, it was in the area of oncology nursing that the need for a nursing diagnosis for the physiological phenomena of myelosuppression, immunosuppression, and coagulation disorders was first identified. However, this area of concern is not limited to oncology but spans medical diseases and various conditions and ages.

Phase II

The retrospective identification model was used as a guideline (Gordon & Sweeney, 1979). In September 1984, a nursing diagnosis committee at the University of Texas M.D. Anderson Hospital and Tumor Institute was formed. The task was to examine nursing diagnoses as a framework for categorizing information on persons with cancer. An evaluation study was conducted with the purpose of assessing the nursing diagnoses for the hospital's oncology nurses.

A questionnaire was distributed to 100 randomly selected registered nurses. Thirty RNs completed the questionnaire. Consent was implied by return of the questionnaire, and anonymity was maintained.

One of the items in the questionnaire was "List the nursing diagnoses/problems/needs you most commonly use." The most frequent response (50%) was a category of concerns stated as "infection, neutropenia, injury, fever." Concerns with bleeding (20%) and weakness and anemia (23%) were identified in the ten most common categories. The conclusion was that the three areas involving myelosuppression and immunosuppression were of great concern, though respondents used diverse terminology (Table 1).

The significance of the findings is that confusion in terms is an important nursing issue. A recommendation from the study was to develop a nursing diagnosis to label this category. In light of the ONS Standard "protective mechanisms" and based on information collected, "alterations in protective mechanisms" was chosen to research as a possible label for these areas of concern.

Phase III

Identification was also done through a study of oncology nursing experts. A 2% sample of 144 RNs was chosen at random from the Oncology Nursing Society's 1985 membership list (8024 members). The sample pro-

Table 1: Problems identified

Diagnosis, problem, or need	% Responding (N−30)
Infection, neutropenia, fever, injury	50
Fluids, dehydration, electrolytes	40
Nutrition, nausea, vomiting	40
Emotional aspects, anxiety	40
Airway, pneumonia, gas exchange	33
Knowledge deficit, teaching	30
Skin care, wound care	23
Weakness, mobility, self-care	23
Bleeding, hemodynamics, shock	20
Pain, discomfort	20

vided nationwide representation. Consent to participate was implied by return of the questionnaire.

The questionnaire provided defining characteristics of a patient situation (see Box 2), and the participants were asked to formulate the most appropriate diagnosis. Because the identification phase of the diagnosis of protective mechanisms is in beginning stages, several choices for diagnoses were given. The possibilities were bone marrow suppression (the physiological phenomenon), alterations in protective mechanisms (the response to the physiological health problem), and potential for injury (the diagnosis currently used to categorize protective mechanisms). The fourth choice was undefined to allow identification of labels.

Sixty-two questionnaires were returned; the most frequently identified diagnosis (52%) was "alterations in protective mechanisms." The second most frequently identified diagnosis was "bone marrow suppression" (32%). This physiological health problem may have been chosen because of knowledge deficit in the area of nursing diagnosis. "Potential for injury" was identified by only two participants (3%). The

BOX 2 **Patient situation**

History: Twenty-four-year old male with Hodgkin's disease receiving chemotherapy (MOPP)

Lab: Platelets < 20,000/mm³
  WBC < 2,000/mm³
  Hemoglobin < 10 g/dl
  Recall antigen test induration < 10 mm
  Lymphocytes < 1,000/mm³
  Decreased percentage of T cells and B cells

Physical assessment:
  Temperature 38.6° C
  Productive cough
  Pain, local erythema
  Weakness, fatigue
  Skin pallor
  Melena
  Petechiae

Nursing diagnosis: Identify the most appropriate diagnosis: % Responding
  (N−62)

1. Bone marrow suppression	32%
2. Alterations in protective mechanisms	52%
3. Potential for injury	3%
4. Other _____	13%

results may reflect a knowledge deficit of nursing diagnosis or the inadequacy of the category "injury" in labeling the response to myelosuppression and immunosuppression. The participants who choose the "other" category (13%) gave the following responses:

- All of the above
- Potential for infection, potential for hemorrhage, possible potential for injury
- Alteration in hematopoietic and immune system related to side effects of MOPP (mechlorethamine hydrochloride, oncouin, procarbazine hydrochloride, and prednisone)
- Chose #1 and #2 "both equally appropriate for the above situation"
- Impaired mobility
- Hodgkin's lymphoma, pancytopenia, anergy, fever, probable GI bleeding
- Potential of IV drugs to extravasate or cause thrombophlebitis
- Altered immune state secondary to chemotherapy (thrombocytopenia, leukopenia, anemia)

Of the participants who chose alteration in protective mechanisms, several added comments. One participant added the etiology component "related to bone marrow suppression." Another participant added "potential for life-threatening host decompensation." Another participant commented that bone marrow suppression "sounds like a medical diagnosis" and that potential for injury "sounds like a nursing diagnosis, but seems too vague." One participant who chose "potential for injury" added the etiology component "related to alternations in protective mechanisms."

In summary, respondents felt that the

nursing diagnosis "alterations in protective mechanisms" was the most appropriate one for the given patient situation. This finding is further supported by the majority in light of the comments in the "other" category (Box 2).

DEFINITION, DEFINING CHARACTERISTICS, ETIOLOGY

The need for a nursing diagnosis for the physiological phenomena of myelosuppression, immunosuppression, and coagulation disorders was identified, and the term "alterations in protective mechanisms" was preferred. "Protective mechanisms" are defined in the ONS Standards as the "immune, hematopoietic, integumentary, and sensory-motor systems" (Oncology Nursing Society 1979, p. 6). In order to limit the scope of the nursing diagnosis to enhance clarity, the systems involved were limited to the immune and hematopoietic systems. The integumentary system as a protective mechanism is addressed in the diagnosis "skin integrity." The sensory-motor system is categorized with the diagnosis "sensory-perceptual alterations." Therefore, the identified definition of "protective mechanisms" was formulated as, "the mechanisms that maintain physical integrity through the hematopoietic and immune systems."

Goals for the nursing diagnosis, "alterations in protective mechanisms," may include "protect the patient, prevent complications, detect early signs and symptoms of complications." The independent nursing actions for these goals are rated high.

"Alterations in protective mechanisms as a response to a health problem "has as its etiology physiological events, namely, myelosuppression, immunosuppression, and abnormal clotting factors. Defining characteristics involve internal and external factors. The internal factors include abnormal blood profile, abnormal coagulation profile, and delayed hypersensitivity skin reaction.

These factors are identified as major factors in defining characteristics. Other internal factors include signs and symptoms of infection, bleeding, anemia, or immune deficiency. Internal factors include extremes of age (elderly and newborn), stress, and inadequate nutrition. External factors include microorganisms, drugs, and treatments, such as radiation, antineoplastics, immunosuppressants, corticosteroids, anticoagulants, thrombolytic enzymes, and some antibiotics. Another factor may be excessive alcohol intake (Box 3).

TAXONOMY

The NANDA group on taxonomies generated an initial taxonomy for the accepted nursing diagnoses. Blank spaces were built into the taxonomic trees to acknowledge their incompleteness. Bracketed terms were modified or inserted for purposes of clarity (Kritek 1984). In the exchanging pattern, a bracketed concept was "alterations in physical integrity." Included in this category were injury (suffocation, poisoning, and trauma) and impairment (skin). Under impairment, a blank space was inserted to illustrate the incompleteness. I propose that "protective mechanisms" is an area of impairment that threatens physical integrity. Further, I suggest a third category under impairment, that of the sensory-motor system (Figure 1). As Kritek states, "The taxonomy is a beginning, not a conclusion" (1984).

CONCLUSION

The identification of the nursing diagnosis alterations in protective mechanisms, was made in clinical practice, by review of the literature, by nurses in one oncology hospital, and by nurses nationwide in the ONS. The diagnosis is significant, because morbidity and mortality in persons with cancer are often related to their compromised protective mechanisms. The diagnosis is applicable to other patient populations in addition to

BOX 3 **Defining characteristics**

Internal factors
  Biochemical
    Abnormal blood profile (leukocytes, erythrocytes, thrombocytes, lymphocytes, immunoglobulins)
    Abnormal coagulation profile
    Delayed hypersensitivity skin reaction
  Physical, signs and symptoms of:
    Infection: redness, fever, cough, drainage
    Bleeding: hematuria, hemoptysis, melena, petechiae
    Anemia: weakness, pallor, dizziness, fatigue
    Immune deficiency: delayed wound healing, increased frequency of infections
  Developmental
    Newborn
    Elderly
  Psychosocial—stress
  Situational—inadequate nutrition

External factors
  Biologic
    Microorganisms
  Treatments
    Drugs
      Antineoplastics
      Corticosteroids
      Immunosuppressants
      Anticoagulants
      Thrombolytic enzymes
      Antibiotics (penicillin, cephalosporins)
    Radiation
  Alcohol

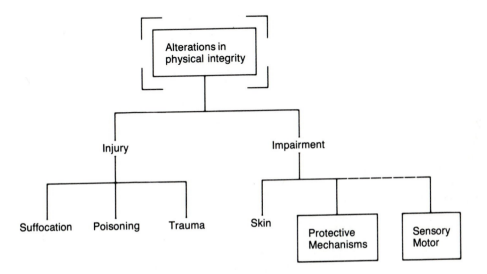

FIGURE 1 Exchanging pattern.

persons with cancer. The independent nursing therapy involved in protecting the patient, preventing complications, and detecting early signs and symptoms of complications is rated high. The physiological nature of the diagnosis also involves interdependent nursing activity. Alterations in protective mechanisms is viewed as a human response to health problems that is a significant area of nursing concern. Further research is recommended.

REFERENCES

Blattner, W., and Hoover, R.: Cancer in the immunosuppressed host. In DeVita, V., Hellman, S., and Rosenberg, S., editors: Cancer: principles and practice of oncology, ed. 2, Philadelphia, 1985, J.B. Lippincott.

Dale, D.: Defects in host defense mechanisms in compromised patients. In Rubin, R., and Young, L., editors: Clinical approach to infection in the compromised host, New York, 1981, Plenum Medical Book Co.

Donham, J., and Denning, V.: Cold agglutinin syndrome: nursing management, Heart and Lung **14:**59-67, 1985.

Donley, D.L.: Nursing the patient who is immunosuppressed, Amer. J. Nurs. **76:**1619-1625, 1976.

Gordon, M.: Nursing diagnoses: process and application. New York, 1982, McGraw-Hill.

Gordon, M., and Sweeney, M.: Methodological problems and issues in identifying and standardizing nursing diagnoses, Adv. Nurs. Sci. **2:**1-15, 1979.

Kim, M.J.: The dilemma of physiological problems. Without colloboration what's left? Amer. J. Nurs. **85:** 281-284, 1985.

Kim, M.J., McFarland, G.K., and McLane, A.M., editors: Pocket guide to nursing diagnoses, St. Louis, 1984, The C.V. Mosby Co.

Kritek, P.B.: Report of the group work on taxonomies. In Kim, M.J., McFarland, G.K., and McLane, A.M., editors: Classification of nursing diagnoses: proceedings of the fifth national conference, St. Louis, 1984, The C.V. Mosby Co.

Oncology Nursing Society, and American Nurses' Association: Outcome standards for cancer nursing practice, 1979, Kansas City, MO, American Nurses' Association.

Pizzo, P.A., and Young, R.C.: Infections in the cancer patient. In DeVita, V., Hellman, S., and Rosenberg, S., editors: Cancer, principles and practice of oncology, ed. 2, Philadelphia, 1985, J.B. Lippincott.

Reich, P.B.: Hematology physiopathologic basis for clinical practice, ed. 2, Boston, 1984, Little, Brown.

Roy, C.: Nursing diagnoses, nursing theory, and framework. In Kim M.J., McFarland, G.K., and McLane, A.M., editors: Classification of nursing diagnoses: proceedings of the fifth national conference, St. Louis, 1984, The C.V. Mosby Co.

Taber, C.: Taber's cyclopedic medical dictionary. Philadelphia, 1968, F.A. Davis.

Wake, M.M., McLane, A.M., and Gotch, P.M.: Nursing diagnosis in critical care: reflections and future directions, Heart and Lung **14:**444-448, 1985.

Injury, potential for, related to sensory or motor deficits: using the stroke scale to validate defining characteristics of this nursing diagnosis

JUDITH A. SPILKER, B.S.N., R.N., C.N.R.N.
RENEE SEMONIN-HOLLERAN, M.S.N., R.N.

Stroke is the third leading cause of death in the United States. In 1983 (American Heart Association, p. 1) over 156,400 people died from stroke and close to 2,000,000 people survived a stroke. A stroke can often leave the patient with multiple chronic disabilities. The incidence of stroke is affected by the combination of expanded life spans, acceptance of high-risk social behavior, geography, and the many stressors of today's society.

Stroke, or cerebral vascular accident, can be the result of either cerebral infarction from vessel thrombosis or emboli, or intracranial hemorrhage (Rudy, 1984). The ischemia and/or necrosis that stroke causes in the brain leaves the patient with neurological deficits that put the patient at risk for injury.

In order to prevent injury from these deficits and to plan and provide care for the stroke patient, nurses need a tool to identify and document sequelae of strokes in a consistent, organized way. The Stroke Scale and its Glossary are such a tool.

PURPOSE

The purpose of this study was to validate the Cincinnati Stroke Scale's ability to measure defining characteristics of "injury, potential for, related to motor/sensory deficits from stroke." Injury, potential for injury, is the state in which an individual is at risk for injury because of physiological deficits (Carpenito 1983).

Defining characteristics of "injury, potential for," include sensory dysfunction, reduced temperature and/or tactile sensation, altered mobility, weakness, hemiparesis and paralysis.

BACKGROUND AND SIGNIFICANCE

In the fall of 1982 the University of Cincinnati and the University of Iowa Neurology Departments were selected to collaborate in the development of a research protocol for the National Institutes of Health to evaluate the drug Naloxone in the treatment of stroke. A tool was needed to measure the effectiveness of the drug treatment regime.

In the winter of 1983, a pilot study was done to determine which specific neurological items would best measure the neurological deficits that result from stroke. This pilot study compared two known neurological scales the Oxbury Neuro Severity Score (Oxbury, Greenhall, and Grainger 1975) and the Toronto Neuro Assessment (Hachinski and Norris, 1985) with a preliminary version of the Cincinnati Stroke Scale. The results of this pilot study contributed to the development of a final version of the Cincinnati Stroke Scale which the investigators believed to be a valid measure of the neurological deficits of stroke (Figure 1).

The design of the Cincinnati Stroke Scale was intentionally directed at time-oriented assessments that are documented on a single page. This was done to better document the trends in the patient's condition as well as to avoid data overload with large amounts of irrelevant data. The Stroke Scale's scoring system was manipulated in order to make the scale as sensitive as possible in detecting changes in a stroke patient's neurological

		* CODE	BASE-LINE	BOLUS	20 MIN.	HOURS 1	6	12	24	26
** 1.a. Level of consciousness	Alert . . . . Drowsy . . . . Stuporous . . . . Coma	0 1 2 3								
** b. LOC questions	Answers both correctly . . . . Answers one correctly . . . . Incorrect	0 1 2								
** c. LOC commands	Obeys both correctly . . . . Obeys one correctly . . . . Incorrect	0 1 2								
2. Pupillary response	Both reactive . . . . One reactive . . . . Neither reactive	0 1 2								
3. Best gaze	Normal . . . . Partial gaze palsy . . . . Forced deviation	0 1 2								
4. Best visual	No visual loss . . . . Partial hemianopia . . . . Complete hemianopia	0 1 2								
5. Facial palsy	Normal . . . . Minor . . . . Partial . . . . Complete	0 1 2 3								
6. Best motor arm	No drift . . . . Drift . . . . Can't resist gravity . . . . No effort against gravity	0 1-3 4-6 7-9								
7. Best motor leg	No drift . . . . Drift . . . . Can't resist gravity . . . . No effort against gravity	0 1-3 4-6 7-9								
8. Plantar reflex	Normal . . . . Equivocal . . . . Extensor . . . . Bilateral extensor	0 1 2 3								
9. Limb ataxia	Absent . . . . Present in upper or lower . . . . Present in both	0 1-3 4-6								
10. Sensory	Normal . . . . Partial loss . . . . Dense	0 1-3 4-6								
11. Neglect	No neglect . . . . Partial neglect . . . . Complete neglect	0 1 2								
12. Dysarthria	Normal articulation . . . . Mild to moderate dysarthria . . . . Near unintelligible or worse	0 1-3 4-6								
13. Best language	No aphasia . . . . Mild to moderate aphasia . . . . Severe aphasia . . . . Mute	0 1-3 4-6 7-9								
14. Impression	Same; Better; Worse	S B W								

FIGURE 1   Cincinnati Stroke Scale. *, Code 99 for untestable. **, Developed from Glascow Coma Scale.

status. The efficiency of the exam was also a consideration for the tool. The patient participants in the study were very susceptible to fatigue; as a consequence, the design of the exam was geared to an average execution time of 6 to 8 minutes.

INSTRUMENT AND PROCEDURE

The components of the stroke assessment tool, the Cincinnati Stroke Scale, include a modified Glasgow Coma Scale (Teasdale and Jennett 1974) for assessment of level of consciousness and orientation; a partial cranial nerve exam; a motor exam; a sensory exam; an ataxia evaluation; a plantar reflex; a neglect assessment; and a speech and language assessment.

Each item in the assessment was numerically scored, zero representing no deficit. A higher number reflects a greater deficit. The patient is scored on the performance of the "weakest" side if asymmetry is noted. A subjective grade of "S" same, "B" better, and "W" worse is also used to document an impression of the patient's condition since the previous exam.

The Stroke Scale is used with a Glossary that provides specific methods for assessment and instructions on how to score the patient's performance. The Glossary assures that the neurological assessment techniques are used consistently. This was necessary because of the many possible approaches to a neurological exam.

METHODOLOGY

The Cincinnati Stroke Scale was administered to a total of 65 stroke patients at both the Universities of Cincinnati and Iowa as part of the "Late Phase I and II Naloxone Studies in the Treatment of Acute Cerebral Infarction" (Adams and Olinger 1986).* All

*USPHS/NIH/NINCDS Contracts NO1-NS-3-2324, and NO1-NS-32-2326, Primary Investigators C.P. Olinger, M.D. and H.P. Adams, Jr., M.D. drug donated by E.I. DuPont de Nemours Co.).

patients in the study received the drug, and no effort was made toward concealment. The University of Cincinnati entered a total of 30 patients. The authors participated as nurse-researchers in the administration of the stroke scale to Cincinnati's 30 patients.

The initial neurological assessment was done prior to drug administration. The patient was then assessed at timed intervals ranging from 20 minutes to follow-up visits at 3 months after the stroke. There was a total of 10 exams per patient (baseline, after bolus, 20 minutes, 1 hour, 6 hours, 12 hours, 24 hours, 7 days, 1 month and 3 months). The examinations were performed by the two nurse researchers who performed at least one overlapping exam. Each stroke patient was evaluated using examination methods identified in the Glossary (Boxes 1 and 2).

RESULTS

The two nurse researchers evaluated this tool as a means of identifying in stroke patients the patterns that validate defining characteristics of injury, potential for, related to motor and/or sensory deficits. The characteristics were distinguished by the specific components of the Cincinnati Stroke Scale. Data were documented in over 300 examinations. The data follow (Tables 1 and 2):

Table 1: Motor deficit components of the stroke scale

5. Facial palsy
6. Best motor arm
7. Best motor leg

Table 2: Sensory deficits components of the stroke scale

3. Best gaze
4. Best visual
10. Sensory
11. Neglect

BOX 1   **Exam methods and scoring for motor deficits**

1. Facial palsy
   Evaluate the seventh cranial nerve.
      0 = Normal
      1 = Minor
      2 = Partial
      3 = Complete
2. Best motor arm
   The patient is examined with arms outstretched at 90 degrees, if sitting, or 45 degrees, if supine. Request full effort for 10 seconds. If consciousness or comprehension are abnormal, cue patient by actively lifting arms into position as request for effort is verbally given. Only the weaker limb is graded.
      0 = Limb holds 90-degrees for 10 seconds.
      1 = Limb holds 90-degree position, but drifts before 10 full seconds.
      2 = Limb cannot hold 90-degree position for full 10 seconds, but some effort against gravity.
      3 = Limb falls; no effort against gravity.
3. Best motor leg
   While supine, the patient is asked to maintain the weaker leg at 30 degrees for 5 full seconds. If consciousness or comprehension are abnormal, cue patient by actively lifting leg into position as the request for effort is verbally given.
      0 = Leg holds 30-degree position for 5-second period.
      1 = Leg falls to intermediate position before 5 seconds.
      2 = Leg falls to bed by 5 seconds, but some effort against gravity.
      3 = Leg falls to bed immediately, with no resistance against gravity.

CONCLUSIONS AND IMPLICATIONS

The Stroke Scale components in Tables 1 and 2 identify the motor and sensory deficits that may result from a stroke and that impair an individual's ability to interact safely with the environment. The information collected with the tool is then incorporated into the plan of care for the patient in the hospital and possibly in the future planning for discharge of the patient to home. During the hospital phase, motor and sensory deficits could require such nursing interventions as the prevention of aspiration owing to dysphagia; prevention of the complications of immobility secondary to hemiparesis, prevention of IV infiltration of toxic substances owing to decreased sensation in the affected extremity; provision of safe bath-water temperature; and frequent assessment for injuries that the patient may be unable to detect, such as skin breakdown due to altered mobility, sensation and weakness.

During the acute phase of stroke, continuous nursing monitoring of the stroke patient is mandatory. According to Hachinski and Norris, (1985) potential reversible deterioration in acute stroke is identified earlier by an accurate nursing assessment than by any type of machine monitoring. The early detection of these changes can help prevent any further injury to the patient from physiological factors.

BOX 2   **Exam methods and scoring for sensory deficits**

1. Best gaze
   0 = Normal
   1 = Partial gaze palsy. This score is given when gaze is abnormal in one or
   both eyes, but where forced deviation or total paresis are not present.
   2 = Forced deviation, or total-gaze paresis not overcome by oculocephalic
   maneuver
2. Best visual
   Test for hemanopia using moving fingers on confrontation with both of the
   patient's eyes open. Double simultaneous stimulation is also performed.
   Use visual threat if level of consciousness or comprehension limit but
   score only 1 if clear-cut asymmetry is found. Complete hemanopia is
   scored for dense loss extending to or within 5 to 10 degrees of fixation.
3. Sensory
   Test with pin. Where consciousness or comprehension is abnormal, score
   sensory *normal* unless deficit is clearly recognized. Only hemi-sensory
   losses are counted as abnormal.
   0 = Normal
   1 = Mild to moderate. Patient is aware of being touched.
   2 = Severe to total sensory loss; patient is not aware of being touched
4. Neglect
   As this is the last scored item, the data base for judgment will be sufficient if double simultaneous finger touch is now tested.
   0 = No neglect
   1 = Visual, tactile, or auditory hemi-inattention
   2 = Profound hemi-inattention to more than one modality

Continuous nursing assessment and nursing care planning also can prevent the secondary complications of stroke that may contribute to injury to the stroke patient. These complications include pneumonia, pulmonary embolism, thrombophlebitis, decubiti, and sudden death from myocardial infarction.

The identified defining characteristics of motor and/or sensory deficits provide an initial framework upon which the Nursing Diagnosis, Potential for Injury can be applied to the stroke patient's discharge. The neurological impairments identified by the Stroke Scale can be used to help plan the appropriate safety measures needed for each individual stroke patient. The patient and his family can then be involved in identifying and making dwelling changes needed to provide a safe environment for the patient when discharged.

In summary, the care of the patient with a stroke needs to be based upon numerous factors. The physiological changes that occur due to a stroke alter an individual's ability to interact with the environment whether it be within the hospital or the home. Specifically, the Stroke Scale components in Table 1 and Table 2 include the motor/sensory deficits that may result from a stroke and decrease an individual's ability to interact safely with the environment. Nursing needs an organized, efficient, and workable tool to identify the patterns that could put the patient at risk for injury. On the basis of the reported observations, the Cincinnati Stroke Scale is a nursing tool that can meet these requirements. Additional research is needed, however, to further establish its validity as a neurological assessment tool.

REFERENCES

Adams, H.P., Olinger C.P., and others: A dose-escalation study of large doses of Naloxone for treatment of patients with acute cerebral ischemia, Stroke **18.** (In press).

American Heart Association: 1986 stroke facts, Dallas, 1986, American Heart Association National Center.

Carpenito, L.: Nursing diagnosis application to clinical practice, Philadelphia, 1983, J.B. Lippincott.

Hachinski, V., and Norris, J.W.: The acute stroke, Philadelphia, 1985, F.A. Davis.

Oxbury, J.M., Greenhall, R.C., and Grainger, K.M.: Predicting the outcome of stroke: acute stage after cerebral infarction, Brit. Med. J. **3:**125-127, 1975.

Rudy, E.B.: Advanced neurological and neurosurgical nursing, St. Louis, 1984, The C.V. Mosby Co.

Teasdale, G., and Jennett, B.: Assessment of coma and impaired consciousness: a practical scale, Lancet **2:**81-83, 1974.

Diagnosing self-harm in the elderly: a descriptive study

WANDA B. RUTHVEN, M.S., M.S., R.N., P.H.N.

Self-inflicted harm has been known since the beginning of recorded history (Shneidman 1978, p. 542). Descriptions have ranged from accounts of people slightly out of step with society to the ultimate self-harm that ends in suicide.

Self-harm from a more indirect perspective is becoming recognized as a different way of shortening the life span in certain aged people. Theories abound as to the causes of harm to the self by the elderly. These include losses of aging, physical disease and psychiatric disorders, to name a few (Burnside 1973, Mancini and Quinn 1981, Weiss 1968). According to psychologists such as Frankl (1963, p. 105) and Miller (1978), interactions with those who are significant to us are vital to health and support our feelings of self-worth throughout life.

Many elders of 70 years or more have good mental acuity and in general manage their own affairs. Even so, some have chosen to discontinue participation in their communities, even in their lives.

In district community health nursing (CHN) caseloads, more and more such individuals are being recognized. In the course of this recognition process by nurses, questions have arisen as to what treatment strategies, if any, might be appropriate for these elderly people. In addition, the characteristics that make up such persons are unknown, as are their numbers in the community. Therefore, it seems logical, in order to diagnose a typical patient liable to harm himself, that devising a list of defining characteristics would be useful.

PURPOSE
The study

The purpose of the study was to develop a diagnostic definition of self-harm in the elderly by identifying observable characteristic behaviors and their correlates that constitute self-harm.

A nursing diagnosis utilizing factor-isolating theory is considered a useful tool for nursing research. According to Gordon (1982), nursing diagnosis is also clinically useful when specific enough to provide the basis for a plan of care as well. When making a nursing diagnosis, the nurse, after assessment, places the client in a diagnostic category to determine therapy (p. 334).

From guidelines developed, a diagnostic category has three parts: (1) the term describing the problem, (2) the probable cause of the problem (the etiological category) and (3) the defining characteristics (Gordon 1982, p. 334). Accordingly, when formulating the diagnosis of self-harm as a health problem that a nurse can treat, it is proper to ask oneself what characteristics of these clients need to be noted (Radovich-Price, 1980). A number of such characteristics associated with reduced function and health of elders have been examined in the literature.

The earliest study found on self-harm was "Suicide" by Emil Durkheim (1897). Later studies of suicide, specific to elders, discussed the institutionalized aged and men in retirement (Weiss 1968, Weisman 1970, Miller 1978).

Studies of self-injury, as a more indirect way of shortening life, addressed problems of institutionalized diabetic men and other groups in self-destructive crises (Mishara, Robertson, and Kastenbaum 1973, Farberow and Moriwaki 1975, Kastenbaum and Mishara 1971, Nelson and Farberow 1980).

During the time interval, 1968 to the present, health workers offering care to the aged in their homes, such as community

253

health nurses, were encountering self-harm with disconcerting frequency in the form of inadequate nutrition and reduced self-care in formerly fastidious clients (Healthy People 1979, Storz 1972, O'Rawe 1982, Weg 1978). In addition accident-prone environments and reduced safety in general were observed (Steffl 1976).

Inability to perform the activities of daily living (ADL) owing to reduced mobility, either from disease or disuse, and pain, along with other etiologies, have combined to induce fear of abandonment, attack and death in some elders (Burnside 1976, Buzzell 1981, Healthy People 1979, Norton and Denbigh, 1981). When care systems collapsed, as they are prone to do, abuse, sometimes by family members unable to cope with daily care, resulted in self-harm on the part of the elder such as failure to eat (Block and Sinnot 1979, Lau and Kosberg 1979, Steinmetz 1978, Treas 1977).

Multiple chronic conditions requiring complicated care regimens were common. Coping with the resulting isolation and loss, depression often played a major role in self-harming behaviors (Abrahams and Patterson 1978/1979, Burnside 1973, Burnside 1976, DSM III 1980, Eliopoulos 1981).

Non-compliance with medication or other medical recommendations such as exercise programs, along with the negative attitudes of care givers, especially physicians, were cited as having a marked self-harming effect (Cooper, Love, and Raffoul 1982, Miller 1978). Strategies for elevating self-esteem by supporting the rights of patients, especially those in nursing homes, were advocated by Taft in 1985 and included increased life control through collaborative decision making and self-direction. Such actions on behalf of patients, when implemented by hospital staff in the future, should increase voluntary adherence. Non-compliance in many aspects of self-care is such a common concern of primary care nurse-practitioners that formal alliances with communication experts have been suggested, the objective being to increase understanding between client and provider (Kasch and Knutson 1985).

Treatment plans using reinforcement of positive health behaviors have successfully addressed self-harm in both institutions and the home. These are presented in studies by Dapsich-Miura and Hovell (1979) and Mishara et al. (1973).

Methods

The method of acquiring and examining data for this study was a retrospective, descriptive, survey design. Fourteen nurses provided anonymous data on fourteen elderly clients.

The sample

The fourteen community health nurses who provided retrospective data for this sample were County Health Department employees. Individual work experience of these nurses as public employees ranged from 5 to 20 years.

The rationale for using data based on the experience and cooperation of community health nurses, particularly public health nurses, who work with this group included:

- They work, supported by community funds, to offer health services based on need
- They must respond to health requests from within an assigned part of the community
- They assist on the spot with complex problems of health and age
- They have had extensive experience and education in chronic disease, counseling and social resources
- They see numerous aged people, some of whom are alone and ill
- They need scientific assessment tools stated in terms common to nurses to help identify and treat elderly clients' complex problems
- Since the likelihood of encountering and caring for individuals as noted is high,

the community health nurse is the most logical health worker to provide the client profile information sought by the investigators.

Representative clients. The community health nurses chose their representative client on the basis of their perception. They were asked to think of a self-harming elder person cared for by them within the last 5 years and then to check off those characteristics on the questionnaire that described that person.

The average age of subject under study was 70 years, the range being 60 to 89 years. Ninety-three percent had one or more chronic diseases. Those diseases specified included: arthritis, hypertension, gout, post-myocardial infarction, polymyalgia rheumaticus, blindness, renal disease, post-CVA, cardiac (other), paranoia, diabetes, ruptured disc, chronic alcoholism, colitis, and cancer with laryngectomy. Only two of the cases carried psychiatric diagnoses.

The questionnaire

The purpose of the study was to define self-harm in the community. A brief tool, in the form of two checklists, was devised to examine self-harm by frail, elderly people living in the community. The questionnaire consisted of 88 items for the defining characteristics and etiological categories. The defining characteristics were limited self-care, nutrition deficit, failure to follow medical recommendations, reduced environmental safety and accident-proneness. The etiological categories included depressive mood, social system deficit losses, chronic illness, abuse or neglect, fears, reduced mobility, care-system collapse, and pain.

Etiological categories were not isolated before the questionnaire was administered, but they were sequentially numbered 1 to 88. This technique was used to reduce bias in and to avoid distraction of the nurses completing the form. In addition, the defining characteristics and etiologies were arrayed in sequential order in appropriate categories.

Data were reported by using descriptive statistics consisting of frequencies and percentages of persons possessing each defining characteristic. Further, the frequencies and percentages of persons with and without the defining characteristic who nevertheless demonstrated the etiological factors were included. Because of the small sample, no further analysis was undertaken (Tables 1 through 4).

FINDINGS

The characteristics that appear to define elderly clients as self-harming, according to community health nurses' perceptions were: failure to follow medical recommendations (100%), accident-proneness (86%), having nutritional deficits (71%), and having reduced environmental safety (71%). It was of interest that just 29% of those seen as self-harming reportedly had limitations in self-care. Loss (100%), chronic illness (93%), social system collapse (79%), and depression (64%) were reported in a majority of cases. The incidence of abuse, neglect, fears, reduced mobility, care-system collapse, and pain were reported differently for those with and without the major characteristics of limited self-care, reduced environmental safety, nutritional deficits and accident-proneness. The differences reported were a higher incidence of abuse or neglect, fears, reduced mobility, care-system collapse, and pain for those possessing the potentially limiting or harmful characteristics of limited self-care, reduced environmental safety, nutritional deficits, and accident-proneness.

ANALYSIS
Profile of a typical self-harming client

A representative profile of a typical client based on this study would be as follows: The client would be a *white* female who *lived alone* and who had *few social interactions*. She would be *70 years old*, and have *at least*

Table 1: Relationship of self-care to etiological categories

	Depressive mood	Social system collapse	Losses	Chronic diseases	Abuse/neglect by others	Fears	Reduced mobility	Care system collapse	Pain
Limited self-care	3*	4	4	4	3	4	3	3	2
N=4 (29%)	75%	100%	100%	100%	75%	100%	75%	75%	50%
Self-care not limited	6	7	10	9	3	2	2	2	1
N=10 (71%)	60%	70%	100%	90%	30%	20%	20%	20%	10%

*Three of the 4 limited self-care clients met the criteria for depression, that is, endorsed 4 or more of the depression items. Thus, 75% (3 out of 4) could be considered to have a depressive etiology.

Table 2: Relationship of nutrition deficit to etiological categories

	Depressive mood	Social system collapse	Losses	Chronic diseases	Abuse/neglect by others	Fears	Reduced mobility	Care system collapse	Pain
Nutrition deficit	7	8	10	10	5	6	3	5	2
N=10 (71%)	70%	80%	100%	80%	50%	60%	30%	50%	20%
Nutrition not limited	2	3	4	3	1	0	2	0	1
N=4 (29%)	50%	75%	100%	75%	10%	0%	50%	0%	10%

one impairing chronic illness. She would be either *widowed* or *divorced* and, in addition, would be seen as *depressed*. She would have had a *loss* within the last year. She would be *non-adhering* as far as medical recommendations, and her *nutritional status* would be *poor*. She would be seen as having *difficulty maintaining a safe environment* for herself and be *prone to accidents at home*. In addition, she would be in constant *pain* and experiencing some type of *abuse or neglect* by others, probably psychological. She would have *limited mobility* and *no care assistance at home*. It is this client who would be at high risk for self-harm, according to the observations of community health nurses.

The extent to which the chosen measurement tool reflects the selected client's true representation of the characteristics and etiologies studied here must be determined in future work. The tool and the method should be used with more clients to establish its reliability and validity.

Table 3: Relationship of environmental safety reduced to etiological categories

	Depressive mood	Social system collapse	Losses	Chronic diseases	Abuse/neglect by others	Fears	Reduced mobility	Care system collapse	Pain
Environmental safety reduced	7	8	10	10	6	6	5	4	3
N=10 (71%)	70%	80%	100%	100%	60%	60%	50%	40%	30%
Environmental safety not reduced	2	3	4	3	0	0	0	1	0
N=4 (29%)	50%	75%	100%	75%	0%	0%	0%	25%	0%

Table 4: Relationship of accident-proneness to etiological categories

	Depressive mood	Social system collapse	Losses	Chronic diseases	Abuse/neglect by others	Fears	Reduced mobility	Care system collapse	Pain
Accident prone	8	9	12	11	6	6	5	4	3
N=12 (86%)	67%	75%	100%	92%	50%	50%	42%	33%	25%
Not accident prone	1	2	2	2	0	0	0	1	0
N=2 (14%)	50%	100%	100%	100%	0%	0%	0%	50%	0%

The purpose of the study was to develop a diagnostic definition of self-harming elder. This was achieved by identifying observable characteristics and associated factors that, in the perception of the community health nurse, constitute self-harm.

Findings from this early study utilized by community health nurses may well contribute to more rapid diagnosis of the self-harming elder. Scrutinizing clients for observable characteristics and etiologies descriptive of self-harm should aid in devising preventive actions and treatment plans for this population.

REFERENCES

Abrahams, R.B., and Patterson, R.D.: Psychological distress among the community elderly: prevalence characteristics and implications for service, Internat. J. Aging Human Develop. **9**:1-18, 1978-79.

Block, M.R., and Sinnot, J.D., editors: The battered elderly syndrome: an exploratory study, College Park, Maryland, 1979, Center on Aging, University of Maryland.

Burnside, I.M.: Multiple losses in the aged: implications for nursing care, Gerontologist **13**:157-162, 1973.

Burnside, I.M.: The special senses and sensory deprivation: nursing and the aged, New York, 1976, McGraw-Hill.

Buzzell, E.M.: So very vulnerable, J. Gerontol. Nurs. **7**:286-287, 1981.

Comptroller General's Report to the Congress: The well-being of older people in Cleveland, Ohio, Washington, D.C., 1975, U.S. Government Printing Office.

Cooper, J.K., Love, D.W., and Raffoul, P.R.: Intentional prescription nonadherence (noncompliance) by the elderly, J. Amer. Geriat. Soc. **30**:329-333, 1982.

Dapcich-Miura, E., and Hovell, M.: Contingency management of adherence to a complex medical regimen in an elderly heart patient, Behav. Ther. **10**:193-201, 1979.

American Psychiatric Association: Diagnostic and statistical manual of mental disorders, ed. 3, Washington, D.C., 1980, American Psychiatric Association.

Durkheim, E.: Suicide, New York, 1951, Free Press (Original edition, 1897).

Eliopoulos, C.: Chronic care and the elderly: impact on the client, the family, and the nurse, Topics Clin. Nurs. **3**:71-83, 1981.

Farberow, N.L., and Moriwaki, S.Y.: Self-destructive crises in the older person, Gerontologist **15**:333-344, 1975.

Frankl, V.E.: Man's search for meaning: an introduction to logotherapy, New York, 1963, Washington Square Press.

Gordon, M.: Nursing diagnosis: process and application. New York, 1982, McGraw-Hill.

Healthy People, DHEW (PHS) Publication No. 79-55071. Washington, D.C., 1979, Superintendent of Documents, U.S. Government Printing Office.

Kasch, C.R., and Knutson, K.: Patient compliance and interpersonal style: implications for practice and research, Nurse Pract. **10**:52-64, 1985.

Kastenbaum, R., and Mishara, B.: Premature death and self-injurious behavior, Geriatrics, **26**:71-81, 1971.

Lau, E.E., and Kosberg, J.I.: Abuse of the elderly by informal care providers, Aging (Sept.-Oct.) 10-15, 1971.

Mancini, A., and Quinn, W.H.: Dimensions of health and their importance for morale in old age: a multivariate examination, J. Commun. Health **7**:118-128, 1981.

Miller, M.: Geriatric suicide: the Arizona study, Gerontologist **18**:488-495, 1978.

Mishara, B.L., Robertson, B., and Kastenbaum, R.: Self-injurious behavior in the elderly, Gerontologist **13**:311-314, 1973.

Nelson, F.L., and Farberow, N.L.: Indirect self-destructive behavior in the elderly nursing home patient, J. Gerontol. **35**:949-957, 1980.

Norton, L.E., and Denbigh, K.: Medical and social factors associated with psychological distress in a sample of community aged, Canad. J. Psych. **26**:244-250, 1981.

O'Rawe, A.M.: Self-neglect . . . a challenge for nursing, Nurs. Times **78**:1932-1936, 1982.

Radovich-Price, M.: Nursing diagnosis: making a concept come alive, Amer. J. Nurs. **80**:668-671, 1980.

Shneidman, E.S.: Suicide. In Psychology, ed. 2, New York, 1978, Worth Publishers.

Steffl, B.M.: Prevention measures and safety factors for the aged. In Burnside, I., Nursing and the aged, San Francisco, 1976, McGraw-Hill.

Steinmetz, S.K.: Violence in the American family, New York, 1978, Doubleday-Anchor.

Storz, R.R.: The role of a professional nurse in a health maintenance program, Nurs. Clin. North Amer., **7**:207-223, 1972.

Taft, L.B.: Self-esteem in later life: a nursing perspective, Adv. Nurs. Sci. **8**:77-84, 1985.

Treas, J.: Family support systems for the aged: some social and demographic considerations, Gerontologist **6**:486-491, 1977.

Weg, R.B.: Nutritional adequacy. Nutrition and the later years. University of Southern California, 1978, The Ethel Percy Andrus Gerontology Center.

Weisman, A.D.: Suicide, death and life-threatening behavior, Paper presented at Suicide Prevention in the Seventies, Phoenix, Arizona, 1970.

Weiss, J.M.: Suicide and the aged. In Resnik, H.L., editor: Suicidal behaviors: diagnosis and management, Boston, 1968, Little, Brown.

Nursing diagnosis in the hospitalized chronic obstructive pulmonary disease patient: a pilot study

LYNNE ANN DAPICE, M.S., R.N.
MARY V. HANLEY, M.A., R.N.
JOY WONG, M.S.N., R.N.

Chronic obstructive pulmonary disease (COPD) describes a group of diseases all of which cause some type of air-flow obstruction. Diseases categorized as COPD are emphysema, chronic bronchitis, bronchiectasis, bronchial asthma, and cystic fibrosis. All told, they affect more than 16 million people in the United States (Cherniack and Cherniack 1983, p. 278) and are the second leading cause of permanent disability after the age of forty (Hodgkin et al. 1975). The diseases may occur singly or in combination. They are not curable but have an ongoing course over many years.

The American Nurses' Association, in its Social Policy Statement (1981), defined nursing as the "diagnosis and treatment of human responses to actual or potential health problems" (p. 9). Because a large portion of the treatment of COPD is aimed at responses to the disease, it is particularly appropriate that pulmonary-care nurses develop expertise in the identification and treatment of those responses in the COPD patient. The development of nursing diagnosis and defining characteristics is in process. Many of the diagnoses and their related defining characteristics have not been validated in the clinical setting. This study is intended to contribute to the beginning body of knowledge related to nursing diagnosis in general and nursing diagnoses of the COPD patient in particular.

GENERAL PROBLEM

The questions asked in this study are as follows:

- What defining characteristics are most often recorded for the hospitalized COPD patient?
- What clusters of defining characteristics are seen in the hospitalized COPD patient?
- Do those clusters of defining characteristics correlate with the nursing diagnoses as developed in the standards of the American Thoracic Society (ATS) Nursing Group (Abraham, Atkinson, Boyce, Briggs, and Kim 1981)?
- Do those clusters of defining characteristics correlate with the nursing diagnoses as developed by the Nursing Diagnosis Classification (NDC) Group at the Fifth National Conference of Nursing Diagnosis (Kim, McFarland, and McLane 1984)?
- What possible nursing diagnoses can be generated from those clusters of defining characteristics?

DEFINITION OF TERMS

Nursing diagnosis: "Nursing diagnosis made by professional nurses describes actual or potential health problems that nurses, by virtue of their education and experience, are capable and licensed to treat" (Gordon 1976, p. 1299). For this study, nursing diagnoses recorded in the American Thoracic Society Standards (Abraham et al. 1981) were used.

Defining characteristics: "The defining characteristics of a diagnostic category are signs and symptoms specified by convention. They are official, formal definitions usually published in a taxonomy manual for use by diagnosticians within the particular profession" (Gordon 1982, p. 138). In this study, defining characteristics developed by the ATS Group (Abraham et al. 1981) and by the NDC Group (Kim et al. 1984) were used.

Defining characteristics cluster: A cluster of defining characteristics is composed of two or more defining characteristics related to a specific nursing diagnosis by the ATS Group (Abraham et al. 1981) and/or by the NDC Group (Kim et al. 1984).

Hospitalized COPD patient: For the purposes of this study a patient is an adult of at least 18 years of age who is hospitalized and who has as one medical problem the diagnosis of COPD, chronic bronchitis, or emphysema.

Chronic bronchitis: "Chronic bronchitis is characterized by a chronic cough with excessive mucus in the bronchial tree that is not due to known specific causes, such as bronchiectasis or tuberculosis, and that is present on most days for at least 3 months of the year for 2 years" (Cherniack and Cherniack, 1983, p. 282).

Emphysema: A disease characterized by loss of elastic recoil of lung tissue (Snider 1985, p. 36-S) leading to "permanent overdistension of air spaces distal to the terminal nonrespiratory bronchioles accompanied by attenuation and destruction of alveolar walls" (Cherniack and Cherniack, 1983, p. 286).

METHOD

Design. The design for this study was retrospective and descriptive and used a cross-sectional survey.

Sample. Charts of eight male patients aged 53 to 65 with a mean age of 61.25 years who had as one of their diagnoses, the medical diagnosis of COPD, chronic bronchitis or emphysema were reviewed. There was no limit to the numbers of concomitant problems a patient could have. Length of hospitalization ranged from <1 week to >1 year.

Setting. The study was conducted in a Boston-area hospital on a 20-bed Respiratory Unit with both acute and chronic patients.

Procedure. The study utilized a check-list of 214 defining characteristics as developed for 12 nursing diagnoses by the American Thoracic Society (ATS) Nursing Group and for 14 nursing diagnoses by the Nursing Diagnosis Classification (NDC) Group at the Fifth National Conference.

FINDINGS

The chart review of hospitalized COPD patients revealed the presence of only 52 defining characteristics (Table 1) from the 214 possible defining characteristics that were identified in the literature. Twelve defining characteristics were found to have greater frequency of occurrence and accounted for 51% of the total.

All of the charted defining characteristics related to those identified by both the NDC group and the ATS nursing group. A greater percentage of ATS defining characteristics was noted (Table 2).

Clusters of defining characteristics were also noted. These clusters were compared to the defining characteristics of 14 nursing diagnoses. The nursing diagnoses seen most frequently were airway clearance, ineffective; breathing pattern, ineffective; and gas exchange, impaired (Tables 3 through 5).

Based on all the clusters of defining characteristics found in the sample it was possible to generate 11 nursing diagnoses (Table 6). Again, the three most frequent diagnoses were airway clearance, ineffective; breathing pattern, ineffective; and gas exchange, impaired.

DISCUSSION

The defining characteristics identified in this chart review partially validate, clinically, the defining characteristics identified and related to nursing diagnoses by the NDC group and the ATS nursing group. Biophysical characteristics were dominant. The paucity of psychosocial, cognitive-perceptual, and cultural-spiritual defining characteristics and diagnoses may imply that they are not clinically relevant. However, one possible reason for their low incidence could be the absence of a comprehensive assessment tool, which is essential for data collection from patients and their families, and validation of defining characteristics and nursing diagnoses that are holistic in nature. In addition, defining characteristics lack specificity in differentiating between critical and supportive indicators.

Table 1: Defining characteristics identified in COPD patients (N=8)

Defining characteristics	Frequency #	%	Rank
Sputum, change in	8	100	1
ABG, abnormal [PO_2 <70; PCO_2 >48]	7	87.5	2
Shortness of breath	7	87.5	3
Hypercapnia [PCO_2 >48]	6	75	4
Wheezes	6	75	5
Decreased PO_2 [PO_2 <70]	5	62.5	6
Hypoxemia [PO_2 <70]	5	62.5	7
Bathing, inability to wash body or body parts	4	50	8
Bathing, inability to get to or obtain water	4	50	9
Tachycardia [heart rate >100]	4	50	10
Tachypnea [respiratory rate >22]	4	50	11
Weight, excessive loss	4	50	12
Depression	3	37.5	13
Dyspnea	3	37.5	14
Fatigue	3	37.5	15
Rales	3	37.5	16
Activity, decrease daily	2	25	17
Anxiety	2	25	18
Bowel pattern change	2	25	19
Cough	2	25	20
Cyanosis	2	25	21
Divorce or separation	2	25	22
Dyspnea with exertion	2	25	23
Edema	2	25	24
Movement, impaired ambulation	2	25	25
Rhonchi	2	25	26
Shortness of breath with exertion	2	25	27

Continued

Table 1: Defining characteristics identified in COPD patients—cont'd

Defining characteristics	Frequency #	%	Rank
Skin integrity, poor	2	25	28
Fatigue, verbal report of	2	25	29
A-P diameter, increased	1	12.5	30
Arrhythmias	1	12.5	31
Congestion	1	12.5	32
Control or influence, verbal report of not having	1	12.5	33
Dehydration	1	12.5	34
Depression related to physical deterioration in spite of compliance with regime	1	12.5	35
Discomfort	1	12.5	36
Exercise tolerance, decreased	1	12.5	37
Prolonged expiration	1	12.5	38
Hopelessness, increased	1	12.5	39
Mental acuity, decreased	1	12.5	40
Movement, imposed restriction	1	12.5	41
Movement, inability to transfer	1	12.5	42
Muscle tone, decreased	1	12.5	43
Muscle wasting	1	12.5	44
Physical activity, limited	1	12.5	45
Polycythemia [hematocrit >52]	1	12.5	46
Range of motion, limited	1	12.5	47
Role change, incapacity to resume former role	1	12.5	48
Temperature, elevated [=or >100°F.]	1	12.5	49
Toileting, inability to flush or to empty commode	1	12.5	50
Weakness	1	12.5	51
Withdrawal-family interactions	1	12.5	52

Total diagnoses for all 8 patients: 125

Range: 9–29   Median: 15   Mean: 15.6

CONCLUSIONS AND RECOMMENDATIONS

Defining characteristics as developed by the NDC group and the ATS nursing group were found individually and in clusters in patient charts. The clusters of defining character- istics can be used to hypothesize the nursing diagnoses.

The investigators recommend the devel- opment of a holistic nursing assessment tool specific to pulmonary patients, which can be tested for validity and reliability, to generate

Table 2: Analysis of defining characteristics identified in 8 patient charts

Group	Total possible	Actually identified	*O/S	BP	PS	CP	CS
NANDA	137	15	10/5	12	3	0	0
ATS	42	20	15/5	14	5	1	0
NANDA/ATS**	20	10	10/0	10	0	0	0
Combination***	15	7	5/2	7	0	0	0
Total	214	52	45/12	43	8	1	0

*O/S = objective/subjective; BP = biophysical; PS = psychosocial; CP = cognitive-perceptual CS = cultural-spiritual
**Defining characteristic related to same nursing diagnosis by both NANDA and ATS
***Defining characteristic related to more than 1 nursing diagnosis. The defining characteristic for each nursing diagnosis may have been developed by a combination of NANDA and/or ATS

Table 3: Cluster of characteristics associated with airway clearance, ineffective

Cluster	Frequency	Cluster	Frequency
Sputum, wheeze, dyspnea, fatigue	2	Sputum, wheeze, hypoxemia, cyanosis, rhonchi	1
Sputum, wheeze	1		
Sputum, hypoxemia, cough	1	Sputum, wheeze, hypoxemia, dyspnea, cough, rhonchi fatigue, fever	1
Sputum, hypoxemia, cyanosis	1		
Sputum, wheeze, hypoxemia, congestion	1		
Range: 2–8	Median: 4	Mean: 4.12	

Table 4: Cluster of characteristics associated with breathing pattern, ineffective

Cluster	Frequency	Cluster	Frequency
Abnormal ABG, shortness of breath, hypoxemia, tachypnea, rales cyanosis	2	Abnormal ABG, shortness of breath hypoxemia, tachypnea, dyspnea, cough	1
Abnormal ABG, dyspnea	1	Abnormal ABG, shortness of breath hypoxemia, increased A-P diameter, prolonged expiration, cough	1
Abnormal ABG, shortness of breath dyspnea	1		
Abnormal ABG, shortness of breath hypoxemia, tachypnea, rales	1		
Range: 2–6	Median: 6	Mean: 4.86	

Table 5: Cluster of characteristics associated with gas exchange, impaired

Clusters	Frequency	Clusters	Frequency
Arrhythmia, decreased mental acuity	1	Hypercapnia, decreased P_{O_2}, tachycardia, tachypnea, dyspnea, fatigue	1
Hypercapnia, dyspnea, fatigue	1		
Hypercapnia, dyspnea, fatigue, weakness	1	Hypercapnia, decreased P_{O_2}, tachycardia, tachypnea, cyanosis, polycythemia	1
Hypercapnia, decreased P_{O_2}, tachycardia, tachypnea	1		
Hypercapnia, decreased P_{O_2}, tachycardia, tachypnea, cyanosis	1		
Range: 2–6	Median: 4	Mean: 4.29	

Table 6: Nursing diagnosis generated from defining characteristics (N=8)

Diagnoses	Frequency #	%	Rank
Airway clearance, ineffective	8	100	1
Breathing pattern, ineffective	7	87.5	2
Gas exchange, impaired	7	87.5	3
Nutrition, alteration in, less than body requirement	5	62.5	4
Fluid volume, alteration in, excess	4	50	5
Self-care deficit	4	50	6
Activity intolerance	3	37.5	7
Mobility, impaired	3	37.5	8
Self concept, disturbance in	2	25	9
Sleep pattern disturbance	2	25	10
Powerlessness	1	12.5	11
Total nursing diagnoses for 8 patients = 46			
Range: 3–9	Median: 5.5	Mean: 5.75	

frequencies of defining characteristics and to distinguish between critical and supportive characteristics. A prototype of this tool would begin to establish the data base for nursing diagnoses and etiologies in the pulmonary patient population.

REFERENCES

Abraham, M., Atkinson, M.L., Boyce, B., and others: Standards for nursing care of patients with COPD, Amer. Thoracic Soc. News 7:31-38, 1981.

American Nurses' Association: Nursing: a social policy statement, Kansas City, 1980, American Nurses' Association.

Cherniack, R.M., and Cherniack, L.: Respiration in health and disease, ed. 3, Philadelphia, 1983, W.B. Saunders

Gordon, M.: Nursing diagnosis and the diagnostic process, Amer. J. Nurs. **76:**1298-1300, 1976.

Gordon, M.: Nursing diagnosis: process and application, New York, 1982, McGraw-Hill.

Hodgkin, J.E., Balchum, O.J., Kass, I., and others: Chronic obstructive airway diseases: current concepts in diagnosis and comprehensive care, JAMA **232:**1243, 1975.

Kim, M.J., McFarland, G.K., and McLane, A.M., editors: Pocket guide to nursing diagnosis, St. Louis, 1984, The C.V. Mosby Co.

Snider, G.L.: Distinguishing among asthma, chronic bronchitis, and emphysema. Chest, **87**(Supplement): 35S-39S, 1985.

Validation studies: abstracts

Sample selection effects on validation studies

ANN MARIE VOITH, B.S.N., R.N.
LOU ANN MADSON, R.N.
DEBORAH ANN SMITH, B.S.N., R.N.
PAMELA JO YOUNGBAUER, B.S.N., R.N.

A source of frequent discussion at the sixth conference of NANDA was the appropriate selection of samples for validation studies. All agreed that experts should be the participants, however, just who the experts are was uncertain. The purpose of this research was to empirically investigate the question: Is identification of signs and symptoms functionally dependent upon nurse education, role, or expertise?

An instrument was developed to help identify individuals with knowledge of the specific diagnoses to be tested. The instrument contained seven true-false and multiple choice questions concentrating on contributing factors, nursing interventions, and a self-assessment of level of knowledge on a Likert Scale of 1 to 5. The instrument was created by the investigators and reviewed by three expert nurses to confirm content validity. Registered nurses from three units of a 350-bed hospital in Milwaukee were then asked to complete the instrument to establish reliability. In order to determine knowledge level from the instrument, self-rating was given two thirds the weight of the high-est possible score on the objective questions. This method provided a classification that produced a curve similar to a normal distribution. The reliability coefficient for the final instrument was 0.78.

Each nurse was classified as knowledgeable if she had a questionnaire score above +1 standard deviation from the mean, and not knowledgeable if the questionnaire score was below −1 standard deviation from the mean. All other nurses were average, and were discarded from the group comparisons used to help answer the research question.

A sample of approximately 1500 registered nurses from across the country working in a variety of settings were asked to participate. Part One of the questionnaire requested demographic information, including knowledge level as determined by the instrument. Participants were classified according to education, nursing experience, work setting, role, and knowledge level. Part Two asked the participants to rank signs and symptoms by strength of association to five nursing diagnoses. Means, standard deviations, and frequencies were calculated. ANOVA was used to determine differences in identification of signs and symptoms based on each of the factors identified.

Preliminary results indicate that there is some difference in identification of signs and symptoms as a function of the factors investigated. Complete analysis will enable us to describe these differences and determine whether they are statistically significant. If statistically significant, future validation studies should consider these factors in sample selection.

Decisional conflict: A phenomenological description from the points of view of the nurse and the client

ELIZABETH HILTUNEN, M.S., R.N.

Purpose: The purpose of this study was to describe the nature of the phenomenon of difficult decision making as a lived experience.

Assumptions: Human beings face many decisions which are consequential and involve important life events. These decisions can involve difficult choices and can be stressful. Identification of the features of difficult decision making has significance in development of nursing knowledge to guide nursing interventions.

Research question: What are the features of the experience of difficult decision making in clients in a home health setting?

Methodology: A qualitative, phenomenological methodology was employed. A convenience sample of five people in family units was drawn from the caseload of 85 clients in a home health agency. The supervisor and staff nurses identified each of these persons as experiencing, or having experienced, difficult decision making. The nurses described the home situation and the difficult decision making of the families. Taped interviews with the subjects were conducted in their homes. The interviews were transcribed and analyzed.

Results: All five subjects care for a significant other in the home. Two subjects were male and three were female. Their ages ranged from 49 to 76 years. From the analysis of the transcribed interviews, two stages of decision making were isolated: decisional conflict and decisional resolution. In addition, a subtype, blocked decisional resolution, was isolated. The theme of "lacks," or stated personal losses, was identified as etiological. Factors of etiological problems were categorized into levels. Characteristics of decisional conflict, such as physical signs of distress and tension, moving between alternatives, diminished self-concept, and self-focusing were identified. Themes of "control" or "lack of control" of self or other and "togetherness" with the significant other were embedded in the subjects' stages of decision making. Comparisons of the nurses' descriptions of persons experiencing difficult decision making and the researcher's findings found very little difference between the two. This may have implications for future methodology.

Significance: This study lends support to the label of "decisional conflict" as a new category for nursing diagnosis classification. In addition, support is given to the term which has been viewed as a concept that is useful in clinical practice.

Recommendations: Further development and validation of the stages and characteristics of difficult decision making are recommended in a variety of client populations.

Toward a nursing diagnosis in wellness

PATRICIA deSILVA, M.S., R.N.
GERI L. DICKSON, M.S.N., R.N.
NANCY FALCONER, M.S., R.N.
MARILYN FRENN, M.S.N., R.N.
HELENA LEE, M.S.N., R.N.
KAREN M. MILLER, M.S.N., R.N.
KATHLEEN A. STRONG, M.S., R.N.

The purpose of this study was to identify categories of client health behavior responses that arise in the context of nursing care delivered in nurse-managed wellness centers. In the changing health care system, wellness centers have become new arenas in which professional nurses give care with a focus on health promotion. Since the current list of nursing diagnoses of the North American Nursing Diagnosis Association was derived primarily from the practice of nurses caring for individuals who were ill, hospitalized, or dealing with a health crisis, it has been inadequate to describe the phenomena of nursing practice when the focus is wellness. Health belief models and health promoting behaviors have begun to be explored, but not in the context of nursing care.

In this research, the investigators examined the responses expressed by clients during an interaction between the nurse and the client in a wellness setting. The objective of this study was to describe in a systematic manner the characteristics of the wellness process. Subjects were healthy adults seeking nursing care at nurse-managed centers. The subjects agreed to participate by having their interactions with the nurse tape recorded. Two nurse-managed centers were the settings for the study. The data were transcribed audio-taped interactions of the nurse-client appointments. Through comparative analysis, using a grounded theory approach, categories of clients' verbal responses during the nurse-client interactions were identified and categorized. The seven researchers used group consensus in the process of data analysis. The categories of the client responses were used to define characteristics of the wellness process. Findings from this study can help to isolate wellness process variables that may form the basis of nursing diagnoses for clients seeking nursing care in wellness centers.

A study to examine the validity of the nursing diagnosis, potential for physical injury for the alcohol detoxification client

LAURIE RUFOLO, M.S., R.N.

The purpose of this descriptive study was to determine whether the nursing diagnosis, potential for physical injury or (potential for injury: trauma) was selected as a valid nursing diagnosis by the staff nurses caring for a client who was admitted to an alcohol detoxification unit.

The 40 clients' ages ranged from 18 to 54, 95% male, and they were from all ethnic backgrounds. The average drinking history was 15 to 20 years duration. The clients must voluntarily request admission to the program.

Within 24 hours of admission to the alcohol detoxification unit, the clients' charts were examined for the selection of nursing diagnoses. Nursing histories and progress notes were reviewed for the defining characteristics of the diagnosis, potential for physical injury, and recorded on an evaluation scale developed by the researcher. The researcher also observed the clients for the defining characteristics of the diagnosis.

Prior to data collection, each of the five nurses in the alcohol detoxification unit was presented with preprinted or standardized care plans for seven nursing diagnoses with defining characteristics, patient outcomes, and nursing interventions in an inservice program. The seven nursing diagnoses represented the most frequently encountered client problems as observed by the nursing detoxification staff and the researcher, and for which there was evidence in a review of the literature. The nurses were given the choice of using the preprinted care plans or writing their own to accurately represent the client's nursing problems.

The diagnosis, potential for physical injury, was determined to be valid for the alcohol detoxification population by 97.5% agreement between the researcher and the staff nurses in the selection of the diagnosis. Using chi square the probability of chance was $p = / < .01$. Alcohol on breath (AOB) and intoxicated (a cluster of signs and symptoms) were most frequently documented as defining characteristics by the nursing staff, followed by history of seizures, weakness, and dizziness. Impaired tactile sensation, disorientation and reduced hand/eye coordination were not found in this sample. This study suggests refining the defining characteristics on the list. The diagnosis has been retained as relevant for the alcohol detoxification client on this unit and will guide inservice education programs and standard care plan and standards development.

Validating a nursing diagnosis, disturbance in self-esteem: a comparison of studies

BARBARA GIBB, B.S.N., R.N.
PATRICIA KRAYNICK, R.N.
MARY BIEBEL, R.N.

Nursing diagnoses must be continually updated to assure practicing nurses that they have a valid and clinically practical nursing tool to assist them with interventions and to document care. Every nurse involved in patient care has some degree of expertise on the subject of disturbance in self-esteem. The purpose of this study was to verify whether a given set of defining characteristics and etiologies describe the diagnosis pertaining to a client's self-concept.

The descriptive design for this project was adapted from work by Fehring (1986). A questionnaire was developed using a list of defining characteristics and etiologies taken from a Nursing Care Plan Guide (NCPG) developed by hospital nursing personnel. Content for the NCPG on disturbance in self-esteem was derived from a review of the pertinent literature, experiences of nurses working in clinical areas, and input from a psychiatric-mental health nurse consultant. The questionnaire asks participants to rate, on a five-point Likert-type scale, the degree to which each of the defining characteristics and etiologies are related to the nursing diagnosis, disturbance in self-esteem.

The questionnaire was sent to 300 registered nurses in a 400-bed hospital with a 41% return, and to 541 nurses in the community including public health agencies, extended care facilities, and universities with a 44% return. The educational background of the community sample consisted of 78% B.S.N.'s of these 31% were master's prepared, and 6% held a doctorate. Sixty-four of the nurses had 10 or more years of nursing experience. The educational background of the

hospital sample consisted of 46% B.S.N.'s; of these 6% were master's or doctorally prepared. Forty-three percent of the hospital nurses had 10 or more years of nursing experience.

Frequency distributions, means, and standard deviations were compiled for each etiology and defining characteristic to determine relevancy. Those with a mean rank of 4.0 or greater were labeled critical indicators. Those with a mean rank greater than 3.0 but less than 3.95 probably have a high degree of relevance for the diagnosis.

Ten of the total (N = 34) number of defining characteristics were ranked as critical indicators (4.00 or greater) by both hospital and community groups. Examples include: lack of self-confidence, fear of failure, and fear of rejection. One additional defining characteristic, difficulty in defining own needs, was ranked greater than 4.00 by the community group. Both groups rated 11 of a total of 18 etiologies 4.00 or greater indicating they were considered highly related to the diagnosis. Examples include: body image, feelings of inadequacy, and real or anticipated loss of body part. The hospital group gave a rank of greater than 4.00 to one additional etiology, loss of personal resources.

Disturbance in self-esteem was defined on the questionnaire as "negative feelings about self which are associated with evaluation of one's qualities, abilities, and performance." Satisfaction with the definition was ranked 3.9 by the hospital group and 3.8 by the community group on a scale of 1 to 5. The most frequent suggestion was to add the word *self* before evaluation to clarify that the evaluation was by oneself rather than by others. Use of the word *negative* was troublesome to some participants. A repeated suggestion was made to substitute the word *alteration*. Usefulness of the diagnosis within the realm of nursing was rated 4.00 by the hospital group and 4.10 by the community group.

As this information is compiled, combined with past and future research projects on self-concept, and added to studies from other geographic areas with different demographic characteristics, we will be able to determine whether a diagnostic validity gap exists between the diagnoses on the NANDA list and those used in clinical practice. Use of well-defined, generally accepted diagnoses will enable nurses to communicate through use of a common taxonomy.

Clinical validations of decreased cardiac output: differentiation of defining characteristics according to etiology

LINDA L. LAZURE, M.S.N., R.N.
JANET CUDDIGAN, M.S.N., R.N.

Current research efforts concerning the nursing diagnosis of decreased cardiac output focus upon validation of defining characteristics and etiologies; and identification and classification of relevant nursing interventions. Interdisciplinary research indicates that the defining characteristics of decreased cardiac output may vary according to the etiology (i.e., cardiogenic, increased preload or hypovolemic, decreased preload).

This study was designed to answer the question, "Are there significant differences in the occurrence of the defining characteristics between these two etiological groups?" This is an important clinical consideration when assessing properly and intervening on a patient's behalf.

The purposes of this study include: differentiation between the defining characteristics for the etiologies, cardiogenic *vs.* hypovolemic, within a known diagnostic group, decreased cardiac output; for further validation of defining characteristics and the nursing diagnosis, decreased cardiac output.

An inductive approach was used. Medical charts were reviewed for demographic data, evidence of defining characteristics (Kim 1984, Gordon 1985), and related physiologic and laboratory data. Two samples of 20 subjects each were deliberately selected to represent two distinct etiologies for the nursing diagnosis, decreased cardiac output. As members of a known group displaying decreased cardiac output, all subjects had a cardiac output of less than 4 l/min or a cardiac index of less than 2.5 l/min as measured by Swann-Ganz catheters. The sample population was subdivided into two groups: Group I (cardiogenic, increased preload etiology) also had pulmonary artery wedge pressure (PAWP) or pulmonary artery diastolic pressure (PADP) of greater than 18 mm Hg and evidence of an acute myocardial infarction. Group II (hypovolemic, decreased preload etiology) also had a PAWP or PADP of less than 10 mm Hg and/or a CVP of less than 5 mm Hg in the absence of cardiac disease with left ventricular dysfunction.

Defining characteristic data were analyzed for frequencies within each group and significant differences between groups. Physiologic and laboratory data were analyzed for means within each group and significant differences between groups. Data analysis revealed that the following characteristics occurred with significantly greater frequency in the cardiogenic group: increased pulmonary artery wedge or diastolic pressure ($p < .0000$), jugular vein distension ($p < .0001$), rales ($p < .0007$), oliguria ($p < .0011$), angina ($p < .0193$), restlessness/anxiety ($p < .0211$), and gallop ($p < .0479$). The presence or absence of these characteristics may help the nurse differentiate between high preload and low preload etiologies for decreased cardiac output, and make subsequent appropriate adjustments in fluid intake.

Validation study of the nursing diagnosis: decreased cardiac output

ANNETTE KAMINSKY, R.N.
MARY MOLITOR, B.S.N., R.N.

Gordon and Sweeney's operational definition of nursing diagnosis, which identifies a structural, conceptual, and competency component (1979), was used to devise a study to validate a comprehensive plan of care developed by the Nursing Care Plan Committee, Columbia Hospital, Milwaukee, Wisconsin, for the nursing diagnosis, decreased cardiac output. The following questions were proposed: (1) Are the defining characteristics developed by the Nursing Care Plan Committee, critical indicators of the nursing diagnosis, decreased cardiac output? (2) Are the interventions developed by the Nursing Care Plan Committee dependent, independent, or collaborative actions?

Competency was identified by using a pretest and self-rating scales to determine an expert population. From a sample of 54 nurses employed at the hospital, 13 were identified as experts and 41 as non-experts. Twenty-five participants listed themselves as critical care nurses and 29 as general medical/surgical nurses.

To test the structural component of this diagnosis, we used a method developed by Fehring and reported at the sixth national conference. Subjects were asked to rate defining characteristics on a scale of one to five (one meaning not characteristic and five meaning characteristic). Signs and symptoms with a mean rating of greater than 4.0 were labeled critical indicators of decreased cardiac output. Twenty of the 29 defining characteristics were rated by all groups as critical indicators with mean scores greater than 4.0. An additional five characteristics were rated as critical indicators with mean scores greater than 4.0 by the experts and critical care nurses.

To test the conceptual component, participants were asked to rate 19 interventions on a scale of one to five. Interventions with a mean rating of less than 2.0 were identified as dependent nursing actions requiring a physician's order. Interventions with a mean rating greater than or equal to 2.0 and less than or equal to 4.0 were designated as collaborative. Interventions with a mean rating greater than 4.0 were classified as independent actions within the scope of nursing practice that do not require a physician's order. Thirteen interventions were rated as independent and six were rated as collaborate by all groups.

On a scale of 1 to 5, all groups rated this diagnosis useful to nursing practice with a mean score greater than 4.0.

Defining the characteristics and interventions for the nursing diagnosis of decreased cardiac output

CYNTHIA M. DOUGHERTY, M.A., R.N.

Nursing diagnosis has been described in the literature since the 1950's and in the last decade has become a more important second step of the nursing process. The National Conference Group on Classification of Nursing Diagnoses introduced decreased cardiac output as a possible diagnosis in 1975. It was accepted as a diagnosis in 1980, but the etiology and defining characteristics remain incompletely defined. The purposes of the study were to: (1) describe the etiology and defining characteristics for the nursing diagnosis of decreased cardiac output; (2) develop and test an assessment tool that can be used to make the nursing diagnosis of decreased cardiac output; and (3) outline nursing interventions related to the nursing diagnosis of decreased cardiac output.

An exploratory design was used to describe the etiology and defining characteristics of the nursing diagnosis, decreased cardiac output, and to outline nursing interventions associated with the diagnosis. A cardiac output assessment tool and a nursing intervention check-list were used as data collection instruments. Nursing interventions were classified as independent, collaborative, or dependent, according to the opinions of both nurses and physicians. Data collection was carried out primarily by reviewing concurrent patient records.

The population included 33 patients, 20 who had the medical diagnosis of congestive heart failure, and 13 who had the medical diagnosis of cardiogenic shock. The sample was limited to adults with no other serious medical problems other than their cardiac diagnosis.

Results of the study are in agreement with the defining characteristics outlined by the National Conference Group for decreased cardiac output and the nursing interventions outlined by Wessel (1981). The etiological factors were not previously identified and are suggested from this study. Additional defining characteristics not on the list previously formulated by the national group are outlined. The cardiac output assessment tool was shown to discriminate between patients with congestive heart failure and cardiogenic shock, lending support to the construct of decreased cardiac output. Nursing interventions were found to be independent (77%) or collaborative (18%) with no dependent nursing interventions identified.

Potential for infection related to invasive intravascular devices in the shock patient

PAUL F. LANGLOIS, M.S.N., R.N.

There is a dearth of information available on the nursing diagnosis, potential for infection related to invasive intravascular devices in the shock patient. Since nurses are usually responsible for inserting and maintaining the intravascular device, they must be aware of the sources of potential contamination and be able to intervene appropriately.

The purpose of this descriptive study was to validate the nursing diagnosis, potential for infection related to invasive intravascular devices in the shock patient. Questions used to guide this research included: (1) What are the defining characteristics of this diagnosis? (2) What are the etiologic factors of this nursing diagnosis?

Two models were used to validate the diagnosis, the retrospective identification model and the clinical model. Using a Delphi technique, six clinical nurse specialists generated five etiologies and seven characteristics using the retrospective identification model.

Data from the clinical model were obtained from 16 adult patients who entered an Emergency Room with a medical diagnosis of shock (except septic shock). The patient must have had an intravascular device inserted in the emergency by a registered nurse to be included in the study.

Data collection was done by research assistants. Inter-rater reliability was greater than .95 for all research assistants. Data were tabulated by the primary investigator, and descriptive statistics were used for data analysis.

The retrospective identification model generated the following etiologies: organisms on the nurse's hands prior to assembly and insertion of the intravascular device; organisms on the skin of the patient prior to insertion of the intravascular device; length of time the same tubing, filter, and fluid bag were attached to the patient; insertion technique; and length of time the same catheter remained in the patient without being removed or dressed. The characteristics from this model included: leukopenia with a low differential; immunocompromising therapy; alteration in the liver, spleen, or bone marrow; alteration in the skin or mucous membranes; alteration in nutritional status; recent history of infection; and extremes of age.

Findings from the clinical model were similar. Four of the 16 patients developed an infection. All of the etiologies and characteristics reported in this study could be assessed and managed by a registered nurse.

Clinical validation of the nursing diagnosis of inability to wean from ventilator

PAT CHAMBERS, R.N.
BETH ANDERSON, R.N.
KAREN A. YORK, M.S.N., R.N.
DRUE STEELE, R.N.

Problem statement and purpose. Critical care nurses have identified a need for nursing diagnoses that address patient problems specific to their area. One of these problems is inability, or potential inability, to wean from mechanical ventilation. The main research questions is whether there is a pattern of defining characteristics associated with patients who are experiencing difficulty in being weaned from mechanical ventilation. A second research question is whether there are specific nursing interventions for this problem. Gordon (1982) called for clinical validation and testing of nursing diagnoses and their defining characteristics. This project is one way of determining a pattern of defining characteristics of patients with inability to wean from the ventilator.

Design and sample. Chart review was done to identify signs and symptoms (defining characteristics) which characterize patients who had difficulty in being weaned from mechanical ventilation (defined as at least two unsuccessful attempts to wean from the ventilator). Demographic data were collected to identify other characteristics that might affect weaning. Subjects were 20 patients on mechanical ventilation who experienced difficulty in being weaned from the ventilator. These difficulties included respiratory system pathology, physical or psychological dependence on the ventilator, and/or nutritional deficits. Ten subjects were selected for retrospective chart review, and 10 patients were reviewed concurrently as they developed the weaning problems. This permitted retrieval of data that might not be recorded in the medical record.

Data collection. Data collection included demographic data, medical history, laboratory findings, respiratory parameters, vital signs, medications prescribed, and psychological assessment data. Also included were the Adverse Factor Scores and Ventilator Scores used by Morganroth, et al. (1984). Nursing care plans and nursing interventions were recorded when appropriate.

Data analysis and major findings. Data were analyzed by frequency counts and percentages. Factors most likely to be abnormal in patients who were unable to wean were: total protein levels below normal (85%), albumin below normal (95%), low hemoglobin and hematocrit (95%), and elevated white blood counts (80%). Nursing interventions were essentially limited to assessment parameters, airway maintenance activities, and psychological support.

Significance. The findings indicate major physiologic abnormalities in patients who are unable to wean, abnormalities not limited to the respiratory system. Four of the abnormal findings may indicate inadequate nutritional intake, a potentially remediable problem. Nursing interventions that promote nutritional intake may help patients wean from mechanical ventilation.

Validation of the defining characteristics for sleep pattern disturbance

LAURA ROSSI, M.S., R.N.
JOAN B. FITZMAURICE, Ph.D., R.N.
MARY ANN GLYNN, M.B.A., R.N.
KATHLEEN CONNORS, B.S.N., R.N.

The purpose of this study was to examine the incidence and nature of the nursing diagnosis, sleep pattern disturbance in cardiac patients. The convenience sample consisted of 43 subjects (29 male, 14 female) hospitalized on a progressive coronary care unit. Mean age of the subjects was 58.7 years (range 29–81). The primary medical diagnoses included coronary artery disease (N=18), complex ventricular arrhythmias (N=16), congestive heart failure (N=4), atrial arrhythmias (N=3). Following a consent to participate, a 45-minute structured interview designed to elicit information on the defining characteristics and etiologies of sleep pattern disturbance was conducted. Findings showed that 91% of the patients (N=39) described a disturbance in sleep. Interrupted sleep pattern was the most frequent characteristic occurring in 85% (N=33) of the subjects with a sleep pattern disturbance. The average uninterrupted sleep time was 4.9 hours (±1.7) during the hospitalization which was relatively unchanged from the preadmission uninterrupted sleep time (4.7±2.3). Other symptoms included difficulty falling asleep (N=32, 82%), not feeling well rested (N=11, 28%), and early awakening (N=9, 24%). Of the patients describing a disturbance in sleep, (N=36, 92%) presented with two or more defining characteristics.

In conclusion, this study did show a relatively high incidence of sleep pattern disturbance in this patient population. Continued investigation into the nature of these symptoms may show that it would be clinically useful to delineate more specific diagnostic categories, thus directing the development of more effective intervention strategies.

Validation of fatigue as a nursing diagnosis

ANNE MARIE VOITH, B.S.N., R.N.
ANN M. FRANK, B.S.N., R.N.
JANICE SMITH PIGG, B.S.N., R.N.

Fatigue can be a particularly severe and longstanding problem for certain patient populations, including those with rheumatic diseases. Nursing observations have stimulated interest in fatigue as a possible nursing diagnosis. Before nurses' potential impact on fatigue can be examined, validation that fatigue exists as a nursing diagnosis must occur. This study sought to identify the defining characteristics of fatigue as the first step toward acceptance of this common patient problem as a nursing diagnosis.

Validation was sought using previously developed methods. A questionnaire was sent to a random sample of 1000 nurses representing concentrations in care of rheumatic disease, cardiac, rehabilitation, and other types of patients. Participants were asked to use a Likert-type scale to rank (1–5) the degree to which possible defining characteristics are associated with the diagnosis of fatigue. The list of defining characteristics was compiled from the literature and experience. The return rate was 27.3%. Means and standard deviations were calculated. Items with a mean greater than 4.0 were considered defining characteristics of fatigue.

The study produced a list of defining characteristics specific to fatigue including: verbalizes fatigue; inability to maintain usual activity level; poor task performance; impaired ability to concentrate; irritability; and increased physical complaints. Development of this list is the first step toward acceptance of fatigue as a nursing diagnosis and can aid nurses in recognition, assessment, and treatment of fatigue as a patient problem. The study also brought into focus the important issue of diagnostic chains, where a label can represent a diagnosis, etiology, or defining characteristic, depending upon the problem. Perhaps careful definition of the problem is our best solution.

Validation of nursing diagnoses regarding alterations in urinary elimination

ANN MARIE VOITH, B.S.N., R.N.
DEBORAH ANN SMITH, B.S.N., R.N.
LOU ANN MADSON, R.N.
PAMELA J. YOUNGBAUER, B.S.N., R.N.

The Taxonomy Committee of NANDA described a category of alterations in urinary elimination and suggested that further development of the category was possible. Five diagnoses based on literature review and clinical observation were identified in an attempt to describe patterns of alteration in urinary elimination. These five diagnoses are: stress, urge, reflex, uncontrolled, and environmental incontinence. A sixth diagnosis, urinary retention, had been previously identified using a similar methodology. The purpose of this project was to establish content validity of the five diagnoses.

Assumptions made include: nurses' retrospective review of clinical observations can provide a reliable source of information. Consensus can be determined statistically by pooling responses to a questionnaire. Consensus is an acceptable method to begin to establish validity for a diagnosis and its signs and symptoms.

A questionnaire was designed that combines research models from Fehring (1984) and York and Martin (1984). The questionnaire was distributed to 1500 registered nurses throughout the country working in acute, long-term, and community-based health care agencies, and nurses employed as educators. Part I of the questionnaire asks for demographic/background information. Differences in identification of defining characteristics based on demographic data were sought using ANOVA. Opinions and comments about each proposed diagnosis were requested, including their usefulness and clarity. Part II of the questionnaire asks participants to rate the degree of association of signs and symptoms to each of the diagnoses. The list of signs and symptoms was formed through literature and group review in the development of the book *Applied Nursing Diagnosis* (Gettrust 1985). Frequencies, means, and standard deviations were calculated to identify patterns of signs and symptoms for each diagnosis. Part III asks participants to label a cluster of defining characteristics identified in the earlier research of urinary retention.

Preliminary results include a list of critical indicators for each of the diagnoses in the category alteration in elimination: incontinence plus confirmation of the label "urinary retention." It is expected that validation of the diagnoses will increase nurses' awareness of the types of alterations in urinary elimination; lead to more effective nursing interventions, and provide a basis for acceptance of a more specific taxonomy by NANDA.

Epidemiologic studies: poster presentations

The occurrence of nursing diagnoses in ambulatory care[*]

ANN F. COLLARD, M.S., R.N., A.N.P.
DOROTHY A. JONES, Ph.D., R.N.C., F.A.A.N.
MARGARET A. MURPHY, M.S., R.N.C.
JOAN B. FITZMAURICE, Ph.D., R.N., F.A.A.N.

In 1980, the American Nurses' Association (ANA) Congress for Nursing Practice developed Nursing: A Social Policy Statement. This document describes nursing's phenomena of concern as those actions that deal with "... human responses to actual or potential health problems" (ANA 1980 p. 9). While this definition has generated both applause and concern, it does provide a framework that helps to describe nursing practice more clearly to the consumer and other health care providers. In addition, the work of the North American Nursing Diagnosis Association (NANDA) has generated a taxonomy to begin classifying nursing phenomena. The nursing community has utilized this taxonomy in a variety of clinical settings in an effort to expand the list of nursing diagnoses, refine the labels, and validate distinguishing signs and symptoms of the diagnoses as reflecting the realities of practice.

Several studies have documented the usefulness of nursing diagnoses in assessing, planning, carrying out and evaluating patient care (Jones and Jakobs 1982, Simmons 1986) and for establishing a data base that reflects nursing's contribution to the care of clients within the health care system (Halloran 1980, and Simmons and Ryan 1982). As Gordon (1985) states in her summary, the literature mainly reflects studies of acutely ill, adult populations. Clinical validation of the presence of nursing diagnosis in ambulatory care remains to be established.

The purposes of this descriptive research were (1) to identify the nursing diagnostic labels used to describe nursing problems found in ambulatory clients; (2) to clinically validate the congruence of the signs and symptoms observed and those listed by NANDA; and (3) to determine the co-occurrence of frequently occurring nursing and medical diagnoses in the ambulatory client group studied.

[*]This research was partially supported by Grant #(5-D23-NU 00160-03) Bureau of Health and Human Services, Advanced Nurse Training.

Within the context of these purposes the following research questions are asked:

- What are the nursing diagnoses frequently observed in ambulatory care practice settings?
- Which signs and symptoms support the nursing diagnoses frequently found in the ambulatory care practice setting?
- What is the frequency of critical sign or symptom used in support of nursing diagnoses frequently found in the ambulatory care setting?
- What patterns of co-occurrence are observed between frequently occurring nursing and medical diagnoses in the ambulatory care setting?

DEFINITION OF TERMS

Nursing diagnosis. A term recorded on a client record and designated as a nursing diagnosis.

Signs and symptoms. Subjective and objective client data listed with the nursing diagnosis or found in the narrative write-up.

Critical sign or symptom. Client data as above that predicts with a high probability that a particular nursing diagnosis is present.

Medical diagnosis. A term recorded on a client record and designated as a medical diagnosis.

METHOD

Retrospective chart review was employed to study nursing diagnoses in six ambulatory care settings. The nurse validation model proposed by Gordon and Sweeney was used as a framework for the study (1979). The model is concerned with validating clusters of signs and symptoms that define the diagnoses. Clusters of signs and symptoms to which the problem labels refer are then standardized as their actual occurrence as clinical entities is noted.

Sample

A convenience sample of 113 (n = 113) nursing records was reviewed in six ambulatory care clinics. Sample records came from five primary care clinics and one employee health clinic. Clients included in the sample were healthy ambulatory clients as well as those with simple acute problems and stable chronic illnesses.

Procedure

Clients' records included in the study were generated by master's degree students in the second semester of study in a clinical nurse specialist-primary care program. Signs and symptoms listed as clusters and labeled as a nursing diagnosis were recorded and sorted into one of the eleven functional health patterns described by Gordon (1982a).

These were then compared to the NANDA taxonomy (Kim and Moritz 1982) and to those additional diagnostic categories described by Gordon as clinically useful (1982b). Additional data concerning age, sex, marital status, race and medical diagnosis were gathered in order to describe the sample and answer the co-occurrence research question.

In factor isolating research the reliability of the data involves some measure of consistency and equivalence agreement on the presence of the same diagnosis by two nurses (Diers and Schmidt 1977). The nurse who wrote the record and at least one of the investigators agreed that use of the diagnostic label was appropriate, given the cluster of signs and symptoms recorded by the care giver. No other inter-rater reliability studies were attempted on the judgments of the nurses. In this study no attempt was made to establish the level of reliability at the point of nurse-client encounter. Other research methodologies presented at the fifth and sixth National Conferences on Nursing Diagnosis provide a mechanism for establishing the reliability of the diagnostic process (Fehring 1986, Hoskins, et al. 1984).

RESULTS

The study sample reflected a client population ranging in age from 18 to 90 years of age.

Within the sample, 38% were male and 62% female. Racial mix and national origin included 50% black, 34% white, 16% Spanish, oriental and other.

Table 1 indicates, as percentages, the total number of nursing diagnoses made and those made within each pattern area. The most common dysfunctional patterns found within this ambulatory care population were cognitive/perceptual (35%), nutrition/metabolic (20%), and health perception/health maintenance (9%). In all, 316 individual nursing diagnoses were recorded in the sample population of 113 clients. The mean number of nursing diagnoses per client was 2.8. Overall 42 diagnostic labels were utilized by the graduate students. Table 1 shows the ten nursing diagnoses that occurred most frequently in the records which were reviewed. These data are contained in the column marked *RANK*. The remaining 32 diagnostic labels occurred in less than 10% of the clients.

Results of nurse validation of the clinical occurrence of signs and symptoms in the three diagnoses selected for analysis are listed in Table 2. They are tabulated by frequency of occurrence and percentage of the subsample in which these characteristics were observed.

To answer the second research question the nursing diagnoses non-compliance (specify), sleep pattern disturbance, and ineffective individual coping were chosen for further analysis for the following reasons: (1) they had approved definitions (many of the diagnoses do not); (2) they occurred frequently in the study population; and (3) each of these diagnoses had signs and symptoms designated as critical (most do not). The use of NANDA defining characteristics with the label sleep pattern disturbance was 60%, with non-compliance 67% and with ineffective individual coping, 70%. Further analysis noted use within these three diagnostic categories of those signs and symptoms which have been designated by NANDA as

critical to the presence of the diagnoses (critical cue). Recorded data were again compared with the NANDA list to determine to what extent these critical defining signs and symptoms occurred in these three labeled symptom clusters. One or more critical signs or symptoms was identified in 100% of cases of sleep pattern disturbance. Analysis of non-compliance showed use of at least one sign or symptom identified by NANDA as critical in 93% of cases. Only 12 of 20 clients (60%) with ineffective individual coping exhibited a sign or symptom identified as critical by NANDA for this diagnosis.

In all, 187 medical diagnoses were recorded from the 113 client records resulting in a mean of 1.7 medical diagnoses per client. Thirteen medical diagnoses occurred in four or more clients and accounted for 59% of all the medical diagnoses in the sample. The high-frequency medical diagnoses in this ambulatory client group were hypertension (n=36), diabetes mellitus (n=16) and arthritis (n=8).

Further analysis of these data revealed that patterns of co-occurrence of nursing and medical diagnoses could be identified. Those clients with the medical diagnosis hypertension averaged 2.4 nursing diagnoses per client. Obesity, knowledge deficit, discomfort, non-compliance and ineffective individual coping accounted for 54% of the nursing diagnoses found in the individuals with hypertension. Clients with diabetes were noted to have the nursing diagnoses: obesity, knowledge deficit and non-compliance. Clients with arthritis averaged 4.38 nursing diagnoses per client. These included diagnoses such as alteration in comfort; pain, decreased activity tolerance and pain management deficit.

DISCUSSION

Use of the functional health pattern assessment format for gathering data and the NANDA taxonomy for clustering signs and symptoms within diagnostic labels indicate

Table 1: Occurrence of nursing diagnoses by pattern area and rank order of 10 most frequent diagnoses

Nursing diagnosis	Freq	%	Freq	%	Rank
1. Cognitive-perceptual pattern			108	34	
Comfort, alterations in: pain	60	19			1
Knowledge deficit (specify)	38	12			2
Sensory perceptual alterations	6	2			
*Pain-self management deficit	3	1			
*Short-term memory deficit	1	0			
2. Nutrition-metabolic pattern			64	20	
Nutrition, alteration in: obesity	36	11			3
Skin integrity, impaired (potential)	3	1			
Nutritional deficit (specify)	11	3			8
+Fluid volume excess	3	1			
Skin integrity, impaired	11	3			9
3. Health perception-health management p.			28	9	
Non-compliance	15	5			6
*Non-compliance, potential	4	1			
−Non-productive illness perception	4	1			
*Health management deficit	1	0			
Potential for trauma	3	1			
*Potential for infection	1	0			
4. Activity-exercise pattern			25	8	
Activity intolerance	18	6			5
Mobility, impaired physical	2	1			
Self-care deficit (specify)	2	1			
Airway clearance, ineffective	2	1			
Diversional activity deficit	1	0			
5. Coping/stress tolerance pattern			21	7	
Coping, ineffective individual	20	6			4
Coping, ineffective family	1	0			
6. Sleep-rest pattern			13	4	
Sleep pattern disturbance	13	4			7
7. Elimination pattern			11	3	
Urinary elimination, altered	9	3			10
Bowel elimination: constipation	2	1			
8. Self perception-self concept pattern			8	3	
Fear (specify focus)	5	2			
*Situational depression	3	1			
9. Role-relationship pattern			7	2	
Grieving, dysfunctional	2	1			
−Unresolved role conflict	2	1			
+Social isolation	2	1			
*Dependence-independence conflict	1	0			
10. Sexuality-reproductive pattern			1	0	
Sexual dysfunction	1	0			
11. Value-belief pattern			0	0	
			286		
−Labels not listed by NANDA/Gordon did not aggregate	30	9	30	9	
Totals	316	99	316	99	

*Described by Gordon, (1982)
+Added from 'to be developed'
−Developed by students

Table 2: Frequency of occurrence of signs and symptoms and percent of subsample in which observed for selected nursing diagnoses

Non-compliance N = 15	FREQ	%
*Direct observation of non-compliance or statements by client or significant other regarding non-compliance	14	93
Physiological indicators of non-compliance	8	53
Development of complications	1	7
Exacerbation of symptoms	2	13
		+

Ineffective individual coping N = 20		
*Verbalization of inability to cope or to ask for help	11	56
*Inability to problem solve	1	5
Inability to meet role expectations	2	10
Inability to meet basic needs	1	5
Alteration in social participation	2	10
Destructive behavior toward self and others	8	40
Inappropriate use of defense mechanisms	1	5
High illness rate	5	10
Anxiety, fear or anger (verbalization of or appearance of)	6	30
		+

Sleep pattern disturbance N = 13		
*Difficulty falling asleep (sleep onset)	9	70
*Interrupted sleep	4	31
Restlessness	1	8
Lethargy	1	8
Listlessness	1	8
		+

*Critical cue
+Does not sum to 100% since clients had more than 1 each

the occurrence of nursing diagnoses within this ambulatory client sample.

The frequency of nursing diagnoses made in ambulatory care clients further indicates that diagnostic categories reflect the realities of practice in the ambulatory care setting. Of the 316 diagnoses made, 266 (84%) were from the list approved for testing by the Fourth National Conference on Classification of Nursing Diagnosis, including 5 designated as 'to be developed' (Kim and Moritz 1981). There were 50 nursing diagnoses found that were not on the NANDA list. Of those not on the list, 14 have been described by Gordon

(1982b) as clinically useful. In this study, 11% of the labels used to describe clusters of signs and symptoms were chosen by the nurses because in their judgment they did not find diagnostic categories on the NANDA list that adequately described the clusters of signs and symptoms they observed in clients. This seems to indicate the need for further replication of this study, expansion of the present list, and further refinement of existing labels. Additionally, perhaps a lack of experience by students in using the taxonomy can also explain their need to use other labels. The finding that ten diagnostic categories accounted for 73% of the nursing diagnoses made remains to be tested in other ambulatory populations with more sophisticated diagnosticians as it could indicate under-assessment or limited use of labels. A plan for inter-rater reliability estimates as suggested by Fehring (1985) is also recommended.

Findings concerning the utility of critical defining characteristics predictive of nursing diagnoses indicate that their use is high but it is not consistent (see Table 2). Use of ineffective individual coping is problematic and supports the findings of Vincent (1985) in her clinical validation study of that nursing diagnosis.

Frequently occurring nursing diagnoses found in this population represent client conditions which nurses must be prepared to diagnose and treat in ambulatory care settings. Nursing diagnoses provide a systematic way for nurses to document nursing's unique contribution to the health and welfare of the primary care population.

Results of this investigation supported the existence of patterns of co-occurrence of specific nursing and medical diagnoses in ambulatory care clients. It is not surprising to find the nursing diagnoses of knowledge deficit, discomfort, pain and noncompliance in conjunction with chronic medical diseases. Nurses have long claimed expertise in

these patient care areas and nursing diagnoses can serve to validate the focus of nursing practice in these settings. Results further suggest that nursing diagnoses take into account responses of the whole person not only to actual or potential health problems but to other life processes as well.

CONCLUSIONS

- Use of the clinical validation model proposed by Gordon and Sweeney for standardization of nursing diagnoses demonstrated the clinical occurrence of nursing diagnoses that reflect the realities of practice in this ambulatory care population.
- Use of the functional health pattern format for gathering and organizing patient data, generated labels associated with clusters of signs and symptoms as identified by NANDA. Alteration in comfort: pain, knowledge deficit, non-compliance and ineffective individual coping occurred most frequently in this ambulatory care sample.
- Analysis of the critical defining characteristics in three diagnostic categories demonstrated high agreement with NANDA for use of at least one critical cue for sleep pattern disturbance (100%) and non-compliance (93%); only moderate agreement (60%) for ineffective individual coping.
- Patterns of co-occurrence of medical and nursing diagnoses can be identified, and can serve as indicators of high probability nursing diagnoses.
- Phenomena not yet described in the ambulatory setting may exist, as indicated by use of non-accepted labels. Further clinical testing is indicated.

REFERENCES

American Nurses' Association: Nursing: a social policy statement, Kansas City, MO, 1980, American Nurses' Association.

Deirs, D., and Schmidt, R.: Interaction analysis in nursing research. In Veronick, P.J., editor: Nursing research, vol. 2, Boston, 1977, Little, Brown.

Fehring. R.J.: Validating diagnostic labels: standardized methodology. In Hurley, M.E., editor: Classification of nursing diagnoses: proceedings of the sixth conference, St. Louis, 1986, The C.V. Mosby Co.

Gordon, M.: Nursing diagnosis: process and application, New York, 1982, McGraw Hill.

Gordon, M.: Manual of nursing diagnosis, New York, 1982, McGraw Hill.

Gordon, M.: Practice-based data set for a nursing information system, J. Med. Systems **9**:46-52, 1985.

Gordon, M., and Sweeney, M.A.: Methodological problems and issues in identifying and standardizing nursing diagnoses, Advances Nurs. Sci. **2**:1-15, 1979.

Halloran, E.J.: Analysis of variation in nursing workload by patient medical and nursing condition, Dissert. Abstr. Internat. **42**:3385B-3386B, 1980. (University Microfilms No. 81-06-567).

Hoskins, L.M., Begley, C.S., McFarlane, E.A., and others: Nursing diagnoses in the chronically ill. In Kim, M.J., McFarland, G.K., and McLane, A.M., editors: Classification of nursing diagnoses: proceedings of the fifth national conference, St. Louis, 1984, The C.V. Mosby Co.

Jones, P.E., and Jacobs, D.F.: The definition of nursing diagnoses: phase 3 and final report, Toronto, 1982, University of Toronto.

Kim, M.J., and Moritz, D.E.: Classification of nursing diagnoses: proceedings of the third and fourth national conferences, New York, 1981, McGraw Hill.

Simmons, D.A.: Implementation of nursing diagnosis in a community health setting. In Hurley, M.E., editor: Classification of nursing diagnoses: proceedings of the sixth national conference. St. Louis, 1986, The C.V. Mosby Co.

Simmons, S., and Ryan, L.: The implementation of nursing diagnosis using a computerized information system. In Kim, M.J., McFarland, G.K., and McLane, A.M., editors: Classification of nursing diagnoses: proceedings of the fifth national conference, St. Louis, 1984, The C.V. Mosby Co.

Vincent, K.G.: The validation of a nursing diagnosis: a nurse consensus survey, Nurs. Clin. North Amer. **20**:631-640, 1985.

A field study to identify nursing diagnoses for childbearing families

VIRGINIA AUKAMP, M.S., R.N.

The concept of nursing diagnosis has been recognized as being of special significance to the profession of nursing, and the growing need for a formulation of a system to promote the use of a common terminology in the practice of nursing has been advocated by the North American Nursing Diagnosis Association (NANDA; Gebbie and Lavin 1975). Over the last 25 years, a variety of definitions have been suggested for nursing diagnosis. From these, the desired definition of nursing diagnosis for this paper is "a statement of actual or potential altered-health-related responses by individuals and families which can be influenced, improved, or alleviated by nursing interventions that are included in the domain of nursing science" (Aukamp 1984, p. 3).

In a review of the literature, no studies were found about nursing diagnosis and childbearing families. Therefore, a field study design was used to identify the human responses that occur in childbearing families.

The assumptions for this study were: (1) There are identifiable predictable human responses in any specialized area of nursing practice. (2) All nursing care is planned.

The research question for this study was, "What are the identifiable human responses among childbearing families that indicate a nursing diagnosis?"

One hundred-eighty-nine families participated in this study over a 4-year period. Data were collected by doing a family assessment (Friedman 1979), a risk factor analysis (Hobel et al. 1975), and a detailed nursing history. Extensive prenatal, intrapartum and postpartum records are kept. By the use of the diag-nostic process, human responses as signs and symptoms were listed and then categorized into the format of a nursing diagnosis. The list of nursing diagnoses identified is shown in Box 1.

A content analysis was done and frequency counts were made for each nursing diagnosis. By far, the nursing diagnosis which occurred most often with childbearing families was knowledge deficit. This diagnosis was used with every family and frequently more than once for different etiologies.

Discomfort was the nursing diagnosis that had the second greatest number of frequencies. Alteration in comfort occurred in all three trimesters of pregnancy, during labor, and the postpartum period, but had decreas-

---

BOX 1: Nursing diagnoses for childbearing families

Knowledge deficit
Discomfort
Alteration in nutrition
Anxiety
Alteration in fluid balance
Alteration in sleep/rest patterns
Alteration in elimination
Alteration in breathing patterns
Alteration in self-concept
Potential for dysfunctional attachment
Potential for dysfunctional relationships
Potential for role conflict
Potential for family dysfunction
Potential for alteration in involution
Potential for infection
Ineffective breathing patterns
Family dysfunction

---

ing frequency in the 6-week follow-up period.

Every family had a nursing diagnosis relating to alteration in nutrition. The two etiologies were additional requirements for normal maintenance during pregnancy and additional requirements needed during lactation. Newborn needs through formula feeding were also common.

At the completion of the content analysis, there were 49 nursing diagnoses with varying etiologies based on 127 low-risk childbearing families. There were 47 nursing diagnoses based on 62 high-risk families.

Further research on the use of nursing diagnosis with childbearing needs to be done in other geographic regions and with various multi-cultural groups. Since some diagnostic labels have been identified, clinical validation studies with childbearing families during each trimester, labor, and family integration would add to the body of knowledge for maternity nursing.

REFERENCES

Aukamp, V.: Nursing care plans for childbearing families, East Norwalk, CT, 1984, Appleton-Century-Crofts.

Friedman, M.: Family nursing, New York, 1981, Appleton-Century-Crofts.

Gebbie, K.M., and Lavin, M.A.: Classification of nursing diagnoses: proceedings of the first national conference, St. Louis, 1975, The C.V. Mosby Co.

Hobel, C.J., Huvarinen, M.A., Ohada, D.N., and others: Prenatal and intrapartum high-risk screening, Amer. J. Ob. Gyn. **117:**1-9, 1973.

Epidemiologic studies: abstracts

Acute confusion in the hospitalized elderly: patterns and early diagnosis

MARY CHAMPAGNE, Ph.D., R.N.
VIRGINIA NEELON, Ph.D., R.N.
ELEANOR McCONNELL, M.S.N., R.N.

Acute confusion, a term commonly used by nurses, is a subcategory of the diagnostic category sensory-perceptual alterations. Acute confusion is differentiated from chronic cognitive impairments such as dementia by its rapid onset and is characterized by global cognitive impairments, including disorders of perception, memory and thinking; disordered attention and wakefulness; and disordered psychomotor behavior. Etiological factors related to the development of acute confusion reported in the literature include environmental factors, altered sensory reception, transmission and integration, chemical alteration, and psychological stress. For the most part, however, these factors have been identified retrospectively, after the development of acute confusional behavior; and few of the factors have been examined in the hospitalized elderly population. Yet studies of acute confusion in the hospitalized elderly report an incidence of 16 or 55%. The study reported here was designed to identify and examine prospectively those factors related to the development of acute confusion in the hospitalized elderly.

My colleagues and I developed a frame-work for disturbed information processing and the development of acute confusion that described functional integrity (cognitive and physical) as dependent on a hierarchy of interactive levels—three primarily physiological factor levels (oxygen-energy level, autonomic response level, sensory-motor level) and a fourth level involving the external environment (physical, interpersonal). From this framework, six factors or independent variables were identified: blood oxygen saturation level, nutritional intake, autonomic instability, activity, functional ability, and character of the external environment. A time series, repeated measures descriptive study explored the relationship of those six factors to the development of acute confusion in hospitalized elderly patients over 69 years of age admitted to the general medical services in a large teaching hospital. Patients were followed throughout hospitalization with factor variables measured on admission and daily or every other day until discharge. The dependent variable, acute confusion, was measured on admission and daily by staff nurse report, on admission and every other day by patient self-report, and on admission and every other day by the researchers using the NEECHAM Confusion Assessment Scale. The NEECHAM was developed to permit rapid bedside documentation of cues indicating the early onset of acute confusion behavior. Data were also collected on the patient's general health status and mental health status on admission and discharge; and data related to treatments, such as drug therapy, were collected daily.

Preliminary analysis suggests that factors related to the occurrence of acute confusion involve the presence or absence of key variables interacting across processing levels: critical periods of caloric deprivation; auto-nomic instability on admission; assertive family advocacy; "cognitive protecting behavior" by the patient, new medications; and nursing-medical interventions that minimize the patient's ability to control body position and movement. Three patterns of confusion development were documented: (1) early onset, environmentally provoked episodes; (2) physiologically unstable, fluctuating episodes; and (3) delayed onset-toxic provoked episodes. This paper discussed the patterns of acute confusion and relationships to the etiological factors found in this elderly hospitalized population.

Generating nursing diagnoses from clinical records with rheumatoid arthritis as the predictor variable

MARY ANN KELLY, Ed.D., R.N.
JESSE E. GREENE, B.S.N., R.N.

Knowing the confluence of nursing diagnoses and other variables advances diagnostic sensitivity (Gordon 1982). A priority for research is identification of predictor variables. Do specific nursing diagnoses co-occur with specific medical diagnoses?

The purpose of this study was to explore the relationship between selected nursing diagnostic and medical diagnostic categories. Rheumatic disease, specifically rheumatoid arthritis was selected as the primary medical diagnosis. Diagnostic categories associated with rheumatic diseases as identified by Carpenito (1984) were selected as the nursing diagnoses. An additional purpose of the study was to test the use of a computer model in identifying nursing diagnoses from data on client records in which nursing diagnoses as recognized by NANDA have not been used.

A descriptive, retrospective record review of 20 client records with the primary medical diagnosis of rheumatoid arthritis is planned to reveal demographic data and defining characteristics as documented by nurses in the data base and care plan sections of a home health agency's medical records. A pilot testing of the computer model was completed using five client records. Collected data were tabulated in the computer model instrument and analyzed by SAS procedures of sort, transpose, and array coding. To differentiate between defining characteristics of the nursing diagnoses Carpenito predicted and the defining characteristics found in the clinical records, a match-merge procedure was used for further analysis, and nursing diagnoses were generated from the sample data.

Of the 14 possible nursing diagnoses, an average of six nursing diagnoses were confirmed from the data found documented in the pilot sample of records. Although rheumatoid arthritis was found to be a predictor of certain nursing diagnoses, an even more interesting finding was that of the repetitious nature of the nursing diagnoses generated from the sample.

Sensitivity to co-occurring, predictor variables strengthens nurses' diagnostic ability and better represents practice realities.

Nurse reported patient problems in alcoholism

ANN POLITYKA FITZGERALD, M.N., R.N.
JEAN KRAJICEK BARTEK, M.S.N., M.S., R.N.
MARLENE G. LINDEMAN, M.S.N., R.N.
MARIAN NEWTON, M.N., R.N.
JANE HOKANSON HAWKS, M.S.N., R.N.

An estimated 9 to 10 million persons in the adult population are problem drinkers or alcoholics. The numerous physiological and psychosocial problems present in the hospitalized alcoholic patient create complex challenges for nurses who provide care to these patients. Although the professional nurse commonly provides interventions for patients with these alcohol-related problems in medical-surgical hospital setting, there is a paucity of research for such interventions. The major objective or purpose of this exploratory study was to determine what nurses themselves view as difficult patient problems in caring for the alcoholic person, the factors affecting the resolution of the problems, and the nursing interventions utilized for the identified problems.

Two hundred and thirty-six full-time-employed registered nurses who work in medical-surgical settings were randomly selected for participation in this study. Eighty-three subjects completed and returned the questionnaire. Respondents were asked in an open-ended questionnaire to list physiological and psychological patient problems, factors that made care difficult, and the interventions used to care for the problems found in alcoholic patients. Selected demographic and biographic data were also collected. The researchers developed a coding log identifying 15 problem categories, 11 factor categories, and 12 intervention categories. The nursing diagnosis classifications described by Kim and Moritz (1982) and Lunney (1982) served as a basis and were adapted for the patient problem categories. Nominal data were analyzed using frequency distributions and percentages.

Subjects identified the categories of: potential for injury related to neurological changes; and deficits in blood volume as the most difficult physiological problems in caring for alcoholic persons. The categories of: alterations in coping; alterations in relationships with family or significant others; and non-compliance in self-management of health comprised the most difficult psychosocial patient problems. Alterations in coping was identified as the most frequently cited difficult patient problem overall. A majority of the subjects reported having had limited classroom and clinical experience with alcoholism content. Eighty percent of the subjects in this study expressed a need for additional inservice education on the topic of nursing intervention in alcoholism. Seventy-one percent of the subjects reported a close personal relationship with an alcoholic person.

Implications for nursing education and practice are: inclusion of additional content hours and experience in both basic nursing programs and continuing education offerings, specifically in the area of family dynamics, communication and management skills, and content as it relates to the most difficult patient problems cited.

Co-occurrence of nursing and medical diagnoses in hospitalized patients

ELVI N. RIGBY, M.S.N., R.N., C.S.
ELINORE HOWARD, M.S., R.N.C.

Statement of the problem. Is there a relationship between nursing diagnoses and medical diagnoses in a selected population of medical-surgical patients?

Purpose of the study. The purpose of the study was to describe the relationship between nursing diagnoses and medical diagnoses in a selected population of medical-surgical patients.

METHODOLOGY

Design. A descriptive study was done utilizing a convenience sample. A tool was developed to record those nursing diagnoses meeting the criteria for inclusion in the study. Inter-rater reliability was established for those diagnoses selected. Cronbach's alpha was computed to establish tool reliability. Significance levels and correlation coefficients were computed for the medical and nursing diagnoses.

Description of subjects and sample size. Patient records were selected from four medical-surgical units in a 300-bed community teaching hospital south of Boston. Criteria were established regarding length of stay and medical diagnosis. Eighty-six patient records were accepted by eight nurse data collectors for inclusion in the study.

Methods of data collection. Data were collected by eight nurse research assistants from November 1984 to July 1985.

Analysis of data. Descriptive statistics were computed for the selected diagnoses, medical and surgical. Medical diagnoses were classified using the Merck Manual system. Inferential statistics were computed for those nursing and medical diagnoses meeting the established criteria.

Major findings. There is a relationship between nursing diagnoses and medical diagnoses in a selected population of adult medical-surgical patients.

Significance of the study. Description of co-occurrence between nursing and medical diagnoses facilitates prediction of nursing diagnoses for DRG categories, as well as identification of staffing and budgetary needs.

PART A

Diagnostic reasoning studies: paper presentations

Hypothesis evaluation: a component of diagnostic reasoning[*]

KAREN P. PADRICK, M.N., R.N.
CHRISTINE A. TANNER, Ph.D., R.N., F.A.A.N.
DEE-J PUTZIER, Ph.D., R.N.
UNA E. WESTFALL, M.S.N., R.N.

Diagnostic reasoning is an essential cognitive ability that nurses must use to provide safe and effective patient care. Although nurses are called upon to make accurate judgments about a patient's condition, there is a paucity of nursing research in this area. To help students and nurses improve their problem solving abilities, a systematic analysis of how novice and experienced clinicians move from clinical data to diagnoses to management must be undertaken.

One theoretical model that assists in providing a framework for this analysis is information processing theory (Newell and Simon 1972). Briefly, this theory describes problem solving as an interaction between an information processing system (the problem solver) and a task environment (the task as described by the researcher). The major assumption underlying the theory is that the human information processing system capacity is limited. Effective problem solving depends upon the individual's ability to adapt the information processing resources to the requirements of the task environment.

In the instance of diagnosis, the diagnostic reasoning model describes strategies that individuals use in that adaptation. Generally, this model includes the following components: (1) narrowing the search field or problem sensing; (2) activation of diagnostic hypotheses that explain some or all of the cues presented; (3) systematic data gathering related to each hypothesis; and (4) evaluation of the hypotheses. The processes of diagnostic reasoning have been studied extensively in medicine using medical students and physicians as subjects (Barrows and Bennett 1972, Ekwo 1977, Elstein, Shulman, and Sprafka 1978, Feightner 1977, Kassirer and Gorry 1978, Neufeld, Norman, Feightner and Barrows 1981). The extent to which this model is descriptive of diagnostic strategies used by nurses is unknown, as research efforts in this area are limited. There is reason to believe,

[*]Partially funded by the Northwest Area Foundation

based on information processing theory, that there are some generic strategies employed in diagnostic reasoning (Gordon 1980, and Tanner, 1977).

This study is part of a larger project exploring the extent to which the proposed model of diagnostic reasoning applies to nurses and nursing students. The focus of this report will be the fourth component of the model: hypothesis evaluation. The specific research question that was investigated is, How do subjects use data to evaluate hypotheses?

METHODS
Subjects

A convenience sample of 43 subjects was used in this study. It was comprised of 15 junior students, 13 senior students and 15 practicing nurses from a health sciences university hospital.

Instruments

Subjects diagnostic reasoning strategies were elicited in response to 11 video-taped patient situations. Two of these video tapes were used for training. The vignettes were developed to be representative both of diagnostic tasks frequently encountered by nurses in the care of adult patients and of task characteristics thought to influence reasoning strategies. Examples of these task characteristics included use of subtle cues, low reliability of the cue and irrelevant cues.

Summaries of the vignettes used in this portion of the study are displayed in Box 1. Because the nursing diagnosis taxonomy was

---

BOX 1   **Descriptions of vignettes**

Vignette 1

This is a 51-year-old female admitted 14 days ago for an excision of a recurrent malignant histiocytoma on the right lateral thigh. The surgical procedure was a wide excision of the tumor with removal of tissue to the femur. A Jackson-Pratt drain, inserted at the time of surgery, continues to be connected to low suction. The video tape portrayed a woman who is feeling nauseated, anorexic, fatigued, short of breath and too sick to ambulate. Further assessment reveals that she feels warm to the touch and is complaining about pain in her affected leg.

Vignette 2

This is a 54-year-old male with a 10-year history of COPD. He was diagnosed with cor pulmonale 18 months ago. He has been on medical disability for 6 years. The video tape portrayed a man in his home who is complaining of increasing shortness of breath and an 8-pound weight gain in 3 days. He had been to the clinic four days ago with complaints of not feeling well and had been started on prednisone. He had been eating at the burger place across the street because he was too tired to walk to the store 10 blocks away.

Vignette 3

This is a 70-year-old male admitted to the hospital 3 days ago for a work-up of abdominal pain. He is an insulin-dependent diabetic and has a history of alcoholism. One day ago, he developed a fever and was diagnosed with viral pneumonia. The video tape portrayed an elderly man, lying supine in bed, with an intravenous infusion running. He was obviously disoriented and did not respond coherently to the nurse's attempts to orient him. Shown on the bedside table were glasses and hearing aids.

---

not universally accepted by all subjects, both medically oriented and nursing diagnoses were included in the study.

Procedures

After hearing a change of shift report and viewing the video tape, subjects were instructed to ask for additional information about the patient as they would in actual practice. For example, they might ask for additional history, physical examination data or laboratory test results. As they asked for information, they were prompted to "think aloud," describing their thinking and their subsequent interpretation of the patient information provided. This thinking aloud was tape recorded and transcribed for later analysis.

RESULTS

Based on three of the nine vignettes, six clear categories of outcome regarding hypothesis evaluation were generated. These categories were based on two dimensions, the accuracy of the decision to accept or reject the hypothesis, and the sufficiency of information to make an informed judgment. Using these dimensions, it was possible to describe how the subjects used the information gathered to evaluate hypotheses generated. The outcomes were: (1) accept a correct hypotheses appropriately; (2) reject an incorrect hypothesis appropriately; (3) accept an hypothesis without sufficient data to support the decision; (4) reject an hypothesis without sufficient data to support the decision; (5) accept an incorrect hypothesis with sufficient data to reject it; and (6) reject a correct hypothesis with sufficient data to accept it.

A summary of subjects who were classified into each category by each of the three vignettes is shown in Table 1. The summary is displayed by vignette, because it has been found that the subject's ability to problem solve differs according to the task. The percentages for each of the categories were calculated using the number of subjects who were classified into the outcome category, divided by the number of subjects who activated an appropriate hypothesis for the outcome. For example, in Vignette 2, 36 subjects activated at least one accurate hypoth-

Table 1: Hypothesis evaluation category by vignette (n=43)

	Vignette						
	1			**2**		**3**	
Category	No./Hyp	%		No./Hyp	%	No./Hyp	%
Accept appropriate	7/7[1]	100		29/36[1]	80	16/29[1]	55
Reject appropriate	14/36[2]	40		2/17[2]	12	30/31[2]	97
Accept without data							
Correct	0	0		12/36[1]	33	13/29[1]	45
Incorrect	15/36[2]	42		13/17[2]	76	5/31[2]	16
Reject without data							
Correct	8/36[2]	25		2/17[2]	12	6/31[2]	19
Incorrect	0	0		0	0	1/29[1]	3
Accept with data to reject (incorrect)	10/36[2]	28		1/17[2]	6	5/31[2]	16
Reject with data to accept (incorrect)	0	0		1/36[1]	3	2/29[1]	7

[1]Denominator is the number of subjects who activated an accurate hypothesis.
[2]Denominator is the number of subjects who activated a plausible hypothesis.

esis related to the patient situation. Of those 36 subjects, 29 made at least one correct decision about an activated hypothesis. Since more than one accurate hypothesis could be generated related to the patient situation, one subject could be classified into more than one category. Hence, the number of subjects in each category does not necessarily equal the number of subjects who activated an hypothesis. Only subjects who made definite decisions were included in the analysis.

Hypotheses were classified into two categories, accurate or plausible. An accurate hypothesis was a correct explanation for cues of immediate concern presented in the situation. A plausible hypothesis was a possible but incorrect explanation for cues of immediate concern presented in the situation.

The first outcome, accepting a correct hypothesis appropriately, was achieved by a majority of subjects who activated an accurate hypothesis in all situations. Subjects who were categorized into this group activated an accurate hypothesis, gathered data to rule in this possibility and then made the decision to accept it. For example, the accurate hypothesis in Vignette 1 (see Box 1) was that the patient was hypokalemic. A subject in this first category would have activated the hypothesis of hypokalemia, asked for the serum potassium level, found that the value was 2.8, and then decided that the cause of the patient's signs and symptoms was the hypokalemia.

The second outcome, rejecting an incorrect hypothesis appropriately, occurred at varying frequencies according to the situation. Subjects who were placed in this category activated a plausible hypothesis, gathered data to rule out the possibility and then decided to reject the hypothesis. For example, one of the plausible hypotheses in Vignette 1 was that the patient had an infection. A subject in the second category would have activated the hypothesis of infection;

asked about the wound, cultures, temperature, and white blood count; found that all of these parameters were within normal limits; and rejected infection as the etiology of the patient's signs and symptoms.

Accepting an hypothesis without sufficient data to support the decision was the third category identified. This category had two subcategories, the decision was either correct or incorrect. A subject could accept an accurate hypothesis without supporting data, and the decision would be correct. However, a subject could accept a plausible hypothesis without supporting data, and the decision would be incorrect. The percentage of subjects who made a correct decision even though they did not have the data to support it ranged from 0% to 45%. An example of a subject who made a correct decision without sufficient data in Vignette 3 is as follows:

I saw them hang a medication there. Could it be Tagamet? A lot of times that can cause confusion in elderly people. If it is Tagamet, I think I'd stop it right away.

In Vignette 3, the patient was receiving tagamet which was an accurate hypothesis. This subject, however, did not find out how long the patient had been receiving the medication so did not have all the data needed to arrive at the conclusion that the medication was causing the patient's signs and symptoms.

A subject could make an incorrect decision by accepting a plausible hypothesis without sufficient information. The percentage of subjects who made incorrect decisions ranged from 16% to 76%. Generally, this type of subject would make a decision without very much data. For example, in Vignette 2, some subjects decided that the patient with chronic obstructive pulmonary disease was having increased shortness of breath because of his smoking. The subjects would see a cigarette in the video tape but would many times not ask if it belonged to the patient. They also might not ask about the patient's smoking habits. Although the patient did smoke, smoking was not the correct etiology for his increased shortness of breath. Thus, because subjects did not ask for information, they made errors in their problem solving.

The fourth category of hypothesis evaluation was rejecting an hypothesis without sufficient data to support the decision. Once again, this category contained two subcategories; the decision was either correct or incorrect. Subjects made incorrect decisions in this category very infrequently. In other words, the correct decision was made more frequently. The subject who made the incorrect decision in Vignette 3 rejected the possibility that the patient's signs and symptoms could be caused by the lack of sensory input because he does not have on his hearing aides and glasses. If the subject would have gathered more data about the cues, it would have been discovered that the patient could see and hear very little without his prostheses. Thus, an incorrect decision was made because sufficient data were not collected.

Subjects could make a correct decision to reject a plausible hypothesis without sufficient data. For example, in Vignette 3, the patient's signs and symptoms could have been caused by hypoglycemia or hyperglycemia. One subject who was classified into this category asked for the patient's past medical history related to his diabetes mellitus. When it was discovered that the patient was adequately controlled at home on 15 units of NPH insulin, the hypotheses related to his diabetes were rejected. This was a correct decision; however, the information gathered was insufficient to make the decision. If the subject would have probed further, it would have been discovered that the patient was on a sliding scale for his insulin, that he did not have glucosuria and that his last fasting blood glucose was 220.

Thus, the outcome of this subject's problem solving was correct, but the process lacked comprehensiveness.

The fifth category of hypothesis evaluation outcomes was accepting an hypothesis with data to reject it. This occurred infrequently (6% to 28%). A subject in this category activated a plausible hypothesis, gathered data about the hypothesis, interpreted the data, and then accepted the plausible hypothesis. In Vignette 3, the subjects are told in the change of shift report that the patient has a history of alcoholism. Some subjects generate an hypothesis that alcohol withdrawal could be causing the patient's signs and symptoms. An example from a subject's transcript who accepted the hypothesis of alcohol withdrawal is as follows:

Subject: "It looks like Mr. Seymour is disoriented. With the information I got from report, with his history of alcohol disease, it's possible he could be having some DT's. Do we have any information about when he last had a drink?"

Tester: "He states and the nurse at the retirement center where he lived also stated that he's been dry for the last 10 years."

At the end of the transcript, the subject summarizes the patient's problems:

Subject: "I think he's definitely disoriented and because he has an alcohol history, it could be related to that."

Thus, this subject was unwilling to reject a plausible hypothesis even though the data to reject it had been obtained.

The final category was rejecting an hypothesis with data to accept it. Once again, this occurred infrequently. The subjects who were in this category activated an accurate hypothesis, gathered data about the hypothesis, interpreted the data and decided to reject the accurate hypothesis. The three subjects who were in this category, all gathered the data needed to accept the hypothesis but decided that the time frame was too short for the hypothesis to occur. For example, in Vignette 3, a plausible hypothesis to explain the patient's signs and symptoms was that the patient was taking cimetidine. The subject asked about the cimetidine, found that the patient had been taking 300 mg intravenously every 8 hours for 3 days and decided that it was too soon for the side effect to occur. Thus, this subject's interpretation of the data led to a conclusion that was incorrect.

DISCUSSION AND CONCLUSIONS

Based upon the results of the analysis thus far, the following conclusions can be delineated:

1. In general, subjects correctly accept hypotheses if they collect the appropriate data. They seldom make incorrect decisions if they have the necessary information.

2. In cases in which subjects had not collected sufficient data, they were much more willing to accept incorrect hypotheses than to reject incorrect hypotheses. This phenomenon may be related to the desire of the subject to solve the problem. By accepting an incorrect hypothesis, the subject at least had an answer, although it was wrong. However, if subjects rejected a hypothesis without data to support the decision, they were left without an answer. This situation made many subjects uncomfortable. Other investigators have found that it is more difficult to reject hypotheses than to accept them. Matthews and Gaul (1979) found that subjects had more difficulty using disconfirming than confirming data. Tanner (1977) also found this to be true.

3. Rejecting hypotheses correctly appears to be related somewhat to the task environment. It was much easier to reject hypotheses correctly in the third vignette than in the second one. This may be related to the availability of more definitive data to reject the hypotheses in the third vignette. There is evidence that tasks in each vignette had

varying degrees of difficulty based on the variation that subjects displayed in their ability to work through the problem. Further analysis on this aspect of the study needs to be conducted.

Based on the analysis of three vignettes, a tentative hypothesis may be advanced. It appears that most subjects were able to make correct decisions if they obtained appropriate data. Currently there is little research to support methods used to teach students and practitioners clinical decision making. There is a need to conduct research to determine whether efforts should be directed toward helping students and practitioners to learn to gather appropriate information. Education needs to assist clinicians in their efforts to focus on relevant cues and determine and use the definitive information that will assist in their problem solving process.

The results of this study indicate the need for further research on the diagnostic reasoning process used by beginning and experienced nurses. Future research related to the present study and hypothesis evaluation includes determining whether there is consistency in the manner in which a subject uses data to evaluate hypotheses and whether there are differences among groups based on experience. Continued efforts to determine functional and dysfunctional approaches which clinicians use to make decisions regarding a patient's condition should aid in the instruction and continuing education of both students and nurses.

REFERENCES

Barrows, H., and Bennett, K.: The diagnostic (problem solving) skill of the neurologist, Arch. Neurol. **26:** 273-277, 1972.

Ekwo, E.: An analysis of the problem solving process of third year medical students. In Proceedings of the 16th annual conference of research in medical education, Washington, DC, 1977, Association of American Medical Colleges.

Elstein, A., Shulman, L., and Sprafka, S.: Medical problem solving: an analysis of clinical reasoning, Cambridge, 1978, Harvard University Press.

Feightner, J.: Clinical methods of physicians: a comparison of primary and secondary care physicians. In Proceedings of the 16th annual conference on research in medical education, Washington, DC, 1977, Association of American Medical Colleges.

Gordon, M.: Predictive strategies in diagnostic tasks, Nurs. Res. **29:**39-45, 1980.

Kassirer, J., and Gorry, C.: Clinical problem solving: a behavioral analysis, Ann. Inter. Med. **89:**245-255, 1978.

Matthews, C.A., and Gaul, A.L.: Nursing diagnosis from the perspective of concept attainment, Adv. Nurs. Sci. **2:**17-26, 1979.

Neufeld, V., Norman, G., Feightner, J., and others: Clinical problem solving by medical students: a cross-sectional and longitudinal analysis, Med. Educ. **15:**315-322, 1981.

Newell, A., and Simon, H.: Human problem solving, Englewood Cliffs, NJ, 1972, Prentice-Hall.

Tanner, C.: The effect of hypothesis generation as an instructional method on the diagnostic process of senior baccalaureate nursing students, Unpublished doctoral dissertation, University of Colorado, 1977.

The nursing diagnosis of population groups*

EILEEN JONES PORTER, M.A., R.N.

It has been proposed that the North American Nursing Diagnosis Association's approved diagnoses can be applied to communities as well as to individuals (Kim, McFarland, and McLane 1984). Yet, uncertainty exists as to whether a community-of-place can be the client of a nurse (Hamilton 1983). There are other conceptual difficulties inherent in the development of community nursing diagnoses. A phrase such as "increased infant mortality rate" (Andrews 1982, p. 125), propounded to be a diagnosis, is instead a fact about a health trend. In contrast, a diagnosis is an *analysis* of facts or a "type of scientific construct . . . used to label the phenomena that nurses identify and treat" (Barnard 1983, p. 223).

The problems of community diagnosis might be circumvented by diagnosing the population groups that comprise the community. According to a recent survey of community health nurses, educators, and administrators, the diagnosis of population groups was the responsibility of community-nurse-administrators (Anderson 1983). Because the actual diagnoses made by these nurses have not been described, an inductive study was warranted to isolate the fundamental concepts (Field and Morse 1985) of their diagnostic reasoning process.

METHOD

Data pertaining to diagnostic strategies were gathered and analyzed concurrently using the grounded theory or constant comparative method. Incidents that were applicable to each category of analysis were compared. The categories and their properties were integrated into a hypothesis that directed further data-gathering and analysis (Glaser and Strauss 1967). Finally, a factor-isolating theory (Dickoff and James 1968) of community-nurse-administrator diagnosis was delineated.

Questionnaire

The open-ended questionnaire was designed according to the assumption that the community-nurse-administrator's diagnostic decisions could be understood from descriptions of the rationale for changing agency services. In the questionnaire, a request was made for: a list of agency services that had been started or discontinued within the last 3 years; an explanation of population group health needs to be met by each service; and a description of the information used to confirm existence of health needs. Opinions were also solicited about the significance of the nurse's role in community health planning in relation to the roles of other decision-makers. Two community nurses with administrative experience confirmed the face validity of the questionnaire.

Subjects

The informed consent of a convenience sample of 34 community-nurse-administrators was secured before they completed the questionnaire. The information about each agency service described on the questionnaire was called a *datum incident*. Theoretical sampling was used so that the responses which could "most facilitate the development of the emerging theory" (Field and

*This paper is based on a research study supported by a Faculty Development Grant from the University of Wisconsin-Oshkosh to Eileen Jones Porter.
I gratefully acknowledge the assistance of Kathleen A. Baldwin, R.N., M.S.N., and Annette G. Lueckenotte, R.N., M.S., in data coding.

Morse 1985, p. 95) were selected for analysis. Of the 208 datum incidents, 33 were discarded because of a focus on staffing change rather than service change. The 31 subjects who cited at least one relevant datum incident participated in one or two telephone interviews. The subjects were of various educational and experiential levels; they were directors of either city or county health departments in one state.

DATA GATHERING AND ANALYSIS
Phase 1: Development of categories and properties from questionnaires

As the completed questionnaires were received, the datum incidents were compared to generate categories of the rationale for changing agency services. Concurrent with preliminary data analysis, a review of the literature related to population group diagnosis was initiated to ensure familiarity with prevailing theories (Field and Morse 1985).

The data-gathering function of the community-nurse-administrator was described as the identification of health-related data about population groups and the entire community (Anderson 1983). Therefore, it seemed that a diagnosis could result from judgments about the characteristics of a group, the status of the environment, or the interaction between a group and its environment.

Based on the datum incidents and the literature, three categories of rationale for service change were identified: personal characteristics of population group members, environmental conditions, and a combination of group characteristics and environmental conditions. The categories and their properties are shown in Figure 1. A hypothesis was generated at the conclusion of Phase 1: The rationale for changing an agency service is based upon a nursing diagnosis pertaining to the characteristics of a population group, environmental conditions, or a combination of group characteristics and environmental conditions.

Phase 2: Telephone interviews

From the perspective of the hypothesis, additional information needed to fully understand the decision-making relative to each datum incident was determined. Based on the requisite information, a semi-structured interview guide was sketched for each subject prior to conducting a telephone interview. All of the subjects' remarks were documented. The interviews were an invaluable source of data, enabling refinement of the categories and properties during Phase 3.

During Phase 2, the data pertaining to the significance of the subjects' health planning roles were also analyzed. Because forced-choice responses were used, the results were computed in percentages.

Phase 3: Data coding and theory refinement

To avoid bias in refining the theory, two community nurses with experience in inductive research and the investigator independently coded the questionnaire and interview data. The specific data used by the subjects to justify each service change were coded according to the three categories established in Phase 1. During the coding, additional properties were identified for each category (see Fig. 1). Of the 208 items coded, complete agreement among the coders was reached for 68% of the items; two coders agreed on the other 32% of the items. This level of agreement was deemed satisfactory.

By comparing how the incidents had been categorized, it was determined that none of the new services had been coded under the category of group member characteristics. A property of the environmental conditions category—lack of needed health care service—ensured that new services would be coded under either the *environmental con-*

PHASE 1	PHASE 3	FACTOR-ISOLATING THEORY OF COMMUNITY-NURSE-ADMINISTRATOR DIAGNOSIS
QUESTIONNAIRE	DATA CODING AND THEORY REFINEMENT	
CONCEPTUAL CATEGORIES OF RATIONALE FOR CHANGE IN AGENCY SERVICES	CONCEPTUAL CATEGORIES OF RATIONALE FOR CHANGE IN AGENCY SERVICES	CONCEPTS: • NEED-RELATED CUE PROCESSING • POPULATION GROUP DIAGNOSIS • DIAGNOSTIC-STAGING • HEALTH CARE SYSTEM DIAGNOSIS • DIAGNOSTIC-BASED MANAGEMENT

1 PERSONAL CHARACTERISTICS OF GROUP MEMBERS
Properties:
• Age
• Personal Medical History
• Family Medical History
• Income
	1 PERSONAL CHARACTERISTICS OF GROUP MEMBERS
	Properties:
	• Age
	• Developmental Status
	• Racial/Cultural Heritage
	• Family Medical History
	• Personal Medical History
	• Lifestyle
	• Social History
		FIRST STAGE DIAGNOSIS
		
		DIAGNOSIS:
		VULNERABLE POPULATION GROUP
		   Defining Characteristics:
		   Properties refined for Category #1 in Phase 3.

2 ENVIRONMENTAL CONDITIONS
Properties:
• Unsanitary Environment
• Communicable Disease Prevalent
• Lack of Needed Health Care Service
	2 ENVIRONMENTAL CONDITIONS
	Properties:
	• Unsafe Environment: Air, water, noise pollution
	• Environmental Deficiency: Lack of flouride in water
	• Communicable Disease Endemic or Epidemic
	• Unsanitary Environment
	• Threats to Safety
	• Crowded Living Conditions
		DIAGNOSIS:
		POPULATION-AT-RISK
		   Defining Characteristics:
		   Properties refined for Category #2 in Phase 3.

3 COMBINATION OF PERSONAL CHARACTERISTICS OF GROUP MEMBERS AND ENVIRONMENTAL CONDITIONS
Properties:
One or more of properties of Category #1 in conjunction with one or more properties of Category #2.
	3 COMBINATION OF PERSONAL CHARACTERISTICS OF GROUP MEMBERS AND ENVIRONMENTAL CONDITIONS
	Properties:
	One or more properties of Category #1 in conjunction with one or more properties of Category #2.
		DIAGNOSIS:
		VULNERABLE POPULATION GROUP-AT-RISK
		   Defining Characteristics:
		   Properties refined for Category #1 in combination with properties refined for Category #2 in Phase 3.

PHASE 2
 	
TELEPHONE INTERVIEWS
	4 MISMATCH BETWEEN GROUP HEALTH NEED AND HEALTH CARE SERVICES
	Properties:
	• Duplication of Services by Agencies
	• Lack of Coordination among Agencies Who Provide a Service Cooperatively
	• No Existing Program to Meet Need
	• Need No Longer Exists, but Service Continues
	• Service Format Ineffective in Meeting Need
	• Service Format Inefficient
		SECOND STAGE DIAGNOSIS
		
		DIAGNOSIS:
		NEED-SERVICE MISMATCH
		   Defining Characteristics:
		   Properties refined for Category #4 in Phase 3.

	5 MATCH BETWEEN GROUP HEALTH NEED AND HEALTH CARE SERVICES
	Properties:
	• Appropriate Service Exists to Meet Need
	• Agencies Cooperate to Meet Need
	• Existing Service can be Modified to Meet Need
		DIAGNOSIS:
		NEED-SERVICE MATCH
		   Defining Characteristics:
		   Properties refined for Category #5 in Phase 3.

FIGURE 1   The development of the factor-isolating theory of community-nurse-administrator diagnosis.

ditions category or the *combination* category. A second conflict with the hypothesis was that datum incidents of service discontinuation were often characterized by a nurse's decision that the health care system was meeting the need in some other way. Thus the coding results for both new and discontinued services pointed to a two-stage diagnostic process, with the first stage focused on the population group and its environment and the second stage focused on the health care system.

For this reason, the emerging theory was modified by deleting the property *lack of needed health service* from the environmental conditions category and adding two additional categories: match (congruence) and mismatch between health needs and health care system resources. These categories and their properties are shown in Figure 1. An additional hypothesis was developed. The rationale for changing an agency service is based upon a second-stage diagnosis pertaining to the degree of match between the health needs of the population group and health care system services. Each datum incident was recoded to establish its congruence first with Category 1, 2 or 3 and then with Category 4 or 5 (see Fig. 1).

Review of relevant literature

During Phase 3, the review of the literature was continued to guide the derivation of "explanations from previous research results" (Field and Morse 1985, p. 35). Information was sought about the familiar term, population-at-risk, which community-nurse-administrators could feasibly use as a label for a specific group.

A population-at-risk had been defined as one that engages in certain activities or has a characteristic that increases its potential for contracting an illness, injury, or health problem (Clemen, Eigsti, and McGuire 1981). However, risk was recently redefined as a element within the environment that is hazardous to health. A companion term, vulnerability, was attributed to groups that possess certain personal characteristics "that interact with the environment to influence health" (Rose and Killien 1983, p. 61). With risk redefined as an environmental hazard, population-at-risk could be modified to mean a group whose health status is threatened by an environmental hazard. Furthermore, it seemed plausible that a population group could be both vulnerable due to its personal characteristics and at-risk due to an environmental hazard.

Therefore, any one of three diagnoses could be made about the health status of a population group: vulnerable population group, population-at-risk, and vulnerable population group-at-risk. One of these diagnoses would constitute the first-stage diagnosis; this would be followed by a second-stage diagnosis pertaining to the degree of match between the group need and health care services.

Content analysis

A content analysis was performed on each of the categorized health needs to determine whether the five categories of rationale for service change coincided with the five proposed diagnoses. Although this analysis revealed a great variety in the terminology used to describe health needs, it could be inferred that each health need corresponded not only to one of the population group-environment diagnoses but also to one of the need-service diagnoses. Thus Phase 3 resulted in the articulation of a nursing diagnosis based on each of the five conceptual categories of data. The defining characteristics of the diagnoses were the refined properties of the categories, which originated from the data about the type of information used to confirm the existence of health needs.

Telephone interviews

The congruence of the theory with the substantive situation—the actual role of the community-nurse-administrator—was determined by a second series of telephone interviews with a random sample of five subjects. They were asked to use the concepts of the theory to explain one of their decisions about service change. Each of the subjects was able to successfully complete this task. They related that the theory was congruent with their decision-making activities.

RESULTS

Significance of subjects' health planning role

Twenty-four subjects (77%) stated that their involvement in health planning was significantly greater than that of other decision-makers in their communities, and 7 subjects (23%) described their contributions as similar to those of other decision-makers. Thus the subjects believed that nursing decision-making was an important feature of community health planning.

Content analysis of health needs: terminology and diagnostic classification

There was great variety in the terminology used to state the health needs of the groups. About 30% of the needs were clearly stated, such as "prevention of hearing problems" or "screening for infectious diseases." However, the remainder were stated as one of the following: (1) the name of the group ("jail inmates"), (2) a cue of a need ("dental caries"), (3) a nursing goal or action ("to offer health education"), or (4) an inadequacy of the health care system ("lack of a formal system for educating children about safety").[1] It is conjectured that the clarity with which the nurse phrases the group's health need may have implications for the success of the ensuing attempt to alter agency services.

---

[1]The idea of categorizing the health needs in this way was borrowed from M.O. Mundinger, who categorized mislabeled nursing diagnoses using similar terminology in her book, *Autonomy in Nursing*.

Table 1 cites examples of the health needs as stated by the subjects; the classification for each diagnostic stage is also shown. For the first diagnostic stage, the majority (53%) of the health needs were related to the diagnosis of vulnerable population group, while 37% pointed to the label of vulnerable population group-at-risk. Although relatively few needs correlated with the diagnosis of population-at-risk, they were considered significant in their impact on the public's health. For the second diagnostic stage, 88% of the health needs were related to need-service mismatch, while only 12% indicated the diagnosis of need-service match.

Statement of theory

Community-nurse-administrators make a series of two diagnoses prior to proposing change in agency services. The first diagnosis is made about the specific health status of the population group, and the second diagnosis is made about the degree of the match between the group's need and health care services.

The concepts of need-related cue processing, population group diagnosis, diagnostic-staging, health care system diagnosis, and diagnostic-based management exemplify the diagnostic activities of the community-nurse-administrator. The evolution of the factor-isolating theory is shown in Figure 1. An example of how the theory can be used to explain a datum incident is shown in Box. 1.

Concepts of the theory

Need-related cue processing. The term *cue* has been defined as the initial signal to the cognitive action that results in a diagnosis (Gordon 1982). The data illustrated that a cue signifies a group's health need. For example, the cue, inadequate natural flouride in the water supply, indicated the need for supplemental flouride. The name *need-related cue processing* was given to the sequential recognition of the cue and the corresponding need, which preceded diagnosis of a group's health status. The cues could be differentiated according to whether they had been passively received or actively sought by the nurse. For example, listening to a service request can be contrasted with conducting studies of the group or the environment to determine if need-related cues emerge. The outcome of need-related cue processing was apparently dependent on the nurse's ability to generalize from the concerns of one per-

Table 1: Categorized health needs and corresponding diagnoses

Health needs stated by subjects/corresponding Phase 3 categories	Inferred first and second stage diagnoses
1. High mortality rate from stroke/Categories 1 and 5	Vulnerable population group (elderly), in need of cardiovascular screening; need-service match, related to existing cardiovascular screening service
2. Physical exams for preschoolers/Categories 1 and 4	Vulnerable population group (preschoolers), in need of well-child screening; need-service mismatch, related to lack of well-child screening service
3. Protection from nitrates/Categories 2 and 4	Population-at-risk, in need of safe water supply; need-service mismatch, related to lack of well-water testing service
4. To prevent influenza/Categories 3 and 5	Vulnerable population group at-risk (elderly, disabled) in need of influenza vaccination; need-service mismatch, related to lack of flu vaccination program

BOX 1   **Vulnerable population group at-risk/need-service mismatch**

Need-related cue processing
    Cue: dental caries in school children
    Need: "dental caries", as stated by subject
First diagnostic stage
    Hypothesis: vulnerable population group-at-risk
    Data: higher local caries incidence than state or nation
    Diagnosis: vulnerable population group at-risk (school children), in need of
        caries prevention
Second diagnostic stage
    Hypothesis: questionable degree of need-service match
    Data: analyzed amount of natural flouride in water; compared caries
        incidence of those who did/did not drink fluoridated water at school;
        no existing supplemental flouride program in the schools
    Diagnosis: need-service mismatch, related to lack of supplemental flouride
        program for school children
Diagnostic-based management
    Analyses: new agency service appropriate, feasible; assistance available
        from state officials; need is a priority
    Decision: seek approval from County Board of Health
Outcome
    Flouride mouthrinse program for Grades K-8 implemented

son to the concerns of others with similar characteristics. Conversely, the nurse had to be aware of the health problems that might affect a particular group to diagnose the members of the group residing within the agency's jurisdiction.

Population group diagnosis. In some cases, the nurses identified that a population group had characteristics that increased the possibility of specific health problems. The investigator inferred that the diagnosis of vulnerable population group had been made in these situations. A second diagnosis, population-at-risk, was indicated when an environmental hazard threatened the health of a population group. The third diagnosis, vulnerable population group-at-risk, was defined as a group that is innately vulnerable and faces an environmental hazard.

Diagnostic staging. A series of two nursing diagnoses was made before service change was considered. The first diagnostic stage culminated in the confirmation or rejection of a hypothesized nursing diagnosis about a group's health status. If the diagnosis was confirmed, the nurse proceeded to a second stage when a diagnosis was made about the degree of the match between the group's need and the existing services that might meet the need.

Health care system diagnosis. A diagnosis of need-service mismatch was confirmed before a change in services was proposed. On the other hand, a diagnosis of need-service match was made when an existing community service either could meet or was meeting the need. For example, after the need of local elderly for cardiovascular screening was confirmed, a nurse found that the required services were being provided by physicians' office nurses. The need for continued nursing intervention (Gordon, 1982) justifies the atypical phrasing of the diagnosis in positive terms. In cases of need-service match, the nurse periodically evaluated the situation to ensure that the group's need continued to be met.

Diagnostic-based management. When the diagnosis of need-service mismatch was made, the appropriateness and feasibility of a service change was considered. The nurse evaluated the priority of taking action to upgrade the health status of that particular population group, vis-à-vis the priorities of continuing other agency services. The nurse then presented the diagnostic judgments to the agency's governing body, because its approval was required prior to most service changes. Frequently, the nurse had to educate the governing body about the significance of the group's need and the gap between the need and the agency's services. After approval of the change, service delivery was altered to increase the likelihood of need-service match, thereby positively affecting the group's health status. If the governing body did not approve a critical service change, the nurse would often attempt to impact upon the need-service mismatch by facilitating another agency's efforts to upgrade a similar service. In some cases, the nurse implemented change without seeking the approval of the governing body, by streamlining the parameters of the vulnerable or at-risk group. For instance, rather than continuing to make home visits to the families of all firstborns, one agency began to visit only the high-risk newborns.

DISCUSSION

The results of this study are the product of inductive analysis which began with examination of actual events and proceeded to the development of a theory which isolates concepts that explain the events. Further study is required to enable complete development and refinement of the theory. The diagnoses and defining characteristics should be validated with other samples of community-nurse-administrators. Because some health needs are met in ways other than direct service (Hamilton 1983), the diagnostic origins of these interventions should also be studied.

After the factor-isolating theory is more fully developed, factor-relating theory, situation-relating theory, and predictive theory could be generated by deductively testing hypotheses based on the factor-isolating theory (Dickoff & James 1968). This factor-relating hypothesis could be tested: Nurses who actively seek cues of needs develop more accurate population group diagnoses than nurses who passively receive cues. Situation-relating theory could be developed from the study of the impact of community staff nurses upon the administrator's diagnostic reasoning. Delving into this issue would help to clarify the role of the community staff nurse in the care of population groups. Predictive theory could result from a study of the impact of the practical use of the theory on the health states of population groups, as measured by standard indices of health. Ultimately, the value of the theory of community-nurse-administrator diagnosis must be determined by its effect on the health of the populace.

However, all studies that focus on the community-nurse-administrator can result only in the derivation of the substantive theory described by Glaser and Strauss (1967). Although such a theory fits the substantive situation, its scope is limited. Nurse-administrators of hospitals and other institutions should also be studied, because they may be employing diagnostic strategies as a basis for administrative intervention with population groups. Based on such studies, the substantive theory that explains the diagnostic strategies of community-nurse-administrators could be upgraded to a formal grounded theory of administrative diagnosis.

Several aspects of the theory derived through this study warrant discussion because of their divergence from traditional nursing diagnosis theory. Articulation of specific diagnoses for population groups violates the premise that the same diagnoses can be used for communities and individuals (Kim, McFarland, and McLane 1984). Gen-eral defining characteristics will suffice if the label of alteration in health maintenance is used for a group (Jakob 1984). However, specific data collection and analysis are essential if one is to diagnose a population group as vulnerable, at-risk, or both vulnerable and at-risk. Such specificity of diagnostic reasoning is desirable (Gordon and Sweeney 1979).

The probable cause of a nursing diagnosis has been cited as an appropriate basis for nursing intervention (Barnard 1983). Yet, the population group diagnoses shown in Table 1 are related to a health need rather than a probable cause, because the nature of the diagnostic judgment could be inferred from the health need of the population group. Because "causality for all theoretic and practical purposes is multifactorial" (Forsyth 1984, p. 70), the etiologies of a group's health state are likely more diverse and complex than those of an individual. The group's health need may also provide a more precise direction for nursing intervention than would an etiology of its health state.

Finally, the concept of health care system diagnosis does not coincide with orthodox diagnosis theory. Although this diagnostic focus is central to the role of the community-nurse-administrator, it is conjectured that every nurse evaluates the status of the health care system in relation to clients' needs. Thus, the diagnoses of need-service match and mismatch may have broader applicability than the realm of community nursing administration.

There are several practice-related implications of the theory. Because of its congruence with the practice setting, it can be used as a guide for practice by the community-nurse-administrator, enabling some "control over the structure and process" (Glaser and Strauss 1967, p. 237) of events. The theory explains how the nurse diagnoses population groups and the health care system and makes management decisions based on the diagnoses, so integrating nursing theory and management theory. The nurse's health planning role can be explained to members of population groups and other decision-makers using the theory. Finally, this empirically based theory reveals the critical contributions of the community-nurse-administrator to quality health care.

REFERENCES

Anderson, E.: Community focus in public health nursing: whose responsibility? Nurs. Outlook **31**:44-48, 1983.

Andrews, P.B.: Nursing diagnosis. In Griffith, J.W. and Christensen, P.J., editors: Nursing process: application of theories, frameworks and models, St. Louis, 1982, The C.V. Mosby Co.

Barnard, K.: Nursing diagnosis: a descriptive method, Amer. J. Mat./Child Nurs. **8**:223, 1983.

Clemen, S.A., Eigsti, D.G., and McGuire, S.L.: Comprehensive family and community nursing, New York, 1981, McGraw-Hill.

Dickoff, J., and James, P.: A theory of theories, Nurs. Res. **17**:197-203, 1968.

Field, P.A., and Morse, J.M.: Nursing research: the application of qualitative approaches, Rockville, 1985, Aspen Systems Corporation.

Forsyth, G.L.: Etiology: in what sense and of what value? In Kim, M.J., McFarland, G.K., and McLane, A.M., editors: Classification of nursing diagnoses: proceedings of the fifth national conference, St. Louis, 1984, C.V. Mosby.

Glaser, B.G., and Strauss, A.L.: The discovery of grounded theory: strategies for qualitative research, Chicago, 1967, Aldine Publishing Co.

Gordon, M.: Nursing diagnosis: process and application, New York, 1982, McGraw-Hill.

Gordon, M., and Sweeney, M.A.: Methodological problems and issues in identifying and standardizing nursing diagnoses, Adv. Nurs. Sci. **2**:1-15, 1979.

Hamilton, P.: Community nursing diagnosis, Adv. Nurs. Sci. **5**:21-36, 1983.

Jakob, D.F.: Nursing care of school children in the community. In Kim, M.J., McFarland, G.K., and McLane, A.M., editors: Pocket guide to nursing diagnoses, St. Louis, 1984, The C.V. Mosby Co.

Kim, M.J., McFarland, G.K., and McLane, A.M., editors: Pocket guide to nursing diagnoses, St. Louis, 1984, The C.V. Mosby Co.

Mundinger, M.O.: Autonomy in nursing, Germantown, 1980, Aspen Systems Corporation.

Rose, M.H., and Killien, M.: Risk and vulnerability: a case for differentiation, Adv. Nurs. Sci. **5**:60-73, 1983.

Nurses' use of cues in the clinical judgment of activity intolerance[*]

JOAN B. FITZMAURICE, Ph.D., R.N., F.A.A.N.

The movement within nursing to adopt a standardized nomenclature of problems amenable to nursing therapy is rapidly gaining momentum. The North American Nursing Diagnosis Association (NANDA) has existed for a little over a decade, yet the published "accepted" nursing diagnoses have been adopted by increasing numbers of health care agencies in North America.

Widespread utilization of the nomenclature may be premature before further clinical validation of the diagnostic labels. At this stage of development, many nursing diagnoses are not well defined. Diagnostic categories, defining characteristics, and etiologic subcategories need refinement and clinical validation. More specific criteria may be necessary for clinicians to achieve agreement. Defining characteristics, also known as signs and symptoms, may take on different values. Some require precise measurement (heart rate), while others are subjective impressions of quality and quantity (fatigue).

The identification and encoding of clinical knowledge is a complex task (Duda and Shortcliffe 1983). Attempts to build or develop a knowledge base often disclose gaps in the understanding of the underlying domain, since much knowledge is stored in forms unavailable to conscious awareness (Johnson, 1983). Characteristics of nursing problems need to be specified and standardized. Data on the prevalence and distribution of nursing problems will provide a base for research on prediction, comparison of interventions, and varying preventative approaches.

The current taxonomy of nursing diagnoses represents an initial stage in the developing of a clinical knowledge base. The major purpose of this study was to examine a methodological approach for the study of nursing diagnosis. A particular nursing diagnosis, activity intolerance, was selected as the focus. This diagnosis commonly occurs in the cardiovascular patient population (Hubilak and Kim 1984, Kim 1984, Rodgers 1985), and the defining characteristics include subjective and objective data.

The generic question in studies of clinical judgment is to determine how individuals combine information in multiple-cue probability judgment tasks. The research questions of this study were:

1. How good is the prediction of activity intolerance using the defining characteristic of NANDA?
2. How do nurses use and weigh defining characteristics to judge the likelihood of the nursing diagnosis?

Definition of terms

Judgment. A phenomenon or cognitive process using information which is available to estimate or evaluate (Newell & Simon 1972). It is not simply the application of a given rule, nor is it the simple transduction of information. Judgment adds information.

Nursing diagnosis. A clinical judgment about an individual, family or community which is derived through a deliberate systematic process of data collection. It provides the basis for prescriptions for definitive therapy for which the nurse is account-

[*]Partial support for this study was received from Alpha Chi Chapter, Sigma Theta Tau

able. A nursing diagnosis is expressed concisely and includes the etiology of the problem when known (Shoemaker 1982).

Activity intolerance. Abnormal responses to energy-consuming body movements involved in required or desired daily activities (Gordon 1985).

Cue. Units of information about a patient that can readily be perceived by the nurse in a judgment situation. Cues are assumed to account for the greatest amount of variation in the judgment (Hammond, Hursch, and Todd 1971). In this study, the cues are the verbal report of fatigue, weakness, exertional discomfort, or dyspnea, and abnormal heart rate or blood pressure response (Kim et al. 1984).

Weights. The weight indicates the importance a person places on the cue when making a judgment. This study will consider two types of weights: (1) standardized beta weights obtained by statistical analysis of data using multiple regression; and (2) subjective weights, self-reported percentage of importance placed on each of the cues in making the judgment (Rothert 1982).

METHOD

Subjects. Twenty-five nurses were recruited from three sources: members of a conference group on the Classification of Nursing Diagnoses; alumnae of a graduate program in medical-surgical nursing at an Eastern university; and members of the local affiliate of the American Heart Association. Criteria for selection of nurses subjects were: (1) master's degrees in nursing, (2) current practice with adult cardiac patients, and (3) routine use of nursing diagnoses in verbal and written communication. Sixteen subjects majored in cardiovascular nursing. The majority of the subjects were currently practicing in an inpatient setting. Eighty-five percent of the subjects rated themselves a 5 or highly experienced (on a scale of 1 to 5) when asked to describe their experience

with cardiac patients. Thirteen subjects were currently or previously held membership in a local, regional, or national Nursing Diagnosis Organization.

The selection criteria were designed to create a homogeneous group. In this fashion, variability in attitudes, values, experience with similar tasks and clinical knowledge was intended to be minimized (Tanner 1984).

Materials for the study consisted of a set of hypothetical patient vignettes and a subject demographic profile. The vignette technique has been used successfully to study a variety of problems, where the objective was to uncover the collective preference schedule concerning a domain. It seemed reasonable to assume that this method would be applicable to the study of judgment in nursing.

Format

Subjects were directed to read each vignette and then to make a judgment of the likelihood of each hypothetical patient having the nursing diagnosis of activity intolerance. A 5-point rating scale was used, 1 being the absence of activity intolerance, and 5, the definite presence of activity intolerance.

The vignettes utilized six of eight defining characteristics or cues contained in the official NANDA diagnosis list. They are: verbal report of fatigue, weakness, exertional dyspnea, exertional discomfort, and abnormal heart rate or blood pressure response to activity. The two remaining cues from the official list, development of arrhythmias or ischemia, were not included. Observation of these characteristics would require the patient's attachment to an electrocardiographic (EKG) device with the capability of continuous monitoring of the heart rate and rhythm. Frequently, these data are not available to the nurse; in addition, the interpretation of an EKG is a skill requiring special training.

Dependent variables. Criteria and scales for measurement of the six cues or defining characteristics were developed through a combination of approaches: personal clinical experience, literature review, and communication with content specialists. Clinical data about the patient's physical findings and symptoms are often regarded as soft, because specific rating scales have not been created for expressing the observations as data. Paradoxically, these data are often cited as the characteristics of the phenomenon or diagnosis. In order to conduct this study, some measurement scales were created to provide gradation criteria to demarcate such entities as the severity of weakness, dyspnea, or discomfort. Each cue has five levels, with one assigned to the absence of the characteristic and five given the most or highest level.

Intervening variables. Day of hospitalization (1-5), age, and level of activity were utilized as intervening variables. The age ranged from 47 years to 67 years at 5 year intervals. Five activities were selected; each activity represented a different energy requirement. The particular level of age, activity and admission date were randomly assigned to each case.

Research design. An experimental design was utilized. A full factorial design would have included 18,750 cases. Therefore a rotated Box-Wilson fractional factorial design was employed (Box and Wilson 1951) utilizing 125 unique cases. One of the limitations of this approach is the need to assume that interactions beyond the quadratic are negligible. However, in behavioral research it is uncommon that higher order interactions are significant or as important or explainable. Therefore it was felt that risk was justified.

Probability sampling was used to create 25 packets. Each case was utilized six times, yet no subject received the same case twice. A table of random numbers was also used to select the five cases per subject to be repeated. A second entry into the random numbers table was made to direct the placement of the five replicates.

Intrarater agreement. Three statistics were employed to assess the level of intrarater agreement: observed percentage of agreement (Po), Kappa (K), and the Pearson product moment correlation coefficient (r).

Percentage of agreement is the proportion of agreement in classifications on both measurement occasions (Subkoviak 1980). Kappa provides a more conservative estimate, since it is the proportion of agreement beyond that expected by chance (Cohen 1960). Both of these statistics assume the data are measured at the ordinal level.

In this study, 0.75 or 75% of the judgments on both occasions were in agreement. However, 0.75 may be an overestimate of intrarater agreement, since 46% of the agreement can be expected by chance (Subkoviak 1980). A more conservative estimate of stability is Kappa. The calculated K of 0.53 indicates a moderate intrarater agreement within the entire sample.

The judgment of likelihood of Activity Intolerance may also be considered as an interval measure. The computed Pearson correlation coefficient of 0.78, $p < .01$ indicates a moderately high degree of stability between judgments on two presentations.

Interrater agreement

Consensus or consistency of judgments was evaluated by examining the means and standard deviations for 125 vignettes. Each vignette was judged approximately six times by different subjects. Total consensus among the nurses would be reflected by standard deviations of zero. In this study, there was total agreement across 18 of the vignettes. In the remaining 107 cases, the standard deviations ranged from 0. to 1.5.

MODEL SPECIFICATION STRENGTH OF ASSOCIATION

The research question examined how nurses use and weigh the information in making judgments of activity intolerance. A multiple regression analysis was conducted to determine the strength of association between the six independent variables and the diagnostic judgment, likelihood of activity intolerance. The calculated squared multiple correlation (R^2) indicates the amount of variation in the dependent variable that is accounted for or explained by a linear combination of the independent variables.

Preliminary analyses

Descriptive statistics are presented in Table 1. Of note is the negatively skewed distribution of the judgments regarding activity intolerance.

Pearson correlations were calculated among the cues, the intervening variables of age, admission day, and activity level, and the dependent variable, likelihood of activity intolerance (see Table 2). As anticipated, the correlations among the independent variables were near zero, owing to the orthogonal design. The one exception is the correlation between fatigue and weakness ($r = 0.42$, $p < .0001$). An error in the development of the initial packets accounted for this spurious relationship.

Table 1: Means and standard deviations of variables in the equation

	M	**SD**
Independent		
Fatigue	2.88	0.97
Weakness	2.37	0.74
Dyspnea	2.99	0.99
Discomfort	2.99	0.98
Heart rate	3.01	0.98
Blood pressure	3.01	0.98
Intervening		
Days since admission	2.94	1.36
Activity level	3.04	1.35
Age in years	56.42	6.95
Dependent		
Activity intolerance	4.37	1.01

All variables except age are measured on a scale of 1–5.

Table 2: Intercorrelations among the 10 variables

Variables	AI	FTGE	WKNS	DYS	DISC	HR	BP	AGE	ADM	ACT
Activity intolerance	—	.08*	.07	.10*	.24*	.04	.20*	−.08*	−.01	−.01
Fatigue		—	.42*	.01	.01	.00	.00	.14*	−.10	.03
Weakness			—	.00	.01	.00	.00	−.02	−.19	−.05
Dyspnea				—	.01	.01	.01	.04	−.04	−.01
Discomfort					—	.01	.01	−.10*	−.10	.00
Heart rate						—	.00	−.12*	.03	−.07
Blood pressure							—	−.03	.00	.18
Age								—	.02	−.10
Admission day									—	−.10
Activity level										—

$N = 748$, 2 missing values
p values are 2-tailed
*$p < .05$

Multiple regression

The research design allowed for 125 unique cases, or combinations of the independent and intervening variables. Each case was used six times, with the restriction that no subject received a duplicate in her packet. This approach yielded 750 judgments of activity intolerance for the main analysis.

Goodness of fit. A multiple regression analysis using the Statistical Analysis System (SAS) was conducted on the pooled data from the 25 subjects using six independent or predictor variables. The R square indicates that proportion of the variance in the diagnostic judgment that can "be accounted for" by the regression equation. Approximately 12% of the nurses' judgments were explained by the characteristics as postulated by NANDA (see Table 3).

When the influence of the intervening variables of patient age, level of activity, and number of days following admission was considered in the equation, the increase in R^2 was minimal, and not statistically significant, $F = 0.02$, p $<.05$ (see Table 4).

A second goodness-of-fit statistic is the standard error (SE) of estimate of the dependent variable, activity intolerance, used to construct a confidence interval for the predicted judgments. Using the full model, the SE of activity intolerance is 0.013, and the 99% confidence interval ranges from 4.336 to 4.404. This range is quite narrow, indicating the model provides a relatively good estimate of activity intolerance.

Defining characteristics

The six cues (fatigue, weakness, dyspnea, discomfort, heart rate, and blood pressure) were each defined on five levels ranging from 1-5. These were the independent variables in the study. The intervening variables, patient age, level of activity, and days since admission to the hospital, were also defined on five levels. Each hypothetical case presented to the subjects consisted of descriptions of one level of each of the nine cues. This was followed by a question asking for a judgment on that case. Multiple regression analysis was used to examine the linear relation of the independent variables to the dependent variable, and to examine relations among the independent variables. This analysis yielded a beta coefficient or partial

Table 3: Regression model (A) including the 6 defining characteristics

Source	df	Sum of squares	Mean square	R SQ	F
Model	6	90.150786	15.025131	.1183	16.574*
Error	741	671.746	.906540		

*p $<.001$

Table 4: Regression model (B) including six defining characteristics and three contextual variables

Source	df	Sum of squares	Mean square	R SQ	F
Model	9	94.519596	10.502177	.1241	11.614*
Error	738	667.377	.904306		

*p $<.0001$

regression coefficient for each variable while other independent variables in the equation were held "constant." A simultaneous inclusion (SAS 1982) method was used, and all variables were entered into the equation. This approach was considered the representation of the simulated diagnostic process of this study. The unstandardized beta coefficients for the cues are presented in Table 5. These beta coefficients can be interpreted as the relative importance of each cue across all subjects. The betas are comparable, since similar scales were utilized in measuring the variables.

A less conservative significance level of $p < .15$ was chosen in examining the utilization of cues. This was done to reduce the risk of Type II error, and was believed justified in light of the exploratory nature of the research. Four defining characteristics contributed significant information to the explanatory model; discomfort, blood pressure response, dyspnea, and fatigue. Two of the intervening variables also influenced the judgments, age of the patient and the level of activity.

Table 5: Beta coefficients, standard errors, t values for independent and intervening variables

Variable	beta	SE	t	p
Fatigue	.061	.04	1.54	.1230*
Weakness	.060	.05	1.12	.2643
Dyspnea	.104	.04	2.95	.0033*
Discomfort	.248	.04	6.88	.0001*
Heart rate	.029	.04	0.82	.4139
Blood pressure	.215	.04	5.94	.0001*
Age	−.007	.01	−1.44	.1495*
Activity level	−.038	.03	−1.44	.1499*
Admission	.024	.03	0.92	.3598

*$p < .15$

DISCUSSION
Strength of association

The research question asked how the subjects used and weighed the information to make judgments of the likelihood of activity intolerance. The strength of association was addressed by studying the squared correlation (R^2) between judgments of likelihood of activity intolerance and the defining characteristics. This squared correlation was computed on judgments from all subjects. Twelve percent of the variation in the judgments could be explained by a weighted linear combination of the cues. In examining the nurses' judgment policy, the R^2 indicates the responses from the cues. To the extent that the judgments are explainable, the resulting regression equation is said to represent or "capture the policy" that subjects used in making the judgment.

This representation measures the extent to which the subjects' control of execution of knowledge, or cognitive control. Cognitive control is statistically independent of the individual's knowledge (Hammond and Summers 1972). Subjects in this study may have had knowledge of the cues important in their judgments of the likelihood of activity intolerance, but not used this knowledge accurately or consistently. The R^2 has a relation to the test-retest reliability coefficients which in this study were moderate. To the extent that a person is inconsistent in judgments, the R^2 is decreased.

Subjects in this study were not comparable to other studies reviewed with different tasks. Most report an R^2 of greater than .50 (Ashton 1974, Dawes 1979, Einhorn, Kleinmuntz, and Kleinmuntz 1979, Lane, Murphy and Marques 1982). Curry and Menasco (1983) suggest that one reason for a poorly fitting linear model may be a misunderstanding of the task. The task in this study may not have been as familiar to the subjects as admission judgments are to admissions committee members. Nurses do not commonly make a scaled judgment. Comments from two subjects following completion of the study did indicate they found the task difficult.

One of the assumptions underlying multiple regression analysis is that the judgment variables are measured without error, and error in the independent variable may be responsible for a low R^2 (Cochran 1970). Clinical data are acknowledged as difficult to quantify, and the reliability of many diagnostic judgments has never been studied (Koran 1975). Another explanation for a poorly fitting linear model is that subjects either do not cooperate with instructions or they use a different diagnostic strategy (Curry and Menasco 1983). Three strategies for making diagnoses are: pattern recognition, multiple branching techniques, and the hypothetical-deductive approach. The task in this study most closely represented pattern recognition. If subjects did not utilize this diagnostic scheme, this may account for the low explanatory power of the model.

The presentation of vignettes without complete background or contextual information made the task less realistic for subjects, and the results may not be generalizable to other contexts (Farrand, Holzemer, and Schleutermann 1982). However, the multiple regression approach was quite useful in uncovering the differences among the nurses, and further investigation is needed before drawing the conclusion that the diagnosis is invalid.

Cue utilization. Four of the six cues described by the NANDA as defining characteristics of activity intolerance were supported in the regression model. Abnormal heart rate response and weakness did not contribute unique information to the explanation of activity intolerance.

Heart rate. Two possible explanations for the non-contributory nature of heart rate are: (1) unfamiliarity with the usual responses of the patient with congestive heart failure, and (2) inadequate patient data to make a judgment regarding the meaningfulness of the changes in heart rate.

One of the major adaptive mechanisms of the heart is to increase the heart rate to meet the increasing demands of the body during exercise (Hellerstein and Franklin 1984). Guidelines for appropriate response to low-level early ambulation activities include a heart rate response less than 120 beats/min or 20 beats/min above the resting heart rate in patients receiving beta-adrenergic-blocking drugs (Wenger 1984). Some studies suggest that patients with congestive heart failure may not manifest this tachycardia (Conn, Williams, and Wallace 1984, Fareeduddin and Abelmann 1969, Wilson, Ferraro, and Wiener 1985). Insufficient information may have been given to the subjects regarding the pharmacologic management of the hypothetical patients. Also, many guides for judging tolerable heart rate responses to exercise have been based on patients recovering from myocardial infarction (heart attack).

Weakness. The second characteristic that contributed no substantive information to the regression model was weakness. Authors often make a subtle distinction between weakness and fatigue. Weakness is a symptom in the movement of the affected muscle or diminished strength in contracting muscles (Blacklow 1983). Fatigue is more commonly defined as a subjective response on a continuum from tiredness to exhaustion, which is a protective homeostatic mechanism (Piper 1986). One author actually directs the clinician to distinguish muscle weakness from fatigue (Minden and Reich 1984.)

The descriptors of weakness utilized in this study referred to a general subjective feeling. It is obviously not possible to focus on the subjective perception of the strength of the cardiac muscle. The parameters selected to gauge the level of activity intolerance theoretically should provide as direct information as possible regarding the critical organ (Gordon 1973). In the context of a cardiac disorder, weakness may not be a defining characteristic of the diagnosis. Weakness may be a quite important discriminator in judging activity intolerance in patients with neuromuscular disorders.

CONCLUSIONS

Clinical judgment is a complex process that is the essence of the health professional. Judgments involve such processes as recognizing cues, classifying information, and weighing alternatives. As an end product, judgment involves assigning phenomena to one of the multiple categories such as no activity intolerance, possible activity intolerance, definite activity intolerance or severe activity intolerance.

Subjects in this study were not explicitly trained (educated) in the recognition of the diagnosis of activity intolerance, owing in part to the recent emergence of nursing diagnoses as a framework for curriculum development. An assumption within the nursing profession in general and NANDA in particular is that the nursing diagnoses described at the national conferences are representative of real patients. If one accepts this assumption educators need to develop teaching strategies which focus on the detection of a cue and the assignment of the cue to a category other than normal. Attention must be directed toward examining how a cue pattern for a given nursing diagnosis varies within the context of various factors such as medical condition, age, gender, and associated nursing diagnoses.

A concern within nursing practice today is the need to make decisions about allocation of resources while assuring the quality of nursing care. The emergence of computerized information systems as a method of collecting data for these decisions assumes the utilization of valid and reliable terms. Several information systems have been developed using nursing diagnoses as a primary data source. However, the evidence regarding validity of nursing diagnoses may be insufficient to warrant their use for this purpose. Diagnostic validation means that defining characteristics occur as a cluster, and that expert nurses recognize this cluster and use a common label for description. Empirical findings from this study did not support the theoretical model of the diagnosis activity intolerance.

REFERENCES

Ashton, R.H.: Cue utilization and expert judgments, J. Appl. Psychol. **59**:437-444, 1976.

Blacklow, R.S.: MacBryde's signs and symptoms, ed. 6, Philadelphia, 1983, J.B. Lippincott.

Box, G.E.P., and Wilson, K.B.: On the experimental attainment of optimum conditions, J. Roy. Stat. Soc. (Series B) **13**:1-45, 1951.

Cochran, W.G.: Some effects of errors of measurement on multiple correlation, J. Amer. Stat. Assoc. **65**:22-34, 1970.

Cohen, J.: A coefficient of agreement for nominal scales, Educ. Psychol. Meas. **20**:37-46, 1960.

Conn, E.H., Williams, R.F., and Wallace, A.G.: Physical conditioning in coronary patients with left ventricular dysfunction. In Wenger, N.K., and Hellerstein, H.K., editors: Rehabilitation of the coronary patient, ed. 2, New York, 1984, John Wiley.

Curry, D.J., and Menasco, M.B.: On the separability of weights and brand values: issues and empirical results, J. Consumer Res. **10**:83-95, 1983.

Dawes, R.M.: A case study of graduate admission: application of three principles of human decision making, Amer. Psychol. **34**:571-582, 1979.

Duda, R.O., and Shortcliffe, E.H.: Expert systems research, Science **220**:261-268, 1983.

Einhorn, H.J., Kleinmuntz, D.N., and Kleinmuntz, B.: Linear models and process-tracing models of judgment, Psychol. Rev. **86**:465-485, 1979.

Fareeduddin, K., and Abelmann, W.H.: Impaired orthostatic tolerance after bed rest in patients with myocardial infarction, New Engl. J. Med. **280**:345-351, 1969.

Farrand, L.L., Holzemer, W.L., and Schleutermann, J.A.: A study of construct validity: simulations as a measure of nurse practitioners' problem-solving skills, Nurs. Res. **31**:37-42, 1982.

Gordon, M.: Assessing activity tolerance, Amer. J. Nurs. **76**:72-75, 1976.

Gordon, M.: Manual of nursing diagnosis, New York, 1985, McGraw-Hill.

Hammond, K.R., and Summers, D.A.: Cognitive control, Psychol. Rev. **64**:438-456, 1972.

Hammond, K.R., Hursch, C.J., and Todd, F.J.: Analyzing the components of clinical inference, Psychol. Rev. **64**:438-456, 1971.

Hellerstein, H.K., and Franklin, B.A.: Exercise testing and prescription. In Wenger, N.K., and Hellerstein, H.K.: Rehabilitation of the coronary patient, ed. 2, New York, 1984, John Wiley.

Hubalik, K., and Kim, M.J.: Nursing diagnosis associated with heart failure in critical care nursing. In Kim, M.J., McFarland, G.K., and McLane, A.M.: Classification of nursing diagnoses: proceedings of the fifth national conference, St. Louis, 1984, The C.V. Mosby Co.

Johnson, P.E.: What kind of expert should a system be? J. Med. Phil. **8**:77-97, 1983.

Kim, M.J., Amoroso-Seritella, R., Gulanick, M.: Clinical validation of cardiovascular nursing diagnoses. In Kim, M.J., McFarland, G.K., and McLane, A.M., editors: Classification of nursing diagnoses: proceedings of the fifth national conference, St. Louis, 1984, The C.V. Mosby Co.

Koran, L.M.: The reliability of clinical methods, data and judgments, New Engl. J. Med. **293**:642-646, 695-701, 1975.

Lane, D.M., Murphy, K.R., and Marques, T.E.: Measuring the importance of cues in policy capturing, Org. Behav. Human Develop. **30**:231-240, 1982.

Minden, S.L., and Reich, P.: Nervousness and fatigue. In

Blacklow, R.S.: MacBryde's signs and symptoms, Philadelphia, 1983, J.B. Lippincott.

Newall, A.N., and Simon H.A.: Human problem solving, Englewood Cliffs, N.J., 1972, Prentice Hall.

Piper, B.F.: Fatigue. In Carrieri, V.K., Lindsey, A.M., and West, C.M.: Pathophysiological phenomena in nursing, Philadelphia, 1986, W.B. Saunders.

Rodgers, C.D.: Incidence of nursing diagnoses in a cardiovascular population, Paper presented at the Second Northeast Regional Conference on Nursing Diagnosis, Mystic, CN, June, 1985.

Rothert, M.L.: Physicians' and patients' judgments of compliance with hypertensive regimen, Med. Decision Mak. **2**:179-195, 1982.

SAS user's guide: statistics, Cary, NC, 1982, SAS Institute Inc.

Shoemaker, J.: Essential features of a nursing diagnosis. In Kim, M.J., McFarland, G.K., and McLane, A.M., editors: Classification of nursing diagnoses: proceedings of the fifth national conference, St. Louis, 1984, The C.V. Mosby Co.

Subkoviak, M.J.: Decision-consistency approaches. In Berk, R.A., editor: Criterion-referenced measurement: the state of the art, Baltimore, 1980, Johns Hopkins University Press.

Wenger, N.K., and Hellerstein, H.K., editors: Rehabilitation of the coronary patient, New York, 1984, John Wiley.

Wilson, J.R., Ferraro, N., and Wiener, D.H.: Effect of the sympathetic nervous system on limb circulation and metabolism during exercise in patients with heart failure, Circulation **72**:72-81, 1985.

Nursing diagnostic skills: a content analysis of spontaneously generated nursing diagnoses

JUDITH L. MYERS, M.S.N., R.N.
MARTHA A. SPIES, M.S.N., R.N., C.C.R.N.

Since 1973, there has been a concerted national effort to identify and develop a standard classification of nursing diagnoses. Books and articles have been written, classes and workshops have been conducted and special interest groups have been formed to disseminate information concerning the nature of diagnostic statements, the correct format for diagnostic statements and what mistakes to avoid in writing statements. The cognitive skills necessary for diagnostic reasoning have been investigated and described. These activities have been utilized to provide guidance for nurses as they utilize nursing diagnostic statements in clinical practice. But this information is often conflicting. The current research was done to study the degree to which nurses do accurately identify and formulate nursing diagnostic labels.

LITERATURE REVIEW

The act of diagnosis is the process of inferring from a series of observable cues an internal, unobservable state of the patient. A diagnostic label is a concise term representing that cluster of signs and symptoms (Gordon 1982). Mundinger and Jauron (1975) have stated that a nursing diagnostic statement has two parts that are linked together by a phrase that indicates the relationship of the parts to each other. The nursing diagnosis consists of a statement of the client's potential or actual health problem or response. This is followed by the phrase "related to" and the etiology or reason(s) for the client's problem or response. Although "due to" is a shorter phrase, Mundinger and Jauron (1975) have recommended avoiding it since legal counsel preferred "related to" because it does not necessarily signify a causal relationship and decreases some legal hazards. Ziegler (1984) conducted a study to determine the extent to which nursing diagnosis statements generated by graduate nursing students met the criteria for nursing diagnosis statements. The nursing diagnoses were evaluated in terms of specific criteria concerning the entire diagnosis and each component of the diagnosis. Only 10 (6%) met all the research criteria. It was concluded that the state of the art of nursing diagnosis is not well developed, because the nursing diagnosis statements generated by this sample would not lead to the goals of accountability, autonomy, or individualized care.

Warren (1984) conducted a descriptive study of graduate nursing students' problems in using nursing diagnosis. One of the areas studied was the students' ability to formulate correctly stated nursing diagnoses using the PES format (problems, etiology, symptoms). It was found that 30% of the diagnostic statements were correctly written. Use of symptoms instead of a problem or response statement occurred in 45% of the statements. Medical diagnoses were used in 15% of the statements. Castles (1982) studied whether assessment of the same patient at approximately the same time by more than one nurse results in the same nursing diagnosis, i.e., whether the nomenclature of diagnoses can be standardized. In this study, no evidence that nurses evaluating the same patient make the same diagnosis was found.

A number of personal variables could be postulated as having an effect of an individual nurse's diagnostic ability. Three of these: level of education, years of experience and education in the formulation of nursing diagnoses, have the most obvious relationship to diagnostic skills. These three variables would seem to differentiate the novice from the expert diagnostician.

Meade and Kim (1984) described a study that indicated that even when the concept of nursing diagnosis and the diagnostic process are learned, application of the knowledge in a clinical setting may not be apparent. They also found no significant difference in clinical documentation of nursing diagnoses based on years of experience as a nurse. In a related study by Carstens (1984), a case study was used to validate the degree of learning that resulted from an inservice presentation. It was found that the inservice program did not have any statistically significant effect on the nurses' ability to identify valid nursing diagnoses.

QUESTION

This study was designed to identify the terminology utilized by nurses in generating nursing diagnostic labels. A secondary focus of the study was to identify the frequency with which nurses used diagnostic labels approved by the North American Nursing Diagnosis Association (NANDA).

METHODOLOGY

In order to study this question, a content analysis of 332 spontaneously generated diagnostic labels was done. These labels were generated by nurses participating in a previous study by Myers, Perry, Wessler, Becker, Resler, Spies, and Metheny (in press). The labels were generated by 54 staff nurses employed in eight critical care units throughout a large midwestern city. The nurses generated the diagnostic statements after viewing a video taped patient care situation depicting a patient admitted to a coronary care unit. The video tape contained cues

to seven nursing diagnoses identified by Rossi and Haines (1979) as occurring in clients experiencing acute myocardial infarctions (Box 1). The validity of the content of the 10-minute video tape was established by five nurse educators and five cardiovascular nurse-clinicians. The video tape simulation ensured that all subjects were exposed to the same patient situation when asked to identify nursing diagnoses.

Each spontaneously generated label was assigned to one of seven categories (Table 1). These categories were established utilizing terminology and definitions proposed by Gordon (1982) and Carpenito (1983) which identify terms included and excluded from the concept of nursing diagnosis as well as common errors in nursing diagnostic statements. Each statement as originally written by the staff nurses was assigned to one category. Then all the labels assigned to each category were examined for homogeneity. Seventeen (5%) of the original assignments were changed at this point and final category assignment was reached by consensus between the two researchers.

Subcategories within each of the seven categories were developed by examining the data and identifying commonalities. State-

---

BOX 1: Nursing diagnoses portrayed in the video tape

1. Alteration in comfort level (pain)
2. Alteration in cardiac output/activity intolerance
3. Altered sleep patterns
4. Knowledge deficit
5. Ineffective coping
6. Non-compliance
7. Alteration of self-concept/body image

Adapted from: Rossi, L.P., and Haines, V.M.: Nursing diagnoses related to acute myocardial infarction, Cardiovasc. Nurs. **15:**11-15, 1979.

Table 1: Descriptions of categories

Category name	Criteria for assignment
1. Correct nursing diagnoses	Labels approved by the North American Nursing Diagnosis Association and portrayed in the video tape
2. Non-nursing statements	Medical diagnoses, disease pathology, descriptions of physiological functions
3. Nursing (therapeutic) needs	Nursing action problems, risk factors amenable to nursing intervention, equipment, nursing needs, therapeutic needs
4. Signs and symptoms	A single cue that is a defining characteristic of a diagnostic label
5. Correct but not portrayed in the video tape	Labels approved by NANDA but not intended to be portrayed in the video tape
6. Correct labels used as etiology	Labels approved by NANDA used as the etiology in a two-part diagnostic statement
7. Miscellaneous	Responses that could not be classified

Table 2: Label frequency by category

Category	Absolute frequency	Relative frequency
1. Correct	75	22.6%
2. Non-nursing statements	34	10.6%
3. Nursing needs	54	16.3%
4. Signs and symptoms	76	22.9%
5. Correct, not in video	64	19.3%
6. Correct as etiology	28	8.4%
7. Miscellaneous	1	.3%
Totals	332	100%

ments in categories 1, 5, and 6 were assigned to subcategories as identified by labels on the National Conference List of Nursing Diagnoses. Statements in categories 2, 3, and 4 were assigned to subcategories appropriate to each area.

RESULTS

The 54 coronary care unit nurses in this sample spontaneously generated 332 diagnostic statements that were assigned to one of seven categories (Table 2). Seventy-five of the diagnostic statements were assigned to Category 1. This category represents correct identification and labeling of diagnoses portrayed in the video tape simulation. Only six of the seven diagnoses portrayed in the video tape simulation, were recorded at least once by the subjects (Table 3). Alterations in comfort level: pain was identified most often, followed by diagnostic statements that described alterations in self-concept/body image. Non-compliance was the only diagnostic label intended to be portrayed in the video tape simulation that was not spontaneously recorded by any of the subjects.

Table 3: Category 1 (correct in video tape) by subcategory

Diagnosis	Absolute frequency	Relative frequency
Comfort/pain	32	42.7%
Self-concept/body image	18	24.0%
Sleep/rest	11	14.7%
Knowledge deficit	11	14.7%
Ineffective coping	2	2.6%
Cardiac output/activity tolerance	1	1.3%
Totals	75	100%

Additional use of labels approved by NANDA is represented by statements in categories 5 and 6. Sixty-four (19.3%) of the spontaneously generated statements were assigned to Category 5, because they were NANDA-approved terms but not portrayed in the video tape. There were 13 different subcategories of NANDA labels in this category. Anxiety and fear account for 39 (60.9%) of the labels in this category. Other labels that occurred with less frequency (less than 8%) include alterations in nutrition and alterations in mobility.

In 28 (8.4%) of the statements a NANDA-approved diagnosis was used as the etiology. In these cases the statement of the problem did not use an accepted label. There were ten subcategories of labels used as etiology. Alterations in comfort: pain accounted for 50% of the statements in this category. Four statements (14.3%) were assigned to the subcategory of knowledge deficit. The remaining eight subcategories had absolute frequencies of one or two each. Included in this group were the diagnoses of impaired gas exchange, alterations in sleep, and alterations in mobility.

Thirty-four statements were assigned to Category 2 (non-nursing statements). Most of the labels in this category were statements describing alterations in physiological function of a specific body system. Changes in respiratory or cardiovascular function ac-

counted for 27 of the statements. Only three diagnostic statements in this category were written as medical diagnoses: depression, angina and infection.

Category 3 (nursing needs) contained 54 statements. Most of the statements in this category began with the words *need for*. The subcategory with the highest frequency included statements related to the patient's need for teaching. Subjects identified the need for teaching in relation to the patients' disease process and cardiac rehabilitation. The need for additional assessment of the patient was included in seven of the diagnoses. Only eight diagnoses in this category identified needs related to preventing complications. These included statements about preventing urinary tract infections, arrhythmias and IV complications.

The 76 statements in Category 4 were divided into 25 different subcategories of signs and symptoms. There were 19 statements (25%) that represented signs and symptoms related to the respiratory system. Statements describing a dependence/independence conflict accounted for another 23.7% of the labels in this category. Adjustments to alterations in lifestyle were included in nine statements (9.2%). Signs and symptoms related to changes in self-concept, knowledge deficit and myocardial infarction were some of the other subcategories.

The one statement assigned to the miscellaneous category was written in the form of a nursing progress note. It described the admission of the patient in the Intensive Care Unit and went on to make statements about some of the changes in his condition during the several days portrayed in the simulation.

Three hundred and thirty-one (331) of the diagnostic statements were sorted into categories as one-part or two-part labels. (The one statement written as a nursing progress note was not used in this part of the data analysis.) The category of two-part statements was further sorted as to type of linkage used: related to, due to, or other. The other category included terms such as associated with, secondary to and those statements written by the same nurse where linkage terms were used inconsistently.

One hundred and sixty-one (161) of the statements were one-part and 170 were two-part statements. The phrase *related to* was utilized in 52 (30.6%) of the two-part statements. *Due to* was utilized 65 (38.2%) times, more than any other single phrase. Other phrases such as *associated with, result of/resulting in* and *secondary to* were used with less frequency.

The nurses in the sample represented all three levels of basic educational preparation. The sample also included nurses with master's degrees in nursing as well as nurses with bachelor's and master's degrees in other fields.

No significant difference was found between years of clinical experience and the type of diagnostic statement generated. There was a significant relationship found between the highest level of formal education completed and the type of diagnostic statement. Nurses with an MSN wrote no statements in the form of nursing needs, and 72.4% of their statements utilized NANDA-approved terminology. Of the correct statements generated, nurses with MSN's had the highest percentage of correct diagnoses within the diagnoses they generated.

Nurses who reported no preparation in the use of nursing diagnosis demonstrated indiscriminate use of terminology in writing diagnostic statements. In contrast, nurses who reported some type of preparation in nursing diagnosis were less likely to write diagnostic labels in terms of medical diagnoses, signs and symptoms or nursing needs.

DISCUSSION

The results of this study are similar to those found by Silver et al. (1984) in a content analysis of nursing diagnoses identified in actual patient care situations. In that study 23% of the labels were classified as NANDA-approved labels from the National Conferences on the Classification of Nursing Diagnoses. The diagnosis identified most often was alterations in comfort: pain. Statements of signs and symptoms accounted for 25% of the diagnostic statements in that sample of 1344 diagnoses taken from 377 patient records.

It would be expected that alterations in comfort: pain would be identified most often by nurses in this study, since the patient portrayed in the video tape had just experienced an acute myocardial infarction. Early in the simulation the patient has a pain episode while in the Intensive Care Unit. Many of the defining characteristics for this diagnosis are presented in the video tape. This finding parallels the findings of Miaskowski, Spangengberg and Garofallou (1984) that pain is a diagnosis identified by nurses in a variety of medical-surgical settings.

It is a positive statement for nursing that only 34 diagnostic statements in the entire sample of 332 were non-nursing statements that included pathophysiologic alterations or medical diagnoses. These findings contradict Davidson (1984) who has stated that many nurses in acute care settings organize care around medical diagnoses or medical care plans to the exclusion of other dimensions. Of the NANDA-approved labels in this sample, those related to pain, changes in self-concept, sleep alterations and knowledge deficit were identified more often than alterations in cardiac output. However, many of the statements of signs and symptoms were representative of physiologic changes in body systems. This finding supports the work of Kim (1984) about the importance of physiologic diagnoses in a taxonomy to represent all domains of nursing practice.

Gebbie (1984) has stated that nurses continue to react to each presenting concern of the patient as if it should be treated independently. This may help to explain the frequency with which nurses in the sample recorded signs and symptoms as nursing diagnoses. The use of signs and symptoms as diagnostic labels may also represent a deficiency in the current diagnostic labels approved for clinical testing. It could be that many of the cues that were identified as specific diagnoses in fact may be defining characteristics of diagnoses yet to be developed and tested. An example would be the number of times statements related to a dependence-independence conflict were identified in the sample. Gordon (1985) has suggested that such a diagnosis is useful in clinical practice, although it is not on the list of diagnoses from NANDA approved for clinical testing.

Using statements of nursing needs or therapeutic patient needs by nurses as diagnostic labels may represent a vocabulary problem rather than a diagnostic skill problem. Carnevali (1983) discusses the influence of vocabulary on the nurse's ability to notice and describe phenomena. The type of diagnostic vocabulary, general or precise, a nurse uses might influence the detail of data gathered about a client. Many of the statements in this category are related to the diagnoses portrayed in the video tape. Need for teaching is related to a diagnosis of knowledge deficit. Need for relief of pain would relate to the diagnosis of alterations in comfort.

The limited use of NANDA-approved labels may be the result of limited knowledge or infrequent use of a formal diagnostic classification system by the nurses in the sample. However many of the diagnostic statements that were written use terminology such as *alterations in* and *related to* suggested by the National Conferences on Classification of Nursing Diagnoses and found in the literature.

The failure of nurses in the sample to spontaneously identify non-compliance as a diagnosis may represent an aversion on the part of the nurses in the sample to using the term. It has been suggested that as a diagnosis, non-compliance is unacceptable, because it conveys a negative, value-laden connotation about the patient (Stanitis and Ryan 1982). Nurses in this sample may find the term unacceptable as a diagnosis to describe the patient's lack of cooperation with the therapeutic program. Other terms such as knowledge deficit or changes in self-concept may better explain the phenomenon of non-compliance.

Tanner (1984) asserts that biases that tend to influence the assessment of likelihood of diagnoses and ease with which diagnostic categories are retrieved include (1) frequency of occurrence in our own experience, (2) recency of experience, and (3) profoundness of memory (we tend to recall more easily the dramatic rather than the typical experience).

The novice diagnostician sees a perfect relationship between the presence of a cue and a given diagnosis. Observations and inferences are treated equally by the novice who has little tolerance for uncertainty of a diagnosis. The novice possesses little range and depth of experience to be used to assign probabilities. The novice has limited categories and subcategories in long-term memory (LTM) with few links between categories. There is usually a single cue-single diagnostic category inference present and retrieval from LTM often takes the form of memorized lists.

In contrast, the expert diagnostician recognizes the fallibility of cues as diagnosis indicators and seeks multiple cues for inferences. The expert has a high tolerance for uncertainty. The expert can draw on a wide range and depth of experience to reduce the chance for bias. When making a diagnosis the expert uses a hierarchical organization of categories and subcategories in LTM with complex linkages among categories. Multiple cross-referencing of cues to diagnostic categories also occurs.

From the data in this study it could be implied that nurses are novice diagnosticians. The nurses demonstrated limited ability in clustering cues and applying a diagnostic label. The frequency with which nurses in the sample recorded diagnoses not portrayed in the video tape using NANDA labels could represent a process in which the nurses responded to only one cue portrayed in the video tape simulation. Both Carnavali (1983) and Gordon (1982) described as part of the diagnostic process the prediagnostic activity of hypothesis testing. At this level the nurse generates one or several possible diagnoses based on the cues that are available from the data base. The cues are stored in short-term memory and compared to diagnostic categories in long-term memory. Available data are compared to those labels that best fit. Limitations of a video tape would not allow the nurses to validate hypotheses through additional assessment.

Sources have offered differing directions to nurses about the exact phrase to use in connecting the two parts of a nursing diagnostic statement. Mayers (1983) used *due to* in examples of nursing diagnostic statements. Carnevali (1983) used symbols such as arrows to show relationships and change. Ziegler (1984) and Resler (1982) both suggested the use of *related to* as the linking phrase. Textbooks of fundamental nursing skills or medical-surgical nursing such as Potter and Perry (1985) and Kozier and Erb (1983) suggested the use of *related to* or used *related to* in the examples of nursing diagnostic statements given. Phipps, Long and Woods (1983) suggested the use of *related to* or *associated with* during the period when there is uncertainty concerning the etiology of the response and then suggested the use of *because of, due to,* or *secondary to* when certainty concerning the etiology is present. Sorenson and Luckmann (1979) directed the student to use *due to* or *related to.* Most authors did not offer a rationale for the use of one term or set of terms over another.

Based on a study of the diagnostic skills of senior baccalaureate nursing students, Deback (1981) questions whether faculty members are prepared to teach the skills of nursing diagnosis. The study also questions whether practicing nurses have the skills needed to generate workable nursing diagnosis statements on which to base patient care. A recommendation was made that a massive education program in the generation of nursing diagnoses is indicated for practicing nurses.

There is a need to continue research in nursing diagnosis to develop appropriate labels that communicate the domain of nursing practice. All nursing education programs need to include activities that will help nurses develop diagnostic skills in the nursing domain.

REFERENCES

Carnevali, D.L.: Nursing care planning: diagnosis and management, ed. 3, Philadelphia, 1983, J.B. Lippincott.

Carpenito, L.J.: Nursing diagnosis: application to clinical practice. Philadelphia, 1983, J.B. Lippincott.

Carstens, J.R.: The effects of an in-service program on nurses' ability to identify valid nursing diagnoses. In Kim, M.J., McFarland, G.K., and McLane, A.M., editors: Classification of nursing diagnoses: proceedings of the fifth national conference, St. Louis, 1984, The C.V. Mosby Co.

Castles, M.R.: Interrater agreement in the use of nursing diagnosis. In Kim, M.J., and Moritz, D.A., editors: Classification of nursing diagnoses: proceedings of the third and fourth national conferences, New York, 1982, McGraw-Hill.

Davidson, S.B.: Nursing diagnosis: its application in the acute-care setting, Adv. Nurs. Sci. **6**:50-56, 1984.

Deback, V.: The relationship between nursing students' ability to formulate nursing diagnoses and the curriculum model, Adv. Nurs. Sci. **3**:51-66, 1981.

Gebbie, K.M.: Nursing diagnosis: what it is and why does it exist? Topics Clin. Nurs. **5**:1-9, 1984.

Gordon, M.: Nursing diagnosis: process and application, New York, 1982, McGraw-Hill.

Kim, M.J.: Physiologic nursing diagnoses: its role and place in nursing taxonomy. In Kim, M.J., McFarland, G.K., and McLane, A.L., editors: Classification of nursing diagnoses: proceedings of the fifth national conference, St. Louis, 1984, The C.V. Mosby Co.

Kozier, B.B., and Erb. G.L.: Fundamentals of nursing: concepts and principles, Menlo Park, CA., 1983, Addison-Wesley.

Mayers, M.G.: A systematic approach to the nursing care plan, Norwalk, Conn., 1983, Appleton-Century-Crofts.

Meade, C.D., and Kim, M.J.: The effect of teaching on documentation of nursing diagnoses. In Kim, M.J., McFarland, G.K., and McLane, A.M., editors: Classification of nursing diagnoses: proceedings of the fifth national conference, St. Louis, 1984,The C.V. Mosby Co.

Miaskowski, C., Spangenberg, S., and Garofallou, G.: An evaluation study of the implementation of nursing diagnosis. In Kim, M.J., McFarland, G.K., and McLane, A.L., editors: Classification of nursing diagnoses: proceedings of the fifth national conference, St. Louis, 1984, The C.V. Mosby Co.

Mundinger, M.O., and Jauron, G.D.: Developing a nursing diagnosis, Nurs. Outlook, **23**:94-98, 1975.

Myers, J.L., Perry, A.G., Wessler, R., and others: Staff nurses' identification of nursing diagnoses from a simulated patient care situation. (In press.)

Phipps, W.J., Long, B.C., and Woods, N.F., editors: Medical-surgical nursing: concepts and clinical practice, St. Louis, 1983, The C.V. Mosby Co.

Potter, P.A., and Perry, A.G.: Fundamentals of nursing: concepts, process, and practice, St. Louis, 1985, The C.V. Mosby Co.

Resler, M.M.: Formulation of a nursing diagnosis. In Carlson, J.H., Craft, C.A., and McGuire, A.D., editors: Nursing diagnosis, Philadelphia, 1982, W.B. Saunders.

Rossi, L.P., and Haines, V.M.: Nursing diagnosis related to acute myocardial infarction, Cardiovasc. Nurs. **15**: 11-15, 1979.

Silver, S.M., Halfmann, T.M., McShane, R.E., and others: The identification of clinically recorded nursing diagnoses and indicators. In Kim, M.J., McFarland, G.K., and McLane, A.M., editors: Classification of nursing diagnoses: proceedings of the fifth national conference, St. Louis, 1984, The C.V. Mosby Co.

Sorenson, K.C., and Luckmann, J.C.: Basic nursing: a psycho-physiologic approach, Philadelphia, 1979, W.B. Saunders.

Stanitis, M.A., and Ryan, J.: Noncompliance: an unacceptable diagnosis? Amer. J. Nurs. **82**:941-942, 1982.

Warren, J.: Problems in using nursing diagnoses: a descriptive study of graduate nursing students. In Kim, M.J., McFarland, G.K., and McLane, A.M., editors: Classification of nursing diagnoses: proceedings of the fifth national conference, St. Louis, 1984, The C.V. Mosby Co.

Ziegler, S.M.: Nursing diagnosis—the state of the art as reflected in graduate students' work. In Kim, M.J., McFarland, G.K., and McLane, A.M., editors: Classification of nursing diagnoses: proceedings of the fifth national conference, St. Louis, 1984, The C.V. Mosby Co.

Diagnostic reasoning studies: poster presentation

Analysis of distinctions between nursing diagnosis-related judgments and disease-related nursing judgments

KATHERINE L. GARTHE, M.S.N., R.N.

As the concept of nursing diagnosis is developed, distinctions between nursing diagnoses and medical judgments made by nurses are proposed and opposed. Because nursing and medicine both work with people in relation to the health-illness continuum, make plans, and intervene in relation to the health and illness of people, distinguishing between judgments made for the purpose of nursing care and those made for the purpose of medical care can be difficult. Making clear boundaries between nursing and medical judgments even more difficult is the lack of consensus among nurses regarding what constitutes nursing's domain. Differences of opinion about the nature of nursing's domain lead to differences of opinion as to what judgments can be labeled nursing diagnoses. This is apparent in the work of Gordon (1982), Kim (1984), and others (Aspinall 1967, Carpenito 1983, Guzzetta and Dossey 1983, Hubalik and Kim 1984) as they struggle to make the term *nursing diagnosis* operable for the nursing profession. One place this is evident is in the questioning of the legitimacy of certain proposed nursing diagnoses. Specifically,

the proposed nursing diagnoses of *decreased cardiac output, fluid volume deficit, altered tissue perfusion, impaired gas exchange,* and *ineffective breathing pattern* have been questioned (Gordon, 1982) for legitimacy to nursing. This study did four things: (1) identified the model of nursing's domain suggested by placing *disease-related* nursing judgments under *medically-delegated* nursing activities, (2) identified the model of nursing's domain suggested by the legal and social responsibilities of nurses, (3) examined whether or not patient care situations developed from a group of proposed nursing diagnoses were more in line with one model or the other, and (4) identified the factor structure underlying the patient care situations and compared it to the two models.

METHODS

Models of nursing's domain were developed through review of the literature on differences between nursing diagnoses and other judgments nurses make, social responsibilities of nurses, and legal responsibilities, and by identifying the assumptions about nursing's responsibilities and relationship with medicine in these writings. The identifying characteristics of 15 nursing diagnoses which have been proposed to the North American Nursing Diagnosis Association (NANDA) were used to produce 20 patient care situations which a nurse might encounter in a hospital. Fourteen situations were based on nursing diagnoses which had not been questioned for legitimacy to nursing. Five situations were based on nursing diagnoses which had been questioned (Gordon 1982), and one situation was based on a diagnosis which had not been specifically questioned but had defining characteristics similar to those of the questioned diagnoses.

Design and procedures

The investigation of the fit between the patient care situations and factor analysis and the models was a descriptive field study. The 20 patient care situations were placed in a questionnaire. Registered nurses involved in hospital-based medical-surgical practice were asked to identify those situations in which the nurse carried responsibility for the care plan and those in which the physician had the responsibility. If a shared responsibility for determining the care plan seemed to exist, the nurse was asked to identify the extent to which the responsibility was a shared one. Responses were given on a scale with 100% nurse responsibility for determining the care plan at one end and 100% physician responsibility at the other. Responses of all nurses were used to calculate means and standard deviations on each patient care situation item. These means were then used to identify to what extent the nursing diagnosis represented by that patient care situation was a nursing or medical responsibility. The means, or placement of responsibility, were then examined to see if they indicated a clear distinction between those situations in which a nurse was responsible for determining the care plan and those in which a physi-

cian was responsible. Finally, a factor analysis was performed. This allowed for identification of the factors operating in the patient care situations which help to account for the responses given by the nurses. The factors identified were then compared to the two models of nursing's domain to measure the fit between the nurse-respondents' view of responsibility for patient care situations and the view put forth by the two models.

Development of models

It has been proposed that nursing judgments can be divided into those that are nursing diagnosis-related and those that are disease-related (Gordon 1982). In this approach, the distinction between the two types of nursing judgments can be made by identifying who is responsible for determining the care plan, nurse or physician. Elsewhere, it has been proposed that nursing judgments can be divided into those for which the nurse is responsible, those for which the nurse shares responsibility with the physician, and those for which the physician is responsible (Carpenito 1983). In this approach, only those judgments for which the nurse carries complete responsibility are said to be nursing diagnoses; the other judgments made by nurses are said to be clinical problems or medical diagnoses made by nurses. Certain assumptions are apparent in these approaches: (1) Nursing diagnosis judgments and disease-related judgments can be distinguished from each other by identifying who is responsible for determining the care plan (Gordon 1982). (2) Nurses make independent as well as interdependent and medically dependent judgments (Carpenito 1983, Gordon 1982). (3) Although nurses make judgments for the purposes of referral to a physician or for initiation of medical orders or protocols, the nurse must think like a physician and for the physician, and so is not exercising independent nursing judgment (Gordon 1982). (4) The interdependent judgments, when nursing and medicine share responsibility for determining the care plan, are not within nursing's independent domain, since nursing cannot independently prescribe all the interventions which follow (Carpenito 1983, Gordon 1982). This model can be diagrammed as in Figure 1, and is called the Nurse Dependence Model (NDM).

Literature on the legal and social responsibilities of nurses suggests a model of nursing's domain different from the NDM. According to the American Nurses' Association (ANA 1980), nurses are "ethically and legally accountable for actions taken in the course of nursing practice" (p. 20). The Michigan Public Health Code (1978) emphasizes nursing as the "care ... of individuals ... experiencing changes in normal health processes" (p. 46), and medicine as the "diagnosis, treatment, prevention, cure or relieving of human disease" (p. 40). Other legal responsibilities of nurses include the responsibility to find another physician for a critically ill patient if that patient's physician does not respond to the nurse's call (Diosegy 1983), an obligation to report what seems to be inadequate medical care (Fiesta 1983, Katz 1983), communicating relevant information regarding a patient's history or condition to the physi-

cian (Fiesta 1983, Herrman 1982, Katz 1983, Who's responsible..., 1983), recognizing when a patient's complaints are unusual and demand special attention (Fiesta 1983, Fortin and Rabinow 1979, Katz 1983, Who's responsible ... 1983), and making judgments based on observation and assessment of patient condition (Fiesta 1983). At one time there was a tendency to hold the physician responsible for negligence of a nurse in the execution of a medical order, but the present trend is to "require that the physician have actually exercised control over the details of the work performed" (Walker 1983, p. 55).

Examination of the literature on nursing's legal and social responsibilities suggests certain assumptions about nursing's domain. (1) Nursing judgments and actions which have been identified in the nursing diagnosis literature as "interdependent" and "dependent" (Carpenito 1983), or as "delegated" activities and judgments (Gordon 1982) are actually independent nursing judgments and actions, *though associated with greater or lesser medical input.* When the nurse initiates a protocol or refers a patient condition to a physician, the nurse still retains responsibility for his or her own judgments and actions in relation to that patient condition (ANA 1980, Diosegy 1983, Fiesta 1983, Fortin and Rabinow 1979, Walker 1983). (2) Nursing and medicine each have responsibilities for determining care/treatment plans, and the involvement of one does not relieve the other of responsibility. (3) Nursing and medicine have related though different focuses of concern in their care/treatment plans. Nursing is concerned with the care of the ill person and promotion of health; medicine is concerned with the diagnosis and treatment of human disease. These concerns are separate, though interfacing. (4) Patient conditions require differing ratios of medical and nursing input, though the responsibility of each professional is present throughout his or her involvement with the patient. This model is

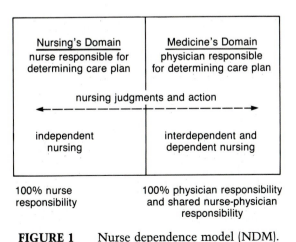

FIGURE 1   Nurse dependence model (NDM).

called the Professional Interface Model (PIM), and can be diagrammed as in Figure 2.

RESULTS

The patient care situation questionnaire was completed by 95 registered nurses involved in hospital-based medical-surgical practice. The nursing diagnoses used to develop the situations, mean responses (the average amount of responsibility assigned to each professional), and the scale along which the responses were placed can be seen in Table 1. Three questions were asked: (1) Does the responsibility for determining the care plan in different patient care situations lie along a continuum (as it would in the PIM), or is it dichotomous (as in the NDM)? (2) Do nursing diagnoses which have been questioned for legitimacy to nursing consistently carry large amounts of physician responsibility for determining the care plan? (3) Do those proposed nursing diagnoses which have not been questioned for legitimacy consistently carry large amounts of nursing responsibility for determining the care plan? In response to the questions, data analysis revealed: (1) The re-sponsibility for determining the care plan for the diagnoses studied falls along a continuum, and so is best accounted for by the PIM. (See Figure 3 for pattern of means for patient care situations and compare with the models in Figures 1 and 2). (2) The nursing diagnoses questioned for legitimacy to nursing do not consistently carry large amounts of physician responsibility for determining the care plan. In fact, in some cases the same diagnosis carries greater nurse responsibility in one situation and greater physician responsibility in another, though the nursing diagnosis remains the same (Figure 3 and Table 1). (3) The proposed nursing diagnoses which have not been questioned for legitimacy were also found to vary greatly in amounts of nurse versus physician responsibility identified by the nurse-respondents, from approximately 40% to 95% nurse responsibility for determining the care plan in different situations (Figure 3 and Table 1).

Factor analysis

Four factors were identified which accounted for 47.1% of the variance. The factors identified were: high physical distress needing quick intervention and potentially responsive to medication, high psychosocial distress needing quick intervention and potentially responsive to medication, physical and emotional needs, less immediate intervention required, and further assessment required (Table 2). The overall means of the factors were examined in relation to the two models of nursing's domain (Figures 4 and 5). First the means of the factors were placed along the nurse-physician responsibility scale of the NDM (Figure 4). With the factors arranged in this way, all factors are found to be within medicine's domain, since none are 100% nursing responsibility. Even if the midpoint between nurse and physician responsibility is taken as the line of demarcation between nursing's and medicine's do-

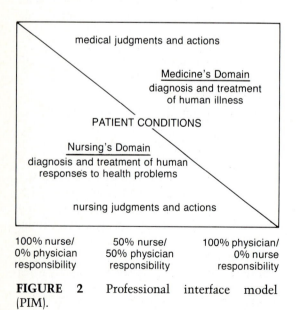

| 100% nurse/ 0% physician responsibility | 50% nurse/ 50% physician responsibility | 100% physician/ 0% nurse responsibility |

FIGURE 2 Professional interface model (PIM).

mains, to place either Factor I or IV in either domain would appear to be arbitrary, since each profession carries only slightly greater responsibility than the other for determining the care plan. Then, the overall means of the factors were placed along the nurse-physician responsibility scale of the PIM (Fig. 5). With the means of the factors arranged in this way, all factors are found to be within nursing's domain of responsibility for determining the care plan, though associated with varying amounts of physician responsibility. For example, Factor I represents those proposed nursing diagnosis situations with high level of physician as well as nurse responsibility for determining the care plan. The individual responsibility of each professional is taken into account.

Table 1: Nursing diagnoses represented by patient care situations and their currently suggested domains, means (assignment of responsibility for determining care plan), and nurse-physician responsibility scale used by nurse-respondents*

Item #	Nursing diagnosis	Domain	$\bar{x}$
1	Altered bowel elimination: constipation	N	4.1
2	Ineffective breathing pattern	M	5.6
3	Alteration in comfort: pain	N	6.5
4	Alteration in comfort: pain	N	3.5
5	Self-care deficit	N	7.7
6	Activity intolerance	N	4.2
7	Anxiety	N	6.4
8	Altered bowel elimination: incontinence	N	6.8
9	Decreased cardiac output	M	3.1
10	Impaired verbal communication	N	7.1
11	Diversional activity deficit	N	7.6
12	Sleep pattern disturbance	N	6.6
13	Actual fluid volume deficit	M	2.7
14	Decreased cardiac output	M	3.0
15	Impaired skin integrity	N	6.0
16	Ineffective airway clearance	NC	3.0
17	Actual fluid volume deficit	M	6.4
18	Ineffective individual coping	N	6.1
19	Sleep pattern disturbance	N	5.4
20	Anxiety	N	5.9

8	6	4	2	0
100% nurse		nurse-physician responsibility scale		100% physician

*Domain refers to domain suggested in nursing diagnosis literature (Gordon 1982). N=nursing, M=medicine, NC=not clear, $\bar{x}$ =mean, 4 on the nurse-physician responsibility scale = 50% nurse/50% physician responsibility for determining the care plan.

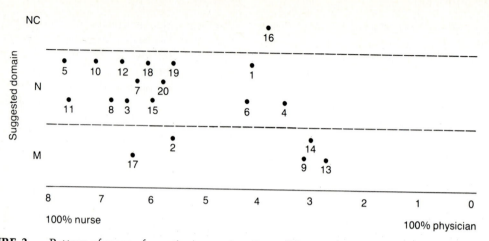

FIGURE 3   Pattern of means for patient care situations. (The numbers in the figure refer to the item number—see Table 1 for the nursing diagnosis associated with any particular item. N = nursing domain, M = medical domain, NC = not clear. 6 = 75% nurse/25% physician responsibility for determining care plan, 4 = 50% nurse/50% physician responsibility, 2 = 25% nurse/75% physician responsibility.)

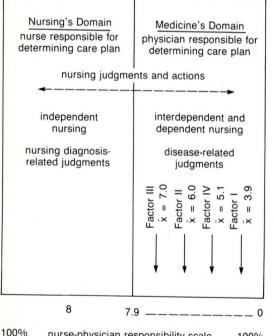

FIGURE 4   Factor placement within the nurse dependence model (NDM). (8 = 100% nurse responsibility for determining the care plan. Because interdependent and dependent judgments of nurses are placed within medicine's domain in the NDM, any factor with an overall means less than 8 falls within medicine's domain. x̄ = overall mean of the factor.)

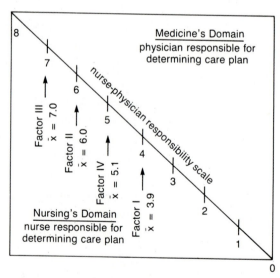

FIGURE 5   Factor placement within professional interface model (PIM). (8 = 100% nurse responsibility for determining care plan, 4 = 50% nurse/50% physician responsibility, 0 = 100% physician responsibility.)

Table 2: Factors operating in patient care situations*

[a]Item #	Characteristics of situation	Domain	$\bar{x}$
Factor I: High physical distress needing quick intervention, potentially responsible to medication.			
9	Difficulty breathing, disoriented, rales	M	3.1
16	Rales, cyanosis, shortness of breath	NC	3.0
6	Weak, vital sign change, fatigue with walking	N	4.2
14	Dyspnea, restlessness, medical diagnosis of CHF	M	3.0
3	Pain and osteoarthritis	N	6.5
4	Pain and osteoarthritis, requests aspirin	N	3.5
			overall $\bar{x}$ = 3.9
Factor II: High psychosocial distress needing quick intervention, potentially responsive to medication			
20	Numerous emotional stressors, nervous	N	5.9
18	Nervous about chemotherapy	N	6.1
7	Pre-op, nervous	N	6.4
19	Pre-op, unable to sleep	N	5.4
15	Open raw area on hip	N	6.0
			overall $\bar{x}$ = 6.0
Factor III: Physical and emotional needs, less immediate intervention required			
5	Unable to feed, bathe, or dress self	N	7.7
10	Pre-op, unable to speak dominant language	N	7.1
11	Patient in traction, complains of boredom	N	7.6
2	Patient with COPD, dyspnea, nervousness	M	5.6
			overall $\bar{x}$ = 7.0
Factor IV: Further assessment required, quick response not required			
12	Cannot sleep at night	N	6.6
8	Recent stroke, incontinent of stool	N	6.8
1	Abdominal pain, infrequent, hard stools	N	4.1
13	Decreased urine output, decreased fluid intake, increased hematocrit, increased serum sodium	M	2.7
			overall $\bar{x}$ = 5.1

*Domain refers to domain suggested in nursing diagnosis literature. N=nursing, M=medicine, NC=not clear, $\bar{x}$=mean.
[a]Nursing diagnoses corresponding to the item numbers can be found in Table 1.

CONCLUSION

The findings of this study suggest that there is a shared responsibility for determining the care plan in all proposed nursing diagnoses included in the study. In addition, the responsibility for determining the care plan will vary from situation to situation depending on factors present in the situation and cannot be fixed for any given proposed nursing diagnosis. Varying responses to different situations developed from the same diagnosis (see items 3 and 4 in Table 1) provide evidence that there is not a consistent distribution of nurse versus physician responsibility for determining the care plan in different situations developed from the same diagnosis.

The varying amounts of nurse versus physician responsibility for determining the care plan found in different patient care situations brings to light the way in which assigning physician responsibility to judgments made by nurses results in giving away legitimate nursing responsibility. If, in one case, alteration in comfort: pain requires a high degree of medical intervention, and is excluded as a legitimate nursing diagnosis on that basis, then nursing has failed to recognize what is, in many other cases, a legitimate nursing diagnosis. It would seem that ANA's original statement that nurses diagnose and treat "human responses to actual and potential health problems" (1980, pp. 9-10) is a more helpful guideline than one which attempts to eliminate nursing judgments for which a physician may have interventions and planning responsibilities.

REFERENCES

American Nurses' Association: Nursing: a social policy statement (ANA Publication Code: NP-63 35M 12/80), Kansas City, MO: American Nurses' Association.

Aspinall, M.J.: Nursing diagnosis—the weak link, Nurs. Outlook **24:**433-437, 1976.

Carpenito, L.J.: Nursing diagnosis: application to clinical practice, Philadelphia, 1983, J.B. Lippincott.

Diosegy, A.J.: A lawyer answers 10 legal questions about current nursing practice, NursingLife, **3:**30-36, 1983.

Fiesta, J.: Breach of duty: how to recognize it before it happens, NursingLife, **3:**19-22, 1983.

Fortin, J.D., and Rabinow, J.: Legal implications of nursing diagnosis, Nurs. Clin. North Amer. **14:**553-561, 1979.

Gordon, M.: Nursing diagnosis: process and application, New York, 1982, McGraw-Hill.

Guzzetta, C.E., and Dossey, B.M.: Nursing diagnosis: framework, process, and problems, Heart Lung **12:**281-291, 1983.

Herrman, F.: Four kinds of carelessness that can send you to court, NursingLife, **2:**62-63, 1982.

Hubalik, K., and Kim, M.J.: Nursing diagnoses associated with heart failure in critical care nursing. In Kim, M.J., McFarland, G.K., and McLane, A.M., editors: Classification of nursing diagnoses: proceedings of the fifth national conference, St. Louis, 1984, The C.V. Mosby Co.

Katz, B.F.: Reporting and reviewing of patient care: the nurse's responsibility, Law Med. Health Care **8:**76-79, 1983.

Kim, M.J.: Physiologic nursing diagnosis: its role and place in nursing taxonomy. In Kim, M.J., McFarland, G.K., and McLane, A.M., editors: Classification of nursing diagnoses: proceedings of the fifth national conference, St. Louis, 1984, The C.V. Mosby Co.

Michigan Public Health Code, Public Act 368 of 1978, Article 15.

Walker, D.J.: Legal rights and responsibilities of the nurse. In Chaska, N.L., editor: The nursing profession: a time to speak, New York, 1983, McGraw-Hill.

Who's responsible here? (Court case column), NursingLife. **3:**80, 1983.

Diagnostic reasoning studies: abstracts

Errors committed by nurses and nursing students in the diagnostic reasoning process

UNA E. WESTFALL, M.S.N., R.N.
CHRISTINE A. TANNER, Ph.D., R.N., F.A.A.N.
DEE-J PUTZIER, Ph.D., R.N.
KAREN PADRICK, M.N., R.N.

Diagnostic reasoning is a crucial part of professional nursing practice. While some nurses think of diagnostic reasoning only in terms of the final diagnosis, it is actually a chain of activities at any point in which errors can occur. Because diagnostic reasoning is a process, it is necessary to examine sequences and activities that lead to the final judgment when analyzing diagnostic errors. No one questions the importance of nurses making sound clinical judgments. However, little is known about the thought processes nurses use to reach such conclusions, because research efforts in this area are very limited. A large descriptive study designed to investigate the cognitive processes used by nursing students and nurses in situations requiring clinical nursing judgment was conducted at a Western university. The study is grounded in information processing theory. As part of that larger study, the research reported in this paper is a qualitative description of the kinds of errors that occur in the process of diagnostic reasoning and the consequences of those errors to the final judgment. Among the results, investigators found that not all errors inevitably led to wrong conclusions. In fact, the correct conclusion was strengthened for some subjects by at least one error.

The convenience sample consisted of 43 subjects—15 beginning junior and 13 beginning senior nursing students, and 15 practicing nurses from one large health science center. Each subject viewed videotaped clinical nursing simulations in individual sessions. Subjects were asked to respond aloud to each situation, articulating their thinking, additional information gathering, and conclusions drawn. The thinking aloud was tape-recorded and transcribed for later analysis.

Each subject's transcripts from three cases were content analyzed for errors. An error was defined as failure to meet any of the following requirements of competent performance: use of available data; generation of reasonable conclusions based on known relationships between presented data and inferences; and efficient use of time. Errors have been identified in each of the major components of a diagnostic reasoning model: (1) problem sensing (e.g., errors of inaccurate recall of information, and not moving beyond data to its meaning); (2) hypothesis activation (e.g., errors of mismatch between data and hypotheses, and lack of focus on priority areas of nursing concern); (3) data gathering related to each hypothesis (e.g., errors of use of knowledge or experience that do not fit data clusters, and inefficient use of time between exposure to data and final judgment); and (4) hypothesis evaluation (e.g., errors of not using confirming or disconfirming data when available, and leaping to a conclusion without testing it. Errors differed in seriousness, consequence to the final judgment, and timing in the process. Examples of errors and resulting consequences from each category were presented.

The patterns identified from these data suggest that clinical diagnostic reasoning is far more complex than has traditionally been thought. Understanding both the processes used by clinicians and the nature of errors occurring in diagnostic reasoning should place us in a better position to help both students and practicing nurses improve their clinical judgment.

Cognitive processes nurses use in diagnosing patients' problems

MARY E. KERR, M.N.Ed., R.N.

The skill with which a nurse is able to diagnose a patient's problems influences the quality of care that a patient receives. This descriptive study was conducted to discover the cognitive processes nurses utilize in diagnosing the problems of their patients. A random sample of five baccalaureate-prepared nurses, working on medical-surgical units in a 600-bed community hospital reviewed two case studies of patients from medical-surgical units, and diagnosed the problems of these patients.

The definition of thinking as a covert activity does not lend itself easily to objective data collection. In order to collect data on internal cognitive activity involved in any type of thinking process, the technique must force the subject to externalize internal thoughts without disturbing the structure of the thoughts. The most effective method of having the personal externalize thoughts is to ask the individual to "think aloud" while performing the specified task. This is known as verbal protocol analysis. Ericcson and Simons (1980) explained the use of verbal protocols and the types of data that may be useful in collecting data based on information processing theory.

In this study, the subjects were asked to "think aloud" while they were reviewing the case studies and diagnosing the patients' problems. These verbalizations were tape recorded and transcribed into verbal protocols. The analysis of the protocols led to the identification of seven distinct cognitive processes which were labeled: recode, search, inference, problem identification, hypothesis generation, validation, and prejudgment. Search, inference, and hypothesis generation were the processes that occurred most frequently during the subjects' diagnostic process.

By increasing the understanding of the cognitive processes nurses currently use to diagnose, researchers can build and expand that knowledge to help nurses help patients in the most complete, efficient, and effective ways possible.

The relatedness of cues with diagnostic labels following use of a patient care planning program

KENNETH L. CIANFRANI, Ph.D., R.N.

Research studies have shown that nurses have not been able to distinguish the importance of cues (Hammond 1966) even though highly relevant cues increase accuracy in diagnosing (Cianfrani 1982). The purpose of this study was to investigate the effects of a computerized patient care plan program on how strongly nurses relate cues to nursing diagnosis labels. The objective of the study was to determine if cues were identified as more or less related to diagnostic labels by staff nurses after use of the computer program. The program required nurse to read a computer screen with a list of cues in order to verify their hypothesized diagnosis. The hypothesis for this study was that there would be either an increase or decrease in the relatedness of cues to a specific diagnostic label after the use of a computerized patient care planning program.

The experiment was a pretest/post-test design with a paired sample. The investigator compared the relatedness score of each cue before the computer program was initiated with the relatedness score of each cue after the program was used by nurses for 6 months. Seventy-five nurses were randomly selected from the scheduling list of the nursing service department of a midwestern hospital of approximately 250 beds. A questionnaire had a return rate of 65% (N=49) for the first collection period and 52% (N=39) for the second collection period. Questionnaires were used from 29 nurses who returned the data collection tool both times. The questionnaire was composed of 20 randomly selected nursing diagnosis labels from a list of 50 labels approved by NANDA. Five cues were also randomly selected for each diagnostic label resulting in a questionnaire of 100 cues. The nurses were asked to rate on a Likert-type scale how strong or weak each cue was related to the label. A two-tailed test for paired samples was used for data analysis of the scores for each cue.

Results of the study showed that there was a significant difference between the relatedness of cues before and after using a computer program (p<.001). Results of the study show that after using a computer program nurses improved in their ability to distinguish the relatedness of cues to diagnostic labels. This is in contrast to previous findings that nurses had confidence in all data received for identifying health problems. Limitations of the study are that nurses from various services were asked to identify relatedness of cues to diagnostic labels which they may not use in clinical practice. As nurses are taught to use cues specific and relevant to the nursing diagnosis labels, they will be able to distinguish which cues are more relevant and become more accurate in identifying nursing diagnoses.

Identification of the assessment cues used by cardiac nurses to diagnose chest pain

SHERRIE L. GOLDSBERRY JUSTICE, M.A., R.N.

Cardiac nurses are responsible for differentially diagnosing the cause of patients' chest pain. The assessment process used has not been documented. The purpose of this study was twofold: (1) to identify the assessment cues used by cardiac nurses to differentially diagnose patients with chest pain and (2) to determine the relationships of subjects' diagnostic accuracy and their educational and practice background to their use of assessment cues.

A descriptive survey approach was used. The convenience sample was comprised of 42 female registered nurses who were practicing in either a coronary care unit or a step-down unit. Data were collected at two moderately sized private hospitals in a midwestern city.

The data collection instrument was composed of biographic data, a diagnostic task, and a questionnaire. The diagnostic task was a simulated patient situation. Each subject was told that a fictitious patient in the coronary unit was complaining of chest pain. The subject's task was to diagnose the cause of the pain. The subjects had to recall the cues needed to diagnose chest pain and request them from the interviewer who provided them from a prepared list of cues. The questionnaire also sought the subjects' confidence in their diagnosis, identification of those cues that were most beneficial in determining the diagnosis, and chest pain etiologies. Analysis of data was accomplished via the use of frequencies, chi-square analysis, Spearman rank correlations and Kruskal-Wallis one-way analysis of variance.

One hundred twenty-two cues were requested. Only nine were requested by at least 50% of the subjects. Two were significantly related to obtaining the correct diagnosis. Only 50% of the subjects accurately diagnosed the pain as being of gastroesophageal origin. The inaccurate diagnosers cited myocardial ischemia as the etiology.

The results indicated that a uniform chest pain assessment procedure did not exist. They also exhibited an unacceptable diagnostic accuracy rate. Nursing must be concerned about the failure to reach an accuracy rate of greater than 50%. The act of diagnosing is now mandated in several practice acts.

Nursing process studies: poster presentations

Nursing assessment of the patient with a nursing diagnosis of alteration in comfort: chronic pain

GAIL C. DAVIS, Ed.D., R.N.

Pain is one of the most frequent problems which nurses assess, treat, and evaluate. The many variables that affect pain contribute to the difficulty of accurate clinical assessment and ongoing evaluation. This complexity is further complicated by the subjective nature of pain.

The division of the major category of pain into acute and chronic pain would facilitate nursing assessment and treatment. "Alteration in comfort: pain" was identified as a nursing diagnosis by the National Conference for Classification of Nursing Diagnosis in 1978 and accepted in 1980 (Kim and Moritz 1982). While this group has not yet divided the pain diagnosis into acute pain and chronic pain, Carpenito (1983) does make this division for purposes of application to clinical practice. Acute pain is defined as

This study was conducted by the author as a participant in The Measurement of Clinical and Educational Nursing Outcomes Project sponsored by The University of Maryland, School of Nursing and supported by the Division of Nursing, Department of Health and Human Services.

The author gratefully acknowledges the assistance of Peggy M. Mayfield, M.S.N., R.N.,C., A.N.P. for her assistance in data collection.

"pain that can last from 1 second to as long as 6 months. It subsides with healing or when the stimulus is removed" (Carpenito 1983, p. 117). Chronic pain is "persistent or intermittent pain that lasts for more than 6 months" (p. 122). Duration is noted as the key element of difference in most definitions of pain. This prolonged and unknown duration leads to increased complexity of effects. This pain which "exists without a known time limit . . . becomes a constant companion, to be controlled if possible but always to be lived with" (Johnson 1977, p. 141).

Nurses need a better understanding of the characteristics of chronic pain, as well as the desired outcomes of its treatment. Identification of the characteristics is essential to evaluation of outcomes. An assessment tool is needed to serve two different functions: (1) to collect information for the further research required for establishing the characteristics and outcomes of chronic pain and (2) to provide an effective and efficient approach to patient assessment.

The major purpose of this study was to determine the adequacy of the McGill Comprehensive Pain Questionnaire (Monks and Taenzer, 1983) for use in assessing the clinical outcomes of the patient with a nursing diagnosis of alteration in comfort: chronic pain. The MCPQ was selected because of its comprehensive approach to the measurement of chronic pain.

RESEARCH QUESTIONS

The MCPQ's adequacy for measuring the characteristics and outcomes of chronic pain was tested through study of the following research questions:

1. Is the MCPQ valid for evaluating clinical outcomes of patients with a nursing diagnosis of alteration in comfort: chronic pain?
   a. Do the tool's quantitative components discriminate between two groups of patients, e.g., those with acute pain (postsurgical) and those with chronic pain (rheumatoid disease)?
      (i)   Present pain intensity (PPI)
      (ii) Pain rating index (PRI)
      (iii) Number of words chosen (NWC)
      (iv) Dimension subscales: sensory, affective, evaluative, miscellaneous
   b. Is there a good correlation between the patient's pain intensity score when measured concurrently by the pain intensity scale of the MCPQ and the visual analogue scale (VAS)?
2. What areas of daily living (work, leisure, sleep, weight, habits, mood, attitudes) are most affected by chronic pain?

METHODOLOGY
Sample

The major sample population was comprised of patients with a projected nursing diagnosis of alteration in comfort: chronic pain. Thirty subjects were selected through a purposive, non-random sampling procedure. These subjects met the following criteria for selection: (1) had a projected diagnosis of alteration in comfort: chronic pain; (2) had a medi-

cal diagnosis of rheumatoid disease; (3) were at least 21 years of age; and (4) had a medical treatment plan for rheumatoid disease.

A second sample group was selected from patients admitted to the hospital for general surgery. Again, a purposive, non-random sampling procedure was used to select 30 patients who met the following criteria: (1) had a potential nursing diagnosis of alteration in comfort: acute pain related to a general surgical procedure; (2) were at least 21 years of age.

Procedures

The procedures used in this methodological study focused on validity assessment of the quantitative portions of the McGill Comprehensive Pain Questionnaire (MCPQ) with an added intent of identifying those areas of qualitative data which are most often related to chronic pain for further development of the instrument.

Instrumentation

The MCPQ expands the pain description of the original McGill Pain Questionnaire (MPQ) developed by Melzack (1983) at McGill University by adding additional questions related to pain history, past medical history, medication, pain modifiers, effects of pain, personal history, and patient expectations. Most of these are open-ended questions, providing qualitative data. The MCPQ was modified for this study by combining two parts of the original MCPQ, the patient questionnaire and the interview guide. The original version of the tool is organized so that the questionnaire (Part 1) can be sent to the patient for completion prior to being seen in the Pain Center of the Montreal General Hospital where Part 2 (the interview portion) is used (Monks and Taenzer 1983). In addition to combining items within the tool, some items were eliminated.

One of the advantages provided by the MPQ/MCPQ is that it provides quantitative information which can be treated statistically (Melzack 1975). Three different types of quantitative data are available: (1) pain rating index (PRI) obtained by adding the rank order value for each dimension and dividing the sum by the total possible dimension score (Kremer, Atkinson, and Ignelzi 1982); (2) the total number of words chosen (NWC), which refers to the total number of words selected in the sensory, affective, and evaluative dimensions; and (3) the present pain intensity, based on a scale of 0 to 5, with 0 representing "no pain" and 5 representing "excruciating pain". The McGill Pain Questionnaire is a "start . . . toward the measurement of clinical pain and permits research on the effects of experimental and therapeutic procedures on pain in clinical rather than laboratory conditions" (Melzack, p. 294).

The visual analogue scale (VAS) was also used. The VAS is a line (vertical or horizontal) with clearly-defined boundaries. Usually the line is 10 centimeters in length; and the patient is asked to make a mark on the line at a point which describes the intensity of his pain. The distance of the mark from the end of the line represents the pain intensity score. Several studies have shown the VAS to provide a reliable method of measurement (Aitken 1969, Huskisson 1983).

Data collection. The investigator administered the VAS and the modified version of the MCPQ, using the interview method, to all 30 subjects in the chronic pain group. Each interview took approximately 1 hour.

The investigator and another nurse administered the quantitative portion of the MCPQ to the 30 subjects in the acute pain group. The sample was selected from patients admitted to a large private hospital for surgery. The same nurse administered the questionnaire to the patient prior to surgery and again on the second postoperative day. The VAS was also used with this group to evaluate pain intensity preoperatively and postoperatively.

RESULTS

The student t test was used to test for significant differences (p<.05) between the chronic and acute pain groups in relation to all of the quantitative data. The study demonstrated that one of the word description subscales, the affective dimension, discriminated between the chronic and acute pain patients. Specific words, used by the chronic pain group, which also discriminated between the two groups were *hot, tingling,* and *fearful.*

The pain intensity rating scale of the MCPQ and the VAS were compared using the Pearson product moment correlation procedure. This comparison (r=.5753) demonstrated concurrent validity for measuring pain intensity at a given time.

The qualitative data were studied for the indications they might provide for further refinement of the instrument. Descriptive statistics—frequencies and percentages—were used for analysis. Those qualitative areas which demonstrated an occurrence of at least 75% were noted: (1) location of pain was the joint, (2) pain was continuous, (3) some hobbies could no longer be continued because of pain, but participation was maintained in those which they could do, (4) no new activities started since onset of pain, (5) did not drink alcohol, (6) people available with whom pain could be discussed, (6) religion helped in coping with pain, (7) modifiers which increased pain were standing, walking, and fatigue, and (8) modifiers which decreased pain were heat, enjoying things, talking with others, and rest. These indicators would seem to give direction for areas of further tool development and for further study in identifying the characteristics associated with chronic pain.

The word descriptors were evaluated to determine which were selected by the chronic pain patients at least one-third of the time. These were *exhausting, sharp, throbbing, shooting, burning, penetrating, nagging, cramping, aching, tender, tiring, fearful,* and *numb.*

DISCUSSION

The major purpose of this study was to determine the adequacy of the MCPQ for use in evaluating the clinical outcomes of the patient with a nursing diagnosis of chronic pain. The tool's various quantitative components were evaluated for discriminant validity and concurrent validity. Qualitative portions were studied in order to determine those indicators which occurred most frequently in relation to chronic pain.

The affective subscale of the MCPQ's word descriptors, which includes 5 word groups, discriminated between the acute and chronic pain groups. This finding, in relation to the outcomes of earlier studies, supports the discriminant validity of the MCPQ's word scales. This finding is also consistent with a review of pain language and affective disturbance (Kremer and Atkinson 1983, p. 120) which indicated that "affective distress influences pain language in a systematic fashion, and that the MPQ is a reliable, valid and unobtrusive measure of emotional disorder in chronic pain patients." Several researchers (Kremer and Atkinson 1983, Lindsay and Wyckoff 1981, Phillips 1983) have questioned whether the affective distress experienced by the person with chronic pain might be indicative of depression and/or anxiety. McCreary (1983) further questions whether the affective pain description indicates that anxiety and depression occur as state or trait measures.

Chapman (1978 p. 179) discounts the association of anxiety with chronic pain, stating that "patients with chronic pain have relatively low anxiety levels." The uncertainty and surprise of pain has dissipated for the person to whom pain is constant. Exceptions to this might be the cancer patient to whom pain recurrence could indicate the spread of disease or to the cardiac patient to whom successive onset of pain might indicate a fatal heart attack. These exceptions would more likely involve intermittent rather than constant pain.

The MCPQ's pain intensity rating demonstrated good reliability with the VAS, indicating concurrent validity of these two pain measurements. This is consistent with previous studies which have shown correlations from 0.39 to 0.10 between the MPQ and verbal and visual analogue rating scales (Reading 1983).

The length of the interviews (approximately 1 hour) reinforced the purpose of developing an efficient and effective tool for the clinical measurement of chronic pain. The qualitative data were carefully examined to determine (1) what areas seemed related to the chronic pain patient with rheumatoid disease and (2) where reorganization of these data might occur within the tool as modified for this study. In further evaluating these data, a question which deserves further consideration is whether one tool can efficiently assess the chronic pain of patients with differing medical diagnoses.

Eighty percent of the acute patients and 83% of the chronic patients described their pain as being "constant." In light of questions which have been raised concerning anxiety and depression in chronic pain patients, the pain time element (constant, intermittent, or transient) should be retained as a part of measurement, even though it does not discriminate between types of patients.

The major implication of this study is that the MCPQ does provide a good beginning measure of the characteristics and outcomes of chronic pain. It provides a valid measure of pain intensity, and the word descriptors differentiate between chronic and acute pain. The qualitative portion of the tool identifies those areas of the patient's daily living which are most affected by chronic pain. These provide indicators which can be tested further.

REFERENCES

Aitken, R.C.B.: Section of measurement in medicine: a growing edge of measurement of feelings: measurement of feelings using visual analogue scales, Proc. Roy. Soc. Med. **62:**989-993, 1969.

Carpenito, L.J.: Nursing diagnosis: application to clinical practice, Philadelphia, 1983, J.B. Lippincott.

Chapman, C.R.: Perception of noxious events. In Sternbach, R.A., editor: The psychology of pain, New York, 1978, Raven Press.

Huskisson, E.C.: Visual analogue scales. In Melzack, R., editor: Pain measurement and assessment, New York, 1983, Raven Press.

Johnson, M.: Assessment of clinical pain. In Jacox, A.K., editor: Pain: a sourcebook for nurses and other health professionals, Boston, 1977, Little, Brown.

Kim, M., and Moritz, D.A., editors: Classification of nursing diagnoses: proceedings of the third and fourth national conferences, New York, 1982, McGraw-Hill.

Kremer, E.F., and Atkinson, J.H., Jr.: Pain language as a measure of affect in chronic pain patients. In Melzack, R., editor: Pain measurement and assessment, New York, 1983, Raven Press.

Kremer, E., Atkinson, J.H., and Ignelzi, R.J.: Measurement of pain: patient preference does not confound pain measurement, Pain **10:**241-248, 1982.

Lindsay, P.G., and Wyckoff, M.: The depression-pain syndrome and its response to antidepressants, Psychosomat **22:**571-577, 1981.

McCreary, C.: Pain description and personality disturbance. In Melzack, R., editor: Pain measurement and assessment, New York, 1983, Raven Press.

Melzack, R.: The McGill Pain Questionnaire: major properties and scoring methods, Pain **1:**277-299, 1975.

Melzack, R.: The McGill Pain Questionnaire. In Melzack, R., editor: Pain measurement and assessment, New York, 1983, Raven Press.

Monks, R., and Taenzer, P.: A comprehensive pain questionnaire. In Melzack, R., editor: Pain measurement and assessment, New York, 1983, Raven Press.

Phillips, C.: Chronic headache experience. In Melzack, R., editor: Pain measurement and assessment, New York, 1983, Raven Press.

The relationship between a structional-functional health/illness pattern (SHIP) tool and the generating of nursing diagnoses: a qualitative and quantitative study

CAROL A. SOARES-O'HEARN R.N., Ph.D., et al[*]

The profession's essential features of nursing practice: assessment, diagnosis, intervention and evaluation have been clearly identified (ANA 1973). All of these features of practice rely upon the quality of initial assessment data. The problems one is able to generate are significantly related to the type and frequency of assessment data analyzed. These in turn are influenced by the type of assessment tool used.

If the identification of nursing diagnoses is central to the scope of clinical practice (ANA, 1980), then the quality and type of tool used to generate diagnoses is even more essential to the scope of practice.

PURPOSE

The purpose of this study was twofold: (1) to develop and expand the categories and parameters within the Gordon Functional Health Pattern assessment tool using qualitative methods, and (2) to investigate the relationship between the developed tool (SHIP), routine tools and the generating of nursing diagnoses using quantitative methods.

[*]Students contributing were: Jean Ayer, R.N. B.A., Gail Bemis, R.N., Mary Beth Collins, R.N., Sharon Ann LaMond, R.N., Kathleen LeBrun, R.N., Judith McGuire, R.N., Elizabeth O'Brien, R.N., Karen Petty, R.N., Michelle Raposa, R.N., Laura Raymond, R.N., Tove Stevens, R.N., and Debra Sullo, R.N.

Leslie (1981) asserts that the use of nursing diagnoses provides a common language for expressing patient problems.

REVIEW OF THE LITERATURE

One tool that is designed to isolate nursing diagnoses is the Functional Health Pattern assessment tool (Gordon 1983). This tool incorporates eleven functional health pattern areas as essential assessment domains. Several studies have examined the frequency of nursing diagnoses and their commonalities using functional health patterns as the assessment format. A common agreed language structure such as nursing diagnoses, also enhances communication among practitioners (Leslie 1981). Continuity of nursing care is promoted by using nursing diagnoses to describe the changes in a patient's functional health patterns (Gould 1983). Gould concurs with Leslie that nursing diagnoses provide a common language for communication among nurses. Overlap in the use of defining characteristics among several nursing diagnoses was identified as a problem area for future investigation (Kim 1984). The need to promote specific terminology to build a common language among practitioners was also recognized (Kim 1984). Toth noted that an established mechanism for defining the domain of nursing practice can be provided through the use of nursing diagnoses. This would also lead to a higher level of professionalism. Nursing diagnoses would also provide a means for documenting the taken-for-granted aspects of the steps taken to prevent complications (Toth 1984: 298).

The literature suggests that the promulgation of a comprehensive system (taxonomy) of accurately developed and defined specific nursing diagnoses and their identifying characteristics would result in higher quality nursing care through enhanced interpractitioner communication, continuity of nursing care, and isolation of the taken-for-granted aspects of preventive actions taken by nurses.

ASSUMPTIONS

Underlying assumptions that were identified are as follows:

1. There is a relationship between the number of problems assessed and the quality of nursing care provided.
2. There is a relationship between the type of tools used and the relevance of data perceived.
3. There is a relationship between methods of data collection and characteristics of data.
4. There is a one-to-one correspondence between assessment tool categories and the nursing diagnoses identified.
5. There is a relationship between systematic data collection and the frequency of problem identification.
6. There is a relationship between use of an assessment tool and cost effectiveness.

STATEMENT OF THE PROBLEM

Is there a relationship between assessment tools used and the frequency and diversity of nursing diagnoses generated?

HYPOTHESES

1. The use of the SHIP assessment tool will lead to greater frequency of nursing diagnoses than will routine assessment tools.
2. The use of the SHIP assessment tool will lead to more diverse types of nursing diagnoses than will routine assessment tools.

OPERATIONAL DEFINITIONS

1. *Nursing Diagnoses*
   a. For the structural-functional tool,
   these were defined as written problem/etiology statements. The diagnoses from the NANDA list were accepted as well as others that the researchers generated.
   b. For the routine tool, all of the above and any health problems or statements that the researchers could infer as NANDA-type problems, e.g., potential for injury could be inferred from "safety concerns."
2. *Structural-functional tool*
   A tool designed to measure structural, functional and developmental areas of health care (see Methodology).
3. *Routine assessment tool*
   Any tool in use at a particular agency which generated health problems.

METHODOLOGY

A combination of inductive and deductive methods was used in developing the SHIP assessment tool. Qualitative and quantitative methods were also incorporated. Definitions of terms were agreed upon from the literature and group consensus.

Four broad domains of classification (Soares 1978) were initially examined as a method of categorizing health problems, (1) biophysical, (2) cognitive-perceptual, (3) psychosocial, and (4) cultural-spiritual. Gordon's (1982) functional health patterns were reclassified under these four broad domains. A decision was then made to examine problems within only two of the broad domains, the biophysical and the psychosocial areas. The latter domain also included cognitive-perceptual.

Background reference materials for the SHIP tool were drawn from the functional health assessment patterns of Marjory Gordon (1982), the classification systems development by Sister Callista Roy (1976), conceptual frameworks of Rogers (1970), Maslow (1954), Jones and Jakob (1977), patterns of functioning of Matthew (1982), ANA generic standards of nursing practice (1973), ANA social policy statement (1980), and other private agency work in diagnosis (Kim 1984).

Based on their clinical interest, two groups were formed to develop the assessment tool. One group of seven worked on the biophysical domain. The other group of seven, worked on the psychosocial domain. Each group developed subcategories for these two dimensions of the assessment tool. The subcategories were generated from the examination of their own nursing experience as well as labels currently used in the nursing literature.

Parameters, grounded in clinical experience, were developed for the subcategories by each group. The biophysical group developed 12 subcategories with parameters for each. The psychosocial group developed four subcategories with parameters for each. Definitions were written for each category and subcategory for the biophysical and psychosocial domains of the assessment tool.

Multiple methods of reliability were reviewed. Consensus agreement (Diers 1979) as a measure of interrater reliability was used. Interrater reliability with 80% agreement for pattern categories, subcategories, parameters, and definitions was decided upon. Content validity was also incorporated.

Questionnaires were designed by each domain group for the purpose of establishing interrater reliability. The biophysical group rated the psychosocial section. Conversely, the psychosocial group rated the biophysical. The rating system categories ranged from 1 (always), 2 (sometimes), 3 (never), 4 (don't know), and 5 (parameter confusing). Revisions were made in the items that did not achieve an acceptable interrater reliability level until at least 80% agreement was attained. The assessment tool was compiled by integrating the biophysical and psychosocial domains. Demographic variables were also included.

The assessment tool was piloted by each member of the group (N = 14) on one client from a convenient population. The pilot study areas needing clarity were identified and revised. The original 16 pattern subcategories were regrouped into the following 12 broad functional health pattern areas:

I.   A. Pattern: Health/illness
     B. Pattern: Health concept/health
        conduct
II. A. Pattern: Nutritional/metabolic
     B. Pattern: Elimination
III. A. Pattern: Sleep/rest
IV. A. Pattern: Cognitive perceptual
     B. Pattern: Self-perception/self-
        concept
V.   A. Pattern: Reproductive/sexuality
     B. Pattern: Role relationships
VI. A. Pattern: Stress/coping
     B. Pattern: Value/beliefs

Regrouping of subcategory parameters was also done. These were further reordered to include parameters that measured (1) structural integrity/alteration, (2) functional/dysfunctional health, and (3) developmental goals for each broad A and B pattern domain areas.

The SHIP tool was also designed to assess structural categories, such as musculoskeletal and neuromuscular functioning. The inclusion of these structural categories was based on the premise that it was necessary to evaluate these particular areas *prior* to assessing activity-exercise functional health patterns. For example, it seemed essential to distinguish between mobility impaired related to *activity intolerance,* mobility impaired 2° *joint contractures* and mobility impaired 2° *altered thought processes.* These parameters were included, since many of the effects of structural alterations are followed by dysfunctional health patterns. In other words, structural assessment as a prerequisite to functional health pattern assessment precedes functional health assessment. Based on its essential features, the tool was entitled the structural-functional/health/illness pattern (SHIP) assessment tool.

SAMPLE

Sample selection criteria were persons of either sex who were 65 to 85 years old, alert, conscious, English-speaking, with enough energy to complete the interview. Each subject had to have recorded a list of nursing problems on an agency's routine assessment tool. From 10 agencies located in Southeastern Massachusetts, a population of 64 was drawn from all available cases meeting the stated sample criteria. A stratified random sample was then drawn, (N=28) from the total population (N=64) meeting the stated criteria within the agencies. The type of agencies used were two community health settings, (N=4) and six medical-surgical settings (N=12) and two nursing homes (N=12).

DATA COLLECTION

Twenty-eight patients were assessed by junior registered nurse baccalaureate students (N = 14). All of the students had completed four courses focusing on nursing diagnoses. Two of these courses had clinical components. All were skilled in functional health assessment. Agency diagnoses were also collected on each subject. Each collector analyzed each case and derived nursing diagnoses, which included presenting problem, etiological problem and characteristics of both.

INTERRATER RELIABILITY

A random sample of 30 nursing diagnoses and characteristics generated from the SHIP tool were rated for interrater agreement. The researchers, in groups of three, were in agreement 73% to 85% of the time. This suggests a fairly high reliability between the characteristics and nursing diagnoses isolated.

ANALYSIS AND RESULTS

A decision was made to examine and compare only the presenting problems at this time (Table 1). The SHIP tool's generated total (N=192) health problems (sample N=28) ranked within the following broad categories: health maintenance *(20%)*, cognitive 5% - perceptual 13% *(18%)*, mobility 9% - activity 5% *(14%)*, nutrition *(13%)*, coping *(13%)*, elimination *(8%)*, skin *(6%)*, respiratory *(5%)*, and circulatory *(3%)*. Fifty-two percent of the SHIP diagnoses and 51% of the routine diagnoses fell into the top three ranking diagnostic clusters. These were: health maintenance deficit, cognitive-perceptual, alterations in, and mobility/activity alterations in. There were 18 sub-diagnoses under these three. The SHIP tool generated a frequency of 100 diagnoses in these three groupings, whereas, the routine tool's frequency was 64. The ranks differ from Leslie's diagnoses in long-term care (Leslie 1981, p. 1012). However, if her data were reordered into similar broad groupings (N=748) perception, alteration in, would result in 12% of her diagnoses (N=184) with a rank order of 2. Fifty percent of Leslie's sample were above 85 years of age (N=210, range = 25–101 years of age). Thus there seem to be similar rankings of perceptual alteration diagnoses between those 65 to 85 years of age and those in long-term care over 85 years of age. Further exploration of the perceptual subcategories by age cohort needs to be explored.

The major health problems of the elderly appear to be related to biophysical energy depletion. In general, the rank order of these problems varied according to their settings. This suggests that diagnoses are contextually determined.

HYPOTHESIS TESTING

H:1 The use of the SHIP tool will generate a higher frequency of nursing diagnoses than the routine assessment tools.

Table 1: Nursing diagnoses, rank order, frequency, and percentage of diagnoses, between SHIP tool and routine tool sample N=28

Diagnoses	SHIP tool		Percentage of diagnoses (N=192)	Cum. percent	Routine tool		Percentage of diagnoses (N=103)	Cum. percent
	Rank order	Frequency			Rank order	Frequency N=103		
HEALTH MAINTENANCE DEFICIT	1	38	20	20	1	22	21	21
Self-care deficit (12)						(10)		
Health management deficit (8)						(3)		
Home maintenance deficit (1)						(0)		
Injury, potential for (13)						(6)		
Infect, potential for (4)						(3)		
COGNITIVE PERCEPTUAL ALTERATIONS	2	34	18	38	3	15	15	36
Cognitive impaired (5)						(5)		
Knowledge deficit (2)						(2)		
Uncompensated short-term memory deficit (1)						(0)		
Communications impaired verbal (1)						(0)		
Perception alteration in, comfort physical (11) pain-sensory deficit uncompensated (5)						(11)		
Sleep-rest disturbance (3)						(0)		
Psychological body image (4)						(1)		
Disturbance sociological						(0)		
Self-esteem (1)						(0)		
Disturbance spiritual distress (1)						(0)		
MOBILITY-ACTIVITY ALTERATIONS	3	28	14	52	4	15	15	51
Mobility impaired physical (16)						(11)		
Joint contractures (12)						(0)		
Activity intolerance (10)						(4)		
NUTRITION ALTERATION	4	25	13	65	2	17	17	68
In less than (12) more than (10)								
Fluid volume deficit (3)								

Table 1: Nursing diagnoses, rank order, frequency and percentage of diagnoses, between SHIP tool and routine tool sample N=28—cont'd

Diagnoses	SHIP tool		Percentage of diagnoses (N=192)	Cum. percent	Routine tool		Percentage of diagnoses (N=103)	Cum. percent
	Rank order	Frequency			Rank order	Frequency N=103		
COPING INEFFECTIVE, INDIVIDUAL (3)	5	24	13	78	8	6	6	74
Conflict unresolved Independence-dependence (2)						(1)		
Non-compliance (3)						(2)		
Depression, reactive (3)						(0)		
Anxiety, mild (1)						(2)		
Family disabling (2)						(0)		
Social, isolation (5)						(0)		
Diversional deficit (5)								
ELIMINATION ALTERATION	6	16	8	86	5.5	9	9	83
Bowel: Constipation (7)						(3)		
Diarrhea (2)						(5)		
Incontinence (1)						(1)		
Urinary: Incontinence (6)								
SKIN INTEGRITY	7	11	6	94	7	8	8	91
Impairment of								
RESPIRATION PATTERN	8	10	5	97	9	4	4	95
Alteration in breathing pattern ineffective (6)						(2)		
Gas exchange impaired (3)						(2)		
Airway clearance ineffective (1)						(0)		
CIRCULATION PATTERN	9	6	3	100	5.5	9	9	104
Alterations in (2)						(3)		
Cardiac output, decreased (3)						(5)		
Hemodynamics alterations in (1)						(1)		
TOTAL	9	192	100	100	9	103	100	104

Table 2: Differences in types of categories between SHIP and routine tools

Types of categories	SHIP	Routine tool	Totals
Same	26 (32)	26 (20)	52
Different	21 (15)	03 (09)	24
Totals	47	29	76

($X^2=8.2$, d.f.=1, $p<.01$.)

The diagnostic frequency generated for both tools combined was 295. Of these, the SHIP tool generated 192, and the routine tools 103 (case N=28). Statistical comparison of the differences between the two group frequencies were made. Using the Sign test (Bush 1985, 113-114) on matched pairs of differences in frequencies 44 pluses and 3 minuses were found. A probability of <0.001 for N=47 (number of differences) and $x \leq 3$ (number of fewer signs) was obtained (Bush 1985, 216). Therefore, the hypothesis (H:1) was supported. The SHIP tool had a significantly greater frequency of diagnoses than did the routine assessment tools.

H:2 The use of the SHIP tool will lead to a greater diversity of types of diagnostic categories than will routine assessment tools. The SHIP Tool generated a total of 47 types of diagnostic categories,* whereas, the routine tools generated 29, $X^2=8.2$, df=1, $p<.01$ (Table 2). Therefore, the SHIP tool generated more different types of diagnostic categories than the routine assessment tools.

This study supported the hypothesis that a systematic method of data collection generated a higher frequency of nursing problems. It also showed that more diverse types of diagnostic categories could be identified.

Of the 47 categories in the SHIP tool, 21 were different (i.e., not used) from the routine categories. Only 3 categories from the routine tool were different from the SHIP. These were: Neurological pattern impaired: Actual (N = 1); Neurological* pattern impaired: Potential (N = 1); and Cardiac Status altered (N = 3). The SHIP analyzers did not use musculo-skeletal and neuromuscular functional alterations as a presenting problem category like the routine analyzers. However, these biophysical categories were used to describe etiological problems.

REFERENCES

American Nurses' Association: Standards of nursing practice, Kansas City, MO, 1973, American Nurses' Association.

American Nurses' Association: Nursing: a social policy statement, Kansas City, MO, 1980, American Nurses' Association.

Bush, C.: Nursing research, Reston, VA, 1985, Reston Publishing Co.

Carpenito, L.: Nursing diagnosis: application to clinical practice, Philadelphia, 1983, J.B. Lippincott.

Diers, D.: Research in nursing practice, New York, 1979, J.B. Lippincott.

Gordon, M.: Manual of nursing diagnosis, New York, 1982, McGraw-Hill.

Gordon, M.: Nursing diagnosis: process and application, New York, 1982, McGraw-Hill.

Gould, M.: Nursing diagnosis concurrent with multiple sclerosis. Amer. Assoc. Neurosci. Nurs. **15:**340-345, 1983.

Jones, D., and Durkin, C.: Medical-surgical nursing: a conceptual approach, New York, 1982, McGraw-Hill.

Jones, D., Lepley, K., and Baker, B.: Health assessment across the life span, New York, 1984, McGraw-Hill.

Jones, P., and Jakob, D.: An investigation of the definition of nursing diagnosis, Report of phase I, Toronto, 1977, University of Toronto.

Kim, M.J., McFarland, G.K., and McLane, A.M., editors: Classification of nursing diagnoses: proceedings of the fifth national conference, St. Louis, 1984, The C.V. Mosby Co.

Kim, M.J., and Moritz, D.A., editors: Classification of nursing diagnoses: proceedings of the third and fourth national conferences, New York, 1982, McGraw-Hill.

Leslie, F.: Nursing diagnosis: use in long-term care, Amer. J. Nurs. **81:**1012-1014, 1981.

Maslow, A.: Motivation and personality, ed. 2, New York, 1954, Harper and Row.

Mathew, D.: Patterns of functioning: Wichita State University curriculum design. A poster presentation at the Midwest Alliance in Nursing annual conference, 1982.

Polit, D., and Hungler, B.: Nursing research: principles

and methods, ed. 2, Philadelphia, 1983, J.B. Lippincott.

Rogers, M.: An introduction to the theoretical basis of nursing, Philadelphia, 1970, F.A. Davis.

Roy, C.: Why are we here? In Gebbie, K., editor: Summary of the second national conference: classification of nursing diagnoses, St. Louis, 1976, The Clearinghouse, National Group for Classification of Nursing Diagnoses.

Soars, C.: Nursing and medical diagnoses: comparisons of variant and essential features. In Chaska, N., editor: The profession: views through the mist, New York, 1978, McGraw-Hill.

Nursing diagnoses along axes: a clinical interview study of prioritizing nursing diagnoses in psychiatric-mental health settings

MARGA S. COLER, Ed.D., R.N., C.S.
KAREN G. VINCENT, M.S.N., R.N., C.S.

Nursing diagnoses are no longer a new discovery. Their use is universal in the nursing profession. Care plans are built around them; patient records address them. Yet, there continues to be a void which is addressed in this paper.

The prioritization of the nursing diagnoses remains an important issue in the implementation of the nursing care plan. Where, when, and whether this takes place has, to date, escaped the literature. It was, therefore, selected as the topic of research conducted toward attaining a goal of expeditious, client-centered nursing care.

The axial model, popularized by the Diagnostic and Statistical Manual-III (DSM-III, 1980) of the American Psychiatric Association (APA) was adopted as the prioritization format for discriminating between those diagnoses that needed immediate intervention and those that could be addressed without urgency.

REVIEW OF THE LITERATURE

The axial concept of diagnosing was introduced in this country by the APA in its DSM-III. Although revolutionary, the method was met with little resistance in the psychiatry-mental health field. Training sessions went quickly, and, within a year, all medical and many non-medical mental health facilities were utilizing the new system. It did not take long for the system to cross national boundaries, and in some cases, replace the traditional diagnostic method of the International Classification of Diseases-9-with Clinical Modifications (ICD-9-CM).

DSM-III not only labels but presents stressors and functional level of the client during the year before his or her help-seeking behavior. Diagnosing along axes, provides a comprehensive view of the psychiatric-mental health system consumer in the following format:

Axis 1 Clinical syndromes
   Conditions that are not attributable to a mental disorder that are a focus of treatment
   Additional codes
Axis 2 Personality disorders
   Specific developmental disorders
Axis 3 Physical disorders and conditions
Axis 4 Severity of psychosocial stressors
Axis 5 Highest level of adaptive functioning past year (APA, 1980)

Although, the coding of diagnostic labels within the axes remains compatible with the ICD-9-CM, Axes 4 and 5, (not being present in the ICD), are coded from 0 to 7 to signify level of severity or impairment. Zero indicates that information is unspecified; 1, that no pathology is present; and 7, shows great impairment or severity. Within this system, it is common to have a client diagnosed in each of the five axes. For example, a person diagnosed in Axis 1 as a major depression, single episode with melancholia (296.23)×; may also have an Axis 2 diagnosis of borderline personality (301.83); a medical diagnosis of asthma; a stressor level of moderate (4); and have functioned at a level that is designated as "good" (3).

Nursing is still a neophyte when it comes to the diagnostic process. Clinicians frequently formulate their own labels or utilize one of many readily available "cookbooks" (Gordon 1982, Lengel 1982, Kim, McFarland, and McLane 1984, Carpenito 1983, Carlson, Craft, and McGuire 1982, etc.) for the labeling process. Such random selection does not lend itself to consistency. It has been the authors' experience that relatively few nurses are aware of the existence of a list of labels that have been validated and approved by the North American Nursing Diagnosis Association (NANDA). This knowledge deficit typifies what Warren (1983) referred to as a communication gap created by the use of "multi-languages."

As with labeling, little has been done to lay a groundwork in the planning phase of the nursing process. Diagnoses are frequently written in a haphazard fashion without a sense of prioritization. Morrison et al. (1985) proposed a sixth axis to the DSM-III to reflect an assessment of basic functioning and a "framework for assessing a patient's longitudinal clinical course" (p. 12). This does not, however, seem to address why one problem should be resolved before another.

One attempt at looking at needs was made by McKibbin et al. (unpublished manuscript), who related nursing diagnoses to nursing care hours. The work also failed to describe a prioritization method to point to what diagnoses (or diagnosis) needed to be addressed at what point in time. Warren (1983), who also addressed client needs, did so in relation to accountability. In short, the subject of prioritization of nursing diagnoses has evaded the authors in their search of nursing literature.

METHODOLOGY

The following project was designed to force a prioritization of nursing diagnoses at the end of a nursing assessment based on Gordon's 11 Functional Health Patterns (1982). The format, appearing on the final page of a Comprehensive Assessment Tool (CAT), developed by Coler and Vincent (unpublished manuscript), appears on axes similar to those utilized in the DSM-III. The first axis is used for listing nursing diagnoses that require immediate intervention, while Axis 2 lists those which may be addressed after the critical problems have been attended to. These generally relate to long-term goals. The tool utilizes Axis 3 for the listing of medical (including psychiatric) diagnoses; Axis 4, to designate stressor level; and Axis 5 to indicate the functional level of the client/patient. Both Axes 4 and 5 evaluate the client's status the year before the help-seeking behavior as in the DSM-III protocol (APA 1980).

The instrument was designed to elicit subjective, objective, physical status and mental status data which may be specifically retrieved for categorical analysis. At the end of each Functional Health Pattern is a Preliminary Assessment Page for the listing of client strengths, weaknesses, and nursing diagnoses from data obtained within the specific category. For example, Gordon's first category, Health Perception-Health Management Patterns would be followed by a page on which the data obtained within that category could be scrutinized in relation to the diagnostic process. Nursing diagnoses emanating from those data would be formulated and entered on this preliminary assessment page. Before arriving at the Final Assessment Page at the end of the CAT, the nurse would have completed eleven preliminary assessments based on each of the functional health patterns.

The study was initiated to assess the prioritization of nursing diagnoses by rejecting the null hypothesis that the frequency of appearance of a diagnosis on preliminary assessments at the end of each functional category would not influence its assigned priority status.

The data were compiled from 46 Comprehensive Assessment Tools: Individual completed in psychiatric inpatient and outpatient settings. A sample of inpatients in a private psychiatric institution were assessed by undergraduate baccalaureate nursing students (N = 36). Sampling was done by student selection of a patient that he or she would like to work with. Patients were of both sexes, and had an age range of 16 to 62. There were 14 females with a mean age of 24, and 19 males whose mean age was 28. The remaining ten assessments were done in outpatient settings by graduate students (N = 4), and by a nurse clinical specialist (N = 6). The same selection criteria were utilized. The outpatients consisted of two women, both of whom were 44 years old, and eight men with a mean age of 34 years. The most frequently identified primary diagnoses which appeared first, if there were more than one diagnosis in DSM-III, Axis 1 diagnostic categories were: schizophrenic disorders (N = 19), affective disorders (N = 15), substance abuse disorders (N = 5), and adjustment disorders (N = 3).

These major DSM-III categories were used for evaluating the prioritization of nursing diagnoses. Nursing diagnoses were also tabulated for each of the functional health categories, and were analyzed according to frequency of appearance. Figure 1 is a representation of the appearance of the four most frequently identified nursing diagnoses: coping, ineffective individual (#11); thought processes, alterations in (#47); self-concept, disturbance in (#39); and sleep patterns disturbance (#44) as identified the DSM-III category, schizophrenic disorders. The numerical code signifies the order of appearance of the diagnosis on the 1982 alphabetical list of nursing diagnoses approved by NANDA.

The most frequently identified nursing diagnosis in the 11 categories was coping, ineffective individual. This appeared 65 times in preliminary assessments of patients

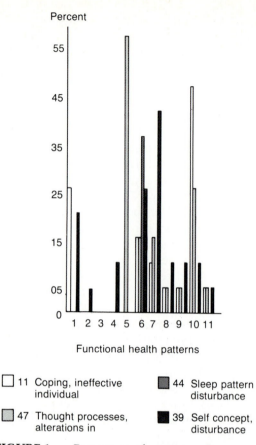

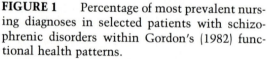

FIGURE 1 Percentage of most prevalent nursing diagnoses in selected patients with schizophrenic disorders within Gordon's (1982) functional health patterns.

across the four identified DSM-III groups. As may be expected, it was most often identified in the functional health pattern of coping-stress tolerance (48%). Thought processes, alterations in, was the nursing diagnosis most frequently identified in a single functional category of the schizophrenic sample. This diagnosis was most prevalent in Gordon's fifth category, cognitive-perceptual patterns (57%, see Fig. 1).

Figure 2 is a graphic representation of the frequency of the four nursing diagnoses within the four most prevalent DSM-III diagnostic categories. Coping, ineffective individual was identified in at least 80% of

SCHIZOPHRENIA (1) AND AFFECTIVE DISORDERS (2)

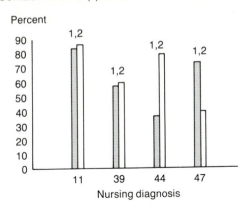

ADJUSTMENT DISORDERS (3)
AND SUBSTANCE ABUSE DISORDERS (4)

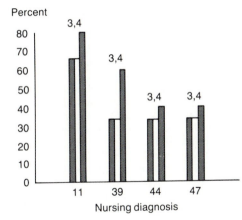

FIGURE 2 Percentage of nursing diagnoses within four major DSM-III categories. Key: Coping, ineffective individual (11); Self-concept, disturbance in (39); Sleep pattern disturbance (44); Thought patterns, alterations in (47).

schizophrenics, affective disorders, and substance abuse disorders.

Sleep patterns, disturbance in was highlighted in 80% of affective disorders, second only to coping, ineffective, individual; while self-concept, disturbance in was the second most prevalent nursing diagnosis identified in the substance abusers.

The prevalent nursing diagnoses were also tabulated in relation to the level of prioriti-

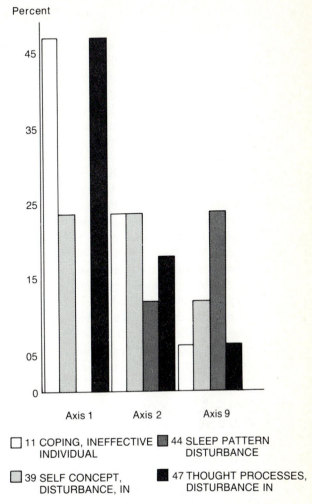

FIGURE 3 Prioritization of selected nursing diagnoses in selected patients with schizophrenic disorders.

zation. Figure 3 is a representation of the level of prioritization in the sample of schizophrenic disorders.

Several factors surface here. Although three diagnoses were identified in the 11 functional categories by at least 80% of the assessors, only 47% gave top intervention priority to any diagnosis. Two nursing diagnoses fell within this percentile: coping, ineffective individual, and thought processes, alterations in. Twenty-four percent of respondents identified coping, ineffective, individual and self-concept, disturbance in as second priority; and an equal number left sleep pattern disturbances in the group of unprioritized nursing diagnoses not identified on the final page (Axis 9).

Of note, also was the identification of the nursing diagnosis, self-concept, disturbance in, in ten of the eleven functional categories of clients with schizophrenic disorders (Figure 3). In the entire sample, it was identified in all of the categories at least once. Coping, ineffective individual, thought processes, disturbance in, and social isolation were identified in all but one of the 11 health patterns.

Inpatient and outpatient priorities differed considerably. Whereas coping, ineffective, individual was identified as a top priority nursing diagnosis for 58% of the inpatients, it was only identified for 20% of the outpatients. Instead, self-concept, disturbance in was the most prevalent for the second category of patients (50%).

DISCUSSION AND RECOMMENDATIONS

The data point to the need for further study of what appears to be an interesting, yet, a possibly alarming phenomenon. The fact that there was a large discrepancy between identification of nursing diagnoses during preliminary assessments and their subsequent prioritization leads us to reject the hypothesis that the frequency of appearance of a nursing diagnosis on preliminary assessments at the end of each functional category will influence its assigned priority status. The pattern we have identified seems to point to factors other than scientific thinking in the process of prioritization. Re-

plication of this study with registered nurses as assessors or with a larger sample of patients is indicated.

Prioritization is important and should not be related to intuition or feelings. Yet, the lack of literature on the subject relegates it to such a realm. It is the hope of the authors that this presentation will stimulate colleagues to further research along this vein.

REFERENCES

American Psychiatric Association: Diagnostic and statistical manual of mental disorders, Washington, 1980, American Psychiatric Association.

Carlson, J., Craft, C., and McGuire, A.: Nursing diagnosis, Philadelphia, 1982, W.B. Saunders.

Carpenito, L.: Nursing diagnosis: application to clinical practice, Philadelphia, 1983, J.B. Lippincott.

Coler, M.: I am nursing diagnosis . . . color me DSM-III green: a comparative analysis of nursing diagnoses and diagnostic categories of the Diagnostic and statistical manual-III of the American Psychiatric Association. In Kim, M.J., McFarland, G.K., and McLane, A.M., editors: Classification of nursing diagnoses: proceedings of the fifth national conference, St. Louis, 1984, The C.V. Mosby Co.

Gordon, M.: Manual of nursing diagnoses, New York, 1982, McGraw-Hill.

Kim, M.J., McFarland, G.K., and McLane, A.M.: Pocket guide to nursing diagnoses, St. Louis, 1984, The C.V. Mosby Co.

Lengel, N.: Handbook of nursing diagnosis, Bowie, MD, 1982, Robert J. Brady Co.

McKibbin, R., Brimmer, P., Clinton, J.G., and others: DRGs and nursing care, (HCFA Grant No. 15-C-98421/7-02). Kansas City, American Nurses' Association Center for Research.

Morrison, E., Fisher, L., Wilson, H., and others: NSGAE nursing adaptation evaluation, J. Psychosoc. Nursing, **23:**10-13, 1985.

Vincent, K.: The validation of a nursing diagnosis: A nurse consensus study, Nurs. Clin. North Amer. **20:**630-639, 1985.

Warren, J.: Accountability and nursing diagnosis, J. Nurs. Admin. **10:**34, 1983.

The computerization of nursing diagnoses: a step into the future for psychiatric/mental health assessment

KAREN G. VINCENT, M.S.N., R.N., C.S.
MARGA S. COLER, Ed.D., R.N., C.S.

The assessment and treatment of the whole person in concert with his world system makes nursing a unique science. All nursing theorists conceptualize nursing as a holistic process, whether the philosophy is discussed from a biopsychosocial perspective or as the nature of unitary man (Vincent 1985, Newman 1984). The synthesis of physical and psychosocial data about a person's health status extends to the assessment and treatment of clients in the psychiatric-mental health setting. However, to date, there have been few assessment tools published which give equal space to physical as well as psychiatric and psychosocial client data (Haggerty 1984, Kneisel and Wilson 1985). Physical assessment skills and needs are often underemphasized in this setting.

The comprehensive assessment tool used in this study does include physical and mental status data in assessing the psychiatric client. The instrument is also adapted for computer entry and retrieval of data. The computer program includes subjective, objective, mental status, and physical assessment material. When these data are entered into a computer, correlations and comparisons can be made between clients with similar psychiatric diagnoses. Additionally, a client's complete health status can be reassessed over the course of treatment to determine progress or lack of movement for specific nursing diagnoses. The clinician can accumulate information about the client's functional level prior to the initiation of treatment and at periods during treatment. In a large sense, these data will also add to the scientific body of knowledge for the nursing care of the psychiatric client.

This poster session focuses on the computer program designed by the authors for use with a Comprehensive Assessment Tool. The purpose of this article is twofold; to introduce use of the computer format and to present an example of its application. The subjective/objective data in the Health Perception/Health Management Pattern are factored out for client's with the Axis 1 diagnosis, schizophrenia, of the *Diagnostic and Statistical Manual III* (DSM-III) of the American Psychiatric Association (APA 1983). The preliminary nursing diagnoses chosen for that pattern area and coding of those nursing diagnoses are presented as well.

COMPUTER TECHNOLOGY IN NURSING

The application of computer technology in nursing will affect each step of the nursing process (Andreoli and Musser 1985, Dawson 1985). The computer can enlarge the potential for research into every clinical setting. The computerization of nursing diagnoses and interventions can also facilitate the scientist's attempt to define the "intuitive" actions in nursing (Soares 1978). An outcome of developing a computer basis for nursing science can be the development of a universal assessment tool; another important step in standardizing nursing's taxonomic language. The current cost containment movement in the United States and centralized regulation of health care underscores the need for nursing to document its efficacy (American Nurse 1983, Gordon 1980). Improved documentation of nursing tasks and services must occur to ensure appropriate reimbursement for nursing services (Martin 1982, Saba 1982).

Andreoli and Musser (1985) reported that most of the nursing literature about computer application to date focuses on administration and management systems. The literature of medical, computer, and engineering literature focuses on the application of computers in the diagnostic process. The computer-assisted diagnostic system (CAD) is one broad-based computer program that is disease specific. It analyzes data about client status, such as hemodynamics, lab values, or cardiac monitoring (Andreoli and Musser 1985). The program is procedurally rigid, unable to handle multiple diagnoses, and lacks the capacity to handle multiple clinical problems. These medical information systems leave no room for identification of client's strengths or potentials for wellness.

The positive result of a computerized assessment tool is the standardization of language and information between nurses (Martin 1982). Lagina (1971) designed a program for nursing assessment that sought to identify different levels of anxiety in hospitalized patients. The program increased the efficiency of the nurses' assessment skills. Wright (1985) describes a program that defines assessment criteria, according to Gordon's functional health patterns. The program covers a broad clinical area in community health nursing. It lists specific symptoms of abnormalities identified within each pattern area for the clinician. The appropriate nursing diagnoses for each functional category are also specified in the program. The program is based on an "if-then" structure of diagnostic branching via the computer. As the above examples show, nursing is beginning the process of developing its own system for documenting and analyzing client behavior, nursing diagnoses, and nursing action via the computer.

DESCRIPTION OF THE PROGRAM

The Comprehensive Assessment Tools designed by the authors is based on Gordon's 11 functional health patterns (Gordon 1982). There are three instruments in all, individual (1), family (2), and community (3). The instrument used in this poster session is the individual assessment. However, the computerization format is the same for all instruments. There are two distinct systems in the instrument. The first system codes the individual assessment items. The first space in the string is constant; it corresponds to the instrument number: individual (1). The second and third number in the string corresponds to the functional health category being assessed. The fourth, fifth, and sixth numbers are variable; they represent the questions and individual responses. See Table 1 for clearer example.

Table 1: Computer entry of items appearing in the comprehensive assessment tool

Digit number (beginning at left of string)	Descriptor
1	*Instrument number*
	Individual - 1
	Family - 2
	Community - 3
2,3	*Functional category**
4,5,6	00-24 = Subjective data
	25-49 = Mental status exam (subjective data)
	50-59 = Measured objective data (lab data, vital signs, other)
	60-75 = Other objective data
	75-99 = Mental status specific (objective data)

*(Gordon 1982)

The second system codes the nursing diagnoses generated at the functional category level and in a five-axis summary of nursing diagnoses located at the end of the assessment tool. The first, at the functional category level, is a summary of the preliminary nursing diagnoses that are arrived at for that functional category. This decision is made after identifying the client's strengths, weaknesses, and defining characteristics in that category. There are no finite diagnoses given for each pattern area, rather the clinician/diagnostician is allowed to choose from the official North American Nursing Diagnosis Association (NANDA) list of nursing diagnoses, which is computerized for this tool.

The code begins with the NANDA code number for that diagnosis (for example, ineffective coping (individual)-011), listed as the first, second, and third numbers. The fourth number represents the code for actual or potential status of the diagnosis in the specific category. The fifth space in the string represents the functional level of the client in the year prior to help-seeking behavior. The final number in the string, six, equals the care level for the client, based on Gordon's code for level of care (1982). Therefore, a client with the diagnosis, ineffective coping (individual), may have the following representation in the summary at the end of functional category, Health Perception/Health Management, 011.1.5.2

Definition: ineffective coping (individual)
Actual status
Functional level: poor
Care level: requires help from other persons (2)

The computer format for the final summary page of nursing diagnoses specifies the priority of intervention for the nursing diagnosis itself. The 5-axis system is explained in another poster session. The first axis represents those nursing diagnoses requiring immediate intervention. The second axis is for those that require secondary intervention or intervention for attainment of long-term goals. The first space indicates the position of the diagnosis on the axis system. The second, third and fourth correspond to the nursing diagnosis number, from the NANDA list. The fifth space is the functional level and the sixth space stands for the care level of the client, similar to the aforementioned string in the functional health category (Table 2). An example follows:

1.011.5.2
Definition:
Nursing diagnosis requires immediate intervention.
Ineffective coping (individual)—011
Functional level—poor
Care level—requires help from others

Table 2: Computerization of nursing diagnoses: the functional category level and the 5-axis summary page

Digit	Classification
1	Priority level: 1 = requires immediate intervention: 2 = requires intervention for attainment of long-term goals
2,3,4	Nursing diagnosis (fifth conference list)
5	Code: 1 = actual; 2 = potential for *Functional*
6	*level;* 1 = superior; 2 = very good; 3 = good; 4 = fair; 5 = poor; 6 = very poor; 7 = grossly impaired; 0 = unspecified*
7	*Care level:* 0 = independent; 1 = requires use of equipment; 2 = requires help from person(s); 3 = requires help from person(s) &/or device or equipment; 4 = completely dependent.**

*Axis 4 criteria as proposed in the DSM-III (1980)
**Gordon, Marjory (1982, p. 17)

This computer program lends itself to adaptation on large hospital-based information systems or for use by clinicians on microcomputers. Future advances in the development of the program are planned. The advantage of this system and program over a computer-assisted diagnostic system is that the system is not disease-related, there is room for evaluation and documentation of wellness diagnoses. Similarly, the program described by Wright (1985) for use in community health nursing contains a finite set of nursing diagnoses to be chosen for a specific functional health category. The program explored here leaves the assignment of diagnoses up to the clinician making the evaluation. This program may therefore lend itself to understanding how nurses make their diagnostic decisions and what behaviors exhibited by the client are necessary for choosing a particular diagnosis.

METHODOLOGY

The Comprehensive Assessment Tool: Individual was tested by undergraduate (N = 36) and graduate (N = 4) students and two psychiatric clinical specialists in the initial assessment process in both outpatient and inpatient mental health settings. Statistical analysis of the data was made via the Statistical Package for the Social Sciences system (Nie et al., 1975). A frequency distribution table was formulated for the nursing diagnoses found most frequently in each functional health pattern. The data were grouped according to DSM-III categories of diagnoses, so that comparisons could be made among clients with similar psychiatric problems.

A total of 46 clients participated in this clinical interview study. Both clinicians and students in inpatient and outpatient settings received approval for the research from the human rights committees in the appropriate facilities. The clients' responses and behaviors observed during the assessment process all serve as clues to choosing the defining characteristics for the nursing diagnoses in each category. The subjective responses and objective assessment made during the evaluation of health perception-health management pattern have been factored out for 17 patients having schizophrenia. This pattern area will be used as an example in showing the computerization format. Additionally, the coding for those actual nursing diagnoses chosen in the pattern area will be presented and discussed. The participants ranged in age from 22 to 44 years, the median age was 22. There were five women participants and 13 men.

RESULTS

The second question in the pattern area showed the first grouping of common responses: 1.1.01 "How do you stay healthy" was open-ended. A pattern of three responses was received. Table 3 contains the representation of those answers. The next question with the most commonality was 1.1.03: "Do you have any illnesses?" Fifty-three percent, (9) of the clients said yes, 47% (8) said no. When asked to describe their illness, 11 (65%) said they didn't know what their illness was. The same was found true for the question 1.1.04 "Have you had any previous hospitalizations?" One hundred percent (17) answered yes but only 4 (24%) of them responded that they were hospitalized for a "nervous breakdown", 11 (65%) responded that they didn't know why they were hospitalized. The clients were most commonly hospitalized for 3 to 4 months (6, 35%) and for an average of two times (7, 41%). Question 1.1.08: "Are you ill now?" Eleven (65%) said yes but the same percentage of clients 11 (65%) could not describe the problem.

The objective assessments by the clinicians were analyzed next. Their determination of the client's (1.1.76) "insight to their problem" was: 47% (8) had some insight into their problem and 5 (29%) had poor in-

Table 3: Client responses and nursing diagnoses for health perception—health management pattern

Nursing diagnoses	Ineffective coping (individual) 011.1.5.2		7
	Knowledge deficit 027.1.5.2		6
	Self-care deficit 038.2.5.2		4
Subjective data			
1.1.01 What do you do to keep healthy?			
	011)	Exercise	5
	012)	Eat right and exercise	4
	013)	Nothing special	4
1.1.03 Do you have any illnesses?			
	031)	Yes	9
	032)	No	8
	033)	Don't know	0
	034)	If yes, describe:	
		Don't know	11
		Nervous breakdown	6
1.1.04 Have you had any previous hospitalizations?			
	041)	Yes	17
	042)	No	0
	043)	For what?	
		Psychiatric service	4
		Don't know	4
		Nervous breakdown	3
	044)	How long?	
		3-4 months	6
		Don't know	
	045)	How many times?	
		Average of 2	7
1.108 Are you ill now?			
	081)	Yes	11
	082)	No	6
	083)	Describe:	
		Don't know	11
Objective data			
1.1.76 Insight to problem			
	761)	Good	6
	762)	Some	8
	763)	Poor	5
1.1.78 General appearance			
	781)	Older than chronological age	6
	782)	Younger than chronological age	0
	783)	Frail	5
	784)	Robust	2
	785)	Rundown	2
1.1.79 Grooming			
	791)	Good	11
	792)	Poor	5
	793)	Odor	0

sight into the cause of their difficulties. For general appearance, 6 (35%) of the clients looked older than their chronological age, 5 (29%) looked frail and 2 (12%) appeared run-down. The majority of clients had blood pressures within normal limits: 4 (24%) had blood pressures within the 120–130/75–80; 6 (35%) were within the range of 110–118/60–70.

The preliminary nursing diagnoses in the health perception-health management pattern were:

Ineffective coping (individual), 7 (41%)
Knowledge deficit, 6 (35%)
Self-care deficit (potential for), 4 (%)

Table 3 illustrates the coding of these diagnoses.

DISCUSSION AND CONCLUSIONS

The results were presented to illustrate the use of a coding system for subjective and objective material in a holistic assessment of the psychiatric client. The nursing diagnoses generated disclosed whether the diagnosis was actually or potentially present. Some correlations may be made between the responses and the preliminary nursing diagnoses. Eleven (65%) of the clients responded that they did have an illness, yet the same number of people could not identify their illness. Similarly, 100% had been hospitalized but 65% did not know why they were in the hospital. Knowledge deficit was an actual nursing diagnosis identified for 35% of the clients.

Ineffective coping (individual) was identified for 41% of the clients. Some defining characteristics of that diagnosis are inability to meet basic needs, inability to meet role expectations, high illness/accident rate (hospitalizations); all of which were identified in the subjective and objective material gleaned from clients. Although the pattern area describes how the person perceives and manages his/her health, it is worth noting that the diagnosis of ineffective coping skills is iden-

tified with high frequency. This diagnostic pattern points to the holistic observations of nurses. Finally, although only five (29%) clients had poor grooming and three (18%) had poor general cleanliness, the diagnosis, self-care deficit, potential for, was listed as a potential problem for this population of clients. An important consideration is that 11 (65%) of these clients were interviewed in an inpatient setting, where hygiene is a part of nursing care.

These data served to introduce the computerization format for a holistic assessment tool for psychiatric/mental health nursing. The assessment instrument incorporates physical and psychiatric data into a complete picture of the patient. Use of a computerization method for data entry, retrieval, and analysis has several implications for suggestions for further research. A research project beyond this pilot study could be the analysis of subjective and objective material for clients in several diagnostic categories. The questions may be: are the defining characteristics similar, are the diagnoses similar, or are there particular nursing diagnoses for specific DSM-III diagnoses? An end result may be the planning of interventions to resolve specific nursing diagnoses within a functional health category. In summary, exploration of all available nursing-oriented computer programs will create a final standardized assessment tool for use by the nurse in the 21st century. It will be a step into the future for psychiatric-mental health assessment.

REFERENCES

American Psychiatric Association: Diagnostic and Statistical Manual of Mental Disorders, Washington, 1983, American Psychiatric Association.

American Nurses' Association: Massachusetts governor sued for bargaining interference, Amer. Nurse **45**:1, 1983.

Andreoli, K., and Musser, L.: Computers in nursing care: the state of the art, Nurs. Outlook, **33**:16-21, 1985.

Dawson, J.: The use of computers in public health nursing: today or tomorrow? Canad. Nurse **4**:40-44, 1985.

Gordon, M.: Determining study topics, Nurs. Res. **29**:83-86, 1980.

Gordon, M.: Nursing diagnosis: process and application, New York, 1982, McGraw-Hill.

Haggerty, B: Psychiatric—mental health assessment, St. Louis, 1984, The C.V. Mosby Co.

Kneisl, C., and Wilson, H.: Handbook of psychosocial nursing care, Reading, MA, 1985, Addison-Wesley Co.

Lagina, S.: A computer program to diagnose anxiety level, Nurs. Res. **20**:484-492, 1971.

Martin, K.: A client classification system adaptable for computerization, Nurs. Outlook **30**:515-517, 1982.

Newman, M.: Nursing diagnosis: looking at the whole, Amer. J. Nurs. **84**:1496-1499, 1984.

Nie, N.H., Hull, C.H., Jenkins, J., and others: Statistical Package for the Social Sciences, ed. 2, New York, 1975, McGraw-Hill.

Saba, V.: The computer in public health: today and tomorrow, Nurs. Outlook **30**:510-513, 1982.

Soares, C.: Nursing and medical diagnoses: A comparison of variant and essential features. In Chaska N., editor: The nursing profession: views through the mist, New York, 1978, McGraw-Hill.

Vincent, K.: The validation of a nursing diagnosis: a nurse consensus survey, Nurs. Clin. North Amer. **20**:631-639, 1985.

Wright, C.: Computer aided nursing diagnosis for community health nurses, Nurs. Clin. North Amer. **20**:487-495, 1985.

Sleep pattern disturbance: nursing interventions perceived by patients and their nurses as facilitating nocturnal sleep in hospital

MARLENE REIMER, M.N., R.N.

Sleep pattern disturbance is a frequent problem among hospitalized patients. Alteration in environment (Thiessen and Lapointe 1983), illness (Williams 1978), invasive procedures (Adam 1982), anxiety (Crisp 1976) and disruption of habits (Adam 1980) have been shown to affect the quality and quantity of night-time sleep. Hospitalization involves varying degrees of all of the above for most patients.

Traditional interventions are discussed in many nursing texts and articles, but there is little research-based evidence as to their effectiveness. In a nationwide study by the American Association of Critical Care Nurses, the question "What are the most effective ways of promoting optimum sleep-rest patterns in the critically ill patient and preventing sleep deprivation?" (Lewandowski and Kositsky 1983, p. 39) was ranked as the top research priority.

PURPOSE

The purpose of this study was to determine what nursing interventions are perceived by patients and nurses as facilitating nocturnal sleep in hospital. Perceived etiologies and congruency of patients' and nurses' perceptions were also examined.

This initial study contributes to the development of testable hypotheses as to the efficacy of selected interventions for sleep pattern disturbance in hospitalized patients.

Conceptual framework

Roy's adaptation model provided the conceptual framework (Roy 1984). Interventions were defined as those actions taken by nurses to modify stimuli identified as affecting sleep in hospital.

METHOD

A descriptive study was designed in which patients and nurses on 13 medical and surgical units of a large general hospital were given self-completion questionnaires. The study was undertaken in three phases: instrument development, pilot study and main study.

Instruments

Separate but similar questionnaires for patients and nurses were developed. Questionnaire design incorporated open-ended questions to elicit etiologies and interventions identified by patients and nurses. Fixed alternative questions followed to facilitate quantitative analysis and measures of internal consistency. The etiologies and interventions included in fixed alternative questions were those identified in the literature as well as those observed and reported by practicing nurses. Questions from the St. Mary's Hospital Sleep Questionnaire (Ellis, Johns, Lancaster, Raptopoulos, Angelopoulos and Priest 1981) were incorporated to compare patients' sleep patterns in hospital and home environments.

Content validity was supported through extensive literature review, blueprinting and a two-stage review panel process. Evidence for construct validity was sought by using the known group technique. During pilot testing 21 volunteers, who had not been hospitalized for 3 or more years, were matched by age and sex with the patient sample. As expected those who had no recent hospital experience differed regarding perceptions of sleep in hospital but were comparable on perceptions of sleep at home.

Reliability on responses to similar questions was 0.84 (Cronbach's alpha). Zero-order correlations on responses to related open-ended and fixed alternative items ranged from 0.6 to 1.00. These questions differed somewhat on content focus as well as format.

Sample

Questionnaires were completed by a stratified, criterion/convenience sample of 143 patients and 157 nurses from 13 medical and surgical units of a large general hospital. All patients had been hospitalized for at least 2 nights and were classified as Level 1 or 2 by the Medicus system. Nurses had to be full-time or permanent part-time employees who rotated onto or worked permanent evening or night shifts. Response rates were 81.7% for patients and 61.6% for nurses.

Procedure

A two-stage process of data collection involved patients the first week and nurses the second week. Two research assistants selected patients meeting the criteria from classification sheets and verification with head nurses. A random numbers table was used if more than 15 eligible patients were identified on a unit. Where fewer than 10 patients were available the process was repeated on subsequent days.

The research assistants delivered questionnaires to selected patients, explained the purpose and emphasized confidentiality and the freedom to refuse. If consent was obtained the questionnaire was left with the patients and collection was arranged for later the same day.

All nursing staff on the involved units who met the criteria and were scheduled to work within the next 96 hours were provided with a nursing questionnaire, consent form and return envelopes.

RESULTS

Patients reported significant differences between hospital and home sleeping patterns. The mean sleep latency in hospital was 39 minutes compared to 21.6 minutes at home ($t(63) = 2.35$, $p < .05$). Time awake during the night in hospital averaged 60.2 minutes in contrast to 17.5 minutes at home ($t(63) = 4.74$, $p < .001$). The number of awakenings during the night while in hospital ($M = 2.4$) was also higher than at home ($M = 1.4$), ($t(89) = 4.33$, $p < .001$). A trend towards longer total nocturnal sleep time at home ($M = 7.19$ hours) was evident, but the difference was not statistically significant ($M = 6.01$, $t(89) = -1.85$, $p < .068$). Daytime sleep in hospital ($M = 1.2$ hours) was over double that at home ($M = 0.5$), ($t(89) = 3.66$, $p < .001$).

Only 20.9% of patients awakened spontaneously in the morning. The majority who were awakened by staff would have preferred to sleep. One-third of those so disturbed believed that the awakening was unnecessary.

Etiologies

Qualitative analysis of responses to questions such as "What was hardest about getting to sleep last night?" suggested four themes: pain and discomfort, worry, inability to relax, and environmental stimuli. The need to void was an additional stimulus cited frequently in questions concerning perceived cause of awakening.

In later fixed-alternative questions patients identified difficulty finding a comfortable position (56.7%) and pain (51.7%) as the most frequent etiologies. When asked to select those stimuli that were most disturbing to sleep in hospital, patients chose pain (44.6%) and position (31.7%) in a reversed order of priority (Table 1). Worry

Table 1: Most frequent etiologies as perceived by patients (XXX) and nurses (////)

	%	50	100
Pain	XXXXXXXX /////////////		
Position	XXXXXX ////		
Fear of dislodging tubing	XXX /		
Dressing, cast discomfort	XXX /		
Worry: tests, surgery	XXXX ////////		
Worry: diagnosis	XXXX ///		
Worry: family, job	XXX /		
Awakening for treatments	XX ///////		
Noise: patients	XXX ////		
Noise: nurses	XX /		
Light	XX		
Uncomfortable bed	XX //		
Temperature	XXX		

Table 2: Percentage of patients and nurses choosing selected interventions as very important

Intervention	Patients %	Nurses %
Pain medication	51.5	91.7
Sleep medication	43.7	56.7
Lights down	60.8	78.3
Back rub	48.0	56.0
Voiding	36.0	87.3
Security (nurse available)	47.6	77.7
Teeth brushed	31.1	43.0
Bedclothes straightened	25.5	61.1

ranked next, both in frequency and importance.

Nurses emphasized pain as an etiology but were less aware of patients' concerns with positional discomfort, attached equipment and personal worries regarding health, family and occupation (Table 1). Nurses chose being awakened for treatments as one of the three most disturbing stimuli three times more often than did patients. Similarly nurses were twice as likely as patients to choose worry about tests and noise from other patients.

Interventions

Qualitative analysis of responses to open-ended questions suggest intervention categories related to: environmental control, medication management, and relaxation.

Fatigue or staying up later was mentioned by 16.9% of the patients as something that would be helpful to improving their sleep in hospital.

The interventions most frequently mentioned by nurses in open-ended responses were back rub and related "comfort measures" (58.8%), medication (50.7%), change of position (31.1%), supportive communication (30%), snack or drink (30%), turning the lights down (27%), and ensuring quiet (18.2%).

Neither patients nor nurses mentioned hygiene care as a sleep-promoting intervention in open-ended responses, yet these activities were among the top eight selected by patients as very important (Table 2).

When given a choice of 20 common interventions both patients and nurses chose pain medication, turning lights down, the security of knowing nurses were available, void-

Table 3: Factor analysis of interventions perceived by nurses as important to patient's sleep

Variables	Factors		
	1	2	3
Back rub	0.26	0.45	0.18
Face wash	0.13	0.10	0.75
Teeth brushed	0.16	0.15	0.71
Bed straightened	0.22	0.74	0.08
Room tidied	−0.13	0.48	0.05
Security (nurse available)	0.46	0.20	0.13
Position changed	0.52	0.13	−0.06
Bathroom/bedpan	0.61	−0.15	0.23
Lights down	0.69	0.28	0.04
Pain medication	0.83	0.00	0.20
. . .			
Eigenvalue	3.69	1.56	1.01
% explained variance	41.2	17.4	11.3

Varimax rotated factor matrix
Principal factor with iterations

ing, a back rub and sleep medication among the eight most important.

These differences were further supported through factor analysis. The three factors that explained 68% of the patient variance represented hygiene measures, medication for pain and sleep, and dimensions of social interaction. A cluster of "settling activities" accounted for 41% of the variance among nurses (Table 3).

DISCUSSION

The prevalence of sleep pattern disturbance in hospital was supported insofar as the defining characteristics of difficulty in falling asleep, awakening earlier than desired and interrupted sleep (Kim, McFarland and McLane 1984) were reported by the majority of patients. The clinical significance of these findings is less clear given the wide range of normal variations among and within individuals (Kripke, Simons, Garfinkel, and Hammond 1979).

Patients who met the criteria were the mild to moderately ill, precluding generalization to all patients on medical-surgical units even in the test hospital. However, it was the investigator's belief that for this descriptive study it was more appropriate to select patients from an accessible population for whom participation was an opportunity for self-expression rather than an added stressor as might have been the case with acutely ill persons.

Patients were most likely to identify the difficulty in finding a comfortable position and pain as disturbing stimuli. DeKonnick, Gagnon and Lallier (1983), in one of the few studies on body position and sleep, found that subjects averaged 30 position changes per night with a mean of 14 minutes per position. Poor sleepers were more likely to spend prolonged periods on their back with their head straight than were good sleepers. The potential relationship between sleep pattern disturbance and impaired physical mobility should be investigated further. In that pain may be an etiology of sleep pattern disturbance or a contributing factor to impaired mobility, the effectiveness of pain management techniques on sleep outcomes needs to be explored.

Environmental stimuli such as light, temperature, noise and quality of bed were cited as disturbing to sleep with sufficient frequency to suggest a clinically important group of patients for whom sleep pattern disturbance may be decreased through simple modifications of the environment. Building on existing research on the effects of noise on sleep, conducted in sleep laboratory (Thiessen and Lapointe 1983), and acute care settings (Minckley 1968, Woods and Falk, 1974), a further quasi-experimental study examining the relationships between selected noise-reducing interventions and patient sleep outcomes is recommended.

Differences between patients and nurses in describing etiologies and interventions for sleep pattern disturbance suggest the need to consider these differences in the design of further studies.

REFERENCES

Adam, K.: Dietary habits and sleep after bedtime food drinks, Sleep 3:47-58, 1980.

Adam, K.: Sleep is changed by blood sampling through an indwelling venous catheter, Sleep 5:154-158, 1982.

Crisp, A.: Sleep, nutrition and mood, Toronto, 1976, John Wiley & Sons.

DeKonnick, J., Gagnon, P., and Lallier, S.: Sleep positions in the young adult and their relationship with the subjective quality of sleep, Sleep 6:52-59, 1983.

Ellis, B., Johns, M., Lancaster, R., and others: The St. Mary's Hospital sleep questionnaire: a study of reliability, Sleep 4:93-97, 1981.

Kim, M., McFarland, G., and McLane, A.: Pocket guide to nursing diagnosis, St. Louis, 1984, The C.V. Mosby Co.

Kripke, H., Simons, R., Garfinkel, L., and others: Short and long sleep and sleeping pills: is increased mortality associated? Arch. Gen. Psych. 36:103-116, 1979.

Lewandowski, L., and Kositsky, A.: Research priorities for critical care nursing: a study by the American Association of Critical-Care Nurses. Heart Lung 12: 35-44, 1983.

Minckley, B.: A study of noise and its relationship to patient discomfort in the recovery room, Nurs. Res. 17:247-253, 1968.

Roy, C.: Introduction to nursing: an adaptation model. Englewood Cliffs, N.J., 1984, Prentice-Hall.

Thiessen, G., and Lapointe, A.: Effect of continuous traffic noise on percentage of deep sleep, waking and sleep latency, J. Acoustic Soc. Amer. 73:225-229, 1983.

Williams, R.: Sleep disturbance in various medical and surgical conditions. In Williams, R., and Karacan, I., editors: Sleep disorders: diagnosis and treatment, Toronto, 1978, John Wiley and Sons.

Woods, N., and Falk, S.: Noise stimuli in the acute care area. Nurs. Res. 23:144-150, 1974.

Documenting nursing diagnosis using focus charting

SUSAN S. LAMPE, M.S., R.N.
ADRIENNE HITCHOCK, B.Ed., R.N.

Accurate and complete documentation is an essential component of quality patient care. The patient chart must reflect the changing patient status, the plan of care, all treatments performed, and the patient's response to medical and nursing interventions. The challenge is to arrange all this information in a logical, organized fashion.

The traditional nurses' notes format is the narrative, block-style note. Limitations of this format include lack of organization, no assistance in analytical problem solving, difficult data retrieval, and no identified relationship to the nursing process.

One attempt to address these shortcomings was presented by Weed (1971) with the introduction of the Problem-Oriented Medical Record (POMR) which organizes the patient record around a list of specific problems. Although this system was designed by a physician for use in episodic care, nursing also began using the system, recording nurses' notes in the SOAP (subjective, objective, assessment, plan) format. Difficulties with nurses using the SOAP format have been documented in the literature (Popkess-Vater 1984 and Flinstein 1973). The most consistent abuse of the system by nursing is limiting the definition of the patient "problem" to the statement of the medical diagnoses. This creates a *medical* record, where patient data are documented from the medical discipline of illness and pathology in preference to the nursing perspective of human response to a health problem.

In 1981, staff nurses at Eitel Hospital in Minneapolis, Minnesota, who had been using POMR for 3½ years, began to voice frustration with it. They formed a committee, with the author as chair, to review the nursing documentation system. The first step in the review process was to develop a standard for patient care notes which was based on the nursing process. The major categories of the standard were:

I. There is documentation of a nursing assessment of the patient's ability to care for himself.
  A. There is a description of the patient's current status at least every 24 hours.
  B. Documentation reflects identification of nursing and medical diagnoses.
II. The nursing plan of care is documented for each concern identified.
III. There is documentation for all nursing care provided to the patient.
IV. Evaluation of the patient response to therapy is documented.

CHART AUDIT

An audit of SOAP notes in 100 randomly selected patient charts was completed to determine whether the content of the notes matched the standard. Medical-surgical and critical care patient charts were included in the audit. The auditors were members of the charting committee who had developed the standard and were most familiar with the intent and definitions of the standard. Records were maintained to insure that 100 separate patient charts were audited.

A variety of deficiencies in the content of the nurses notes were revealed. Implementation was the only step of the nursing process which scored higher than 20% (Table 1).

Analysis of the audited charts disclosed that nurses were "filling in the blanks" in the SOAP format rather than documenting

Table 1: Analysis of the content of nurses narrative notes before and after focus charting

	% Before	% After 6 weeks	% After 8 months	% Before	% After 5 months
Topic identified is a patient concern	12	64	55	17	96
Supporting data present				13	96
Plan of care is documented for each concern identified	18	67	48	17	92
Documentation for all nursing care provided to patient	85	91	77	10	92
The patient response to therapy is evaluated	12	67	51	10	62

N = 100
Eitel Hospital
Minneapolis, Minnesota
100-bed, urban

N = 30
Memorial Hospital
Cambridge, Minnesota
86-bed, rural

the analytical thinking and problem solving which was occurring in patient care. A major weakness was that "problem" was most often a statement of the medical diagnosis. Mixing the documentation of medical and nursing diagnoses caused the notes to be disjointed and disorganized. No logical progression could be made from the problem statement to the documentation of independent nursing activities. Furthermore, there was no "cue" for documentation of the patient response to therapy. This resulted in poor audit scores.

PROBLEM STATEMENT

Nurses notes provide inadequate documentation and communication of patient care due to the absence of a charting system based on the nursing process.

A NEW CHARTING SYSTEM

The Eitel documentation committee chose to handle the problems revealed in the chart audit by developing a new charting format for the care plan and narrative notes. Focus charting features a column format with the heading of FOCUS to organize data in the narrative notes of the patient record and on the care plan. A FOCUS is defined as a current patient concern or behavior, an acute change in the patient condition, or a significant event in the patient's therapy (Lampe 1984). A FOCUS is identified as an outcome of nursing assessment. Thus, one definition for FOCUS is nursing diagnosis.

FOCUS appears on both the care plan and the narrative notes providing a unifying format. Focus charting supports the nurse's documentation of all steps of the nursing process. The body of the notes in Focus charting is organized into the categories Data, Action, and Response. Assessment information becomes Data in the patient care notes. The three-part nursing diagnosis (problem, etiology and defining characteristics) is stated as the Focus on the care plan. A key word or phrase from the nursing diagnosis is carried from the care plan to the Focus column in the narrative notes. The care plan is written in ink and is a permanent part of the patient record. Action documents the nurses' activities in carrying out the plan of care and the delegated medical functions. Response documents the patient response to therapy indicating whether a care plan goal has been reached or a Focus resolved (Fig. 1).

Focus charting was introduced at Eitel Hospital in June, 1981. At that time every member of the nursing staff attended either a 2-hour inservice education class presented by the author, or completed a self-learning workbook in which the principles of Focus charting were presented and practice sessions conducted. Education included review of the nursing process and emphasis on the relationship between the nursing process and focus charting. Both the inservice education attendees and staff who completed the workbook were required to successfully complete a written test. The goal was to teach nurses to evaluate and to document the patient's needs using categories describing human responses rather than language describing nursing tasks or medical diagnoses. Initially, informal language (chest pain, nausea, activity tolerance, appetite) was encouraged to promote ease of understanding and greater flexibility of the system. Introduction of nursing diagnosis terminology was planned as a future activity.

REPEAT CHART AUDIT

Six weeks after the introduction of Focus charting, the chart audit was repeated on 100 randomly selected patient charts using the same documentation standard. The original auditors repeated this task. Records were maintained so that 100 separate charts were audited. The auditor judged whether the FOCUS identified was a patient concern or behavior (rather than a medical diagnosis) and whether the content of nursing notes over one 48-hour period included a plan of action for each concern identified, and the patient response to care provided. Docu-

mentation of nursing actions (care provided) was acceptable if entered on the activities flow sheet or in the text of the narrative notes.

The results of the second audit showed dramatic improvement in documentation of all steps of the nursing process (Table 1). The content of nurses notes in the second audit identified a patient concern 64% compared to 12% in the first audit. Also, information on plan of care and patient response rose from 18% and 12% to 67%. Implementation was recorded in 91% of charts.

After the initial inservice, no formal documentation inservice or management programs were presented. A third audit of 100 randomly selected charts in April, 1982, 8 months after implementation of Focus charting revealed an expected leveling off of scores. However, scores remained much improved over the original, pre-Focus charting audit with the exception of "implementation" (Table 1).

MEMORIAL HOSPITAL EXPERIENCE

In October of 1982, the nursing staff of Memorial Hospital in Cambridge, Minnesota, began an evaluation of their charting system. For several years these nurses also had used the POMR format for documenting nursing care; and they too, experienced frustration. This was evidenced by an increase in negative comments about the nurses' notes from both nursing and medical staff. Nurses demonstrated their frustration with charting by repeatedly leaving it as the last task of the shift.

A chart audit using nursing process criteria similar to Eitel Hospital was conducted with the addition of a category "supporting data are present." Chart entries from 30 different nurses were audited. Scores consistently below 20% were evidence of inadequate documentation even though subjective measures indicated adequate patient care was being delivered (Table 1).

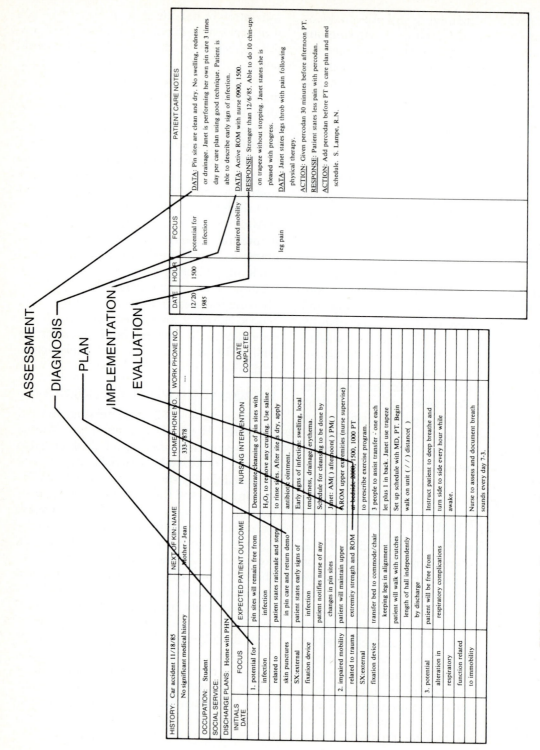

FIGURE 1 Focus charting sample with care plan showing documentation of nursing process.

A task force including head nurses and the education director reviewed a variety of measures for the purpose of improving the content of the nurses' notes. They selected Focus charting. Inservice education was provided for all nursing personnel. The same self-learning materials developed at Eitel Hospital were readily adapted for use at Memorial Hospital.

Five months after the introduction of Focus Charting, the task force at Memorial Hospital conducted a second audit of nurses' notes from 30 different nurses. A marked improvement in documentation of the nursing process was recorded. In the second Memorial Hospital audit, only the category of patient response to therapy showed less than 90% compliance (Table 1).

DISCUSSION

In studying the results of these before and after audits, the initial question is how to separate the effect of the inservice education from the effect of the new system itself (Hawthorne effect). It is believed that the drop in percentages found in the 8-month follow-up audit at Eitel Hospital is related to the drop in attention by management to the specific area of documentation. The figures in the 8-month follow-up audit are believed to more accurately represent the effects of the charting system alone. While the third Eitel Hospital audit represents a considerable improvement in the content of the notes compared to pre-Focus charting levels, it is also clear that documentation is an area which demands constant attention by management with frequent and specific attention to the content of nurses' notes through such mechanisms as inservice education, chart audit and individual staff evaluation during annual performance appraisal.

Focus charting provides two major changes in format from the POMR or SOAP charting. First, Focus charting includes the "cue" *response* which facilitates documen-

tation of the evaluation step of the nursing process. SOAP does not include a cue for documenting evaluation unless the form SOAPE or SOAPIER is adopted. In the Eitel Hospital audit, the percentage of nurses' notes which included statements regarding the patient response to therapy increased from 12% to 51% after 8 months. Documentation of patient response to therapy is the primary purpose of narrative nurses' notes. Whereas other steps of the nursing process may be documented on other chart forms (assessment and implementation on flow sheets and plan on the care plan) there is no other chart form where analysis of care is located. Documentation of patient response is central to relating current patient status to care plan goals. Documentation of the patient response is essential to complete the nursing process cycle. The presence of the *response* "cue" is key to documentation of nursing process.

Secondly, in Focus charting the use of the column title *focus* is significant, because it alters the negative connotation of the term *problem* which usually means something is wrong or abnormal. However, many nursing assessments anticipate potential problems and seek to define nursing interventions that will prevent the development of an abnormal or harmful response to a health problem. For many years the only formal taxonomy for labeling the patient's problem was the medical diagnosis. Today a taxonomy of nursing diagnoses is available that focuses on human responses (Hurley 1986). Some authors (Popkess-Vater 1984, Martens 1986) are calling for nursing diagnosis to be less problem-oriented and to reflect strengths. Changing the identity of the topic on the care plan and in the nurses' notes from *problem* to *focus* can support the education of staff to use the taxonomy of nursing diagnosis and meet the need to identify the patient strengths as well as limitations.

If nursing diagnoses are to become an integral part of patient care, it is essential that a documentation system which facilitates the organization and recording of nursing process and nursing diagnosis be developed. Focus charting provides a flexible format to meet these goals.

CONCLUSIONS

- Changing the title of the column in the narrative notes from *problem* to *focus* assisted staff nurses to identify and document patient concerns.
- Focus charting, including a column format for narrative notes using *focus*, *data*, *action*, *response* and a care plan which is a permanent record, provides a format for documentation of nursing process.

- Implementation of Focus charting resulted in improved content in nurses' notes.

REFERENCES

Feinstein, A.R.: The problems of the problem oriented medical record, Ann. Intern. Med. **78**:751, 1973.

Hurley, M.E.: Classification of nursing diagnoses: proceedings of the sixth conference, St. Louis, 1986, The C.V. Mosby Co.

Lampe, S.: Focus charting: a patient-centered approach, ed. 2, Minneapolis, 1984, Creative Nursing Management.

Martens, K.: Let's diagnose strengths, not just problems, Amer. J. Nurs. **86**:192, 1986.

Popkess-Vater, S.: Strength-oriented nursing diagnoses. In Kim, M.J., McFarland, G.K., and McLane, A.M., editors: Classification of nursing diagnoses: proceedings of the fifth national conference, St. Louis, 1984, The C.V. Mosby Co.

Weed, L.: Medical records, medical education, patient care, Chicago, 1971, Year Book Medical Publishers.

A replication study evaluating the use of a focused data collection tool for the generation of nursing diagnoses

THERESE M. DOWD, M.S., R.N.
ANGELYNN M. GRABAU, M.S.N., R.N.
MARY R. KOLBE, M.S.N., R.N.
DAWNEANE K. MUNN, M.S.N., R.N.
BARBARA W. McCABE, Ph.D., R.N.
DONNA R. SMITH, M.S., R.N.

Nursing diagnosis has been heralded as a means to refine the scientific basis of the practice of nursing. Difficulty in formulating nursing diagnoses that are supported by appropriate data has become an increasing concern among nurses. Historically, this process has been hampered by use of the medical model for nursing assessment. There is a need to identify strategies based on a nursing model which lead to the formulation of valid nursing diagnoses.

A recent study by Levin and Crosley (in press) indicates that a nursing-focused data-collection instrument fosters formulation and documentation of valid nursing diagnoses. In an effort to replicate the findings obtained by Levin and Crosley, a study was conducted that addressed the question: Does the use of a focused data collection tool increase documentation of valid nursing diagnoses?

There is a paucity of literature and research relating the need for focused assessment tools to the development of valid nursing diagnoses. Gordon states, "data must be relevant to areas of nursing concern if the purpose of data collection is nursing diagnosis" (Gordon 1982, p. 216). Cianfrani (1984) supports Gordon. He found that collection of "low-relevant data" resulted in a decrease of accuracy in identification of health problems. He identifies the need for further research to determine cues that are relevant to health problems treated by nurses.

The foundation for the formulation of valid nursing diagnoses is a specific assessment format that promotes the collection of sufficient and relevant data. Problems arise in the development of these diagnoses not because of a lack of nursing knowledge but rather because of assessment tools that do not lead to the generation of sufficient and relevant data. Therefore, the format of the assessment tool is crucial.

METHODOLOGY

An audit of nursing assessment forms from 66 purposively selected charts of two inpatient units of a midwestern veterans' medical center was conducted using a nursing process audit tool developed by Levin and Crosley (in press). Thirty-three charts using the nursing department's original assessment instrument were audited. Standardized teaching sessions were conducted with nursing staff to introduce a focused data collection instrument. The new form was used for 1 month with each patient admitted to the two clinical areas. At the end of the month, 33 chart audits were conducted retrospectively to determine if the focused data collection instrument increased the documentation of valid nursing diagnoses.

The following definitions were assigned to terms/concepts used in this study:

- *Valid nursing diagnosis:* a statement of clinical judgment that describes "actual or potential health problems which nurses, by virtue of their education and experience are capable and licensed to treat" (Gordon, 1976, p. 1229). The valid nursing diagnostic statement must have two components: (1) a NANDA-approved stem and (2) a connecting phrase ("related to").
- *Focused data collection instrument:* a guide used to assist nurses in collecting appropriate data needed to develop a valid nursing diagnosis statement. The instrument was based on Gordon's Functional Health Patterns. These 11 health patterns form a framework for organizing a nursing assessment based on function (Gordon 1982).

The following underlying assumptions were basic to this study:

- A valid nursing diagnosis is derived from an interpretation and analysis of collected data.
- A specific focus facilitates progression toward a goal.
- The focused data collection instrument will cue the individual as to appropriate data needed for valid nursing diagnosis formulation.

The data obtained from this study were nominal in nature. Data were analyzed using statistical measures of frequencies, Friedman's t, and percentages. The level of significance was set at the p≤0.05 level. Interrater reliability for the audit tool was established at .92 based on six consecutive chart audits by six trained data collectors.

DATA ANALYSIS

Descriptive statistics were used to analyze the data. Table 1 presents pretest-posttest results of the frequencies and percentages for the nursing diagnostic statement and its components.

Of the total number of diagnostic statements (n=89) documented in audited patient records, 14 (33%) were found to meet criteria of a valid nursing diagnosis using the original assessment form. The number of valid diagnostic statements increased to 27 (59%) when the focused assessment format was used. This increase was significant at the p≤.01 level (Friedman's t).

Both components of a valid nursing diagnosis showed a significant increase at the p≤.01 level. The standardized stem was present in 100% (n=46) of the diagnostic

Table 1: Comparison of frequencies and percentages for the nursing diagnostic statement and its component with use of the original and focused instruments

	Valid diagnoses	Components	
		Standardized stems	Connecting phrases
Original instrument	14 (33%) N=43	36 (84%) N=43	15 (35%) N=43
Focused instrument	27 (59%) N=46	46 (100%) N=46	27 (59%) N=46
Percentage difference	26% p<.01*	16% p<.01*	24% p<.01*

*Friedman's t

statements made with use of the focused assessment instrument. This was a 16% increase when compared with those diagnoses generated from data collected with the original format, in which 36 or 84% (n=43) of documented diagnoses contained a standard stem.

Of the 43 diagnostic statements audited in patient records using the original form, 15 (35%) contained a "related to" connecting phrase. With use of the focused format for patient assessment the number of diagnostic statements containing a connecting phrase was 27 or 59% (n=46). This increase was significant at the $p \leq .01$ level (Friedman's t).

Patient records were also audited to determine whether diagnostic statements could be validated by data documented in the patient record (Table 2). With the original instrument 38 or 88% (n=43) of nursing diagnoses were found to have data supporting the diagnosis. Validating data were found in 100% (n=46) of patient records using the focused assessment instrument. This increase was significant at the $p \leq .01$ level (Friedman's t).

There was an increase (p=.05) in data supporting diagnoses documented on the focused assessment form. Thirty-seven (80%) of diagnoses made (n=46) with the focused

instrument contained supporting data on that form, while 31 (72%) of diagnostic statements (n=43) made with the original tool were supported by data found on that form.

Although most diagnoses were validated with data obtained from nursing assessment, there were data found elsewhere in the client record that supported the nurses' diagnoses. Seven (16%) of the 43 nursing diagnoses using the original instrument and nine (23%) of the 46 nursing diagnoses using the focused tool were found to be supported by data documented by other health professionals.

Finally, five (12%) of nursing diagnoses (n=43) using the original instrument were made without any documented supporting data. In contrast, all 46 (100%) of the nursing diagnoses made using the focused instrument were validated with documented data from the patient record.

DISCUSSION AND IMPLICATIONS

Analysis of data supports the findings of Levin and Crosley (in press). A focused data collection instrument does increase the number of valid nursing diagnoses generated. The cues which were added to the original assessment form may have led to more specific documented data. It should be noted that nurses at this institution were

Table 2: Comparison of frequencies and percentages for documented data validating nursing diagnoses and their sources

| | Validating data | Data sources | | |
		Nursing assessment	Elsewhere	No supporting data
Original instrument	38 (88%) N=43	31 (72%) N=43	7 (16%) N=43	5 (12%) N=43
Focused instrument	46 (100%) N=46	37 (80%) N=46	9 (20%) N=46	0 (0%) N=46
Percentage difference	12% p<.01*	8% p<.05*	4% p<.05*	12% p<.05*

*Friedman's t

familiar with writing nursing diagnoses using the standardized stem. Thus, it was not surprising that with the use of both assessment forms there was a high percentage of diagnoses made that met the criteria of a NANDA-approved stem.

Documentation of the etiology of the problem based on appropriate data improved significantly with the use of the focused tool. Not all nursing diagnoses had supportive data documented when using the original tool, but all nursing diagnoses were validated with documented data when the focused tool was used.

An unexpected finding, however, showed that although there was an increase in data documented on the focused assessment supporting the diagnosis, some diagnoses were validated by data found elsewhere in the patient record (e.g., physician's history and physical, progress notes and physician's consults). This finding raised the question as to what factors led the nurse to look elsewhere in the patient record for data to validate a nursing diagnosis.

We are unable to explain the reason for an increase in the number of diagnoses validated from sources other than nursing assessment with use of the focused instrument. It may be postulated that: (1) the nurses became increasingly aware of the need to validate a diagnosis and used other sources to do so; (2) the focused tool did not always meet the needs of the nurses and thus they sought validating data elsewhere.

The third postulation concerns the type of patient admitted during use of the focused instrument. Forty-two percent (14) of the patients assessed with the focused format had a hospital stay of less than 5 days. Because the medical diagnoses of those patients admitted during the period when the focused tool was used did not necessitate extensive hospitalization, the nurses may not have done as detailed an admission assessment as they did on patients who were expected to be in the hospital for a more protracted stay and thus, used data from other sources to support their diagnoses. In all cases, however, the researchers found that the nursing assessment history was complete in all areas. It may be wise to assess the need for a less extensive nursing assessment form for those patients whose hospital stay will not be longer than 3 to 5 days.

With continued use of a focused assessment instrument, nurses will be able to sort through the myriad of subjective and objective data found in the patient record and to identify the germane data leading to a valid nursing diagnostic statement. Certainly the focused format will help to generate nursing diagnoses based on fact rather than supposition, and diagnoses will be made from a nursing rather than a medical viewpoint.

In summary, the introduction of a new focused nursing assessment form using Gordon's Functional Health Pattern Areas as an organizing framework for data collection, increased the documentation of valid nursing diagnoses by staff nurses in an acute care setting. In further analysis, the study indicated an increase in the documentation of supporting data found in the nursing assessment form.

The study supports findings of Levin and Crosley (in press) whose results also indicated "that the focus or perspective which nurses use to collect data influences their ability to generate valid nursing diagnoses." The findings underscore the importance of evaluating current instruments used to assess patients. Nurses should also consider using a focused instrument based on a nursing framework to increase identification and documentation of patient problems. The focused tool may increase the accuracy of nursing observations documented for legal and accreditation purposes. Based on the findings of this study, the researchers believe a focused patient assessment instrument has the potential to assist in refining the essential elements of a professional nursing practice.

REFERENCES

Cianfrani, K.: The influence of amounts and relevances of data on identifying health problems. In Kim, M.J., McFarland, G.K., and McLane, A.M. editors: Classification of nursing diagnoses: proceedings of the fifth national conference, St. Louis, 1984, The C.V. Mosby Co.

Gordon, M.: Nursing diagnosis and the diagnostic process, Amer. J., Nurs. **76:**1298-1300, 1976.

Gordon, M.: Nursing diagnoses: Practice and application, New York, 1982, McGraw-Hill.

Levin, R., and Crosley, J.: Focused data collection for the generation of nursing diagnoses, J. Staff Develop. (in press).

Nursing process study: abstract

Organization of patient assessment data and nursing diagnosis

PAULINE T. DION, M.S., R.N.
JOAN B. FITZMAURICE, Ph.D., R.N., F.A.A.N.
CAROL A. BAER, M.S., R.N.

The purpose of this experimental study was to examine the relationship between the organization of patient assessment data and the identification of nursing diagnoses. The specific research hypothesis tested was that there would be a difference in the number and correctness of nursing diagnoses from data organized according to the Functional Health Patterns (FHP) and Biomedical Systems (BMS).

Similar patient data, consisting of 138 cues, were placed into the two formats. Content validity was addressed through expert review. The case study contained sufficient data for six nursing diagnoses, namely, exogenous obesity, fear of dependency, intermittent constipation, potential health management deficit, sleep pattern disturbance, and value conflict.

Following informed consent, 121 full-time registered nurses, employed at a tertiary hospital in eastern Massachusetts, were randomly assigned to receive the FHP (N=62) or BMS (N=59) case study. The groups were similar with regard to years of practice, spe-cialty, and advanced degrees. A higher percentage of the nurses in the BMS group had baccalaureate degrees in nursing ($\chi^2 = 5.4$, $P <.05$), while more of the nurses in the FHP group received their basic education in nursing in an associate degree program ($\chi^2 = 4.1$, $P<.05$).

Subjects completed the task during one 1-hour session, in a classroom setting away from the clinical area. The principal investigator was present during all data collection sessions. Included with the case study (which also contained pertinent data from the physician's history and physical) were preprinted directions and an answer sheet. Each subject was instructed to read the case study and then to list the nursing diagnosis(es) or problem(s).

The major results showed no difference between the two groups. The groups were alike in the mean number of final nursing diagnoses (FHP = 0.6, SD 0.7, Range 0–2, BMS = 0.7, SD 0.7, Range 0–2, t = NS). The most common nursing diagnoses identified were sleep pattern disturbance, potential health management deficit, and intermittent constipation.

Findings suggest that assessment format did not influence the nurses' diagnostic recognition. Further study is necessary before generalization of the findings is warranted. A particularly interesting question would be to examine the data collection process and its influence on the identification of nursing diagnoses.

PART A

Utilization studies: paper presentation

Nursing complexity, the DRG, and length of stay

EDWARD J. HALLORAN, Ph.D., R.N.
MARYLOU KILEY, Ph.D., R.N.
LAURA J. NOSEK, M.S.N., R.N.

INTRODUCTION

Adoption of the DRG to guide prospective payment for hospital care is encouraging nurses toward self-actualization. For years nursing theorists have struggled to define nursing. More recently some effort has been directed toward differentially defining nursing and medicine. The need to measure consumption of nursing resources to estimate nursing care costs for prospective payment focuses attention on correlations between: (a) medicine and nursing, (b) nursing diagnosis and medical diagnosis, and (c) the nursing care of a patient and the patient's prescribed medical diagnosis and treatment regimen.

Exclusive use of medical diagnostic terminology to determine case mix management and hospital reimbursement is based on the premise that all clinical activity directly or indirectly evolves from the medical diagnosis, and is therefore prescribed by physicians. While prescriptions for hospital admission and discharge are written by physicians, there is little agreement by nurses that the care they give their patients is predicated upon there being an established and accurate medical diagnosis. In fact, clas-sic works in nursing do not mention medical diagnosis and treatment at all (Abdellah, et al., 1960; Henderson, 1978; Nightingale, 1969).

The total time nurses spend with patients has been shown to be highly correlated with the length of hospital stay (Caterinicchio and Davies, 1983; Halloran, 1980). If nursing care is prescribed by the medical diagnosis and, therefore, by physicians, then we would expect to find a strong association between medical diagnosis and the amount of time that nurses spend with patients. On the other hand, if nurses practice independently of physicians as suggested in nursing literature, then we can expect nursing time, as measured by length of stay in the hospital, to have a strong association with nursing diagnosis.

It is vitally important to accurately attribute nursing diagnosis and treatment behavior, since nursing accounts for 20 to 30 percent of total hospital expenditure (American Hospital Association, 1983; McKibbin, 1983). If nursing diagnosis and treatment decisions made by skilled nurses are shown to be redundant with medical diagnosis and treatment, then it might be

391

possible to substitute physician protocols for nurses' judgment. If so, non-nurses could simply carry out physician protocols to achieve the same outcomes achieved by nurses using nursing judgment. If, however, nursing care and length of stay are predicted by nursing diagnosis patterns, then it would seem appropriate to shift greater responsibility for hospital length of stay management and for patient discharge prescriptions to nurses.

Purpose

This study examined whether an index of medical diagnosis and treatment patterns differs from an index of nursing diagnosis and treatment patterns in explaining variability in length of hospital stay and, therefore, the time nurses spend with patients.

Hypotheses

The two hypotheses tested in this study were:
H_1: The nursing complexity index predicts length of stay.
H_2: The DRG relative cost weight predicts length of stay.

Definitions

The conceptual and operational definitions used in this study were:
1. *Nursing Diagnosis*—human responses to actual or potential health problems that are identified by nurses and that those nurses, by virtue of their education and experience, are capable and licensed to treat (ANA Congress for Nursing Practice, 1980; Gordon, 1982).

   Operational definition—measured by the patient health conditions identified by nurses on the Nurse/Patient Summary (Fig. 1).
2. *Nursing Complexity*—constellation of different nursing diagnoses assessed for an individual patient (Halloran, 1985).

   Operational definition—measured by the nursing complexity index that is computed by adding the number of different nursing diagnoses present during the hospitalization.
3. *Medical Complexity*—severity of illness, likely outcome, difficulty of treatment, need for timely intervention, and amount and composition of resources used to treat the patient (Luke, 1979).

   Operational definition—measured by the DRG relative cost weight, an index of relative resource consumption assigned to each DRG.

METHOD
Sample

This study used data collected at an urban health science center in the midwestern United States from March through July, 1983. The sample consisted of all patients (n =1294) on four conveniently chosen adult medical and surgical wards. The single criterion for inclusion in the study was that the entire length of stay was within the data collection period.

The sample was heterogeneous in character. The age of the sample ranged from 16 to 97 years, with a mean of 54 years and standard deviation of 19.9 years. There were 611 men and 683 women included. Of these, 605 were treated with some surgical intervention and 623 were treated without surgery. DRGs representing 281 of the 470 DRG categories and 21 of the 23 major diagnostic categories were included. Each nursing diagnosis was identified at least once.

Instruments

The data collected included: (a) the nursing diagnoses identified for each of the 1294 patients by the nurses providing direct nursing care to those patients, (b) the DRG assigned to the case by the GROUPER software program at discharge (Yale University School of

UNIVERSITY HOSPITALS OF CLEVELAND
NURSE/PATIENT SUMMARY

	RN Code Number	Other Code Number	Consultant Code Number
TODAY			
LAST NIGHT			
LAST EVENING			
Primary Nurse Code Number _____			

NAME

HOSP.NO.   DATE

SERVICE

SEX   AGE

DIVISION   ROOM NO.

Date Today_____

DIRECTIONS: Check the items below if Actually or Potentially Present.

HEALTH PERCEPTION-MANAGEMENT

Potential for Injury . . . . _____001
Noncompliance . . . . _____002
Infection/Contagion . . . . _____003
Prolonged Disease/Disability . . . . _____004
Instability . . . . _____005
Impaired Life Support Systems . . . . _____006
Sanitation Deficit . . . . _____007
Socio-cultural-economic Considerations . . . . _____008

NUTRITIONAL-METABOLIC
Fluid
Excess Volume . . . . _____009
Volume Deficit . . . . _____010
Potential Volume Deficit . . . . _____011
Bleeding . . . . _____012
Nutrition
Less Nutrition than Required . . . . . . _____013
More Nutrition than Required . . . . _____014
Potential for Excess . . . . _____015
Skin Integrity
Actual Skin Impairment . . . . _____016
Potential Skin Impairment . . . . _____017
Alterations in Oral Mucous Membrane . . . _____018
Altered Body Temperature . . . . _____019

ELIMINATION
Urinary
Incontinence . . . . _____020
Other Altered Urinary Elim. Pattern 021
Bowel
Constipation . . . . _____022
Diarrhea . . . . _____023
Incontinence . . . . _____024

ACTIVITY-EXERCISE
Activity Intolerance . . . . _____025
Ineffective Airway Clearance . . . . _____026
Altered Breathing Pattern . . . . _____027
Impaired Gas Exchange . . . . _____028
Altered Tissue Perfusion . . . . _____029

Decreased Cardiac Output . . . . _____030
Diversional Activity Deficit . . . . _____031
Altered Health Maintenance . . . . _____032
Impaired Mobility . . . . _____033
Self-Care Deficit . . . . _____034
Impaired Home Maintenance Mgmt. . . . . _____035

COGNITION-PERCEPTION
Altered Comfort
Discomfort . . . . _____036
Pain . . . . _____037
Altered Level of Consciousness . . . . _____038
Altered Thought Process . . . . _____039
Impulsivity/Hyperactivity . . . . _____040
Altered Sensory Perception . . . . _____041
Knowledge Deficit . . . . _____042
Growth and Development Deficit . . . . _____043

SLEEP-REST
Sleep Disturbance . . . . _____044

SELF-PERCEPTION/SELF-CONCEPT
Anxiety . . . . _____045
Disturbed Self-Concept . . . . _____046
Depression . . . . _____047
Fear . . . . _____048
Powerlessness . . . . _____049

ROLE RELATIONSHIPS
Grieving . . . . _____050
Altered Family Process . . . . _____051
Altered Parenting . . . . _____052
Social Isolation . . . . _____053
Impaired Verbal Communication . . . . _____054
Potential for Violence . . . . _____055

SEXUALITY-REPRODUCTION
Sexual Dysfunction . . . . _____056
Rape-Trauma Syndrome . . . . _____057

COPING-STRESS TOLERANCE
Ineffective Individual Coping . . . . _____058
Ineffective Family Coping . . . . _____059
Potential for Growth in Family Coping . . . . . . _____060

VALUE-BELIEF
Spiritual Distress . . . . _____061

FIGURE 1   University Hospitals of Cleveland Nurse/Patient summary.

Organization and Management, 1981), (c) the length of stay generated from the hospital admission and discharge dates using the SAS statistical package, and (d) demographic descriptors of the hospital episode extracted from the inpatient record at the time of discharge. All of the data including the nursing diagnoses were retrieved from computer files.

The tool used to collect nursing diagnosis data (Nurse/Patient Summary) was developed by Halloran and Kiley to describe patients' need for nursing care. The instrument includes the nursing diagnoses approved for clinical testing by the North American Nursing Diagnosis Association (NANDA) in 1982, elaboration of some of the NANDA nursing diagnoses, and terms from the nursing literature hypothesized to describe needs for nursing care. Gordon's (1982) functional health patterns provided the organizing framework for the tool.

Validity

The content of nursing diagnoses can be traced to several classic works on nursing (Abdellah, et al., 1960; Henderson and Nite, 1978; Nightingale, 1969). Nightingale's mid-nineteenth century discussion of the conditions nurses attend to is amazingly congruent with the nursing diagnosis taxonomy, although Henderson (1978) most comprehensively discusses the nursing diagnoses using the nursing intervention perspective. The more recent work conducted by NANDA and others (Gordon, 1985) suggests the content validity of nursing diagnoses. In a study by Jones and Jakob (cited in Gordon, 1985), congruence between the NANDA nursing diagnosis taxonomy and supporting clinical data ranged from 76% in a sample of 2700 diagnostic labels to 95% in a sample of 270 labels. A recent examination of content validity in psychiatric and maternity-gynecology populations found the NANDA nursing diagnoses inclusive of terms nurses use to describe the nursing needs of those populations (Kiley, et al., 1984).

Reliability

Several studies of reliability have been reported. Hoskins, et al. (1984) used five raters to assess 11 interviews for nursing diagnoses and found 91.5 mean percent interrater agreement. Abraham (1984) obtained a reliability coefficient of 0.8 for internal consistency of subjects using nursing diagnoses. An aspect of reliability, efficiency of the estimation of the population mean, was demonstrated by Halloran (1985) in a comparison of 37 nursing diagnoses in a community hospital (n=2560) with 56 nursing diagnoses in a university hospital (n=1294). A total of 16 nursing diagnoses were common to both samples and had incidence in similar proportions (r = 0.91, $p \le 0.01$). Following transformation of the frequencies of the 16 nursing diagnoses to logarithms based on the integer 10 to normalize distribution of the sample, eight of the 16 university hospital means were within the 99 percent confidence intervals of the community hospital sample. A recent study of the Nurse/Patient Summary reliability revealed 90 percent agreement between the nursing diagnoses identified at 8-hour intervals on the same patients (n=185 patient days) (Halloran and Nosek, 1986).

PROCEDURE

This study was completed in preparation for implementation of the Nurse/Patient Summary to collect nursing diagnosis and nurse assignment data on 33 inpatient wards and in ambulatory care settings at the study site. A manual defining each of the nursing diagnoses on the instrument was developed to guide the nurse's selection of nursing diagnoses. Each registered nurse on the participating wards was oriented to the nursing diagnosis concept and literature, use of the manual, and use of the instrument in a series of staff education conferences conducted by the investigators. Data were collected manually each day during the study period by nurses providing direct nursing care to the patients. Nurse compliance with the data collection was over 90 percent.

Nursing diagnosis data were entered in the IBM mainframe computer daily. At the completion of the study period the nursing diagnosis data were merged with the demographic and medical diagnostic and treatment data in the hospital computer files. The DRG relative cost weight was added to the data base for each subject. Statistical analyses were performed on the data base using the BMDP statistical package.

Nursing complexity index

The nursing complexity index was determined for each of the 1294 subjects. The index is the number of different nursing diagnoses present at any time during the hospital stay. The nursing diagnoses approved by NANDA in 1982, and seven nursing diagnoses derived by combining several subcategories of a diagnosis on the instrument, were used for the study. The derived variables were: (a) *bleeding* (internal bleeding plus external bleeding plus oozing from wound plus hemorrhage); (b) *infection* (contagion plus susceptible to infection); (c) *prolonged disease or disability* (prolonged disease plus prolonged disability); (d) *sociocultural–economic considerations* (socioeconomic considerations plus cultural considerations); (e) *impaired skin integrity* (five types of impaired skin integrity); (f) *self-care deficit* (bathing, feeding, grooming, and toileting deficits); and (g) *impaired mobility* (seven stages of immobility). For computation of the index each nursing diagnosis was equally weighted.

The nursing diagnoses identified each day during the hospitalization and the nursing complexity index are illustrated in Table 1 for a patient assigned DRG 278 carrying a relative cost weight of .8096. A second patient with a different DRG yet the same relative cost weight, and a different constellation of nursing diagnoses comprising more than twice the nursing complexity of the patient in Table 1, are illustrated in Table 2. The nursing complexity index for the patient in Table 1 is computed by summing the four different nursing diagnoses present on Day 1 (16, 34, 36, and 45), the new nursing diagnosis that appears on Day 3 (37), and the additional nursing diagnoses noted on Day 5 (60) and Day 6 (17). The complexity

Table 1: Patient's nursing conditions by day

Day of stay	1	2	3	4	5	6	7
Patient	16	16	16	16	16	16	16
Conditions	34	36	36	36	60	17	
	36	45	37				
	45						

DRG 278   Cellulitis   Age 18-60 w/o complications

DRG weight .8096

Nursing Complexity Index 7

See numbers on Nurse/Patient Summary to identify nursing diagnosis

Table 2: Patient's nursing conditions by day

Day of stay	1	2	3	4	5	6	7	8
Patient	4	4	4	10	4	4	21	21
Conditions	5	5	5	19	14	15		
	15	9	10	21	21	21		
	21	15	15	31	22	22		
	42	21	21	32	37	36		
		35	22			37		
		42	35			51		
		60	60			52		
						59		

DRG 294   Diabetes   Age greater than or equal to 16

DRG weight .8097

Nursing complexity index 19

See numbers on Nurse/Patient Summary to identify nursing diagnosis index for the patient in Table 1 is therefore seven. Using the same computational method, the nursing complexity index for the patient in Table 2 is 19.

DRG relative cost weight

This numerical factor is intended to reflect the relative resource cost of treating all cases in the DRG across all hospitals. Multiple diagnoses were taken into account in the data base used at the Health Care Financing Administration to construct mutually exclusive and exhaustive weights and average standardized cost amounts for each DRG. Higher DRG relative cost weights are assigned to DRGs believed to contain sicker patients who are, therefore, expected to consume greater amounts of resources. The actual federal payment rate for each DRG was determined by multiplying the DRG relative cost weight by the standardized costs. The relative cost weights were published in the Federal Register and are in the public domain (DHHS, 1983).

RESULTS

Values for both complexity indexes were broadly dispersed. The possible values for the nursing complexity index were 0 to 61, and the actual values ranged from 0 to 52. The mean nursing complexity index was 14.5 and the standard deviation was 10.54. The actual values for the medical complexity index covered the entire range of possible values, 0 to 6.63. The mean relative DRG cost weight was 1.09 and the standard deviation was 0.69.

The distribution of the nursing complexity index was skewed to the right, a nonnormal distribution. The skewness and kurtosis were 0.94 and 0.36, respectively. The relative cost weight distribution was also non-normal with positive skewness. The skewness of the relative cost weight distribution was 2.16 and the kurtosis was 8.29. In order to meet the mathematical assump-

tions of normality for statistical analysis, all variables were transformed to their logarithms based on the integer 10.

Nursing complexity index

The relationship between nursing complexity and length of stay was explored using the linear regression model

$$Y_i = B_o + B_1 x_{1i} + e_i$$

where $i = 1, \ldots, 1294$.

For this sample 45 percent of the variation in length of stay was explained by the nursing complexity index ($R^2 = .451$, $F(1,1261) = 1037.22$, $p \leq .0001$). In the regression the b coefficient was 0.67, the intercept was 0.04, and the standardized b coefficient (beta weight) was 0.67.

DRG relative cost weight

Using the same linear model, a regression of Log 10 length of stay on the DRG relative cost weight was done. This regression resulted in a coefficient of determination of .2088 ($F[1, 1270] = 355.1$, $p \leq .001$). Thus, the DRG relative cost weight explained 21 percent of the variation in length of stay. In this regression the b coefficient was 0.76, the intercept was 0.75, and the standardized beta coefficient was 0.46. Both regressions showed significant linear relationships, yet the nursing complexity index was more than twice as predictive of length of stay as the DRG relative cost weight.

Nursing complexity index and the DRG relative cost weight

A third regression was done to test the combined explanatory power of nursing complexity and the DRG weight for LOS. The linear model was

$$Y_i = B_o + B_1 x_{1i} + B_2 x_{2i} + e_i$$

where x_1 = nursing complexity index, x_2 = DRG relative cost weight, and $i = 1, \ldots, 1294$.

Nursing complexity entered the regression equation first and explained 45.4 percent of the variation in LOS, while the DRG weight explained 5.3 percent additional variation ($R^2 = .507$, F[2,1245] = 640.62, $p \le .001$). In this regression the b_1 coefficient was 0.585, b_2 was 0.413, and the intercept was 0.142. The beta weights for b_1 and b_2 were 0.582 and 0.248, respectively. The superior explanatory power of nursing complexity over the DRG relative cost weight was again supported.

DISCUSSION

The following admonition, lost for a century, sums the implications of these findings. "Experience teaches me now that nursing and medicine must never be mixed up. It spoils both" (Florence Nightingale, letter to Sir Henry Wentworth Ackland, 1869).

This study showed that nurses' use of a patient's DRG is less effective for management and control of hospital length of stay than use of nursing diagnostic data. The nurse manages such patient circumstances as immobility, pain, and anxiety. These circumstances cut across medical diagnostic categories. Patients need services from nurses that will allow them to be independent of the nurse's help, or will lead to a peaceful death (Henderson and Nite, 1978). These services are substantially different from those obtained from a physician, and impact directly on how long the patient stays in the hospital.

The patient hospital length of stay should ideally be clinically managed by nurses and physicians working together with the patient. Each must have a better understanding of their unique role. Patients need physicians, patients need nurses, and patients need to know what to expect from each. There should be little overlap in the activities and responsibilities of nurse and physician, lest confusion, waste, and untoward results arise. The ideal information base, reflective of a patient's use of health care services, would include nursing diagnosis and treatment information as well as medical diagnosis and treatment information.

SUMMARY

The index of nursing complexity derived from nursing diagnoses describes circumstances that are the targets for resolution through care by nurses. The terms incorporate both psychologic and physiologic conditions for which patients look to nurses for relief. These clinical variables managed by nurses provide an alternative explanation for the length of stay variation heretofore attributed solely to physician behavior. Based on these observations, it is concluded that length of hospital stay is due to the complexity of the demands that patients make on nurses and, to a lesser extent, the medical diagnostic and treatment patterns of physicians.

REFERENCES

Abdellah, F., et al.: Patient centered approaches to nursing, New York, 1960, Macmillan.

Abraham, I.: Social cognitive determinants of clinical inference in mental health: an experimental analysis, doctoral dissertation, University of Michigan, 1984, Ann Arbor.

American Hospital Association. Hospital statistics 1983 edition, pp. xv-xxi, 218, Chicago, 1983, Author.

American Nurses' Association Congress for Nursing Practice: Nursing: a social policy statement, Kansas City, 1980, American Nurses' Association.

Caterinicchio, R., and Davies, R.: Developing a client-focused allocation statistic of inpatient nursing resource use: an alternative to the patient day, Soc. Sci. and Med., **17**:259-272, 1983.

Department of Health and Human Services (DHHS): Federal, register [9/1/83] (Publication No. X-0119990), pp. 39760-39764, 39876-39886. Washington, DC, U.S. Government Printing Office.

Gordon, M.: Nursing diagnosis: process and application, New York, 1982, McGraw-Hill.

Gordon, M.: Nursing diagnosis. In Werley, H.H., and Fitzpatrick, J.J., editors: Annual Review of Nursing Research, vol. 3, New York, 1985, Springer Publishing Co.

Halloran, E.J.: Nursing workload, medical diagnosis related groups, and nursing diagnoses. Res. in Nursing and Health **8:**421-433, 1985.

Halloran, E.J.: Analysis of variation in nursing workload by patient medical and nursing condition, doctoral dissertation, University of Illinois at the Medical Center, 1980, Dissertation Abstracts International 41-09B, University Microfilms No. 8106567.

Halloran, E.J. and Nosek, L.: Interrater reliability on patient assessments using nursing diagnosis, unpublished data, 1986.

Henderson, V. and Nite, G.: Principles and practice of nursing, 6th edition, New York, 1978, Macmillan Publishing Co., Inc.

Hoskins, L., et al.: Nursing diagnosis in the chronically ill. In Kim, M.J., McFarland, G.K., and McLane, A.M., editors: Classification of nursing diagnoses: proceedings of the fifth national conference, St. Louis, 1984, The C.V. Mosby Co.

Kiley, M.: Unpublished data of nursing assessments using nursing diagnosis and record reviews of nurse problem lists, University Hospitals of Cleveland, Department of Nursing, 1984.

Luke, R.D.: Dimensions in hospital case mix measurement, Inquiry, **16:**38-49, 1979.

McKibbin, R.: R.N. wages: only 11% of hospital costs, Amer. Nurse, p. 1, 16, January 1983.

Nightingale, F.: Notes on nursing: what it is and what it is not, New York, 1969, Dover Publications (original manuscript 1860).

Yale University School of Organization and Management: The new ICD-9-CM diagnosis related groups classification scheme: user manual, New Haven, 1981, Author.

Utilization studies: poster presentations

Nursing diagnosis: assessment of use in acute care settings in Iowa

ROSEMARY J. McKEIGHEN, Ph.D., R.N., F.A.A.N
PEG A. MEHMERT, B.A., R.N.C.
CAROL A. DICKEL, R.N.

The use of nursing diagnosis in clinical practice has been the accepted standard for the profession since its inclusion in the Standards of Nursing Practice by the American Nurses Association (ANA) in 1973: "Nursing Diagnoses are derived from health status data" (p. 4). In the 1960s and the early 1970s nursing, in accordance with its developmental history of response to society's needs, focused on expanding the role of the nurse to complement the role of the physician. In 1971 a special committee appointed by the Secretary of the Department of Health, Education, and Welfare (HEW) sanctioned an expanded role for the nurse in a report that stated that there were no legal obstacles to the role extension for nurses. At about this same time nurse theorists began to advocate the use of nursing models to guide practitioners in their clinical practice. However, as a result of nurses serving as extensions of physicians, the focus on nursing as a discipline was obscured. Guided by the 1971 HEW committee decision, 30 states enacted amendments to nurse practice acts which

sanctioned diagnostic and treatment functions for nurses (Bullough, 1976). Iowa, not included in the initial 30, amended its Nurse Practice Act in 1976 to include the terms "nursing diagnosis and nursing treatment." The Iowa Nurse Practice Act states that one of the functions of the nurse is to:

a. Formulate nursing diagnosis and conduct nursing treatment of human responses to actual or potential health problems through services, such as case finding, referral, health teaching, health counseling, and care provision which is supportive to or restorative of life and well-being (Iowa Board of Nursing, 1983, p. 1).

Bullough (1976) clearly documents the debate that arose in some states over the legality of nurses diagnosing and treating patients. Perhaps this debate is the reason that Carnevali (1984) reports that the majority of nursing administrators have not formally promoted the use of nursing diagnosis, even though it has been defined as an essential component of nursing practice by the ANA since 1973, and stated specifically in the

nurse practice acts of many states. Furthermore, Lash (1982) reports, ". . . little evidence exists that the making and the recording of nursing diagnoses have penetrated
into the daily activities of professional
nurses" (p. 45). These facts stimulated the
interest of the authors in exploring the extent of the use of nursing diagnoses by
nurses in clinical practice in Iowa.

Nurses, as well as their educators and administrators, are all concerned with this issue. Nurses academically prepared to use
nursing diagnoses as part of the nursing process have questioned the discrepancy between the prominence of nursing diagnoses
presented in the curriculum and their lack of
implementation in practice settings (Lash
1982). Educators have recognized this gap
between theory and practice and have raised
questions, yet research has not been generated to solve the problem. It would seem
natural that nursing administrators would
be sensitive to nurses' adherence to professional standards within their facilities.

LITERATURE REVIEW

Nursing diagnosis first appeared in the literature in 1950 (McManus). Fry (1953) described nursing diagnosis as a new, creative
activity to be used to plan patient care. At
this point nursing had been conceptualized
as a process by Hall (1955). In 1956 Hornung
defined the word "nursing" as an ethical and
acceptable qualifying adjective of the term
"diagnosis." Abdellah (1957) offered a list of
21 nursing problems, classifying them by
type. McCain (1965) identified 13 functional
areas for nursing assessment, and proposed
them as a beginning effort to establish a universal assessment tool for nursing. These
served as forerunners for the more recent attempts to establish a nursing diagnosis
classification system.

The increasing awareness of nursing diagnosis in the 1960s was the stimulus for beginning research concerning the concept. All
of the research was directed toward nursing
diagnosis as a clinical inference (Hammond,
1966; Kelly, 1966). Hammond's action of defining nursing diagnosis in terms of making
an inference still serves as a basis for nursing
diagnosis research. He stated:

Only recently has formal recognition been made
of the fact that nurses do make inferences about
the state of the patient for whom they provide
care. Recognition of this function is important:
Many of the tasks which the modern nurse
encounters are cognitive for they require that the
nurse make inferences about the state of the
patient (Hammond, 1966, p. 27).

Rothberg (1967) continued the dialogue in
the literature by stating that the function of
the professional nurse is performed when
the patient is assessed, the need of nursing
care is diagnosed, and a course of action is
followed. In other words, she confirmed that
an inference made by nurses requires their
professional intervention.

To date no one theory that interrelates
education, practice, and research has been
universally accepted by the nursing profession. The value of accepting a single theory
at this point in the evolution of the discipline is questioned because of a concern
about premature closure; each of the theories and models has a different conceptual
framework, yet all reflect the structure of
the nursing process as defined by the ANA
in the *Standards of Nursing Practice*. The
standards define the phases of the nursing
process as: assessment, nursing diagnosis,
planning, implementation, and evaluation.
However, even though each of the conceptual models and theories culminates in a
clinical inference statement (nursing diagnosis) as the end product of assessment, few
elucidate how nurses arrive at these conclusions. In addition, the nursing diagnosis concept did not appear in nursing education
texts prior to the 1970s (Gordon 1982). This
lack of consistency for naming the clinical
inferences made by nurses with a standard-

ized terminology results in confusion among nursing practitioners and affects the planning and provision of patient care.

Nursing diagnosis has been identified in the literature as a means to improve both communication and continuity of care by providing a standard terminology for the profession (Dalton 1979, Dodge 1975, Fredette and Gloriant 1981, Gordon 1979, Gordon, Sweeny, and McKeehan 1980, Dossey and Guzetta 1981, Lister 1983, McKeehan 1979, Weber 1979). The consistency inherent in the use of nursing diagnosis could promote a decreased incidence of errors in communication (Gordon 1982). The nurse's decision-making, or the establishment of nursing diagnoses, directs all other components of the nursing process—establishing desired patient outcomes, determining appropriate nursing interventions, and evaluating the nursing care delivered. The use of nursing diagnoses will assist the professional nurse in prescribing patient treatments that are amenable to nursing intervention (Curtin 1984, Halloran and Kiley 1984). It provides a focus for care (Dalton 1979, Demers 1979, Dodge 1975, Dossey and Guzetta 1981, Lister 1983, Rothberg 1967, Shoemaker 1979) and assists in generating an individualized care plan for the patient that may be used by all those nurses caring for the individual (Gebbie 1984). Nursing diagnosis gives structure to the documentation of patient care that is required in practice (Fredette and Gloriant 1981, Hausman 1980, Mundinger and Jauron 1975, Morris 1982, Tilton and Maloof 1982). All of the above functions serve to define the scope of clinical science in nursing (Evans 1979, Gordon and Sweeney 1979), which in turn serves to improve nurse accountability by defining the domain of the profession (Bruce 1982, Dodge 1975, Hausman 1980, Weber 1979).

Nursing diagnosis has also been cited as providing a basis for third-party reimbursement for nursing practice (Dalton 1979, Hausman 1980, Weber 1979). It is anticipated that nurses will be required to justify the care delivered during a patient's hospitalization (Curtin 1983). Holloran's study (1980), an exploratory effort, examined nursing workload according to the patient's nursing and medical condition. His findings provide support for the clinical validity of the use of nursing diagnoses. Using multiple regression analysis, Halloran noted that 52 percent of the variation in nursing workload could be explained by 37 nursing diagnoses. The use of nursing diagnoses in identifying the patient's problems that require the intervention of the nurse could assist the profession in accurately describing the specific nursing care needs of an individual (Curtin 1984, Curtin 1985, Reitz 1985). A complete care plan based on nursing diagnoses will also assist in patient classification (Giovanetti 1978, Gordon 1982, Simmons 1980). Accurate descriptors of patient care elements will foster accuracy in measuring patient acuity and in determining the nursing care hours required by the patient on a shift-to-shift basis (Audette and Tilquin 1977, Curtin 1984). This accuracy will result in providing the nursing units with sufficient staff to deliver nursing care that is based on the patient's actual needs. In turn, with clearly identified nursing care needs, accuracy in predicting staffing requirements will be facilitated. These factors will improve both the quality of care and the cost effectiveness of a nursing department. Nurse managers will have a reliable mechanism to justify the allocation of nursing resources and thereby justify the cost of patient care (Adams and Duchene 1985, Curtin 1984, Gordon 1982, Halloran 1980).

METHODOLOGY

An exploratory descriptive study of the acute care hospitals listed by the Iowa Hospital Association (N=140) was conducted to determine the extent of use in Iowa of nursing diagnosis as defined by the North American Nursing Diagnosis Association (NANDA) classification system. For the purpose of this study the decision was made to limit the study to acute care hospitals, since over 60 percent of all nurses practice in such settings. Facilities included in the study represent both rural and urban hospitals. The proportional ratio of rural/urban hospitals in Iowa is 79/21. Subjects for investigation were directors of nursing or their designees. In early 1985 a survey questionnaire was mailed to each of the subjects, who were asked to respond in five areas: (1) Is nursing diagnosis used in the agency? (2) If not currently in use, is implementation currently in progress? (3) Are there plans to implement nursing diagnosis in the future? (4) Is nursing diagnosis being considered for use? (5) Would the hospital be willing to participate in further study on nursing diagnosis?

The survey response rate following the original and a repeat mailing was 79% (n=111). Eighty-three percent (92) of the hospitals that responded were designated as rural facilities and 17 percent (19) represented urban facilities.

RESULTS

Sixty-seven percent (74) of the respondents reported that they do not use nursing diagnosis as defined by NANDA. Thirty-two percent (35) reported the use of nursing diagnosis, and in 2 percent (2) of the responses the question was not scored. Fifty-eight percent (11) of the urban respondents, used nursing diagnosis, while 26 percent (24) of the rural respondents used the concept.

Of the 67 percent (74) of the administrators reporting that they do not use nursing diagnosis, 20 percent (22) said that plans for use were currently in progress, 24 percent (27) were considering its use for their facility, and 20 percent (22) were not considering the use of nursing diagnosis at all. Five percent (5) did not score the question.

In response to the question of willingness to participate in further study, 50 percent (56) of the nursing administrators responded positively, 36 percent (40) responded negatively, 10 percent (11) gave no response, and 4 percent (4) were undecided.

DISCUSSION

It was reassuring to find that 32 percent (35) of nursing administrators in Iowa have staff nurses who are actively involved in the use of nursing diagnosis in clinical practice. It was also very gratifying to note that the use of nursing diagnosis is based upon the NANDA classification system. This standardization of nomenclature will facilitate communication amongst nurses, provide a universal basis for the planning of patient care, and positively affect patient outcomes.

Of the 67 percent of nursing administrators who reported not using the NANDA classification of nursing diagnosis (74), 20 percent (22) have plans to do so. When this group is added to those who already are using nursing diagnosis for planning care, the number of acute care hospitals in the state that will use the concept is 57 (52 percent). This should affirm a growing agreement amongst nursing administrators who need to be at the forefront in establishing the standards for clinical practice in Iowa. Also, it is commendable that these nursing administrators have taken the risk of implementing the concept in its embryonic stage, a step which must be taken if nursing is to determine the reliability and validity of nursing interventions made in clinical practice areas. It will be interesting to compare the use of nursing diagnosis in Iowa with its use in other states when such studies are reported. This is needed to determine acceptance of the concept at a national practice level.

It is hoped that the 27 (24 percent) who report that they have been considering the use of nursing diagnosis in their hospitals will formulate such a plan and adopt it. In

Iowa this would further increase the number of hospitals using nursing diagnosis to 84 (76 percent). However, one can not make the assumption that consideration is equated with action.

It was perplexing to find that 20 percent (22) of the hospitals were not considering the use of the concept at all. Further examination of the data revealed that 82 percent (18) of this number were rural hospitals. Seventy-three percent (16) of those hospitals have a bed capacity of less than 100 beds, and 9 percent (2) have 101-200 beds. This finding adds support to the uniqueness of the rural practice setting in Iowa. In such a setting, the nurse may be responsible for the delivery of care to a variety of patients on a medical/surgical unit, and also be responsible for staffing the emergency room and supervising the ancillary personnel who deliver care to patients in extended care units. With such diverse responsibilities, time for the conceptualization and writing of a nursing diagnosis and the resulting plan of care may be at a minimum. The remaining 18 percent (4) were urban hospitals ranging from less than 100 to more than 400 beds.

Two percent (2) of the respondents did not answer the question on use or non-use of nursing diagnosis. This non-response is puzzling.

CONCLUSION

Further research needs to be conducted to determine an accurate picture of the scope of the use of the concept at the national level. The variables that exist among nursing administrators and nurses in the practice setting that inhibit or promote the use of nursing diagnosis need to be identified and examined. Situational factors that inhibit the use of nursing diagnosis must be identified and studied. Empirical data that identify the benefits of nursing diagnosis in effecting patient care outcomes have yet to be reported.

The methods that professional organizations successfully use to facilitate the actualization of the concept in nursing practice also need to be isolated and defined. The role that nursing educators play in facilitating the use of nursing diagnosis in the practice of new graduates must be explored. Educators could use the knowledge gained from these studies to implement continuing education programs for the current practitioners who are not using nursing diagnosis.

Further investigation is planned by the authors to identify factors that influence or inhibit the implementation and use of nursing diagnosis, variables that enhance implementation, and benefits of the use of nursing diagnosis in clinical practice.

REFERENCES

Abdellah, F.B.: Methods of identifying covert aspects of nursing problems, Nurs. Res. **6**:4-23, 1957.

Adams, R. and Duchene, P.: Computerization of patient acuity and nursing care planning: new approach to improved patient care and cost-effective staffing, J. Nurs. Admin. **15**(4):11-17, 1985.

American Nurses' Association: Standards of nursing practice, Kansas City, MO, 1973, Author.

Audette, M.C.L. and Tilquin, C.: Patient classification by care required, Dim. in Health Serv. **54**(9):32-36, 1977.

Bruce, J.A.: The legal side—the right and responsibility to diagnose, Amer. J. Nurs. **82**(4):645-646, 1982.

Bullough, B.: The law and expanding nursing role, Amer. J. Public Health, **66**(3):248-254, 1976.

Carnevali, D.L.: Nursing diagnosis: an evolutionary view, Topics Clin. Nurs. **5**(4):10-20, 1984.

Curtin, L.: Determining costs of nursing service per DRG, Nurs. Management **14**(4):16-20, 1983.

Curtin, L.: What we say/what we do, Nurs. Management **15**(1):7-8, 1984.

Curtin, L.: Integrating acuity: the frugal road to safe care, Nurs. Management **16**(9):7-8, 1985.

Dalton, J.M.: Nursing diagnosis in a community health setting, Nurs. Clinics N. A. **14**(3):525-531, 1979.

Demers, B.: How nursing diagnosis helps focus your care: beyond endocarditis, RN **42**(12):51-54, 1979.

Dodge, G.H.: What determines nursing vs. medical diagnosis? AORN J. **22**(1):23-24, 1975.

Dossey, B. and Guzzetta, C.E.: Nursing diagnosis, Nurs. 81, **11**(6):34-38, 1981.

Evans, S.L.: Descriptive criteria for the concept of depleted health potential, Adv. Nurs. Sci. **1**(4):67-74, 1979.

Fredette, S. and Gloriant, F.S.: Nursing diagnosis in

cancer chemotherapy, Amer. J. Nurs. **81**(11):2013-2022, 1981.

Fry, V.: The creative approach to nursing, Amer. J. Nurs. **53**(3):301-302, 1953.

Gebbie, K.M.: Nursing diagnosis: what is it and why does it exist? Topics Clin. Nurs. **5**(4):1-9, 1984.

Giovanetti, P.: Patient classification systems in nursing: a description and analysis, HRA 78-22, Washington, D.C., 1978, U.S. Department of Health, Education and Welfare.

Gordon, M.: The concept of nursing diagnosis, Nurs. Clinics N. A. **14**(3):487-496, 1979.

Gordon, M.: Nursing diagnosis: process and application, New York, 1982, McGraw-Hill.

Gordon, M. and Sweeney, M.: Methodological problems and issues in identifying and standardizing nursing diagnosis, Adv. Nurs. Sci. **2**(1):1-15, 1979.

Gordon, M., Sweeney, M., and McKeehan, K.: Nursing diagnosis: looking at its use in the clinical area, Amer. J. Nurs. **80**(4):672-674, 1980.

Guzzetta, C.E. and Dossey, B.M.: Nursing diagnosis: framework, process, and problems, Heart Lung, **12**(3):281-291, 1983.

Hall, L.: Quality of nursing care, Public Health News, New Jersey State Department of Health, 212-213, June 1955.

Halloran, E.J.: Analysis of variation in nursing workload by patient medical and nursing condition, doctoral dissertation, University of Illinois, 1980, Dissertation Abstracts International, 41, 3385B, p. 166.

Halloran, E.J. and Kiley, M.L.: Case mix management, Nurs. Management **15**(2):39-43, 1984.

Hammond, K.R.: Clinical inference in nursing, a psychologist's viewpoint, Nurs. Res. **15**(1):27-38, 1966.

Hausman, K.A.: The concept and application of nursing diagnosis, J. Neurosurgical Nurs. **12**(2):76-80, 1980.

Hornung, G.: The nursing diagnosis—an exercise in judgment, Nurs. Outlook **4**(1):29-30, 1956.

Iowa Board of Nursing: Extracts pertaining to the practice of nursing, Des Moines, 1983, The State of Iowa.

Kelly, K.: Clinical inference in nursing, Nurs. Res. **15**(1):23-26, 1966.

Lash, A.A.: Nursing diagnosis: some comments on the gap between theory and practice. In McCloskey, J.C. and Grace, H.K., editors: Current issues in nursing, Boston, 1982, Blackwell Scientific Publications.

Lister, D.W.: The nursing diagnosis movement and the occupational health nurse, Occupational Health Nurs. **31**(2), 11-14, 1983.

McCain, R.F.: Nursing by assessment—not intuition, Amer. J. Nurs. **65**(4):82-84, 1965.

McKeehan, K.M.: Nursing diagnosis in a discharge planning program, Nurs. Clinics N. A. **14**(3):517-524, 1979.

McManus, R.L.: Assumptions of the function of nursing: report of work conference at Plymouth, NH, June 12-23, 1950. In Regional Planning for Nursing and Nursing Education, New York, 1950, Bureau of Publications, Teacher's College, Columbia University.

Morris, J.L.: Nursing diagnosis: a focus for continuing education. J. Contin. Ed. Nurs. **13**(3):33-35, 1982.

Mundinger, J. and Jauron, G.: Developing a nursing diagnosis, Nurs. Outlook **23**:94-98, 1975.

Reitz, J.A.: Toward a comprehensive nursing intensity index: part II, testing, Nurs. Management **16**(9):31-42, 1985.

Rothberg, J.S.: Why nursing diagnosis? Amer. J. Nurs. **67**(5):1040-1042, 1967.

Shoemaker, J.: How nursing diagnosis helps focus your care, RN **79**:56-61, 1979.

Simmons, D.A.: Classification scheme for client problems in community health nursing, DHHS Publication No. HRA 80-16, Washington, D.C., 1980, U.S. Government Printing Office.

Tilton, C. and Maloof, M.: Diagnosing the problems in stroke, Amer. J. Nurs. **82**(4):596-601, 1982.

Weber, S.: Nursing diagnosis in private practice, Nurs. Clinics N. A. **14**(3):533-539, 1979.

Testing a nursing diagnosis classification system for pediatric nurse practitioners

CATHERINE E. BURNS, M.N., R.N., P.N.P.
MARY KATHRYN THOMPSON, M.N., R.N., F.N.P.

BACKGROUND

The purpose of this study was to develop a diagnostic classification system applicable to Pediatric Nurse Practitioner (PNP) practice. The need for the study became evident when an Oregon county health department decided to implement the VNA of Omaha classification scheme department-wide (Simmons, 1980). This classification was designed for community health nurses. The PNPs working in the health department were concerned that the system would not reflect their specialized practice accurately, and turned to the faculty of the nearby university with their concern. We were asked to modify and test the system by adding diagnoses for the PNPs while taking nothing away from the VNA scheme. The theoretical context within which the system was developed, the results of its testing, our conclusions, and suggested further revisions are discussed.

THEORETICAL PERSPECTIVES

Theoretical perspectives included definition of the role of PNPs, definitions of nursing and medical diagnoses, and taxonomic theory.

The PNP was viewed as a nursing specialist who provides primary health care to children. The practitioner's care is guided by a process involving nursing assessments and nursing interventions. Additionally, the PNP manages a variety of minor childhood illnesses. For this aspect of practice the PNP uses medical diagnoses to guide interventions. Thus, for a classification system to be of use to PNPs, both a full range of ambulatory pediatric nursing problems and a limited number of pediatric diseases need to be incorporated into the system.

The nursing diagnosis definition of Mundinger and Jauron (1975) as "the statement of a person's response to a situation of illness which is actually or potentially unhealthful and which nursing intervention can help to change in the direction of health" (p. 97) was used. The definition guided formation of new nursing diagnoses. The medical diagnosis definition of Soares (1978) as "the pathologic state of a patient which would identify abnormal organ system disorders or diseases" (p. 269) was used to identify diagnoses for the medical domain.

The criteria for taxonomic organization which are generally recognized (including relevance, completeness, clarity, mutual exclusiveness, usefulness, openness, and compatibility with other systems) were used as the system was modified.

METHODOLOGY
Construction of the classification system

The preliminary classification was constructed from three taxonomies—the VNA of Omaha Classification (Simmons 1980), the Child and Youth Projects Nursing Problem Scheme from Minnesota (U.S. Department of Health and Human Services 1977), and the International Classification of Diseases (Commission of Hospital and Professional Activities 1978).

The VNA taxonomy served as the basic unit since the Health Department planned to use it. This system divides nursing problems into four domains: environmental, psychosocial, physiological, and health behaviors and beliefs. Forty-nine problem labels are distributed among these domains, each with a list of "descriptors" or defining characteristics. Numerical coding allows the system to be computerized. Designed for Community Health Nurses, the system was thought to be incomplete for describing PNP practice because it lacked both specificity in describing pediatric nursing problems and the medical diagnoses needed by PNPs. The Child and Youth taxonomy (U.S. Dept. of Health and Human Services 1977) provided most of the additional nursing diagnoses which were chosen to reflect health promotion aspects of pediatric nursing care as well as child and family oriented nursing problems.

A fifth domain (medical) was added to the system to allow documentation of this aspect of Pediatric Nurse Practitioner work. To keep the system compatible with the ICD system, codes in this domain were given a number 5 prefix, but the remaining digits were standard for these diseases according to the ICD-9-CM system. The other domains followed the VNA numbering system. Finally, an open number was added to

each domain. Use of the open number required a written statement of the problem. Construction of the system is summarized in Table 1.

After construction of a preliminary system we began testing its usefulness for PNP practice. The system was pretested and revised following review of 29 cases and coding of diagnoses of 100 patient encounters. Further revisions were made so that the final outcome appeared as in Table 1.

Sample and settings

Following these revisions, six PNPs with varied educational backgrounds were enlisted to collect data. All had more than 3 years of experience as PNPs. Diagnostic skill was deemed necessary to test the system. The settings for data gathering included a county health department, a hospital outpatient pediatric clinic, and a large health maintenance organization pediatric clinic. The use of these varied settings was considered desirable for testing the adaptability of the system. In all sites the PNPs had their own caseloads, calling for physician consultation when necessary. The problem-oriented medical record system was used in all settings and was essential to the interrater

Table 1: Construction of the classification system

Domain	Sources
I. Environmental	—VNA of Omaha System —1 diagnosis added from the Child and Youth Nursing Problem Scheme
II. Psychosocial	—VNA of Omaha System —4 diagnoses added from the Child and Youth Nursing Problem Scheme
III. Physiological	—VNA of Omaha System —4 diagnoses added from the Child and Youth Nursing Problem Scheme
IV. Health behaviors and beliefs	—VNA of Omaha System —5 diagnoses added from the Child and Youth Nursing Problem Scheme, PNP experience
V. Medical	—57 pediatric diseases added from the International Classification of Diseases, 9th revision-Clinical Modification

reliability testing process used. The PNPs served patients ranging in age from 3 days to 20 years, with a median age of 1.42 years and a mean age of 3.74 years.

Procedure

A code book of diagnoses was compiled and the PNPs were oriented to its use. They were instructed to code all problems managed during patient encounters, and to code to the highest level of understanding. For example, management of a child with obesity due to excessive calories would be coded as a Nutrition problem, rather than in the more general category of Growth Impairment. The PNPs were asked not to force a fit between the problem and available categories. If no existing category seemed appropriate, the open number available in each domain was to be used. The intent was to fit the system to practice rather than forcing practice to artificially fit the available labels.

Data including the patient's name, record number, and age, the date of the encounter, the coder indentification number, and the diagnostic code numbers were recorded on site-coded cards after each patient encounter.

Interrater reliability was checked initially and again midway through the data collection period. The nurses began collecting data when they achieved 85 percent or greater agreement for two consecutive sets of 10 cases. The reliability level was achieved with only one or two practice rounds, and was maintained during the data collection period.

Analysis of the data

One thousand and seventy-four consecutive patient encounters with a total of 2695 diagnoses were coded in 11 weeks. Each diagnosis was described in terms of overall frequency, frequency by site, and frequency by individual coder. Correlations among domains and diagnoses were also done. As another measure of reliability and validity, charts were sampled to determine whether patients with selected commonly-used or new diagnoses were similar in terms of their subjective and objective findings.

FINDINGS AND DISCUSSION

The mean number of diagnoses per patient was 2.5, with a range of 1 to 8. There was no significant difference in number of diagnoses per patient from site to site.

The distribution of diagnoses among the five domains varied greatly. Sixty-nine percent of the children had diagnoses in the medical domain, 51.5 percent in the health behaviors and beliefs domain, 14.6 percent in the physiological domain, 5 percent in the psychosocial domain, and only 1 percent in the environmental domain. Some patients had more than one diagnosis in a domain. Diagnoses used five or more times are listed in Table 2.

Interdomain correlations were not significant except between the medical and health behaviors and beliefs domains. Twenty percent of patients with a diagnosis in one also had a diagnosis in the other. Thus, the PNPs used some patient care encounters for both preventive and curative care, rather than deferring attention to wellness in sick children and vice versa. Here the overlap between medical and nursing functions was demonstrated.

Overall, the three most commonly used diagnoses were *Immunization need, Otitis media,* and the *Nutrition* subproblem of the *Well child: Need for knowledge and guidance* diagnosis.

In examining data from the medical domain it was noted that, as in most pediatric practices, infected ears, rashes, and upper respiratory infections made up the majority of diagnoses. Of interest to the investigators was the tendency among the PNPs to use discrete labels from the medical domain rather than the more general labels from the

Table 2: Frequencies: most commonly used diagnoses for 1074 patient visits

Diagnosis		Frequency
ENVIRONMENTAL DOMAIN:		
+1.041	Parental Health Problem	5
PSYCHOSOCIAL DOMAIN:		
2.011	Communication with Community Resources: Impairment	20
2.111	Parenting Impairment	7
2.121,131	Neglect and Abuse: Child/Adult	12
+2.141	Developmental Lag	10
PHYSIOLOGICAL DOMAIN:		
3.021	Vision: Impairment	29
3.031	Dentition: Impairment	21
3.051	Circulation: Impairment	25
3.071-3	Reproductive Function Problems	42
+3.151	Growth Deficit or Excess	22
3.999	Other	5
HEALTH BEHAVIORS DOMAIN:		
+4.001...	Well child: Need for knowledge/guidance (see subproblems below)	
+4.001.01	Emotional relationships	13
+4.001.02	Physical care	10
+4.001.03	Nutrition	213
+4.001.04	Growth	46
+4.001.05	Development	88
+4.001.06	Behavior expectations	56
+4.001.07	Safety	160
+4.001.08	Social	11
+4.001.09	Sexuality	29
+4.001.10	Dental	70
+4.002	Immunizations	268
+4.003	Screening procedure need	194
+4.004	Fluoride need	132
4.011	Nutrition: Impairment	46
4.021	Sleep/Rest: Impairment	10
4.041	Personal hygiene: Deficit	5
4.063	Therapeutic regimen noncompliance: Meds	15

+ = Addition to the VNA of Omaha scheme (Simmons, 1980)

physiological domain, even when their care was probably more physiological nursing than medical in nature. The medical labels were apparently more meaningful to the nurses in describing the status of patients. The overlap of these two domains is of some concern conceptually, and an alternative arrangement of listings is under consideration for the next revision.

The open number in the medical domain was used 136 times, showing a gap in system comprehensiveness. Additions should include lice, scabies, and a range of infectious diseases including venereal diseases and tuberculosis. The majority of open number additions were single-occurring cases.

In the health behaviors and beliefs domain, the majority of diagnoses used were in

Table 2: Frequencies: most commonly used diagnoses for 1074 patient visits—cont'd

Diagnosis		Frequency
MEDICAL DOMAIN+:		
Accidents:		
5.920	Contusion	6
Allergies:		
5.507	Allergic rhinitis	26
5.493	Asthma	12
5.693.1	Food	8
Dermatology:		
5.692.9	Atopic dermatitis	61
5.112.1	Candida/thrush	48
5.706.3	Impetigo	30
Eyes, Ears, Nose, Throat:		
5.360	Conjunctivitis	23
5.381.1	Otitis media	234
5.462-3	Pharyngitis, tonsillitis	63
5.381.3	Serous otitis media	48
5.528	Stomatitis	5
Gastrointestinal:		
5.280	Anemia	17
5.564	Constipation	11
5.558.9	Diarrhea	19
5.787	Vomiting	12
Genito-urinary:		
5.783.9	Enuresis	18
5.559	Urinary tract infection	16
Respiratory:		
5.490	Bronchitis	5
5.484	Pneumonia	10
5.460	Upper respiratory infection	142
Orthopedics:		
5.754.53	Metatarsus adductus	5
5.737.3	Scoliosis	9
Other:		
5.999	Other (specify)	136

+ = Addition to the VNA of Omaha scheme (Simmons, 1980)

the *Immunization need* and *Well child: Need for knowledge and guidance* areas. Teaching about nutrition, safety, and development were the most commonly used subproblems from a list of 10. Unfortunately, data from 194 cases were sequestered in the *screening procedure* category which was used for such things as school physicals. In retrospect, this was not a valid category. It will be deleted on system revision.

Taxonomically, the labels in the psychosocial domain were not as mutually exclusive as desired, due in part to differences in theoretical perspectives on the problems at hand. For example, one would classify a child's behavior problem differently depending on whether a family theory, intra-psychic, or behaviorist perspective were used.

Throughout the system there were significant differences in diagnosis use among coders, even within the same sites.

CONCLUSIONS

Generally, the scheme described seemed quite workable. Diagnoses needed were available, except for gaps in the medical domain. Ease of use was reflected in both the lack of difficulty in achieving and maintaining interrater reliability and the brief recording time needed. The taxonomic criteria were somewhat more difficult to meet, with overlaps between the medical and physiological domains and some lack of clarity within the psychosocial domain. The system is compatible with the VNA system and the ICD system. Finally, it is open to additional diagnoses with permanent or open numbers.

The VNA system worked reasonably well as a base for the system. However, modification did seem necessary for the following reasons: 1) the environmental domain was rarely used by PNPs, and is probably more relevant to Visiting Nurse/Community Health Nurse practice executed in the home or community setting; 2) the added medical domain was used most commonly by PNPs, and reflects a portion of their specialty practice as primary health care providers; 3) the well-child diagnoses added to the health behaviors and beliefs domain were used in more than 50 percent of cases, indicating the emphasis on health promotion by PNPs.

REFERENCES

Burns, C.E.: Developing a nursing diagnosis classification system for PNPs, Ped. Nurs. **10:**411-414, 1984.

Commission of Hospital and Professional Activities: International classification of diseases: clinical modification, 1, 9th revision, Ann Arbor, MI, 1978, Author.

Mundinger, M., and Jauron, G.: Developing a nursing diagnosis, Nurs. Outlook **23:**94-98, 1975.

Simmon, A.: A classification scheme for client problems in community health nursing, Hyattsville, MD, 1980, U.S. Department of Health and Human Services, Division of Nursing, DHHS Publication Number HRA80-86.

Soars, C.: Nursing and medical diagnoses: a comparison of variant and essential features. In Chaska, N., editor: The nursing profession: views through the mist, New York, 1978, McGraw-Hill.

U.S. Department of Health and Human Services, Public Health Services: Nursing problem classification for children and youth, Rockville, MD, 1977, U.S. Department of Health and Human Services, DHHS Publication Number HSA77-5201.

The usefulness of nursing diagnoses in neonatal intensive care units

MARIBETH STEIN, M.N., R.N.

The Classification System of Nursing Diagnosis proposed by the North American Nursing Diagnosis Association (NANDA) was established to facilitate professional nursing practice. Accordingly, there are reports in the literature that suggest that the diagnoses accepted by NANDA can be successfully implemented and utilized in actual clinical practice (Bruce 1979, McKeehan 1979, Morris 1982). However, implementation and validation of the accepted diagnostic categories have not been researched in every clinical setting as specified in the principles established by the First National Conference Group on the Classification of Nursing Diagnoses.

One particular clinical setting which is totally unexplored regarding the utilization of nursing diagnoses is the neonatal intensive care unit (NICU). The NICU has rapidly developed in response to the need of critically ill and premature newborn infants for specialized, highly technical health care.

The concept of nursing diagnosis and its implementation in neonatal intensive care units presents a substantial challenge to the nursing profession. For many NICU nurses the severity of the patients problems demands that the biophysiologic state of the infant be their primary concern. This is of particular importance, since the primary focus of medicine is also the biophysiologic state of the patient. If the value of a classification system of nursing diagnosis lies in its validity and usefulness to all nursing specialities, even those which are heavily influenced by the medical model, then the issues raised by the practice of nursing in the NICU must be explored.

STATEMENT OF PURPOSE

The purpose of this study was to determine the usefulness of the classification system of nursing diagnoses to nursing practice in neonatal intensive care units. Based on the literature review, questions examined included:

1. Of the 50 diagnoses classified by NANDA, which 10 diagnoses are most useful for nursing practice in a NICU?
2. What defining characteristics do NICU nurses identify for the 10 most useful diagnostic categories?
3. How do NICU nurses treat the 10 most useful diagnostic categories?
4. Excluding the classified diagnostic categories, what problems do NICU nurses identify and treat in their practice?

METHODOLOGY

The research design chosen for this investigation was a descriptive panel study. One group of subjects was asked to provide data at two different points in time.

The sample for this study was one of convenience. It consisted of the 99 nurses who had attended the First National Conference for Neonatal Nurse Clinicians, Practitioners, and Specialists held in April, 1983, as well as two of the nursing colleagues of each participant, for a total N=297. Inclusion of the colleague nurses was to offset the possible bias of the conference group.

In this two-phase study two questionnaires and a biographical data survey were utilized. In phase one, the subjects were given the 50 diagnostic categories classified by NANDA and asked to rank the 10 most

Table 1: The 10 most useful nursing diagnoses for NICU nursing practice

Diagnosis	No. of subjects (n=57) ranking in top 10	Percent of subjects ranking in top 10
Nutrition, alteration in: less than body requirements	51	89.5
Breathing patterns, ineffective	51	89.5
Gas exchange, impaired	49	86.0
Parenting, potential alteration in	37	64.9
Airway clearance, ineffective	34	59.6
Cardiac output, decreased	34	59.6
Parenting, alteration in	29	50.9
Tissue perfusion (chronic), alteration in	28	49.1
Fluid volume deficit, potential	25	43.8
Urinary elimination pattern, alteration in	25	43.8

useful diagnoses based on their nursing practice in the NICU. These data were compiled by the researcher, and the 10 most useful diagnoses were identified. In phase two of the study, ten weeks later, the same subjects were sent a second questionnaire to elicit additional information about the 10 selected diagnoses.

The subjects in the study were contacted by mail. Only those subjects who had returned the first questionnaire were included in the second phase of the study. Total sample size was 297. Response rate for the first questionnaire was 22.2 percent. Response rate for the second questionnaire was 24.6 percent.

Data analysis for this study consisted of descriptive statistics. Measures of central tendencies and frequency distributions were used to determine sample characteristics and to analyze data from both questionnaires.

KEY FINDINGS

In phase one of the study, 10 diagnoses were identified as most useful for neonatal nursing practice (Table 1). In addition, 53 neonatal health problems other than the 50 classified diagnoses were identified by NICU nurses (Box 1).

Phase two of the study yielded numerous data. Neonatal signs and symptoms and nursing interventions for each of the 10 selected diagnoses were obtained.

CONCLUSIONS

The findings suggest that two of the selected nursing diagnoses, "Parenting, potential alteration in" and "Airway clearance, ineffective," are indeed useful and appropriately described by NANDA for NICU nursing practice. Therefore, there two diagnoses are ready for clinical validation in Neonatal Intensive Care Units.

The data also indicate that the remaining eight diagnoses considered to be most useful for NICU nursing practice lack appropriate defining characteristics for neonates. Therefore, in order to adequately meet the needs of nurses in the NICU and prior to testing for clinical validation, the nursing diagnoses require additional defining characteristics which are pertinent to neonates.

BOX 1   **Common health problems that NICU nurses identify and treat in their nursing practice (other than 50 stated nursing diagnoses)**

Hypo/hypertonia
Hyperbilirubinemia
Sepsis
Bronchopulmonary dysplasia
Infant stabilization in delivery room
Persistent fetal circulation
Respiratory distress syndrome
Pulmonary interstitial emphysema
Cardiomyopathies
Dysmorphic infant
Syndrome of inappropriate
    antidiuretic hormone (SIADH)
Renal failure
Small for gestational age (SGA)
Large for gestational age (LGA)
Asphyxia
Congenital heart disease
Thermoregulation/temperature
    instability
Meconium aspiration
Retrolental fibroplasia (RLF)
Pneumothorax
Transient tachypnea of the newborn
    (TTN)
Atelectasis
Pneumonia
Congestive heart failure (CHF)
Patent ductus arteriosus (PDA)
Hypo/hypertension

Acute tubular necrosis (ATN)
Prematurity
Cardio-respiratory collapse
Anemia
Apnea
Bradycardia
Electrolyte imbalances
Necrotizing enterocolitis (NEC)
Surgical problems
Vomiting
Disseminated intravascular
    coagulation (DIC)
(Iatrogenic) blood loss
Blood incompatibilities
Intraventricular hemorrhage (IVH)
Hydrocephalus
Anoxia
Seizures
Family problems
Developmental stimulation
Bonding problems
Drug withdrawal
Feeding problems
Social problems
Ostomy care
Tracheostomy care
Stress intolerance
Acute alteration in tissue perfusion

REFERENCES

Bruce, J.A.: Implementation of nursing diagnoses: a nursing administrator's perspective, Nurs. Clinics N. A. **14:**509-515, 1979.

McKeehan, K.M.: Nursing diagnosis in a discharge planning program, Nurs. Clinics N. A. **14:**517-524, 1979.

Morris, J.L.: Nursing diagnosis: a focus for continuing education, J. Contin. Ed. Nurs. **13:**33-39, 1982.

Nursing diagnosis: incidence and perceived value by nurses

CYNTHIA LEE LESSOW, M.S., R.N.

Nurses are taught about nursing diagnoses and how to use them—but are these diagnoses implemented in practice? Gordon (1976) described nursing diagnoses as an integral part of the nursing process, yet Aspinall (1976) called the nursing diagnosis the "weakest link" of the process. The need for nursing diagnoses to be standardized and classified was identified in 1973 with the formation of a National Task Force which later developed a formal organization, the North American Nursing Diagnosis Association (NANDA) (Kim, McFarland, and McLane 1984a). Since that time the importance of nursing diagnoses has been stressed in the literature.

The literature on nursing diagnoses has been largely that of validating accepted nursing diagnoses as compiled by the National Conference Group from 1973 to 1982. These studies indicated that nursing diagnoses were being used to some degree, and gave direction to the national group for any additions, deletions, or modifications. The results of these and other studies suggest some skill deficits and areas that nursing needs to concentrate on in order to use nursing diagnoses to their full potential. These include: (1) nurses have difficulty in problem solving and using theoretical knowledge (Aspinall 1979, Grier 1976, Matthews and Gaul 1979); (2) nurses lack the ability to carry out the nursing process (Deback 1981); and (3) nurses do not write care plans that conform to the accepted NANDA list (Martin and York 1984, Halloran 1980).

STUDY DESIGN

In 1984, Martin and York conducted a study with three purposes: 1) to validate the assumption that there was a skill deficit in identifying nursing diagnoses; 2) to determine the incidence of nursing diagnoses in order to obtain epidemiologic information for use at national conferences; and 3) to measure the concept of "valuing."

The present descriptive study was a replication of parts of the Martin and York study. The skill deficit assumption was evaluated based on the use of correct terminology when writing nursing diagnoses and noting the most frequently written ones. The nursing diagnoses most commonly used and the incidence of accepted nursing diagnoses were measured, along with the valuing of the nursing diagnosis as perceived by the nurses. A demographic profile was also obtained. For convenience and feasibility, the portion of the original study dealing with assessment of the diagnosis by a panel of experts was not replicated.

The first purpose of this study was to explore and describe the nursing diagnoses written by staff nurses. Information on which nursing diagnoses are being written is important for several reasons. First, it can indicate which nursing problems the nurses feel most comfortable with and capable of diagnosing. Second, if nurses are using nursing diagnoses that are not on the accepted list, then perhaps the nursing diagnoses that *are* being written need to be researched more extensively for the next NANDA conference. This also explains the importance of determining how many of the nursing diagnoses are on the accepted list from NANDA; if nurses are not using the classification system from the National Conference Group, then the whole concept of standardization must be reconsidered or revised.

The second purpose of the study was to explore and describe nurses' perceptions of the usefulness of nursing diagnoses in communicating, giving care, and charting. Steele (1979) contended that valuing the care plans (which contain the nursing diagnoses) would be expressed by using the care plan, and Manthey (1984) stressed that care plans must be useful to the care giver or they do not meet their primary purpose. Therefore, knowing whether or not nurses value nursing diagnoses in all phases of their clinical practice could give direction to educators. If nurses place little or no value on care plans the utilization of the nursing diagnoses would reflect this, and motivation would have become a priority for nurse educators.

RESEARCH QUESTIONS

1. What percent of charts contain nursing diagnosis statements?
2. Of the nursing diagnoses written, what is the representation from the accepted Fifth Conference of the National Group for Classification of Nursing Diagnoses list?
3. How are staff nurses writing nursing diagnoses?
4. Which nursing diagnoses are being used most frequently by staff nurses?
5. How useful do nurses think nursing diagnoses are in giving care?
6. How useful do nurses think nursing diagnoses are in communicating?
7. How useful do nurses think nursing diagnoses are in charting?

STUDY SETTING

The study was conducted in an 850-bed midwestern tertiary care hospital. Eleven

months prior to the data collection, the nurses employed in this hospital attended a mandatory 8 hour workshop on the implementation of nursing diagnoses. They were taught the nursing diagnostic process and how to correctly write a nursing diagnosis using the accepted list of nursing diagnoses from the Fifth National Conference (Kim, McFarland and McLane 1984b). The units participating in the study were 12 medical-surgical units and two maternity units. The critical care, psychiatric, and rehabilitation units were not included in the study.

STUDY METHODOLOGY

A stratified random sampling technique using a random number table was used. For convenience, the sample was separated by units, and five patient care plans per unit were randomly selected for the study. Five care plans from each of 14 units (70 care plans) were examined. The nursing diagnoses on the 70 care plans were recorded verbatim (161 nursing diagnoses), including the problem and etiology clauses. The diagnoses were then separated into three categories: acceptable (those on the Fifth National Conference list of accepted nursing diagnoses), correctly written but not worded as on the accepted list, and unacceptable (problem only, wrong expression of relationship, medical diagnosis, or correct format but not similar to those on the accepted list of nursing diagnoses).

The 41 nurses that were asked to complete a questionnaire were chosen in a similar fashion. A random number table was used to choose a maximum of three nurses from each unit. Only two nurses were on duty on one unit, so both were asked to complete the questionnaire.

ANALYSIS

The demographic data indicated that the age group most represented in this study was between 20-30 (63 percent); 17 percent were between 31 and 40, and 20 percent were 41 and older. Fifty-one percent of the nurses had been in practice from 1 to 5 years, 22 percent had practiced between 5 and 10 years, 22 percent had been practicing for more than 10 years, and 5 percent had one year's experience or less. The majority of the nurses indicated that a BSN was the highest level of nursing education earned (61 percent); 26 percent had a diploma, 12 percent had an associate degree, and none held a master's degree.

The data showed that out of the 70 care plans reviewed, 66 (94 percent) had at least one nursing diagnosis and 4 (6 percent) were blank. The number of diagnoses per care plan ranged from 0 to 22, with the mean being two per care plan.

Of the 161 nursing diagnoses evaluated, 80 (50 percent) were written correctly according to the accepted Fifth National Conference list; 41 (26 percent) were written correctly but not worded exactly as suggested by the Fifth National Conference, and 40 (25 percent) were either written incorrectly or written correctly but were not similar to any of the accepted nursing diagnoses.

Twenty-six percent (41) of the nursing diagnoses had the correct format but were not listed by the Fifth National Conference; 11 percent (9) of the unacceptable diagnoses had the problem statement only; 6 percent (5) either did not include an expression of relationship or did not use related to; 6 percent (5) used a medical diagnosis, and 26 percent (21) were problems that were not similar to those on the accepted list but were written correctly.

Of the 80 acceptable diagnoses, the six most frequently written were: 1) alteration in comfort, 20 (25 percent); 2) anxiety, 13 (16 percent); 3) knowledge deficit, 12 (15 percent); 4) potential for injury, 6 (8 percent); 5) alteration in tissue perfusion, 6 (8 percent), and 6) impairment in skin integrity, 5 (6 percent).

Of the 41 diagnoses that were not worded according to the accepted NANDA listing but were written correctly, the three most prevalent were: 1) alteration in coping, 6 (15 percent); 2) skin breakdown, 5 (12 percent); and 3) alteration in respiratory status, 5 (12 percent). The problems identified by all three are covered by NANDA, but they are worded differently (i.e., "alteration in skin integrity" instead of skin breakdown).

Of the 21 diagnoses that were not similar to those on the accepted NANDA list but were written correctly, the two most prevalent were: 1) potential for infection, 10 (48 percent); and 2) potential for complications, 5 (24 percent). Many of the nursing diagnoses that identified these problems continued the diagnosis with "related to IV therapy."

The results of the questions on valuing suggest that the nurses generally agree that nursing diagnoses are helpful to them in caring for their patients, appropriate for their patients, useful in giving care, and useful in charting. However, they appear to be neutral about how useful the diagnoses are in communicating with other nurses.

DISCUSSION OF FINDINGS

The number of diagnoses that were actually written and the fact that 75% were worded exactly or similarly as on the Fifth National Conference list of accepted diagnoses indicate that the nurses in this institution are writing diagnoses and do have a basic understanding of how to write them; the implementation of nursing diagnoses was successful, and nurses are motivated to write them.

The fact that alteration in comfort, anxiety, and knowledge deficit were used more than any other nursing diagnoses indicates that the nurses believe that these diagnoses are appropriate for their patients and accurately reflect the patient problems they are identifying.

The results show that many of the nursing diagnoses on the list of accepted nursing diagnoses are being used, although there are a few that seem to be either too specific or too broad. For example, the three most prevalent diagnoses suggest several things. For one, the diagnoses on the accepted list that relate to coping might be too specific—the nurses seem to prefer the broad category of "alteration in respiratory status" rather than "ineffective airway clearance" or "ineffective breathing pattern." This is exemplified again with the nursing diagnoses on nutrition and elimination—the nurses preferred "alteration in nutrition" or "potential for malnutrition" and "alteration in elimination" instead of the more specific ones. It seems that the nurses were more prone to generalize the problem clause and become more specific in the etiology clause. However, they also appeared to prefer the specific problem of "skin breakdown" to the accepted broader problem of "alteration in skin integrity." Findings like these aid in the continued development of a valid, standardized taxonomy by encouraging further research on these specific diagnoses.

The most prevalent diagnoses of the 21 that were not similar to those on the accepted list but were written correctly were "potential for infection," "potential for complication," and "potential for bleeding and hemorrhage." This suggests that nurses have a significant need for nursing diagnoses that reflect the problems of potential infections and complications. Therefore, further research in the validation of these nursing diagnoses is indicated.

IMPLICATIONS OF THE STUDY

The data from this study suggests that at this hospital diagnoses are being written on most care plans, and that the majority are on the list of accepted diagnoses. The nurses had only one inservice meeting on nursing diagnoses, yet were able to synthesize the information they were given and incorporate the diagnoses into their daily care planning. This is perhaps an indication that nurses are ready and willing to assume more responsibility for carrying out the nursing process.

On the other hand, although the nurses are writing diagnoses using the acceptable problems, there does seem to be a need to further evaluate what is being written. For instance, many diagnoses repeated the problem in the etiology clause (i.e., ineffective breathing pattern related to SOB) or had inappropriate etiology clauses for the identified problem (i.e., actual knowledge deficit related to OR (surgery) in the AM). Even though this was not measured in the study, a closer look at the etiology phrases and the appropriateness of the problems to patients might indicate that the nurses need additional education.

Another question that arises is: How strict do institutions have to be regarding the use of only NANDA approved nursing diagnoses? There has been some discussion in the literature on this topic (Shamansky and Yanni 1983, Kritik 1985). This hospital was not very specific as to whether or not the nurses should use only the approved nursing diagnoses, yet 50% of those written were on the approved list, and 26% were similar to those listed but with slightly different wording. Thus, the majority of nurses might agree that the accepted nursing diagnoses were really appropriate for their patients. They indicated this on the questionnaire, as well as in the written diagnoses. In light of the many advantages of nursing diagnoses, and because nurses seem to be using the accepted diagnoses anyway, it might enhance nursing if nurses were encouraged to use those diagnoses validated by NANDA. This expectation might also encourage research on nursing diagnoses (so that more could be added to the 50 already approved by NANDA), and would also alleviate the writing of problem clauses that are medical diagnoses or unacceptable in other ways.

Another implication of this study was the lack of NANDA approved nursing diagnoses written by the obstetrical division. On closer examination of the list it became evident that very few of the approved diagnoses pertain to obstetrics. It would appear that the National Study Group needs to develop and research the addition of nursing diagnoses that pertain more specifically to problems of the obstetric patient.

One last implication relates to the fact that nurses were neutral about how useful nursing diagnoses are in communicating with other nurses. This can be attributed to the fact that nurses were taught only to write nursing diagnoses, especially those appropriate to their patients. The communication component of nursing diagnoses was not emphasized, and therefore does not seem to have made much of an impact. This component needs to be emphasized during the education of staff nurses.

REFERENCES

Aspinall, M.J.: Nursing diagnosis: the weak link, Nurs. Outlook 24:433-436, 1976.

Aspinall, M.J.: Use of a decision tree to improve accuracy of diagnosis, Nurs. Outlook 28:182-185, 1979.

DeBack, V.: The relationship between senior nursing students' ability to formulate nursing diagnoses and the curriculum model, Adv. Nurs. Sci. 3:51-56, 1981.

Gordon, M.: Nursing diagnosis and the diagnostic process, Amer. J. Nurs. 76:1298-1300, 1976.

Grier, M.: Investigation of the quantification of selected patient care decisions by registered nurses. Doctoral dissertation, Texas Women's University, 1976. Dissertation Abstracts International, 36:6073B.

Halloran, E.J.: Analysis of variation in nursing workload by patient, medical and nursing condition. Doctoral dissertation, University of Illinois, 1980. Dissertation Abstracts International, 41:3385B.

Kim, M.J., McFarland, G.K., and McLane, A.M.: Classification of nursing diagnoses: proceedings of the fifth national conference, St. Louis, 1984, The C.V. Mosby Co.

Kim, M.J., McFarland, G.K., and McLane, A.M.: Pocket guide to nursing diagnoses, St. Louis, 1984, The C.V. Mosby Co.

Kritek, P.: Nursing diagnosis in perspective: response to a critique, Image 17:3-8, 1985.

Manthey, M.: Nursing care plans, Nurs. Management 12:28, 1984.

Martin, P.A. and York, K.A.: Incidence of nursing diagnoses. In Kim, M.J., McFarland, G.K., and McLane, A.M., editors: Classification of nursing diagnoses: proceedings of the fifth national conference, St. Louis, 1984, The C.V. Mosby Co.

Matthews, S.C. and Gaul, A.: Nursing diagnosis from the perspective of concept attainment and critical thinking, Adv. Nurs. Sci. 2:17-26, 1979.

Shamanski, S.L. and Yanni, C.R.: In opposition to nursing diagnosis: a minority opinion, Image 15:47-50, 1983.

Steele, S.: Values and values clarification. In Steele, S. and Harmon, V.M., editors: Values clarification in nursing, New York, 1979, Appleton-Century-Crofts.

Utilization studies: abstracts

Nursing diagnosis in print: observations and implications

BEATRICE B. TURKOSKI, M.S., R.N.

Following the earliest references to nursing diagnoses (ND) in the 1950s interest in ND grew rapidly, and in 1973 ND was identified as a professional responsibility by the American Nurses' Association. Since that time there have been six National Conferences and several regional conferences specifically addressing the classification and taxonomy of ND. Schools of Nursing are teaching ND, and health care institutions are implementing its use. However, theories, concepts, and practical application of ND differ greatly among academicians and practitioners. Nowhere are these differences so apparent as in published articles referring to ND.

This survey was designed to identify the predominant areas of difference among the ND articles found in professional journals between 1950 and 1985. Literature from the United States, Canada, England, and Australia was reviewed, and 150 articles were chosen for study. Primary criteria for inclusion required that nursing diagnosis, taxonomy, or classification be specifically mentioned in the article title.

Articles were analyzed for author demographics and type of journal. Content was analyzed for specific factors: 1) defense of ND or comparison between ND and medical diagnosis; 2) discussion of ND methodology, theory, and conceptual bases; 3) relating ND to specific health problems; 4) having ND replace nursing assessment in the nursing process; and 5) opposition to ND.

Analysis of content identified a significant ($p<.05$) relationship between nursing position and conceptualization of ND. Nurses in clinical settings were more likely to discuss ND as assessment applied to clinical cases or specific settings. Nurses in academic settings were more inclined to address the conceptual, theoretical, or methodological considerations. More than 50 percent of the articles identified the need for ND research, and yet less than 5 percent of the authors actually reported research directed at validating specific diagnoses or the effect of implementing ND in specific health care settings.

The purpose and need for ND were described from a variety of standpoints, and more than 40 percent of the articles had statements defending or rationalizing the concept of ND. Interestingly, while we know that there is a strong body of opposition to ND within the profession, less than 3 percent of the published articles questioned or attacked ND.

The results of the study support the hypothesis that there are conceptual differences among nurses concerning various aspects of ND and the application of ND to practice. These results indicate a need to develop improved intraprofessional communication between nurse clinicians and nurse academicians. In addition, the small number of articles from outside the United States suggests that, if ND is to provide a taxonomy of nursing applicable to professional nursing as a world wide profession, there must be increased dialog among nurses from all nations. We vitally need international taxonomic discussions and international taxonomic research to develop a valid and acceptable identification of the human responses to disruption in health that are treated by nurses in a variety of settings and geographical locations. We also need to expand our awareness of the influence that differing orientations have on our approach to nursing research, education, and practice. We need to recognize the legitimacy of a variety of paradigms that are used to develop nursing science. An acceptable ND taxonomy must be flexible enough to represent the depth of extant nursing knowledge while also lending itself to worldwide research which seeks to verify the congruence between nursing theory and practice.

Nursing process and nursing diagnosis utilization in South Africa

LINDA SCHWARTZ RABINOWITZ, M.S., R.N.

A descriptive design was used to survey the use of nursing diagnosis and nursing process in programs of university-based nursing schools located in South Africa. American nurses can add to their knowledge about nursing diagnosis by researching the use of the concept in other countries. A demographic and research questionnaire was mailed to 16 South African nursing schools. The sample size consisted of 18 South African nurse educators. Over one-half worked full-time in their nursing program, spent 11 years or more as licensed nurses, taught medical-surgical nursing, and held either baccalaureate or master's degrees in nursing. The major findings included:

1) One hundred percent of the sample reported use of the nursing process in their school's curriculum, while only 11 percent reported consistent use.

2) The nursing process was frequently incorporated in the nurses' notes, the majority of which (83 percent) utilized four or five steps that did not include nursing diagnoses.

3) Only 18 percent did not use nursing diagnoses in their school's curriculum. They reported that the concept was not well understood by the hospital nursing staff and that there were no plans to utilize the concept in the future.

4) Among those nurse educators who utilize nursing diagnoses, over one-half of the diagnostic statements contained one structural component, and one-fourth contained two components accompanied by a phrase connecting the two components.

5) None of the nursing diagnosis definitions were consistent, although the majority included the phrase "patient problem-oriented."

6) None of the subjects reported consistent use of nursing diagnoses in their school's curriculum or patients' charts.

7) The subjects reported use of more American than non-American publications to learn about nursing process and nursing diagnoses.

Conclusions based on the findings were: 1) Nursing process and nursing diagnoses are utilized in countries outside of the United States. 2) Nursing service and nursing education in South Africa utilize nursing process and nursing diagnoses to improve patient care. This study demonstrated the need for continued research in both the classification and operational definitions of nursing diagnoses and nursing process.

The Omaha system and NANDA: similar or different?

KAREN MARTIN, M.S.N., R.N.

Since 1975 the Visiting Nurse Association of Omaha has pursued the following question: What are the essential components of a total community health practice and recording system adaptable to computerization? Three studies have been conducted in the past 10 years. The general purpose of the studies was to positively impact on quality of care and cost benefit by enhancing effectiveness, efficiency, accountability, and evaluation of practice and recording. The specific objectives included identifying and refining a schema of problems of nursing diagnoses, expected outcomes-outcome criteria, and interventions addressed by community health nurses; validating the schema in three additional agencies; preparing a manual to facilitate implementation by others; and developing a client management information system.

A quantitative, descriptive design was used. The studies were based on empirical data collection from more than 1000 actual client records. Approximately 200 staff nurses and supervisors from agencies in Delaware, Indiana, Texas, Iowa, and Nebraska were involved. At various times data analysis has included frequencies, cross tabs, and correlation statistics. The studies have resulted in a compatible schema of problems, expected outcomes, and interventions. The schema is organized into the following four domains: environmental, psychosocial, physiological, and health behaviors.

An ongoing, informal survey has identified more than 80 individuals or agencies in 26 states as users of some part of the system. Staff nurses, supervisors, and management personnel using the system have reported benefits from its use. These range from organizing, retrieving, and computerizing client data to monitoring client progress and facilitating communication between health care providers. The system design integrates clinical data with financial and personnel data, and similarities and differences between the described system and NANDA are elaborated.

Education studies: paper presentation

Can theory improve diagnosis? An examination of the relationship between didactic content and the ability to diagnose in clinical practice

SHEILA LaFORTUNE FREDETTE, Ed.D., R.N.
EILEEN SJOBERG O'NEILL, M.S., R.N.

Although the term "nursing diagnosis" appears in the literature as early as 1950 (McManus), its application to clinical nursing has occurred only since the First National Conference on the Classification of Nursing Diagnosis in 1973. During this developmental period articles have been generated about the concept in general (Gebbie and Lavin 1975, Mundinger and Jauron 1975, Gordon 1976, Gordon 1982a, Henderson 1978, Kritek 1978, Lash 1978), along with a number of articles specific to the clinician (Feild 1979, McKeehan 1979, Dalton 1979, Weber 1979, Bruce 1979, Price 1980, Leslie 1981, Lunney 1982). The linkage between nursing diagnosis and the medical domain has also been described (Henderson 1978, Mundinger 1978, Rossi 1979, Fredette and Gloriant 1981, Tilton and Maloof 1982, Sjoberg 1983, Fredette 1984a).

Throughout the literature a clear message has been put forth by nursing authors: the nursing educator bears the responsibility for understanding, practicing, and teaching the skills of diagnosis (Roy 1976, Aspinall 1976, Gordon 1980, Carnevali 1984). Faculty have responded by integrating the concept of diagnosis into curricula, and a few examples of such curricula have been published (Fredette and O'Connor 1979, McLane 1982, Fredette 1984b).

The belief that the main focus of nursing is the diagnosis of health problems treatable by nurses was recently expressed by Mallick (1983), who stated that the role of diagnostician should be designated and taught as the primary role of nursing. For those in agreement with Mallick's position, a question to be answered is "How should the complex process of diagnosis be taught?" This research studies the effect of one teaching strategy for developing diagnostic ability by examining the performance of students after the introduction of content on the diagnostic process.

REVIEW OF THE LITERATURE

Literature and research have shown that, on the whole, nurses are poor diagnosticians of their patients' problems (Aspinall 1976, Aspinall 1978, DeBack 1981, Mathews and Gaul 1979, McCue 1981). There are possible explanations for this alleged deficiency in the problem solving skills of nurses which are suggestive of research questions. McCue states that nursing theory and nursing practice seem to be poorly linked, with educators presuming that students will automatically synthesize cognitive with affective and psychomotor domains and apply this body of knowledge to patient care. In reference to diagnosis, if the problem solving skills of nurses can be identified, an attempt can be made to improve those cognitive processes. Research can also be conducted on which theoretical framework will provide the most logical basis for diagnosis. Finally, researchers might investigate the most effective strategies for teaching diagnostic skills.

DeBack (1981) found a paucity of literature on problem solving in nursing, an allegation that is easily documented. Although a number of studies were conducted in the 1960s to identify how nurses deal with cues and make clinical inferences (Hammond, Kelly, Schneider, and Vancini 1966, Hammond 1966) little appears in the nursing literature since that work until the mid-1970s. After discovering that most of the nurses in her study lacked both theoretical knowledge of patient problems and strategies for evaluating cues and deriving problems, Aspinall (1979) found that the use of a decision tree increased accuracy in diagnosing.

Gordon's (1980) study determined the influence of inferential ability and restricted-unrestricted information on graduate student's hypothesis-scanning strategies, diagnostic accuracy, and confidence in diagnostic tasks. She found no relationship between inferential ability (as measured on GRE and MAT) and ability to diagnose or confidence in diagnosis. She also found that the subjects used predictive hypothesis testing procedures as part of their diagnostic repertoires. Gordon suggested that nurses be taught a network of propositional inferences which

can be retrieved from memory (i.e., nursing diagnoses) along with the relationships and variables influencing high risk states. She further stated that both skills of inferential reasoning and strategies to increase diagnostic validity need to be learned (1980).

Mathews and Gaul (1979) concluded that the ability to diagnose may depend upon identification of learned discrimination cues for each diagnosis, rather than on critical thinking ability. That is, nurses diagnose by applying theoretical knowledge about specific diagnoses to the diagnosis of patients. These authors say that educators and researchers need to focus on identifying and teaching this cognitive task if diagnostic ability is to improve.

Tanner (1982) found that a major determinant of diagnostic accuracy appeared to be the inclusion of the correct diagnosis in the original set of hypotheses. She suggested further research to examine information-seeking strategies and analyze diagnostic tasks encountered by nurses which affect hypothesis generation.

In analyzing nursing diagnoses in care plans of senior students from 270 baccalaureate nursing programs, DeBack (1981) found that only 28 percent met all expected criteria, and 35 percent met none of the criteria. She cited possible reasons for this deficiency: newness of the concept, lack of professors with knowledge to teach diagnosis, inappropriate teaching framework, students' difficulty applying theory to clinical practice, and lack of consistency and clarity concerning how to teach the concept. DeBack concluded with two questions: "Are there teaching strategies that are more effective in teaching the skills necessary for diagnosis? If so, what are they?" (p. 65).

Mallick (1983) discovered advanced strategies for teaching diagnosis in a number of basic nursing textbooks. She felt that the novice student needs basic principles and rules for diagnosis; that is, "strategies that are simple, yet elegant, to guarantee that nursing diagnosis is taught, not caught" (p. 459).

Initial data on factors influencing diagnostic reasoning and cognitive strategies in nursing students and nurses indicate that there are decided differences in the problem solving of novices versus experts. Examination of diagnostic errors made by novices has led to suggestions for strengthening the teaching of decision making processes (Tanner 1984). When final data from this study are reported, there may be additional insights concerning how to teach the diagnostic process.

In summary, research into the diagnostic processing of nurses is in its infancy. A literature survey revealed minimal suggestions for incorporating diagnosis into nursing theory, and little or nothing was found about how to teach diagnosis clinically (Carpenito and Duespohl 1981, deTornyay and Thompson 1982, O'Shea and Parsons 1979, Schweer and Gebbie 1976, Meleca, Schimpthauser, Witteman, and Sachs 1981).

Although neither the components of the diagnostic process nor the most appropriate strategies for teaching the components have been determined, the literature does urge educators to pay attention to variables which are likely to impact on diagnostic skills.

PURPOSE OF THE RESEARCH

These two studies were conducted over two academic years to investigate how one variable, didactic content, affects the development of diagnostic ability.

The first year of the research served as a pilot study in order to evaluate and reformulate both the research procedure and the didactic content prior to beginning Study II.

The same question was asked in each study: Can the diagnostic skills of the beginning nursing student be improved by increasing the amount of selected theoretical content on diagnosis? The researchers hypothesized that an increased amount of didactic theory about the diagnostic process would result in increased skill in clinical diagnosis. The underlying assumption was that the novice student does, indeed, require a basic set of heuristics in order to adapt innate and acquired problem solving skills to clinical diagnosis.

CONCEPTUAL FRAMEWORK

The theoretical content was derived from Gordon (1982b) and Carnevali, Mitchell, Woods, and Tanner (1984), and is summarized in Box 1. In addition to theory on nursing diagnosis, this content included the principles and rules of diagnosis, which provide the learner with foundation skills for diagnosing. The researchers developed the *Diagnostic Skills Criteria*, which were used as a framework for analysis of students' nursing diagnoses; these are as follows:

Level I Skills:
1. Makes a nursing diagnostic statement
2. Cites supportive assessment data

Level II Skills:
1. Clusters data accurately
2. Identifies a nursing etiology

Level III Skills:
1. Uses multiple etiologies
2. Cites potential diagnoses

We believe that this scheme of increasingly complex skill levels is consistent with the Piagetian Theory of Cognitive Development as described in Ginsburg and Opper (1969).

DEFINITION OF TERMS

Nursing Process: The problem solving methodology of nursing which includes the steps of assessment, diagnosis, intervention, and evaluation.

Nursing Diagnosis: "Nursing Diagnoses, or clinical diagnoses, made by the profession-

---

BOX 1   **Theoretical content on nursing diagnosis**[1,2]

    I. Overview of the Concept of Nursing Diagnosis
       A. As a category
          1. structural definition
          2. conceptual definition
       B. As a process
          1. information collection
          2. information interpretation
          3. information clustering
          4. cluster naming
    II. Assessment—Collecting information
       A. Methods of collecting information
          1. pre-encounter data
          2. information seeking strategies
       B. The nature of clinical information
          1. cue versus inference
          2. types of cues
          3. cue evaluation
          4. probabilistic nature of clinical cues
       C. Tools used in diagnosis
          1. clinical knowledge
          2. recognition of cues
          3. clinical practice experience
   III. Interpreting Information—Clinical Reasoning
       A. Strategies—hypotheses—decisions
          1. early diagnostic hypotheses (functions—dangers)
          2. branching logic—considering the alternatives
          3. focused cue search
          4. single hypothesis testing
          5. clustering cues
       B. Problem formulation—stating the diagnosis
          1. tentativeness of the diagnosis
          2. questioning the diagnosis
       C. Etiologies
       D. Sources of diagnostic error
          1. data collection errors
          2. data interpretation errors
          3. data clustering errors

---

[1]Gordon, M.: Nursing diagnosis: process and application, New York, 1982, McGraw Hill.
[2]Carnevali, D., Mitchell, P., Woods, N., and Tanner, C.: Diagnostic reasoning in nursing, Philadelphia, 1984, J.B. Lippincott.

al nurse, describe actual or potential health problems which nurses by virtue of their education and experience are capable and licensed to treat" (Gordon 1976, p. 1298).

Clustering Data: Combining individual pieces of data which fit together to have a meaning; also called chunking data.

Nursing Etiology: The cause or causes of the nursing diagnosis which can be remedied by nursing intervention.

Clinical Paper: A comprehensive paper concerning the patient assignment; one is required each week of the student's clinical experience. It includes assessment, diagnosis, goal setting, intervention, and evaluation.

Accepted Nursing Diagnoses: Those accepted at the North American Nursing Diagnosis Fifth National Conference on the Classification of Nursing Diagnoses.

METHODOLOGY

Since the sample, setting, and treatment were the same in both studies, these aspects will be discussed together, whereas the procedure and analysis will be presented separately.

Sample and setting

The entire study was conducted over 2 consecutive academic years with junior students in a baccalaureate nursing program that has included nursing diagnosis in the curriculum for over 12 years. The subject pool for study Part I consisted of 108 students, whereas the subject pool for study Part II contained 107 students.

The students began their third year with the same foundational courses in nursing and the natural and behavioral sciences. A sophomore nursing course provided introductory content on nursing process/diagnosis, including basic diagnostic skills. The diagnostic skills are applied during 18 hours of clinical practice, which also focuses on technical skills.

The junior year nursing course, divided into two sections of equal number, provided the structure for the research. Section I became the control group; Section II was the experimental group. Both groups not only shared the same basic courses, but also were representative of the average generic student in nursing (mean age of 21, 98 percent female). A multivariate analysis of variance on each of these sections for both years showed no significant differences between groups on two variables: overall cumulative grade point average and nursing cumulative grade point average. The two semester course for each section included content on all of the nursing diagnoses accepted at the North American Nursing Diagnosis Fifth National Conference. Finally, faculty expectations were similar regarding clinical requirements; all students utilized assessment and diagnosis with reference handbooks by either Gordon (1985), Kim (1984), or Carpenito (1983).

Treatment

At the beginning of 2 consecutive years, both junior class sections were given the usual 2 hour review on nursing process/diagnosis. Additionally, the experimental group was given 5 more hours of content (see Box 1) adapted from Gordon (1982b) and Carnevali, Mitchell, Woods, and Tanner (1984).

For Study I this content was delivered during the first month of the fall semester. Based on the pilot, the researchers felt that the content might be more effectively learned if spaced throughout the academic year. Thus, for Study II, content was begun in September and concluded in March. Although faculty and students knew that research was being conducted, neither knew the exact nature of the study nor the criteria to be examined.

STUDY I
Procedure

Using a post-test with follow-up design, students' clinical papers were examined at two intervals: 1 month and 6 months after completion of the presentation of the extra nursing diagnosis content to the experimental group. Student papers were randomly drawn by a research assistant equally from medical-surgical, obstetric, and pediatric groups of both experimental and control class sections. The researchers' clinical groups were excluded from the sample. The assistant copied and coded each paper and removed all identifying marks; the code was not revealed until after completion of analysis. Thus, neither student name nor group identification were known to the researchers at the time of analysis.

In order to examine individual students' longitudinal development at the 6 month period, papers were matched from the two sampling periods. This resulted in 16 students (32 papers) from the experimental group and 18 students (36 papers) from the control group. These two paired groups again showed no statistically significant differences as reflected by a multivariate analysis of variance on cumulative averages. Each researcher independently analyzed each nursing diagnosis by applying the *Diagnostic Skills Criteria*. After independent analysis, findings were compared and areas of disagreement reconciled. Interrater reliability was .98.

Findings

Differences on sum of the criteria. Overall differences on an aggregate of the criteria showed no significant differences between experimental and control groups for either sampling period.

Differences between groups on each criterion for both sampling periods. Cross tabulation of group membership by attainment of criteria was performed for each criterion for both sampling periods; a significant relationship was found for only one criterion: level 3 criterion 2 in sampling period 2 (potential diagnoses): $x^2 = 4.24$, $p \leq .05$. The experimental group performed better than the control group on this criterion.

Differences within groups for each time period. When individual student clinical papers were examined at the two sampling periods, the experimental group showed no significant change on any of the criteria. The control group, however, showed a statistically significant increase in level 3 criterion 1 (multiple etiologies): $x^2 = 4.0$, $p \leq .05$.

Differences between groups on the average number of diagnoses. In sampling period 1 no significant difference was evident between the groups; however, at sampling period 2 the experimental group identified a significantly higher number of diagnoses ($t = 3.61$, $df = 32$, $p < .001$).

STUDY II

Variations were introduced in the second portion of the research. They are discussed under Part IIa and Part IIb.

Part IIa. Using an experimental design, a case study was given pre- and post-course to students in each section. The case (Appendix), which was written by the researchers and normed by experts in nursing diagnosis, had data for eight actual and 11 potential diagnoses. It was given in a regular 50 minute class period during the first week of fall semester, and again during the last week of spring semester. Students were asked to formulate nursing diagnostic statements that they could derive from the data base in the case. Several response sheets with headings of "data" and "diagnostic statement" were attached to the case (Box 2).

Before giving papers to the researchers, the research assistant removed all identification, coded the papers, and paired the pre- and post-student numbers. The resulting sample included 41 pairs in the experimental section and 29 in the control. An analysis of variance showed no statistically significant difference in overall cumulative averages for these two groups.

Each researcher analyzed each diagnostic statement made by each student relative to each diagnostic skills criterion for the pre- and post-test period. For Level I and II skills the student was given a "yes" if they met the criterion more than 50% of the time. Because Level III skills were not expected of a novice practitioner, any presence of the skill was recorded as a "yes." Additionally, each diagnostic statement made by each student was listed, and the total number was tallied.

Part IIb. The second variation during Part II had to do with analyzing subjects' clinical papers. To further evaluate application of diagnostic skills to actual clinical settings, a random sample of clinical papers was drawn from both experimental and control groups several weeks before the end of spring semester. The same blind review procedure was used, with the same research assistant drawing the random sample and coding papers. Experimental group clinical papers numbered 33, while the control group numbered 20. Researchers once again compared data after first analyzing each paper separately according to the *Diagnostic Skills Criteria*.

Findings

Case study results

Sum of the criteria. The experimental group showed a statistically higher ability on the aggregate of the criteria at the post-test (Tables 1 and 2).

Identification of actual diagnoses. Of the eight diagnoses for which actual data were present, the mean number identified by the experimental group prior to the course was 2.68 and after the course was 4.54. The control group had a pre-course mean of 2.38 and a post course mean of 3.93. The difference between groups was not significant for either period.

Table 1: Pre-course and post-course means and standard deviations for sum of criteria for experimental and control groups

	Exp (n=41)		Control (n=29)	
	Pre-course	Post-course	Pre-course	Post-course
Mean	3.31	3.73	2.31	2.37
S.D.	1.14	.94	1.07	1.65

Table 2: Post-course performance: experimental vs. control

	Ss	df	MS	F value	sig
Between groups	31.06	1	31.06	18.71	p<.05
Within groups	112.87	68	1.6599		
Total	143.94	69			

Identification of potential diagnoses. Of the eleven potential diagnoses, the experimental group made a total of six potential diagnoses pre-course and 19 post-course, whereas the control group made two pre-course and 11 post-course.

Differences between groups on each criterion at pre- and post-course periods. When cross-tabulations of group membership by attainment of criteria were performed on each criterion for both pre- and post-course data, significant relationships were found on the following criteria:

post–course level 1 criterion 1 (diagnostic statements): $x^2 = 6.49$, df = 1, p<.05.

Table 3: Differences between groups on each criterion L1C1* post-course, study II— diagnostic statements

Count
Row %
Column %
Total %

	YES	NO	Row Total
Experimental			
	37	4	41
	90.2	9.8	
	66.1	28.6	
	52.9	5.7	58.6
Control			
	19	10	29
	65.5	34.5	
	33.9	71.4	
	27.1	14.3	41.4
Column	56	14	70
Total %	80.0	20.0	100.0

Exp. - $x^2 = 6.49$, df = 1, p < .05.
*L1C1 = Level 1, Criterion 1.

Table 4: Differences between groups on each criterion L1C2* post-course, study II— supportive data

Count
Row %
Column %
Total %

	YES	NO	Row Total
Experimental			
	41	0	41
	100.0	0	
	68.3	0	
	58.6	0	58.6
Control			
	19	10	29
	65.5	34.5	
	31.7	100.0	
	27.1	14.3	41.4
Column	60	10	70
Total	85.7	14.3	100.0

Exp. - $x^2 = 16.49$, df = 1, p < .05.
*L1C2 = Level 1, Criterion 2.

post–course level 1 criterion 2 (supportive data): $x^2 = 16.9$, df = 1, p < .05.

post–course level 2 criterion 1, (clustering data): $x^2 = 25.68$, df = 1, p < .05.

On all criteria the experimental group scored better than the control group (Tables 3, 4, and 5).

Differences within groups on each criterion—pre- and post-course. When the case study papers were examined for each time period, it was found that they improved significantly on the following criteria:

Experimental group:

Level 2 criterion 1 (clustering data): $x^2 = 9.0$, df = 1, p < .05.

Level 3 criterion 2 (potential diagnoses): $x^2 = 8.0$, df = 1, p < .05.

Control group:

Level 1 criterion 2 (supportive data): $x^2 = 7.0$, df = 1, p < .05.

Level 3 criterion 2 (potential diagnoses): $x^2 = 7.4$, df = 1, p < .05.

Average number of diagnoses at pre- and post-course. No significant differences between the groups were found in pre- and post-course.

Clinical paper data. The experimental group did significantly better than the control group on two of the criteria (Table 6 and 7):

Level 1 criterion 2 (data to support dx): $x^2 = 4.18$, df = 1, p < .05.

Level 2, criterion 1 (clustering data): $x^2 = 4.88$, df = 1, p < .05.

DISCUSSION

The hypothesis (that an increased amount of didactic theory about the diagnostic process would result in increased skill in clinical diagnosis) was not supported when examin-

Table 5: Differences between groups on each criterion L2C1* post-course, study II—data clustering

Count
Row %
Column %
Total %

	YES	NO	Row Total
Experimental			
	40	1	41
	97.6	2.4	
	75.5	5.9	
	57.1	1.4	58.6
Control			
	13	16	29
	44.8	55.2	
	24.5	94.1	
	18.6	22.9	41.4
Column	53	17	70
Total	75.7	24.3	100.0

Exp. - $x^2 = 25.68$, df=1, p<.05.
*L2C1=Level 2, Criterion 1.

Table 6: Clinical papers L1C2* post-course, study II—supportive data

Count
Row %
Column%
Total%

	YES	NO	Row Total
Experimental			
	32	1	33
	97	3.0	
	66.7	20	
	60.4	1.9	62.3
Control			
	16	4	20
	80.0	20.0	
	33.3	80	
	30.2	7.5	37.7
Column	48	5	53
Total	90.6	9.4	100.0

Exp.– $x^2 = 4.18$, df=1, p<.05.
*L1C2=Level 1, Criterion 2.

Table 7: Differences between groups on each criterion L2C1* post-course, study II—clustering data

Count
Row%
Column%
Total%

	YES	NO	Row Total
Experimental			
	31	2	33
	93.9	6.1	
	70.5	22.2	
	58.5	3.8	62.3
Control			
	13	7	20
	65.0	35.0	
	29.5	77.8	
	24.5	13.2	37.7
Column	44	9	53
Total	83.0	17.0	100

Exp. – $x^2 = 4.88$, df=1, p<.05.
*L2C1=Level 2, Criterion 1.

ing individual criteria across the two time periods in Study I. The only significant finding was that the experimental group identified a higher number of correct diagnoses in sampling period 2.

Study II findings are more strongly suggestive of a link between theory and improved diagnostic skills. When aggregating the criteria, the experimental group showed a higher overall ability to utilize diagnostic skills.

It is also important to note that the experimental group excelled at the post-course on three of the individual criteria: diagnostic statements, data supportive of the diagnosis, and correct clustering of data. These findings were supported by sampling and analysis of clinical papers, which showed that the experimental group displayed greater ability on two of the three criteria. This consistency seems to indicate that these students both learned and applied the skills to clinical diagnosis.

Both groups grew in ability to identify diagnoses present in the case study, as well as on certain of the criteria. Such growth can be expected in that each of the sections were in a course that included theoretical content on specific nursing diagnoses. Both groups also had clinical practice in which they collected, sorted, interpreted, and analyzed clinical data. Skill in diagnosis is fostered by such repeated processing of data.

Nursing etiologies were used infrequently by both groups, which may reflect lack of clarity about this aspect of nursing diagnosis. In place of nursing etiologies, students named the medical diagnosis, procedures, and treatments, none of which were accepted by the researchers. Confusion in the literature and among experts on this concept is undoubtedly reflected in both teaching and practice.

Even though the data indicate that both groups had statistical increases in the naming of potential diagnoses, these Level 3 skills were scored only on their presence or absence, rather than on being used over 50 percent of the time. Inability to apply Level 3 skills is most likely related to the beginning learner's developmental stage and theory base.

IMPLICATIONS FOR CURRICULUM

Teaching diagnostic skills according to the three level framework is a useful technique which is adaptable to any nursing curriculum. Student ability to apply the skills can be easily monitored through clinical papers.

While further research is needed, the results of this study suggest that the novice nursing student's ability to diagnose can be influenced by the inclusion of didactic material on the diagnostic process. It also seems that integrating the content throughout a course may be the most effective way to impart these skills. Riley (1983) and Elstein, Shulman, and Sprafka (1976) suggest that problem solving depends largely on having an understanding of the relatonships between the entities in a domain, and that such complexity is lacking in the novice. In other words, the learner may understand diagnostic concepts more thoroughly when they are connected to more concrete information about the various diagnoses. Tanner supports this belief by stating that "the single greatest variable influencing diagnosis is the extent to which the knowledge network is developed in long term memory" (1984, p. 102).

SUGGESTIONS FOR FURTHER RESEARCH

This study should be replicated in other baccalaureate nursing programs to verify and increase the generalizability of findings. It also could be modified for replication in a number of ways. For example, diagnostic skills taught in the classroom to one group could be compared with those of another group taught the same content in a clinical setting with direct patient application. Experimenting with varied data collection tools might prove interesting. In this study no attempt was made to control the clinical assessment tool. Would there be a difference between the diagnostic ability of students who use a biological systems assessment tool versus those who use a functional pattern assessment tool?

Since the effectiveness of nursing intervention hinges on accuracy of diagnosis, educators need to seriously consider ways to improve the teaching of diagnosis. This study, which includes the teaching of principles and rules for diagnosis, has offered one approach for strengthening diagnostic skills. Investigation needs to be conducted to identify how other variables relate to diagnosis. Once effective teaching strategies have been delineated, improved diagnostic skills for nurses can begin to be realized.

REFERENCES

Aspinall, M.J.: Nursing diagnosis—the weak link, Nurs. Outlook **24:**433-437, 1976.

Aspinall, M.J.: Use of a decision tree to improve accuracy of diagnosis, Nurs. Res. **28:**182-185, 1979.

Bruce, J.A.: Implementation of nursing diagnosis: a nursing administrator's perspective, Nurs. Clinics N. A. **14:**509-516, 1979.

Carnevali, D.: Development of diagnostic reasoning skills: implications for nursing practice, education, management, nursing literature, and research. In Carnaveli, D.L., Mitchell, P.H., Woods, N.F., and others: Diagnostic reasoning in nursing, Philadelphia, 1984, J.B. Lippincott.

Carnevali, D.L., Mitchell, P.M., Woods, N.F., and others: Diagnostic reasoning in nursing. Philadelphia, 1984, J.B. Lippincott.

Carpenito, L.: Nursing diagnosis: application to clinical practice, Philadelphia, 1983, J.B. Lippincott.

Carpenito, L., and Duespohl, T.A.: A guide for effective clinical instruction, Aspen, 1981, Aspen Systems Corp.

Dalton, J.M.: Nursing diagnosis in a community health setting, Nurs. Clinics N. A. **14:**525-532, 1979.

DeBack, V.: The relationship between senior nursing students' ability to formulate nursing diagnoses and the curriculum model, Adv. Nurs. Sci. **3:**51-66, 1981.

deTornyay, R. and Thompson, M.C.: Strategies for teaching nursing, 2nd ed, New York, 1982, John Wiley & Sons.

Elstein, A.S., Shulman, L.S., and Sprafka, S.A.: Medical problem solving: an analysis of clinical reasoning, Cambridge, MA, 1978, Harvard University Press.

Feild, L.: The implementation of nursing diagnosis into clinical practice, Nurs. Clinics N. A. **14:**497, 1979.

Fredette, S.L.: When the liver fails, Amer. J. Nurs. **84:**64-67, 1984.

Fredette, S.L.: Patterns for teaching the diagnostic process. In Kim, M.J., McFarland, G.K., and McLane, A.M. editors: Classification of nursing diagnoses: proceedings of the fifth national conference, St. Louis, 1984, The C.V. Mosby Co.

Fredette, S.L. and Gloriant, F.: Nursing diagnosis in cancer chemotherapy: in theory and in practice, Amer. J. Nurs. **81:**2013-2021, 1981.

Fredette, S.L. and O'Connor, K.: Nursing diagnosis in teaching and curriculum planning, Nurs. Clinics N. A. **14:**541-552, 1979.

Gebbie, K.M. and Lavin, M.A.: Classification of nursing diagnoses: proceedings of the first national conference, St. Louis, 1975, The C.V. Mosby Co.

Ginsburg, H. and Opper, S.: Piaget's theory of intellectual development, Englewood Cliffs, NJ, 1969, Prentice-Hall, Inc.

Gordon, M.: Nursing diagnosis and the diagnostic process, Amer. J. Nurs. **76:**1298-1300, 1976.

Gordon, M.: Predictive strategies in diagnostic tasks, Nurs. Res. **29:**39-45, 1980.

Gordon, M.: The diagnostic process. In Kim, M.J. and Moritz, D.A., editors: Classification of nursing diagnoses: proceedings of the third and fourth national conferences, New York, 1982, McGraw-Hill.

Gordon, M.: Nursing diagnoses: process and application, New York, 1982, McGraw-Hill Co.

Gordon, M.: Manual of nursing diagnosis, 2nd ed, New York, 1985, McGraw-Hill Co.

Guinee, K.: Teaching and learning nursing, New York, 1978, Macmillan Publishing Co.

Hammond, K.R.: Clinical inference in nursing: a psychologist's viewpoint, Nurs. Res. **15:**27-38, 1966.

Hammond, K.R., Kelly, K.J., Schneider, R.J., and Vancini, M.: Clinical inference in nursing: information units used, Nurs. Res. **15:**236-242, 1966.

Henderson, B.: Nursing diagnosis: theory and practice, Adv. Nurs. Sci. **1:**75-83, 1978.

Kelly, K.J.: Clinical inference in nursing: a nurse's viewpoint, Nurs. Res. **15:**23-26, 1966.

Kim, M.J., McFarland, G.K., and McLane, A.M.: Pocket guide to nursing diagnoses, St. Louis, 1984, The C.V. Mosby Co.

Kissinger, J.F. and Munjas, B.A.: Nursing process, student's attributes, and teaching methodologies, Nurs. Res. **30:**242-246, 1981.

Kritek, P.B.: The generation and classification of nursing diagnoses: toward a theory of nursing, Image **10:**33-40, 1978.

Lash, A.A.: Re-examination of nursing diagnosis, Nurs. Forum, **17:**332-343, 1978.

Leslie, F.M.: Nursing diagnosis: use in long-term care, Amer. J. Nurs. **81:**1012, 1981.

Lunney, M.: Nursing diagnosis: refining the system, Amer. J. Nurs. **82:**456-459, 1982.

Mallick, J.J.: Nursing diagnosis and the novice student, Nurs. Health Care, **4:**455-459, 1983.

Mathews, C.A. and Gaul, A.L.: Nursing diagnosis from the perspective of concept attainment and critical thinking, Adv. Nurs. Sci. **2:**17-26, 1979.

McCue, H.: Clinical teaching and the nursing process: implications for nurse teacher education, Australian Nurses' J., **10:**36-37, 1981.

McKeehan, K.M.: Nursing diagnosis in a discharge planning program, Nurs. Clinics N. A. **14:**517-524, 1979.

McLane, A.M.: Nursing diagnosis in the master's practicum. In Kim, M.J., and Moritz, D.A., editors: Classification of nursing diagnoses: proceedings of the third and fourth national conferences, New York, 1982, McGraw-Hill Co.

Meleca, C.B., Schimpfhauser, F., Witteman, J.K., and Sachs, L.: Clinical instruction in nursing: a national survey. J. Nurs. Ed. **20**:32-40, 1981.

Mundinger, M. and Jauron, C.: Developing a nursing diagnosis, Nurs. Outlook **23**:94-98, 1975.

Mundinger, M.: Nursing diagnoses for cancer patients, Cancer Nurs. **1**:221-226, 1978.

O'Shea, H.S. and Parsons, M.K.: Clinical instruction: effective/ineffective teacher behaviors, Nurs. Outlook **27**:411-415, 1979.

Price, M.R.: Nursing diagnosis: making a concept come alive, Amer. J. Nurs. **80**:668-674, 1980.

Reilly, D.: Behavioral objectives in nursing: evaluation of learning attainment, New York, 1975, Appleton-Century-Crofts.

Riley, M.: Instructional methods that make a difference: structural understanding and the acquisition of problem-solving skills. Expanded version of paper presented at a meeting of the American Educational Research Association, Montreal, Quebec, 1983.

Rossi, L.P. and Haines, V.M.: Nursing diagnoses related to acute myocardial infarction, Cardiovasc. Nurs. **15**:11-15, 1979.

Roy, C.: A diagnostic classification system for nursing, Nurs. Outlook **23**:90-94, 1975.

Schweer, J. and Gebbie, K.: Creative teaching in clinical nursing, 3rd ed. St. Louis, 1976, The C.V. Mosby Co.

Sjoberg, E.L.: Nursing diagnosis and the COPD patient. Amer. J. Nurs. **83**:244-248, 1983.

Tanner, C.: Instruction on the diagnostic process: an experimental study. In Kim, M.J. and Moritz, D.A., editors: Classification of nursing diagnoses: proceedings of the third and fourth national conferences, New York, 1982, McGraw-Hill Co.

Tanner, C.: Diagnostic problem-solving strategies. In Carnevali, D.L., Mitchell, P.H., Woods, N.F. and others: Diagnostic reasoning in nursing, Philadelphia, 1984, J.B. Lippincott.

Tanner, C.: Factors influencing the diagnostic process. In Carnevali, D.L., Mitchell, P.H., Woods, N.F. and others: Diagnostic reasoning in nursing, Philadelphia, 1984, J.B. Lippincott.

Tilton, C. and Maloof, M.: Diagnosing the problems in stroke, Amer. J. Nurs. **82**:596-600, 1982.

Weber, S.: Nursing diagnosis in private practice, Nurs. Clinics N. A. **14**:533-540, 1979.

APPENDIX: NURSING DIAGNOSIS CASE STUDY

Mrs. Jones is a 59 year old housewife who lives in Fitchburg in a one-family, two-story home with her husband. Mrs. Jones has had five prior admissions to the local hospital for bronchial asthma. Precipitating factors in these attacks include upper respiratory infections (twice), her youngest son leaving for college, her husband's hospitalization for a myocardial infarction 6 years ago, and one admission for which there is no documentation regarding onset.

Mrs. Jones' parents are deceased, her father of C.O.P.D. 4 years ago, her mother of hypertension complicated by congestive heart failure 10 years ago. She has two siblings, both brothers; age 53 and 62. The 62 year old brother has had several hospitalizations for alcohol related problems. The 53 year old is healthy.

Mr. Jones is employed as a press tender in a local paper mill. Six years ago he had a myocardial infarction and recovered without complications. His work schedule has been reduced because of less work available at the mill. He now works three days a week and plans to retire next year at age 62.

The Jones have two children, both married, who live in distant states; one in North Carolina and one in Colorado. The children and their families visit home during the summer.

Mrs. Jones has never been employed outside of the home. She finished two years of high school, leaving to marry. Beside taking care of the home, she has a flower and vegetable garden during the summer. Additionally, she knits, watches television, and visits her next door neighbor, with whom she is friendly. On weekends she and her husband go to a movie or an occasional auction. Mrs. Jones does not drink alcohol and gave up smoking 5 years ago.

On admission at 1 A.M., Mrs. Jones had weight 163 lbs. and height 5'3". She looked anxious, holding onto her husband's hand and sitting upright. Her respiratory rate was 60, rales were heard at the base of both lungs, and she was cyanotic. Heart rate was 112, B.P. 160/102, and T. 99². She had audible wheezing and kept saying "I can't breath."

Her chest x-ray revealed underventilation but no other abnormalities. Epinephrine 0.3 c.c. × 2 was given in the emergency room and Mrs. Jones was admitted for continuing assessment.

It is now the next morning and you are the primary nurse taking care of Mrs. Jones. Her respiratory rate is now 36 and she has wheezing and rales on auscultation. She says she feels better but her breathing is "still not right." She is in high-Fowlers position with oxygen by cannula at 2 L./minute. Her heart rate is 92 and regular; B.P. is 150/94 and T. is 99.

Doctors orders include:

O$_2$ 2L. continuously.

I.P.P.B. with Bronkosol 1 c.c. Q.I.D.

Breathine .5 mg. q 6° P.O.

Chest x-ray this A.M.

Aminophylline 500 mg. in 500 c.c. 5% D/W—I.V. to be infused over 12°.

1500 cal. diet.

B.R.P. with assistance.

Mrs. Jones states that she has not felt well for the last few days. She has noticed some shortness of breath when climbing stairs in her house over the last 2 years, but states that it has increased in the last 4-5 days. Her fatigue level has also increased. She noticed that she had to rest more during her garden work this summer.

She states that she eats well, "too well," and likes to cook. Since her husband's heart attack she has eliminated butter in her cooking and tries to limit their intake of red meat, although she says it is difficult. Mrs. Jones says her husband does not like sweets but she does, so she makes them and shares some with her neighbor.

You, as the primary nurse, must develop Mrs. Jones' care plan.

Directions

This is part of an ongoing nursing diagnosis research project by S. Fredette and E. Sjoberg. Your papers will be handled by a research assistant who will assign numbers to your names and remove the names. Therefore, none of you will be identifiable by the two researchers. Please read the case carefully, identify the data, and write the nursing diagnostic statement(s). Place your name on top of the attached sheets and then begin. Thank you for your cooperation in this project. We will inform you about the findings at the conclusion of our research (Box 2).

BOX 2

Student Name _____

Data	Nursing Diagnostic Statement

Education studies: poster presentations

Nursing diagnosis: crucial link between theoretical knowledge and nursing practice

DEVAMMA PURUSHOTHAM, Ed.D., R.N.

STATEMENT OF THE PROBLEM

Health care in the 1980s includes modern electronic life-saving equipment. However, no machine can save a life without a skilled professional to interpret and utilize the data it provides. Developments in medical electronics and technology have made a tremendous impact on patient care, nursing education, and nursing practice. All knowledge, including medical knowledge, is advancing rapidly. To keep abreast of the accumulating knowledge will require increasing specialization and active participation of professional nurses.

A corollary to the influence of technology on health care services is an increasing realization of the need for nurses to make nursing diagnoses. The diagnostic process is common to many professions. However, the differences in diagnoses arise from the unique nature and knowledge peculiar to the practice of each profession. Making an accurate diagnosis in nursing requires a clear understanding of what data to gather, and an ability to make judgments based on scientific knowledge. Nursing diagnosis as a component of the nursing process provides a concise summary statement of identified patient problems which are amenable to nursing interventions.

Professional nursing utilizes as its methodology the nursing process. The conscious and systematic use of all phases of the nursing process (assessment, nursing diagnosis, planning, implementation, and evaluation) facilitates the professional nurse's performance as an independent decision maker, accountable for his/her nursing practice. In order to make an accurate nursing diagnosis, the nurse must have the knowledge to understand the encountered situation. The nurse must also comprehend the principles underlying the measures to alleviate the problem, and determine the patient's reactions to the problem. Thus, nursing diagnosis as an integral part of the nursing process forms a crucial link between theoretical knowledge and nursing practice.

Currently in Canada there are two types of preparation for registered nurses providing direct nursing services to patients: the diploma and the baccalaureate degree. Advances in the health sciences have been such that today's programs of basic nursing education are hard pressed to offer curricula which address the depth and breadth of theoretical content and related clinical experience for safe and effective practice. The expansion of knowledge required for competent practice and the range of responsibilities expected of the nurse at all levels are matters of concern for nurse educators, administrators, and practitioners.

The question raised by the educationalists is whether there is a need for two levels for professional practice as a registered nurse. They contend that before the end of the century the scope of practice and the depth of knowledge required by the nurse will of necessity warrant a baccalaureate degree. However, there is a dearth of empirical evidence to substantiate this concern.

The present developments in the health sciences and the impact of technology require the acquisition of appropriate knowledge and new skills in providing nursing services. One of the areas where a depth of theoretical knowledge is essential is in making nursing diagnoses. Professional nursing rests on a commitment to the well being of people, which is demonstrated through the provision of nursing care consistent with a professional code of ethics. Nursing activities inherent in providing care result from the exercise of intellectual judgment, and are the responsibility of the individual practitioner. Since the practicing nurses who are required to make nursing diagnoses differ in their educational backgrounds, the present study focuses on the diploma and the baccalaureate degree registered nurses.

The purpose of the study was to determine if there is a difference between diploma and baccalaureate degree registered nurses in ability to make correct nursing diagnoses.

Research question

Is there a difference between diploma and baccalaureate degree registered nurses in ability to make correct nursing diagnoses?

Hypothesis

The baccalaureate degree registered nurses will make more correct and fewer incorrect nursing diagnoses as compared to diploma registered nurses.

REVIEW OF LITERATURE
Literature related to nursing diagnoses

The literature relating to nursing diagnoses deals with: 1) the definition of nursing diagnosis; 2) the classification and taxonomy of nursing diagnosis; and 3) the issues related to nursing diagnosis.

A number of conceptual definitions of nursing diagnosis have appeared in the literature. Gebbie and Lavin (1975) define nursing diagnosis as a statement of a problem derived from a nursing assessment which points to a specific intervention and outcome. While Gebbie and Lavin suggest that it is a product of assessment, Gordon (1976) views nursing diagnosis as a description of "actual or potential health problems" which nurses by virtue of their education and experience are capable and licensed to treat (p. 1299). In addition to a conceptual definition, Gordon (1976) describes a structural definition which serves to clarify the concept of nursing diagnosis. Three structural components of a nursing diagnostic category described by Gordon are the problem, etiology, and signs and symptoms. Campbell (1978) defines nursing diagnosis as "human responses and resource limitations," and labels as nursing diagnoses "signs, symptoms, and processes" that have traditionally been within the realm of the medical profession (p. 6).

Classification and taxonomy of nursing diagnoses

Developing a taxonomy of summary statements is the process of developing a diagnostic classification system. Bircher (1975) notes that a system that involves identifying, naming, describing, stating critical attributes, and then classifying essential phenomena into an ordered category system (the taxonomy) is essential for making nursing diagnoses. Roy (1975) describes the rules for a taxonomy of nursing diagnoses. She states that the category sets must be: 1) relevant to the purpose of the classification system; 2) comprehensive and exhaustive; 3) clearly defined and mutually exclusive; 4) open to allow for insertion of new items into the system; 5) workable and communicable; 6) compatible with related systems; and 7) capable of computerization.

Gebbie and Lavin (1974) describe the basic process for developing a taxonomy for nursing diagnoses. The first step is to identify those things which nurses diagnose in patients. Next, nurses must reach agreement about consistent nomenclature; then identified diagnoses must be grouped into classes and subclasses. Finally, numbers or equivalent abbreviations are substituted for the terminology.

The inductive/deductive approach was used by both Jones (1979) and Gebbie and Lavin (1974). However, the setting in which a deductive methodology was used to derive nursing diagnostic categories varied. At the National Conference on Classification of Nursing Diagnoses (Gebbie and Lavin, 1974) the participants worked in small groups to pool their nursing experience in a project of labelling nursing diagnoses.

In the work of Jones (1979) nursing diagnostic statements were derived from 500 client encounters, reported by more than 50 volunteer practicing clinical nurse specialists and nurse clinicians who had direct patient/client contact. There are approximately 64 diagnoses in this set, with a definition for each diagnosis. There are similarities in the diagnostic categories developed by Jones and the participants of the National Conference on Classification of Nursing Diagnoses, and to a large extent they overlap.

Issues related to nursing diagnoses

The available empirical literature deals with a variety of issues relating to nursing diagnoses. Gordon and Sweeny (1979) are concerned with the methodological problems and issues in identifying and standardizing nursing diagnoses. Two major issues are encountered in attempts to design research in the area of nursing diagnoses. One of the concerns is how the term can be operationalized with the current diversity which exists in the conceptualization of nursing. The second issue concerns the deductive versus inductive approach to identifying diagnostic categories. According to these authors, two types of studies are needed to eventually develop a classification system of clinical diagnoses. Studies focusing on identification and labelling are the first type required. Secondly, research investigations are required to validate the nomenclature as it develops.

A great deal of research is being done on the development of diagnostic categories, etiology, defining characteristics, classification system, and application of nursing diagnoses in nursing practice (by individuals, groups, and the North American Nursing Diagnosis Association). Gordon (1982); Carlson, Craft, and McGuire (1982); and Carpenito (1983) focused on nursing diagnosis and its application to clinical practice. Gordon (1982) described the steps and conceptual framework for the nursing process, diagnostic strategies, classification system, and use of nursing diagnoses in direct care services. Carlson, Craft, and McGuire (1982) provided an overview of historical and theoretical development of the diagnostic process and its relationship to the nursing process. The authors expounded on the advantages and difficulties of using nursing diagnoses in a variety of nursing situations with specific client examples. Both groups of researchers addressed the implications of nursing diagnoses for nursing education, management, and research. Carpenito (1983) described the history of etiology and the concept of nursing diagnosis, with their implications for nursing practice. She differentiated nursing diagnoses from other problems, and described the components of nursing process with clinical illustrations. The author explored the diagnostic categories accepted by NANDA with reference to definitions, etiology, defining characteristics, and assessment criteria rationale for nursing care.

METHODS
Design

The nature of this study was causal comparative in that a comparison was made between two types of programs, one offered a diploma and the other a baccalaureate degree.

Subjects

Two samples of 30 subjects each (one group composed of diploma prepared nurses and a second group composed of baccalaureate degree prepared nurses) who met the predetermined criteria were selected for the study. A cluster sampling technique was used for the selection of the sample.

Demographic data

A questionnaire was devised to elicit relevant information concerning the subjects. The demographic variables included sex, age, year of graduation, type of program, years of experience since graduaton, and area of clinical practice.

Instrument

A case study technique of data collection was used. An instrument consisting of five vignettes with variation in their content was developed. Each vignette described a patient's behavior, and physiological indicators such as pulse, respiration, and blood pressure. The biopsychosocial indicators represented the knowledge required by the practitioner to make nursing diagnoses.

Each vignette was designed to result in five correct diagnoses and had five points as a maximum vignette score. The highest possible score on the instrument of five vignettes was 25 points.

The *validity* of the instrument was determined by a panel of judges.

Reliability was determined by a test-retest method, and a reliability of .84 was obtained, indicating a high reliability of the instrument.

The *independent* variable of educational background was not manipulated in the study. The *dependent* variable was the score on the diagnostic vignette, a paper and pencil simulation test.

DATA ANALYSES AND RESULTS

The data obtained on the instrument (scores on the vignettes) were subjected to a two-tailed t-test for independent samples in order to determine whether there was a difference in the two groups. A t-value of 5.14 was significant at the $p < .05$ level. The baccalaureate degree respondents were able to make more correct nursing diagnoses compared with the diploma respondents, and the difference was significant. This finding supported the stated hypothesis—the baccalaureate degree registered nurses will make more correct and fewer incorrect nursing diagnoses compared with diploma registered nurses.

Demographic variables

The demographic variables were computed to determine their frequency distribution. As shown in Table 1, there is a very slight difference in the two groups in their age and experience in nursing.

However, there were twelve subjects with experience in nursing ranging between 6 to 10 years in each of the two groups. Subsequently, these subjects were matched on the variable of "years of experience," and the data were subjected to a two-tailed t-test for related samples in order to determine whether there was a difference in the two groups. A t-value of 2.10 was obtained, p greater than .05 level of significance. There was no significant difference in performance

Table 1: Demographic variables

	Diploma F	Degree F
Age		
20-24	11	4
25-29	4	6
30-34	5	10
35-39	3	6
40-44	5	3
45-49	—	—
50-over	2	1
Mean age	31.2	32.3
Years of Experience		
Below 1 year	2	2
1-5 years	9	5
6-10 years	12	12
over 10 years	7	11
Mean years of experience	6.9	8.1
Nature of Experience		
Medical-Surgical	19	20
ICU/CCU	16	14
Emergency	2	5
Obstetrics	2	7
Pediatrics	2	11
Psychiatry	3	11
Community Health	4	7
Geriatrics	3	2
Nursing Home	2	4

shown between the two groups based on their years of experience in nursing. It would appear that knowledge is essential to making correct nursing diagnoses irrespective of the number of years of experience. It is generally assumed that years of nursing experience alone without further education are sufficient for adequate performance. However, our findings support the notion that experience can no longer be equated with learning (Rogers, 1970). An individual's learning is enhanced by education and experience. Rogers (1970) views intellectual skill in utilizing nursing's body of scientific knowledge as a determining factor in professional practice.

Responses by Categories of Required Knowledge

The data were subjected to two kinds of analysis to ascertain the difference between diploma and degree subjects in their ability to make correct nursing diagnoses: 1) on each vignette the data were tabulated as correct and incorrect responses with reference to the diagnoses (Tables 2, 3, 4, 5, and 6); 2) the data were further analyzed according to the specific knowledge required of each nursing diagnosis and subjected to a chi-square test of significance. The same results were summarized according to the significant and non-significant results (Tables 7, 8, and 9).

The results of the analysis dealing with knowledge *vs.* responses manifest the following trends: 1) the overall pattern of correct and incorrect responses made by the two sample subjects indicated that the baccalaureate degree subjects were able to make more correct and less incorrect nursing diagnoses compared with diploma subjects (this finding is consistent with the stated hypothesis); 2) further analyses of the data relating to each individual nursing diagnosis using a chi-Square test revealed the following features: a) there were significant differences seen between the two groups when depth of scientific knowledge was a factor in making correct nursing diagnoses (Table 7); b) when a cursory scientific knowledge was necessary for making correct nursing diagnoses, there was no significant difference between the two groups (Table 8); c) the differences between the two groups were not significant when psychosocial knowledge was essential to making correct nursing diagnoses (Table 9).

Table 2: Vignette #1 Responses by categories of required knowledge

		Responses*			
		Degree		Diploma	
Knowledge category	Nursing diagnoses	Correct	Incorrect	Correct	Incorrect
Physiology →	• Pain	25	5	19	11
$x^2 = 2.13^*$, p>.05 level of significance.					
Psychology →	• Anxiety	23	7	19	11
$x^2 = 0.71^*$, p>.05 level of significance.					
Pathophysiology →	• Sensory/perceptual alteration	12	18	2	28
$x^2 = 0.05^*$, p>.05 level of significance.					
	• Inadequate pulmonary ventilation	28	2	25	5
$x^2 = 0.65^*$, p>.05 level of significance.					
	• Circulatory impairment	28	2	13	17
$x^2 = 15.09^{**}$, p<.05 level of significance.					

*Not significant, Critical value = 3.84; **Significant, Critical value = 3.84

Table 3: Vignette #2 Responses by categories of required knowledge

		Responses			
		Degree		Diploma	
Knowledge category	Nursing diagnoses	Correct	Incorrect	Correct	Incorrect
Physiology →	• Fluid volume deficit	28	2	15	15
$x^2 = 11.82^{**}$, p<.05 level of significance.					
Psychology →	• Alteration in mood	18	12	11	19
$x^2 = 2.40^*$, p>.05 level of significance.					
Biochemistry →	• Altered metabolism	27	3	22	8
$x^2 = 1.78^*$, p>.05 level of significance.					
	• Chemical imbalance	28	2	25	5

Table 3: Vignette #2 Responses by categories of required knowledge—cont'd

		Responses			
		Degree		Diploma	
Knowledge category	Nursing diagnoses	Correct	Incorrect	Correct	Incorrect
$x^2 = 0.65^*$, p>.05 level of significance.					
Pathophysiology →	• Altered level of consciousness	28	2	15	15
$x^2 = 11.82^{**}$, p<.05 level of significance.					

*Not significant, Critical value = 3.84; **Significant, Critical value = 3.84

Table 4: Vignette #3 Responses by categories of required knowledge

		Responses			
		Degree		Diploma	
Knowledge category	Nursing diagnoses	Correct	Incorrect	Correct	Incorrect
Psychology →	• Anxiety	23	7	16	14
$x^2 = 2.63^*$, p>.05 level of significance.					
Sociology →	• Inadequate family support	18	12	9	21
$x^2 = 0.23^*$, p>.05 level of significance.					
Biochemistry →	• Chemical imbalance	28	2	14	16
$x^2 = 8.62^{**}$, p<.05 level of significance.					
Pathophysiology →	• Circulatory impairment	30	0	20	10
$x^2 = 9.72^{**}$, p<.05 level of significance.					
	• Inadequate pulmonary ventilation	29	1	24	6
$x^2 = 2.59^*$, p>.05 level of significance.					

*Not significant, Critical value = 3.84; **Significant, Critical value = 3.84

Table 5: Vignette #4 Responses by categories of required knowledge

		Responses			
		Degree		Diploma	
Knowledge category	Nursing diagnoses	Correct	Incorrect	Correct	Incorrect
Pathophysiology → • Knowledge deficit		15	15	10	20
$x^2 = 1.10^*$, p>.05 level of significance.					
Psychology → • Emotional impact of illness		24	6	19	11
$x^2 = 1.31^*$, p>.05 level of significance.					
• Emotional reaction (grieving)		15	15	11	19
$x^2 = 0.61^*$, p>.05 level of significance.					
• Alteration in self-concept		29	1	25	5
$x^2 = 1.67^*$, p>.05 level of significance.					
• Alteration in mood		21	9	19	11
$x^2 = 0.075^*$, p>.05 level of significance.					

*Not significant, Critical value = 3.84; **Significant, Critical value = 3.84

Table 6: Vignette #5 Responses by categories of required knowledge

		Responses			
		Degree		Diploma	
Knowledge category	Nursing diagnoses	Correct	Incorrect	Correct	Incorrect
Physiology → • Alteration in nutrition		18	12	9	21
$x^2 = 4.30^{**}$, p<.05 level of confidence.					
Psychology → • Change in self-concept		16	14	8	22
$x^2 = 3.40^*$, p>.05 level of significance.					
• Anxiety (level)		28	2	24	6
$x^2 = 1.30^*$, p>.05 level of significance.					
Sociology → • Communication barrier (language)		28	2	22	8
$x^2 = 3.0^*$, p>.05 level of significance.					
Pathophysiology → • Alteration in comfort level		22	8	11	19
$x^2 = 6.73^{**}$, p<.05 level of significance.					

*Not significant, Critical value = 3.84; **Significant, Critical value = 3.84

Table 7: Summary of significant responses according to required specific scientific knowledge

Knowledge	Nursing diagnoses	Vignette #	Table #
Pathophysiology →	• Circulatory impairment	1 & 3	2 & 4
	• Altered levels of consciousness	2	3
	• Alteration in comfort	5	6
Physiology →	• Fluid volume deficit	2	3
	• Alteration in nutrition	5	6
Biochemistry →	• Chemical imbalance	3	4

Table 8: Summary of non-significant responses according to required specific scientific knowledge

Knowledge	Nursing diagnoses	Vignette #	Table #
Pathophysiology →	• Sensory/perceptual alteration	1	2
	• Inadequate pulmonary ventilation	1 & 3	2 & 4
	• Knowledge deficit	4	5
Physiology →	• Pain	1	2
Biochemistry →	• Alteration in metabolism	2	3
	• Chemical imbalance	2	3

Table 9: Summary of non-significant responses according to required specific psychosocial knowledge

Knowledge	Nursing diagnoses	Vignette #	Table #
Psychology →	• Anxiety (level)	1, 3, & 5	2, 4, & 6
	• Alteration mood	2 & 4	3 & 5
	• Emotional impact of illness	4	5
	• Emotional reaction	4	5
	• Alteration in self concept	4 & 5	5 & 6
Sociology →	• Inadequate family support	3	4
	• Communication barrier	5	6

DISCUSSION/IMPLICATIONS

The significant results indicating the differences between the two groups suggest that the baccalaureate degree nurses are able to perform better than the diploma nurses under conditions where a greater understanding of psychosocial knowledge is essential in rendering nursing services. On the other hand, when basic theoretical knowledge was necessary in making correct nursing diagnoses, there was no significant difference found between the two groups.

These findings of significant and non-significant differences between the degree and diploma nurses have broad implications. To reflect on the concern stated earlier, the educationalists contend that by the end of the century the scope of practice and depth of knowledge required by the nurse will of necessity justify a baccalaureate degree preparation for "entry to practice." These assertions, however, raise two fundamental questions: 1) What is the scope of nursing practice? 2) What kind of depth of knowledge is required of the nurse to render direct services to the clients?

With respect to the first question, studies are needed to determine the types of required nursing services. The second issue is similar to the concern expressed by the educationalists. They question whether there is a need for two levels of professional practice as a registered nurse. With respect to these matters, the present study results suggest that: 1) there are different types of services that are required by society; and 2) different categories of nurses are needed to provide nursing services.

It is to be noted that the findings of the present study do not imply adequacy of either the two year diploma or the baccalaureate degree nursing program. It is beyond the scope of this study to determine the effectiveness of these programs. The study findings, however, indicate the purpose that the current types of nursing educational programs serve under the present circumstances.

REFERENCES

Bircher, A.U.: On the development and classification of nursing diagnoses, Nurs. Forum, **14:**10-12, 1975.

Campbell, C.: Nursing diagnosis and intervention in nursing practice, New York, 1978, John Wiley Co.

Carlson, J.H., Craft, C.A., and McGuire, A.D.: Nursing diagnosis, Philadelphia, 1982, W.B. Saunders Co.

Carpenito, J.L.: Nursing diagnosis: application to clinical practice, Philadelphia, 1983, J.B. Lippincott Co.

Feild, L.: The implementation of nursing diagnosis in clinical practice, Nurs. Clinics N. A. **14:**497-509, 1979.

Gebbie, K.: Summary of the second national conference: classification of nursing diagnoses, St. Louis, 1976, The Clearinghouse, National Group for Classification of Nursing Diagnoses.

Gebbie, K., and Lavin, M.A.: Classifying nursing diagnoses, Amer. J. Nurs. **74:**250, 1974.

Gordon, M., and Sweeney, M.A.: Methodological problems and issues in identifying and standardizing nursing diagnoses, Adv. Nurs. Sci. **2:**1-15, 1979.

Gordon, M.: Nursing diagnosis and the diagnostic process, Amer. J. Nurs. **76:**1298-1300, 1976.

Gordon, M.: Predictive strategies in diagnostic tasks, Nurs. Research, **29:**39-45, 1980.

Gordon, M.: Nursing diagnosis: process and application, New York, 1982, McGraw-Hill Co.

Jones, P.E., and Jakob, D.P.: The definition of nursing diagnoses: report of phase 2, Ontario, 1980, University of Toronto.

Kim, M.J., McFarland, G.K., and McLane, A.M., editors: Classification of nursing diagnoses: proceedings of the fifth national conference, St. Louis, 1984, The C.V. Mosby Co.

Kritek, P.B.: Commentary: the development of nursing diagnosis and theory, Adv. Nurs. Sci. **2:**73-79, 1979.

Rogers, M.E.: An introduction to the theoretical basis of nursing, Philadelphia, 1970, F.A. Davis Co.

Roy, C.A.: A diagnostic classification system for nursing, Nurs. Outlook **23:**90-98, 1975.

Warren, J.: Accountability and nursing diagnosis, J. Nurs. Admin. **13**(10):43-47, 1983.

A comparison of assessment and diagnostic competencies of B.S. and A.D. nurses

RONA F. LEVIN, Ph.D., R.N.
BARBARA C. KRAINOVICH, M.S., R.N.

Documentation of nursing process, including assessment, diagnosis, intervention, and evaluation, is considered an essential component of nursing practice. Nursing educators agree that nursing process is used as a framework for both professional and technical practice. However, it is suggested that the associate degree nurse demonstrates competence in the implementation or intervention phase, and the baccalaureate degree nurse, who is capable of performing technically, demonstrates competence in the assessment, planning, and evaluation phases of nursing process (Johnson, 1966; Montag, 1951; NLN, 1978a; NLN 1978b; Rines, 1977).

Although many studies (e.g., Gray, Murray, Roy, and Sawyer, 1977; Petti, 1975; Schwirian, 1978; Waters, Chater, Vivier, et al., 1972) have attempted to differentiate the competencies of nurses with varying educational backgrounds, most have used indirect methods of assessing nursing performance. For example, Gray, et al. used open-ended, short essay questions based on nursing care situations to assess differential competencies. Petti (1975) used supervisory personnel's perceptions of staff nurses' performance. None of these studies focused specifically on the differential competencies of baccalaureate and associate degree nurses' documentation of nursing process in the delivery of patient care.

Johnston (1982) compared the preferred nursing process strategies of baccalaureate, diploma and associate degree nurses. Her findings revealed a number of differences in preferred strategies among the groups. Of particular interest is the finding that baccalaureate prepared nurses prefer the formulation of nursing diagnoses as a product of assessment more than do diploma or associate degree nurses. Although Johnston's study supported preferences, the actual use of nursing process in the clinical setting was not studied.

Levin, Brooks, Krainovich, and Fogel (1984) investigated the differences between baccalaureate and associate degree graduates in their actual use of nursing process in the clinical setting at entry into practice and at 6 months post-employment. No significant differences were found on the basis of educational level or time. Since composite nursing process competency scores were obtained for each nurse subject, differences between the groups on the specific competencies of assessment and diagnosis were not ascertained.

Since Johnston's work suggests that the baccalaureate nurse differs from the associate degree nurse in terms of preference for formulating nursing diagnoses, it was deemed important to reanalyze the data from the Levin, et al. study in order to ascertain if differences in assessment and diagnostic competencies between these groups would become apparent.

PURPOSE

The first purpose of the present study, therefore, was to examine the differences in assessment and diagnostic competencies between baccalaureate and associate degree nursing graduates. The second purpose was to determine if these competencies changed over time.

The following hypotheses were formulated for testing:

1. Baccalaureate nursing graduates have higher mean assessment competency scores than associate degree nursing graduates at 1 month and 6 months post employment.
2. Baccalaureate nursing graduates have higher mean nursing diagnostic competency scores than associate degree nursing graduates at 1 month and 6 months post employment.

METHOD

The present study was a secondary analysis of data obtained by Levin, et al. (1984) for their investigation of "Nursing Process Competencies of B.S. and A.D. Nurses." The primary study used a comparative, longitudinal design to examine the documentation of graduate nurses via retrospective audits of patient records.

Sample

The initial sample consisted of 30 graduate nurses from ten different schools of nursing; 15 had baccalaureate degrees and 15 had associate degrees. The nurses were hired for the position of staff nurse in all divisions except psychiatry at a major New York City medical center. In order to participate in the study, graduates could not have been employed in nursing for more than 3 months prior to beginning orientation at the medical center. As it turned out, none of the subjects had previous work experience as a registered nurse. Oral informed consent was obtained from each nurse participant.

Of the original 30 participants, 22 (14 B.S. and 8 A.D.) generated usable data for phase I (entry level) of the study and 17 (11 B.S. and 6 A.D.) continued participation through phase II (6 months post employment). The reasons for subject discontinuation were: state board failure (four), resignation from the medical

center (one), and voluntary withdrawal from the study (three during phase I and five during phase II).

Instrument

The instrument used to measure nursing process competencies was the Baccalaureate Nurse-Associate Nurse Competencies Checklist II (BNANCC II). The BNANCC II is a 21 item checklist which combines selected nursing process competencies of baccalaureate and associate degree nursing graduates.

The selected competencies (the BNANCC II and the accompanying *Data Collector's Manual* are available from the first author upon request) deemed measurable by chart audit are derived from a more comprehensive set of competencies developed by Mitchell and Krainovich (1978). The American Nurses' Association *Standards of Nursing Practice* was used as a framework for competency development. The content validity of the BNANCC II is based on the fact that competencies were drawn from nationally accepted statements of performance expectations of B.S. and A.D. nurses (NYSNA, 1978; NLN, 1978a; NLN, 1978b) and supported by faculty from three different baccalaureate and associate degree programs and representatives from nursing service.

Box 1 depicts the 21 competency statements included in the instrument. Each competency statement has accompanying criteria. An example is provided in Table 1. Data for competencies 1, 4, and 5 were rescored for the present study as follows:

1. Competency 1 has 35 criteria. Each criterion was scored as 1. The total number of criteria met was divided by 35 to obtain an assessment score for each patient chart. Total assessment score for each nurse was obtained by summing individual chart scores and

BOX 1   **Competency statements included in the BNANCC II**

1. Records data obtained from performing nursing health assessment.
2. Records additional data obtained from observation and/or inspection of patient's progress record (PPR).
3. Records an actual patient problem on patient's progress record.
4. Records an initial nursing diagnosis dealing with an actual problem.
5. Records an initial nursing diagnosis dealing with a potential problem.
6. Records initial short term goals (STGs) on nursing care plan (NCP).
7. Records at least one long term goal (LTG) on NCP.
8. Records planned interventions (nursing orders) on NCP.
9. Records additional STGs for an established nursing diagnosis on NCP or PPR.
10. Records nursing protocols* related to additional STGs on NCP or PPR.
11. Records individualized teaching plan on patient's chart.
12. Records initiation of individualized teaching plan.
13. Records information given to patients according to teaching protocol.*
14. Records implementation of planned interventions on PPR.
15. Records data pertinent to the medical/dental regimen.
16. Records intra and/or interdisciplinary referrals on PPR.
17. Records initiation of emergency measures.
18. Records achievement of established STGs on NCP.
19. Revises STGs based on data.
20. Records additional nursing diagnoses on NCP.
21. Discharge summary completed.

*Protocol refers to a standardized procedure.

Table 1: Sample competency and criteria from the BNANCC II

Selected competency	Criteria
#4 Records an initial nursing diagnosis dealing with an actual problem.	1. Includes a statement of an actual patient response.
	2. Includes a statement about the factor(s) which contribute to the response.
	3. There is data in the health assessment to support the nursing diagnosis.

dividing by the total number of applicable charts.

2. Competencies 4 and 5 each have 3 criteria. These were combined to obtain a nurse's total diagnostic score as outlined above.

Procedure

All study participants received the usual 4 week orientation session for newly hired nurses. The first 2 weeks address hospital policies, various technical skills and procedures, and in-depth discussion of and practice in documentation of nursing process. The second 2 weeks consist of clinical orientation related to the assigned area of practice. Study participants were given a special session conducted by one of the investigators during the third week of orientation which included an in-depth discussion of the study, with particular emphasis on the nursing process competencies included in the BNANCC II. All participants received a copy of the instrument.

Study participants were requested to keep a list (data generation sheet) of the medical record numbers of the patients for whom they cared during their second and sixth months of employment. They were also requested to place an "A" next to the medical record number of each patient for whom they performed an initial nursing assessment. These nurses were reminded via written memos and telephone calls prior to the designated months for data generation.

Five patient records for each study participant from each of the two study phases were randomly selected for retrospective audit. A stratified approach was used in order to insure a sampling of charts which contained initial nursing assessments performed by participants. Thus, if possible, two of the five charts were selected from those having an "A" next to the medical record number.

Four independent data collectors, master's prepared nurses, were recruited for data collection. After participating in a 4 day training session and achieving appropriate interrater reliability (greater than 80% agreement), they audited the patient records using the BNANCC II.

RESULTS AND DISCUSSION

Analysis of variance with repeated measures, using BMDP Statistical Software, was performed to test each hypothesis. Results indicated no significant difference in mean assessment or diagnostic scores on the basis of educational preparation or time (Tables 2 and 3). The hypotheses, therefore, were not sup-

Table 2: Anova for effects of educational level and time on assessment competency

Source	Sum of squares	DF	Mean square	F	Probability
Ed level	13.885	1	13.885	0.17	0.693
Error	574.760	7	82.109		
Time	11.485	1	11.485	0.50	0.503
Time/ed level	88.705	1	88.705	3.85	0.090
Error	161.100	7	23.014		

Table 3: Anova for effects of educational level and time on diagnostic competency

Source	Sum of squares	DF	Mean square	F	Probability
Ed level	870.250	1	870.250	2.90	0.133
Error	2103.310	7	300.473		
Time	8.410	1	8.410	0.03	0.860
Time/ed	0.934	1	0.934	0.00	0.953
Error	1717.270	7	245.324		

ported. It is of interest to note that the mean assessment and diagnostic scores for both groups of nurses and for both time periods were relatively low (see Table 4). Note that the maximum obtainable score for each of these competencies was 100.

Due to the limitations of sample selection, sample size, and differential mortality in the present study, these findings cannot be generalized to the entire population of baccalaureate and associate degree nurses. Recent research findings, however, lend credibility to our results. Suhayda and Kim (1984), for example, in evaluating documentation of nursing process in critical care were unable to trace problem identification, nursing action, and patient outcome in such a way as to indicate deliberate and systematic information processing, decision making, or evaluation of patient care. In the 50 randomly selected patient records which they reviewed, patient problems were found in unclustered and unrelated pieces of documentation.

In addition, two studies which explored the relationship between type of basic education of staff nurses and ability to formulate nursing diagnoses found no significant differences on the basis of educational preparation in either simulated or clinical documentation (Meade and Kim, 1984; Myers, et al., 1984).

Table 4: Cell means and standard deviations for assessment and diagnostic competencies

	Means		SD	
	BS	AD	BS	AD
Assessment				
Entry	35.160	28.925	6.438	8.917
6 months	32.300	35.000	8.787	2.751
Diagnostic				
Entry	39.467	53.733	17.601	4.277
6 months	37.533	52.767	18.063	17.374

Finally, the studies of Ziegler (1984) and Warren (1984), both using samples of graduate nursing students, demonstrated that subjects were unable to generate assessment statements upon which measurable goals, individualized care, and evaluation of patient outcomes could be based.

IMPLICATIONS

Considering the emphasis on cost containment and the trend toward costing out nursing services in today's health care environment, nurses must begin documenting the quality services which they provide to patients in order to validate their worth. The first step in accomplishing this goal is to accurately and systematically assess patients' responses to health problems and formulate nursing diagnoses to direct the plan of care. The results of the present study in conjunction with other research findings support a lack of competence in these nursing skills at both the technical and professional level of practice. Thus, this implies the need for critical assessment of our approach to teaching nursing assessment and diagnosis, as well as our approach to implementation of these skills in the service setting.

The contention by nurse educators that the baccalaureate (or professional) nurse demonstrates greater competence in assessment and planning than the technical (or associate) nurse has not been supported unequivocally by research findings. Many questions remain unanswered. Several of these are:

What is the effect of role adjustment on demonstration of competence in assessment and diagnosis?

Would an increase in competence be demonstrated at 1 year or 2 years post-employment?

What is the relationship between competence in documentation of nursing process and communication skills, values, and accountability?

REFERENCES

Gray, J., Murray, B., Roy, J., and others: Do graduates of technical and professional nursing programs differ in practice? Nurs. Research **26:**368-373, 1977.

Johnson, D.E.: Competence in practice: technical and professional, Nurs. Outlook **14:**30-33, 1966.

Johnston, S.C.: The use of the Rines model in differentiating professional and technical nursing practice, Nurs. Health Care **3:**374-379, 1982.

Levin, R.F., Brooks, C.A., Krainovich, B.C., and others: Nursing process competencies of B.S. and A.D. nurses. Paper presented at a meeting of the Southern Council on Collegiate Education for Nursing. Dallas, TX, 1984.

Meade, C.D., and Kim, M.J.: The effect of teaching on documentation of nursing diagnoses. In Kim, M.J., McFarland, G.K., and McLane, A.M., editors: Classification of nursing diagnoses: proceedings of the fifth national conference, St. Louis, 1984, The C.V. Mosby Co.

Mitchell, C.A., and Krainovich, B.C.: Competencies/ skills for B.S. and A.D. graduates. Unpublished working drafts, 1978.

Montag, M.L.: The education of nursing technicians, New York, 1951, Putnam.

Myers, P.A., Perry, A.G., Wessler, R., et al.: Staff nurses' identification of nursing diagnoses from a simulated patient care situation. In Hurley, M.E., editor: Classification of nursing diagnoses: proceedings of the sixth conference, St. Louis, 1986, The C.V. Mosby Co.

National League for Nursing (NLN): Competencies of the associate degree nurse on entry into practice. Publication No. 23-1731, New York, 1978, Author.

National League for Nursing (NLN): Competencies of the associate degree nurse on entry into practice, Nurs. Outlook **26:**457, 1978.

New York State Nurses' Association Task Force on Behavioral Outcomes, Nursing Education Programs: Unpublished working drafts, 1978.

Petti, E.R.: A study of the relationship between three levels of nursing education and nurse competency as rated by patient and head nurse. Doctoral dissertation, Boston University. Dissertation Abstracts International, **35:**12A, 1975.

Rines, A.R.: Development of objectives: program level, course, and unit. In National League for Nursing: preparation of associate degree graduates, New York, 1977, Author.

Schwirian, P.M.: Evaluating the performance of nurses: a multidimensional approach, Nurs. Research **27:**347-351, 1978.

Suhayda, R., and Kim, M.J.: Documentation of nursing process in critical care. In Kim, M.J., McFarland, G.K., and McLane, A.M., editors: Classification of nursing diagnoses: proceedings of the fifth national conference, St. Louis, 1984, The C.V. Mosby Co.

Warren, J.: Problems in using nursing diagnoses: a descriptive study of graduate nursing students. In Kim, M.J., McFarland, G.K., and McLane, A.M., editors: Classification of nursing diagnoses: proceedings of the fifth national conference, St. Louis, 1984, The C.V. Mosby Co.

Waters, V.H., Chater, S.S., Vivier, M.L., et al.: Technical and professional nursing: an exploratory study, Nurs. Research **21:**124-131, 1972.

Ziegler, S.M.: Nursing diagnosis: the state of the art as reflected in graduate students' work. In Kim, M.J., McFarland, G.K., and McLane, A.M., editors: Classification of nursing diagnoses: proceedings of the fifth national conference, St. Louis, 1984, The C.V. Mosby Co.

Effects of education on documentation of nursing diagnoses by school nurses

JOAN DOLCE DUNN, M.S., R.N.C.
FRANCES STEVRALIA CROSBY M.S., R.N.

Author Notes

This research was supported by a grant from the American Nurses' Foundation.

We gratefully acknowledge Adele Pillitteri, M.S., R.N., Charlene McKaig, M.S., R.N., Carol Gutt, Ed.D., R.N., Bernadette Curry, M.S., R.N., Jacquelyn Dietz, M.S., R.N., Frances Wollner, M.S., R.N., and Beverly Shipe, M.S., R.N., for review of the Case Study Instruments; Mary Jane Feldman, Ph.D., for statistical analysis and interpretation; and Donna Radecki, M.S., R.N., for agency support.

At the First National Conference on Classification of Nursing Diagnoses in 1973, the initial nursing diagnoses labels and nomenclature were proposed (Gebbie and Lavin, 1975). Since that time, a list of 42 nursing diagnoses has been approved for clinical testing by the North American Nursing Diagnosis Association (NANDA) (Carpenito, 1984). NANDA advocates the need for research and clinical experimentation of nursing diagnoses to move the concept forward on a sound scientific foundation.

Published studies regarding nursing diagnoses in school practice settings have been minimal. When Levin (1984) conducted a comprehensive review of the literature, she concluded that a total of 75 research studies had been published in the field of nursing diagnosis, with only a small percentage of

these in primary or ambulatory care settings.

Lash (1982) raised concern regarding the gap between the theory of nursing diagnosis and its practice in clinical settings. Two studies that examined the effects of teaching the theory of nursing diagnosis on its documentation substantiate the gap between theory and practice. Both of these studies were conducted in hospital settings. Meade and Kim (1984) found that although there was a significant difference between pre-teaching and post-teaching documentation of nursing diagnoses on case studies following a classroom program regarding nursing diagnosis, no significant difference was found in the clinical documentation in actual practice. Carstens (1984) also analyzed the effects of an inservice program on staff nurses' ability to identify valid nursing diagnoses from a case

453

study. Her conclusions indicated that an in-service program did not have any statistically significant effect on the identification of nursing diagnoses from a case study. These studies suggest the need for further exploration into the effects of teaching the theory of nursing diagnosis on clinical documentation in an ambulatory practice area not previously studied, the school health setting.

METHOD
Sample

A total of 48 school nurses (21 full-time and 27 part-time) were employed by a County Health Department to deliver school health services to the city school population at the time of this study. Twenty-eight volunteered to participate and provided written informed consent. They were asked to complete a Demographic Data Form, and were designated the participant group. Seven of the original 28 became ill or resigned from their jobs as the study progressed. A final total of 21 school nurses remained in the participant group. They were all female and ranged in age from over 20 to under 60 years old. The majority of the nurses had Bachelor's Degrees in nursing. One participant had a Master's Degree in Nursing, and the remaining nurses had diplomas or Associate Degrees as basic nursing education. Nineteen participants received their degrees prior to 1980, while two received their education in the 1980s.

Setting

The 30 elementary and secondary schools to which the participant group of nurses were assigned ranged in student census from 176 to 1315 and served a variety of handicapped students. The number of monthly student–nurse initiated health office encounters ranged from 268 in a large public high school to 35 in a small parochial school.

PROCEDURE
Design

The study design employed a time series pre-treatment post-treatment evaluation with a comparison control group. It was conducted over a 3 month time period. Data collection on Modified Daily Log sheets by both experimental and control groups occurred during 1 month phases prior to and following the treatment, the continuing education program. The cognitive effect of the continuing education program on the experimental group was evaluated pre- and post-treatment by Case Study Instruments One and Two. A two-round consensus by a panel of experts was used to establish the standard of valid NANDA diagnoses within the cases. The experimental group's subjective satisfaction with the continuing education program and opinion regarding clinical application of nursing diagnoses were determined using Feedback Questionnaires A and B. The instruments and the continuing education program were piloted with a group of school nurses employed in a nearby county prior to implementation with study participants.

Sampling procedure. The participant group of nurses was randomly assigned via a table of random numbers into the experimental group (N = 10) and the control group (N = 11), stratifying for full- and part-time employment status. A comparison of the groups applying chi-square analysis to the demographic data which they supplied indicated comparability in all areas.

Data collection procedure—Modified Daily Logs. A form traditionally maintained by the school nurses was the Daily Log. This served as a formal documentation of the nurse-student encounter. Because the nursing diagnosis was not mandated to be recorded on the Daily Log prior to this study, it was necessary to modify the traditional form slightly to include a column entitled "Nursing Diagnosis" to accommodate data collection.

A month's supply of Modified Daily Logs and directions for use and collection during pre-treatment period were distributed to both the experimental and control groups by the investigator at a staff meeting. Dispensing and collecting of the Modified Daily Logs were handled similarly for the post-treatment data collection period, which began 1 month after the completion of the pre-treatment period.

A Diagnostic Category System was established to quantify the responses on the Modified Daily Log Form. A five category system ranging from 0 to 4 was designed to classify the responses in the "Nursing Diagnosis" column. For the purpose of this study, statements of health conditions which interfered with the client's life processes and could be ameliorated by independent nursing practice (Carpenito, 1983) were designated nursing diagnoses.

Categories 0, 1, and 2 represented the variety of responses which could not be defined as nursing diagnoses. Category 0, No Diagnosis, was assigned if the column was left blank or the noted entry was unknown. Category 1 was indicated for a notation that described a Normal Variance, such as "tired." The use of a Medical Statement (a cellular response or one which "identifies and labels the precise pathological disease" (Griffith, 1982, p. 114) such as "conjunctivitis" or "pharyngitis") was noted in Category 2.

Categories 3 and 4 represented responses that could be defined as nursing diagnoses. Category 3 was assigned to notations of Nursing Impressions or nursing diagnoses which did not utilize the NANDA terminology, for example "emotional upset due to family problems." Category 4 was assigned to those nursing diagnoses which utilized the terminology from the approved NANDA list (Kim and Moritz, 1984). The Diagnostic Category System was tested prior to use to determine interrater reliability.

Treatment—the continuing education program with Case Studies One and Two. The five-hour intervention entitled "Nursing Diagnoses in School Nursing Practice" was presented to the experimental group by the investigator. They were requested not to discuss the content with the control group, who received a delayed treatment subsequent to the final data collection period.

Case Study One was distributed to the experimental group just prior to the class. It was used as a pre-test measure of accuracy of usage of NANDA diagnostic labels.

The purpose of the continuing education program was to educate the school nurses on identifying defining characteristics and formulating nursing diagnoses using the nomenclature approved for clinical testing by NANDA. Theoretical content developed from current literature in the field consisted of 1½ hours of background information and terminology clarification. The remaining 2½ hours emphasized application and formulation of nursing diagnoses using the case and vignette approach. A nursing diagnosis handbook, a pocket card with the NANDA list, and continuing education credits were supplied to each participant. Upon completion of the inservice sessions the nurses were requested to complete the post-test Case Study Two and Feedback Questionnaire A. Feedback Questionnaire B was mailed to the experimental group at the conclusion of the study.

RESULTS
Modified Daily Log analysis

During the pre-treatment period, a total number of 2,579 responses were made by the experimental and control groups together on their Modified Daily Logs under the column "Nursing Diagnosis." During the post-treatment period a total of 2,366 responses were noted on the Modified Daily Logs by these nurses. Each response was assigned to one of the five Diagnostic Categories (Figure 1).

Comparison of pre- to post-treatment change. In order to examine the effects of the treatment, the pattern of change from pre- to post-treatment between the experimental and control groups was analyzed. The experimental group's change in documentation from pre- to post-treatment was compared to the control group's change in documentation from pre- to post-treatment.

Change scores were determined individually. To determine the change score the percent of responses documented by the individual in each Diagnostic Category on the Modified Daily Log in the pre-treatment period was subtracted from the percent documented by the individual in the same Diagnostic Category in the post-treatment period. The amount of change in the experimental group was then compared to that in the control group members. T-test analysis was applied to determine if the amount of change differed between the groups for each Diagnostic Category.

The results of the analysis of change scores indicate that the groups changed differently with statistical significance in four of the five categories. Frequency of use of Categories 0, 1, and 2 decreased for the experimental group, whereas minimal change was noted for the control group in these Categories. Also, frequency of use of Category 4 increased dramatically in the experimental group and remained unchanged in the control group. Only Category 3 was the same for both groups. There was no significant change in this Category.

Case studies one and two

The case study measures were examined using a t-test analysis to compare pre– to post–treatment differences of identified valid NANDA diagnoses by Group A. The average number of valid nursing diagnoses identified by each nurse in the experimental group on the pre-test Case Study One was 0.4, as compared to the average valid nursing diagnoses identified by the same nurses on post-test Case Study Two, which was 7.6. A significant increase was identified (t [9] = 7.06, $p = < .05$) from pre– to post–continuing education program measurement.

LIMITATIONS

A limitation of this study was that time constraints prevented conducting measurements over time to evaluate sustained documentation of nursing diagnoses statements. Also, the Modified Daily Log provided frequency information, but quality analysis of the nursing diagnoses using this type of instrument was limited.

DISCUSSION

The ultimate impression resulting from the findings was that the school nurses not only increased their documentation of NANDA diagnoses, but also decreased their frequency of distribution of responses in categories which represented no indication for nursing concern. The experimental group's post–treatment patterns of change representing decreased utilization of the categories No Diagnosis, Normal Variance, and Medical Statements, coupled with their increased usage of the NANDA category, reflect their increased recognition and labeling of student health complaints as nursing concerns. The increased labeling of complaints as concerns which can be ameliorated by nursing intervention suggests that the experimental group clarified their clinical practice boundaries and increased their discrimination of the nursing domain.

Formulating a nursing diagnosis without the use of the NANDA terminology did not significantly differ, however, from pre– to post–treatment. Both the experimental and control groups continued to note only mini-

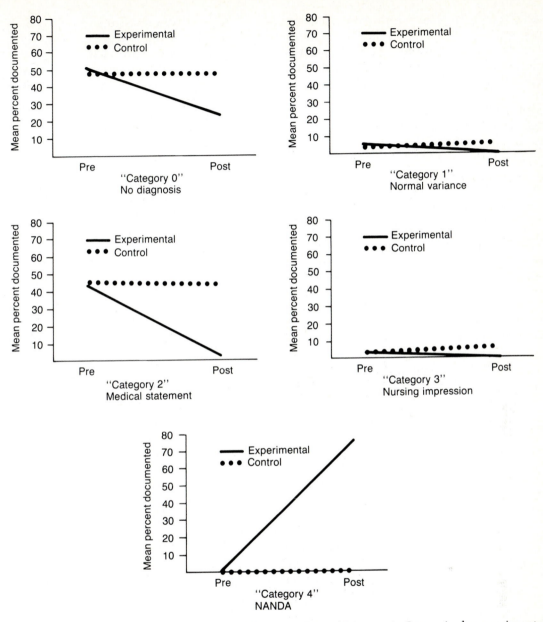

FIGURE 1   Pre to post treatment change in documentation of Diagnostic Categories by experimental (N = 10) and control (N = 11) groups. (t-test analysis, p < .05)

mal Nursing Impressions (nursing diagnoses phrased in non-NANDA language in the post–treatment period. This suggests that the use of the NANDA list facilitated articulation of identified nursing concerns.

CONCLUSION AND RECOMMENDATIONS

Four overall conclusions were drawn from this study:

1. Inservice trainings on nursing diagnoses were both feasible and effective when provided in school health settings. School nurses significantly increased their documentation of NANDA diagnoses both on case studies and in practice settings following a continuing education program entitled "Nursing Diagnosis in School Nursing Practice." The gap between theory and practice was bridged.

2. School nurses increased their ability to interpret student health concerns within the realm of nursing practice. This was reflected by their pattern of change—decreasing usage of categories representing no indication for nursing intervention.

3. The Case Study Instruments with a standard of valid NANDA diagnoses determined by a panel of experts proved to be an effective measure of nurse participants' mastery of the theoretical concepts and accuracy of usage of diagnostic labels. Gordon and Sweeney (1979, p. 8) suggest that "nurse-subjects . . . need to be trained and their reliability as diagnosticians established."

4. The majority of school nurses involved in this study enthusiastically supported the continuing education program and the future documentation of nursing diagnoses in school nursing. Most felt that documentation of nursing diagnoses was important enough that

they would recommend that it be formally incorporated into the student permanent health record.

This study endeavored to educate school nurses and to investigate the results of that education in their clinical practice. It was a preliminary step in the study of the utilization of nursing diagnoses by school nurses as part of the validation process of nursing diagnoses theory. The next step is to generate and validate the diagnoses themselves. The nurse participants in this study are now prepared for further research regarding nursing diagnoses pertinent to ambulatory practice.

REFERENCES

Carpenito, L.: Nursing diagnosis: application to clinical practice, Philadelphia, 1983, J.B. Lippincott.

Carpenito, L.: Handbook of nursing diagnosis, Philadelphia, 1984, J.B. Lippincott.

Carstens, J.: The effects of an inservice program on nurses' ability to identify valid nursing diagnoses. In Kim, M.J., McFarland, G.K., and McLane, A.M., editors: Classification of nursing diagnoses: proceedings of the fifth national conference, St. Louis, 1984, The C.V. Mosby Co.

Gebbie, K. and Lavin, M., editors: Classification of nursing diagnosis: proceedings of the first national conference, St. Louis, 1975, The C.V. Mosby Co.

Gordon, M. and Sweeney, M.A.: Methodological problems and issues in identifying and standardizing nursing diagnoses, Adv. Nurs. Sci. **2:**1-15, 1979.

Griffith, J.W. and Christensen, P.J.: Nursing process application of theories, frameworks, and models, St. Louis, 1982, The C.V. Mosby Co.

Kim, M.J. and Moritz, D.A.: Classification of nursing diagnoses: proceedings of the third and fourth national conferences, New York, 1982, McGraw Hill.

Lash, A.A.: Nursing diagnosis: some comments on the gap between theory and practice. In McCloskey, J. and Grace, H., editors: Current issues in nursing, Boston, 1982, Blackwell Scientific Publications.

Levin, R.: Yesterday, today and tomorrow: nursing diagnosis research. Paper presented at the First Regional Conference on Nursing Diagnosis, Philadelphia, 1984.

Meade, C. and Kim, M.: The effect of teaching on documentation of nursing diagnoses. In Kim, M.J., McFarland, G.K., and McLane, A.M., editors: Classification of nursing diagnoses: proceedings of the fifth national conference, St. Louis, 1984, The C.V. Mosby Co.

Education studies: abstracts

Nursing diagnosis curriculum model for a baccalaureate nursing program

MARITA G. TITLER, M.A., R.N.

The purpose of this paper was two-fold. First, this paper describes a new baccalaureate nursing curriculum model which was designed from the Unitary Human Framework and related diagnostic nomenclature. Second, the paper describes the effectiveness of this model based on data elicited from the program's systematic evaluation plan and results of the N-Clex-RN examination results.

The curricular model described in this paper provides the registered nursing student and the four year basic nursing student an opportunity to study nursing in a nursing diagnosis framework. The nine human/environment interactional patterns of the Unitary Human Framework serve as constructs for course development and implementation, and thus guide students in formulating nursing diagnoses and implementing appropriate nursing care. It is the belief of the faculty that nursing diagnosis is an integral part of nursing practice, and therefore must be integrated into all nursing courses. The major constructs of the curriculum model are: 1) person/environment interaction patterns; 2) health status; and 3) nursing process. A model illustrates the relationships among these three constructs.

The paper further describes each of the constructs and corresponding concepts.

The effectiveness of the curriculum was evaluated through a systematic evaluation plan. Because only one class had graduated from the program (less than 6 months ago) the data are limited to the graduates' results on the N-Clex RN examination and a graduate questionnaire completed at the time of graduation. All 11 basic students passed the N-Clex examination. The scores ranged from 1779 to 2471, with a mean of 2071.63. The graduate questionnaire was returned by six RN advanced placement students and ten basic students immediately following graduation. Based on a scale of 1 (least effective) to 5 (highly effective), graduates rated themselves on how effective they perceived themselves to be in a variety of situations. Of interest is their perceived effectiveness in formulating nursing diagnoses and developing individualized nursing care plans. A 6 month follow-up questionnaire to be distributed in November 1985 will gather additional data on the graduates' current use of nursing diagnoses in the clinical area. The results of the initial questionnaire demonstrate a highly to moderate self-perceived effectiveness in the formulation of nursing diagnoses by a majority of the graduates. The R.N. advanced placement group tended to rate themselves higher for perceived effectiveness in formulation of nursing diagnoses than did the basic student graduates.

The significance of such a curriculum model is yet to be fully realized. The initial data suggest that graduates of such a program use nursing diagnoses in delivering nursing care and perceive themselves as moderately to highly effective in formulating diagnostic statements.

Using nursing diagnoses to describe clinical competence of baccalaureate and associate degree graduating students: a comparative study

HELENA A. LEE, M.S.N., R.N.
KATHLEEN A. STRONG, M.S., R.N.

The purpose of this study was to compare perceptions of clinical competence of professional and technical nursing students with the competence expectations of their nursing faculty, using a nursing diagnosis framework. The research question addressed by this study was: What are the clinical competencies of graduating associate degree (ADN) and baccalaureate (BSN) nursing students using a nursing diagnosis framework to describe clinical practice?

The subjects were graduating ADN and BSN nursing students and their faculties from two midwestern schools of nursing (N=102). Two-part faculty and student questionnaires were developed. Part I included demographic information; Part II contained a listing of the 51 nursing diagnoses from the fifth conference of the National Group for Classification of Nursing Diagnoses. Using a Likert-type scale, faculty indicated degree of expected graduate competence and students indicated degree of perceived personal competence.

Means were calculated and rank ordered for each group. Responses of students and faculty-student groups were compared. Perceptions of their clinical competence as beginning practitioners were similar for the ADN and BSN students. Alteration in bowel elimination: constipation; alteration in comfort: pain; and impairment of skin integrity: actual and potential were among the five (10 percent) top-ranked nursing diagnoses in which both ADN and BSN students perceived themselves as being most competent. Rape-trauma syndrome and spiritual distress were among the areas in which both ADN and BSN students perceived themselves as being least competent. Findings indicated considerable agreement among all four sample groups, with only six diagnoses with 0.5 or more difference in group mean between the ADN and BSN faculty-student groups.

Replication of this study with a stratified random sample is recommended to further describe beginning professional and technical clinical competence using a nursing diagnosis framework.

New diagnoses & submission/review guidelines

New nursing diagnoses approved 1986

PATTERN I: EXCHANGING

1.2.1.1	Infection: Potential for
1.2.2.1	Body Temperature, Altered: Potential
1.2.2.2	Hypothermia
1.2.2.3	Hyperthermia
1.2.2.4	Thermoregulation, Ineffective
1.3.2.1.1	Incontinence, Stress
1.3.2.1.2	Incontinence, Reflex
1.3.2.1.3	Incontinence, Urge
1.3.2.1.4	Incontinence, Functional
1.3.2.1.5	Incontinence, Total
1.3.2.2	Urinary Retention
1.6.2.2	Tissue Integrity, Impaired

PATTERN 3: RELATING

3.1.1	Social Interaction, Impaired
3.3	Sexuality, Altered Patterns

PATTERN 5: CHOOSING

5.1.1.1.1	Adjustment, Impaired

PATTERN 6: MOVING

6.5.1.1	Swallowing, Impaired
6.6	Growth and Development, Altered

PATTERN 7: PERCEIVING

7.2.1.1	Unilateral Neglect
7.3.1	Hopelessness

PATTERN 9: FEELING

9.1.1.1	Comfort, Altered: Chronic Pain
9.2.5	Post-trauma Response

The nursing diagnosis Deconditioning was reviewed by the seventh conference participants but was not approved by NANDA's members (See Appendix G).

Development/submission guidelines for proposed new nursing diagnoses

INTRODUCTION

The North American Nursing Diagnosis Association (NANDA) solicits proposed new nursing diagnoses for review by the Association. Such proposed diagnoses undergo a systematic review process which concludes with a mail ballot vote by the entire membership. Acceptance of a proposed diagnosis by mail ballot establishes the diagnoses for inclusion in NANDA's official list of diagnoses. Such acceptance indicates NANDA's view that the diagnosis shows readiness for use and continuing development by the discipline.

To assist interested parties in submitting proposed diagnoses, the NANDA Diagnosis Review Committee, which is charged with overseeing this process, has prepared a set of guidelines for submission. These guidelines are designed to assure consistency, clarity, and completeness of submissions. Diagnoses submitted which do not meet the guidelines will be returned to the person submitting them for appropriate revision to assure that the review process can be initiated. Proposed diagnoses are reviewed by the Diagnosis Review Committee, the Clinical Technical Review Task Forces, and the NANDA Board prior to General Assembly review, comment, and membership vote.

NURSING DIAGNOSIS DEFINED

Several definitions of nursing diagnoses exist in the nursing literature. The following are provided as four possible ways of conceptualizing a nursing diagnosis.

1. "A nursing diagnosis is a clinical judgment about an individual, family, or community which is derived through a deliberate, systematic process of data collection and analysis. It provides the basis for prescriptions for definitive therapy for which the nurse is accountable. It is expressed concisely and it includes the etiology of the condition when known" (Shoemaker, 1984, p. 94).

2. "Nursing diagnosis is a concise phrase or term summarizing a cluster of empirical indicators representing patterns of unitary man" (Roy, 1982, p. 219).

3. "Nursing diagnosis made by professional nurses describes actual or potential health problems that nurses, by virtue of their education and experience, are capable and licensed to treat" (Gordon, 1976, p. 1299).

4. "A nursing diagnosis is a concise phrase or term summarizing a cluster or set of empirical indicators, representing normal variations and altered patterns (actual or potential) of human functioning which nurses by virtue of education and experience are capable and licensed to treat" (McLane, 1979, p. 33).

PROPOSED NEW NURSING DIAGNOSIS: REQUIRED COMPONENTS FOR SUBMISSION

1. Name: This part provides a name for the diagnosis, a concise phrase, term, or label.

2. Definition: This part provides a clear, precise definition of the named diagnosis. The definition expresses the essential nature of the diagnosis named and delineates it's meaning. The definition should enable one to differentiate this diagnosis from all others.

3. Defining characteristics: This part provides a list of observable cues that the client presents which substantiate the nursing judgment (i.e., that the selected diagnosis appropriately labels and describes the client state, the phenomena of

concern). Cues must be both listed and defined. Cues are separated into two positions or sets: major and minor.

a. Major defining characteristics: those which appear to be present in all clients experiencing the phenomena of concern.

b. Minor defining characteristics: those which appear to be present in many clients experiencing the phenomena of concern.

4. Substantiating and Supportive Materials: This part provides documentation which substantiates the existence, nature, and characteristics of the phenomena of concern. Minimal validation documentation is a listing of references demonstrating a reasonable review of relevant literature. Narrative materials accompanying such a reference list may not exceed 1500 words.

PROPOSED NEW NURSING DIAGNOSIS: OPTIONAL COMPONENTS FOR SUBMISSION

1. Supplemental Information: The following types of supplemental information may be submitted to further clarify the nursing phenomena identified by the proposed nursing diagnosis.

a. Related Factors: In some cases there may be specific factors which appear to show some type of patterned relationship with the phenomena of concern, named as a nursing diagnosis. Where this situation exists it may be helpful to name and describe these. Such factors may be described variously as antecedent to, associated with, related to, contributing to, or abetting.

b. Sources of Variance: In some cases unique sources of variance in the experience of the phenomena may be possible. Where this situation exists it may be helpful to identify these. Such sources of variance may include developmental stage variance, ethnic or cultural variance, levels of risk variance, acuity variance, and multi-diagnosis variance.

2. Supplemental Validation: If it is available, supplemental validation of the nursing diagnosis may be submitted. This may include research abstracts, brief reports of validation projects, or reports of intervention or treatment studies. These must not exceed 1500 words.

REFERENCES

Gordon, M.: Nursing diagnosis and the diagnostic process, Amer. J. Nurs. **76**:1298-1300, 1976.

McLane, A.: A taxonomy of nursing diagnoses: toward a science of nursing, Milwaukee Prof. Nurse **20**:33, 1979.

Roy, C.: Theoretical framework for classification of nursing diagnosis. In Kim, M.J., and Moritz, D.A., editors: Classification of nursing diagnoses: proceedings of the third and fourth national conferences, New York, 1982, McGraw Hill.

Shoemaker, J.: Essential features of nursing diagnosis. In Kim, M.J., McFarland, G.K., and McLane, A.M., editors: Classification of nursing diagnoses: proceedings of the fifth national conference, St. Louis, 1984, The C.V. Mosby Co.

Diagnosis review cycle

The North American Nursing Diagnosis Association (NANDA), in an effort to meet its purpose "to develop, refine, and promote a taxonomy of nursing diagnostic terminology of general use to professional nurses," has developed a formal cycle of diagnosis review as part of the process of incorporation of new diagnoses submitted by interested parties. This process is cyclic in character, assuring continuous development and refinement of the taxonomy.

STEP 1. RECEIPT OF DIAGNOSES

Diagnoses may be entered into the review cycle on the initiative of either NANDA or other individuals or groups.

A. NANDA initiates this process by soliciting diagnoses, advertising its interest in diagnoses, publishing its guidelines for submission, and responding to inquiries concerning such guidelines.

B. Individual nurses or nurse groups initiate this process by submitting a diagnosis for review. When a submission is received by NANDA, it is initially reviewed for compliance with submission guidelines. Those submissions which involve only a suggested name or are only partially developed are returned to the person submitting the recommendation with a request for completion as described in the guidelines. Those submissions which meet criteria of the guidelines then enter the review process. The person submitting the suggested diagnosis receives a copy of the description of the Diagnosis Review Cycle at this time to facilitate an understanding of NANDA's policies and procedures.

STEP 2. DIAGNOSES ENTER THE PUBLIC DOMAIN

NANDA formally recognizes all diagnoses under review as part of the public domain. As such, any diagnosis submitted for review is briefly reported in the NANDA Newsletter when it enters the review cycle. Persons submitting diagnoses are advised of this fact and are asked to indicate in writing their acceptance of the policy on a form provided by NANDA.

It is recognized, however, that individuals have often invested considerable time and energy in an effort to delineate one or more diagnoses. Therefore, the publication of a diagnosis entering the review cycle will include the name of the person(s) submitting this diagnosis, assuring them of recognition of their efforts. This will also improve networking and communicating among members actively engaged in exploring common or comparable diagnoses.

STEP 3. DIAGNOSES ARE REVIEWED BY CLINICAL/TECHNICAL TASK FORCES

The NANDA Diagnosis Review Committee (DRC) is charged with the task of reviewing proposed diagnoses and recommending their acceptance, modification, or rejection to the NANDA Board. This committee's work is guided by the advice and critique of clinical/technical task forces who review diagnoses.

A. Each diagnosis accepted for review is assigned by the Chairperson of the DRC to a member of that committee. This person serves as a primary or lead reviewer of the diagnosis and the Chairperson of the Clinical/Technical Review Task Force which will review the diagnosis.

B. The Clinical/Technical Review Task Force is a panel created to review a specific diagnosis based on individual clinical and technical expertise. Task Force members are drawn not only from the NANDA membership, but also from expert groups in organizations such as the Canadian Nurses' Association and the American Nursing Association. NANDA Board Members who do not serve on the DRC are ineligible to serve on these Task Forces. Task Forces are created as needed by the DRC.

C. Members of the various Task Forces receive diagnoses for critique and review with an evaluation form provided. This evaluation form enables reviewers to assess the degree to which the diagnosis submitted meets the criteria of the submission guidelines. Task Force members are given 2 weeks to respond to a request for a review. These reviews are forwarded to the primary reviewer.

D. Based on Task Force member advice and comments, the primary reviewer prepares a diagnosis proposal for each diagnosis. This is presented at a meeting of the DRC.

STEP 4. DIAGNOSES ARE REVIEWED BY THE NANDA DIAGNOSIS REVIEW COMMITTEE

The Diagnosis Review Committee convenes to review, discuss, and take action on the proposals for new diagnoses prepared by the primary reviewers of the Clinical/Technical Task Forces. Three possible outcomes emerge from this process.

A. The DRC accepts the proposed diagnosis or makes minor changes.

B. The DRC substantively alters the diagnosis as submitted by the original proposer, based on reviewer advice. The DRC then accepts the proposed diagnosis.

C. The DRC rejects the diagnosis and identifies specific reasons for the rejection. In this case the original proposer of the diagnosis is provided with specific recommendations for improvement.

The DRC notifies the original proposer of their action at this time. They concurrently forward their recommendations to the NANDA Board.

STEP 5. DIAGNOSES ARE REVIEWED BY THE NANDA BOARD

The NANDA Board receives the recommendations of the DRC and convenes to review, discuss, and take action on the DRC recommendations. Once more, three possible outcomes emerge from this process.

A. The board accepts the DRC recommendation.

B. The board returns the diagnosis to the DRC with comments for revision and recommendations for change.

C. The board rejects the DRC recommendation and identifies specific reasons for the rejection.

The DRC then notifies the original proposer of the Board's action, and prepares accepted diagnoses for General Assembly review and comment.

STEP 6. DIAGNOSES ARE REVIEWED BY THE GENERAL ASSEMBLY

The General Assembly has the authority to review and comment on proposed diagnoses for the DRC's actions prior to submission to the membership for acceptance. The DRC prepares proposed diagnoses for this review and comment. The DRC therefore engages in the following activities.

A. The DRC groups the diagnoses as possible or appropriate for General Assembly review.

B. The DRC structures time for review and comment by the General Assembly during the National Conference, advising the original proposer of this action.

C. The DRC develops policies, procedures, and protocols for General Assembly review and comment, and conducts these sessions accordingly.

D. The DRC collects General Assembly comments and incorporates these into proposed diagnoses as appropriate and feasible.

E. The DRC reports these changes to the board.

STEP 7. DIAGNOSES ARE VOTED UPON BY THE NANDA MEMBERSHIP

The DRC prepares diagnoses for a NANDA membership vote. This includes several activities.

A. The DRC creates a mail ballot of proposed diagnoses to be distributed to all current NANDA members.

B. The DRC oversees the distribution and tallying of ballots. It records any suggestions for needed subsequent revision of any given diagnosis.

C. The DRC communicates information on the outcome of balloting to the original proposer of the diagnoses. Unapproved diagnoses can be revised and re-enter the cycle. Approved diagnoses become a part of the approved NANDA Taxonomy.

D. The DRC forwards the approved diagnoses to the National Conference Proceedings editor for inclusion in the Proceedings, and to the Taxonomy Committee for inclusion in the NANDA Taxonomy.

E. The DRC prepares a cycle report for the board.

STEP 8. THE CYCLE IS REACTIVATED

The entire diagnosis review cycle is then reactivated. NANDA's Nursing Diagnosis Newsletter is the official vehicle for communication with the membership about the process, guidelines, timelines, changes, and necessary publicity. Changes in accepted diagnoses undergo this same process and utilize the same review procedures.

NANDA Taxonomy I

Guideline observations about NANDA nursing diagnosis Taxonomy I

The nine major category headings in this taxonomy are viewed as nine central human response patterns. The second category level refers to "alterations," used in this context to refer to "the process or state of becoming or being made different without changing into something else." As used here it is essentially a neutral term, and does not connote either a positive or a negative change. Each subsequent lower level of the taxonomy reflects a higher degree of clinical specificity in the phenomena named. Given the incomplete nature of this taxonomy, where a given diagnosis has not yet been identified a more generic category name may have to be used until clinically discrete phenomena are better identified.

Bracketed items in the taxonomy refer to items that have not actually been formally named, described, reviewed, or voted upon, but were viewed as necessary or desirable inclusions to create some degree of conceptual coherence. The "black boxes" or "blank boxes" are included to demonstrate the provisional nature of this first effort and to highlight overt incompleteness. Both the boxes and the bracketed items indicate areas that still must be defined, described, and approved. They are not, however, in any sense exhaustive indicators of incomplete work.

This taxonomy includes all diagnoses formally approved by NANDA up to and including the diagnoses approved by ballot after the Seventh National Conference held in April 1986. A common set of definitions for frequently used diagnosis qualifiers was also approved at the Seventh National Conference. This list of qualifiers, while incomplete at this time, initiates some common definitions to guide further development. In subsequent taxonomies it is anticipated that these qualifiers will be designated by a numerical code. The list of qualifiers and their definitions follows.

It is recognized that several partial conceptual systems or constructs and mutually incompatible principles of classification are currently embedded in portions of this taxonomy. It is anticipated that these complex issues will have to be addressed and resolved in the development of subsequent taxonomies. NANDA Taxonomy II will be presented to the General Assembly in 1988 and will reflect some initial resolution of these issues.

Endorsement of this taxonomy by the NANDA General Assembly indicates an investment by NANDA in a specific taxonomy which can be tested, refined, revised, and expanded.

Diagnosis qualifiers

CATEGORY 1

Actual: Existing at the present moment; existing in reality.

Potential: Can, but has not yet, come into being; possible.

CATEGORY 2

Ineffective: Not producing the desired effect; not capable of performing satisfactorily.

Decreased: Smaller; lessened; diminished; lesser in size, amount, or degree.

Increased: Greater in size, amount, or degree; larger, enlarged.

Impaired: Made worse, weakened; damaged, reduced; deteriorated.

Depleted: Emptied wholly or partially; exhausted of.

Deficient: Inadequate in amount, quality, or degree; defective; not sufficient; incomplete.

Excessive: Characterized by an amount or quantity that is greater than is necessary, desirable, or usable.

Dysfunctional: Abnormal; impaired or incompletely functioning.

Disturbed: Agitated; interrupted, interfered with.

Acute: Severe but of short duration.

Chronic: Lasting a long time; recurring; habitual; constant.

Intermittent: Stopping and starting again at intervals; periodic; cyclic.

Source: Websters New World Dictionary, College Edition. Cleveland, 1959, The World Publishing Company.

NANDA nursing diagnosis Taxonomy I

1. EXCHANGING: A HUMAN RESPONSE PATTERN INVOLVING MUTUAL GIVING AND RECEIVING.

1.1 Alterations in Nutrition
  1.1.1 [Cellular]
  1.1.2 [Systemic]
    1.1.2.1 More than body requirements
    1.1.2.2 Less than body requirements
    1.1.2.3 Potential for more than body requirements
    1.1.2.4
1.2 [Alterations in Physical Regulation]
  1.2.1 [Immune]
    1.2.1.1 Potential for Infection
    1.2.1.2
  1.2.2 Alteration in Body Temperature
    1.2.2.1 Potential
    1.2.2.2 Hypothermia
    1.2.2.3 Hyperthermia
    1.2.2.4 Ineffective Thermoregulation
    1.2.2.5
1.3 Alterations in Elimination
  1.3.1 Bowel
    1.3.1.1 Constipation
    1.3.1.2 Diarrhea
    1.3.1.3 Incontinence
  1.3.2 Urinary Patterns
    1.3.2.1 Incontinence
      1.3.2.1.1 Stress
      1.3.2.1.2 Reflex
      1.3.2.1.3 Urge
      1.3.2.1.4 Functional
      1.3.2.1.5 Total
    1.3.2.2 Retention
  1.3.3 [Skin]
    1.3.3.1
    1.3.3.2
1.4 [Alterations in Circulation]
  1.4.1 [Vascular]
    1.4.1.1 Tissue Perfusion
      1.4.1.1.1 Renal
      1.4.1.1.2 Cerebral
      1.4.1.1.3 Cardiopulmonary
      1.4.1.1.4 Gastrointestinal
      1.4.1.1.5 Peripheral

    1.4.1.2 Fluid Volume
      1.4.1.2.1 Excess
      1.4.1.2.2 Deficit
        1.4.1.2.2.1 Actual
        1.4.1.2.2.2 Potential
  1.4.1.3
  1.4.2 [Cardiac]
    1.4.2.1 Decreased Cardiac Output
    1.4.2.2
1.5 [Alterations in Oxygenation]
  1.5.1 [Respiration]
    1.5.1.1 Impaired Gas Exchange
    1.5.1.2 Ineffective Airway Clearance
    1.5.1.3 Ineffective Breathing Pattern
  1.5.2
1.6 [Alterations in Physical Integrity]
  1.6.1 Potential for Injury
    1.6.1.1 Potential for Suffocating
    1.6.1.2 Potential for Poisoning
    1.6.1.3 Potential for Trauma
  1.6.2 Impairment
    1.6.2.1 Skin Integrity
      1.6.2.1.1 Actual
      1.6.2.1.2 Potential
    1.6.2.2 Tissue Integrity
      1.6.2.2.1 Oral Mucous Membrane
      1.6.2.2.2
      1.6.2.2.3
    1.6.2.3

2. COMMUNICATING: A HUMAN RESPONSE PATTERN INVOLVING SENDING MESSAGES.

2.1 Alterations in Communication
  2.1.1 Verbal
    2.1.1.1 Impaired
    2.1.1.2
    2.1.1.3
  2.1.2 [Nonverbal]
2.2
2.3
  2.3.1
  2.3.2

3. RELATING: A HUMAN RESPONSE PATTERN INVOLVING ESTABLISHING BONDS.

3.1 [Alterations in Socialization]
  3.1.1 Impaired Social Interaction
  3.1.2 Social Isolation
  3.1.3
3.2 [Alterations in Role]
  3.2.1 Role Performance
    3.2.1.1 Parenting
      3.2.1.1.1 Actual
      3.2.1.1.2 Potential
    3.2.1.2 Sexual
      3.2.1.2.1 Dysfunction
      3.2.1.2.2
      3.2.1.2.3
    3.2.1.3 [Work]
  3.2.2 Family Processes
  3.2.3
3.3 Altered Sexuality Patterns
3.4

4. VALUING: A HUMAN RESPONSE PATTERN INVOLVING THE ASSIGNING OF RELATIVE WORTH.

4.1 [Alterations in Spiritual State]
  4.1.1 Distress
  4.1.2
  4.1.3
4.2
  4.2.1
  4.2.2

5. CHOOSING: A HUMAN RESPONSE PATTERN INVOLVING THE SELECTION OF ALTERNATIVES.

5.1 Alterations in Coping
  5.1.1 Individual
    5.1.1.1 Ineffective
      5.1.1.1.1 Impaired Adjustment
      5.1.1.1.2
    5.1.1.2
  5.1.2 Family
    5.1.2.1 Ineffective
      5.1.2.1.1 Disabled
      5.1.2.1.2 Compromised
    5.1.2.2 Potential for Growth
    5.1.2.3
  5.1.3 [Community]

5.2 [Alterations in Participation]
  5.2.1 [Individual]
    5.2.1.1 Noncompliance
    5.2.1.2
    5.2.1.3
  5.2.2 [Family]
  5.2.3 [Community]

6. MOVING: A HUMAN RESPONSE PATTERN INVOLVING ACTIVITY.

6.1 [Alterations in Activity]
  6.1.1 Physical Mobility
    6.1.1.1 Impaired
    6.1.1.2 Activity Intolerance
    6.1.1.3 Potential Activity Intolerance
    6.1.1.4
  6.1.2 [Social Mobility]
    6.1.2.1
    6.1.2.2
6.2 [Alterations in Rest]
  6.2.1 Sleep Pattern Disturbance
  6.2.2
6.3 [Alterations in Recreation]
  6.3.1 Diversional Activity
    6.3.1.1 Deficit
    6.3.1.2
  6.3.2
6.4 [Alterations in Activities of Daily Living]
  6.4.1 Home Maintenance Management
    6.4.1.1 Impaired
    6.4.1.2
  6.4.2 Health Maintenance
  6.4.3
6.5 Alterations in Self Care
  6.5.1 Feeding
    6.5.1.1 Impaired Swallowing
    6.5.1.2
    6.5.1.3
  6.5.2 Bathing/Hygiene
  6.5.3 Dressing/Grooming
  6.5.4 Toileting
6.6 Altered Growth and Development
  6.6.1
  6.6.2

7. PERCEIVING: A HUMAN RESPONSE PATTERN INVOLVING THE RECEPTION OF INFORMATION.

7.1 Alterations in Self Concept
  7.1.1 Disturbance in Body Image

7.1.2 Disturbance in Self-Esteem
7.1.3 Disturbance in Personal Identity
7.1.4
7.2 Sensory/Perceptual Alteration
  7.2.1 Visual
    7.2.1.1 Unilateral Neglect
    7.2.1.2
  7.2.2 Auditory
  7.2.3 Kinesthetic
  7.2.4 Gustatory
  7.2.5 Tactile
  7.2.6 Olfactory
7.3 [Alterations in Meaningfulness]
  7.3.1 Hopelessness
  7.3.2 Powerlessness
  7.3.3

8. KNOWING: A HUMAN RESPONSE PATTERN INVOLVING THE MEANING ASSOCIATED WITH INFORMATION.

8.1 Alterations in Knowledge
  8.1.1 Deficit
  8.1.2
  8.1.3
8.2 [Alterations in Learning]
  8.2.1
  8.2.2
8.3 Alterations in Thought Processes
  8.3.1 [Confusion]
  8.3.2
  8.3.3

9. FEELING: A HUMAN RESPONSE PATTERN INVOLVING THE SUBJECTIVE AWARENESS OF INFORMATION.

9.1 Alterations in Comfort
  9.1.1 Pain
    9.1.1.1 Chronic
    9.1.1.2 [Acute]
    9.1.1.3
  9.1.2 [Discomfort]
9.2 [Alterations in Emotional Integrity]
  9.2.1 Anxiety
  9.2.2 Grieving
    9.2.2.1 Dysfunctional
    9.2.2.2 Anticipatory
    9.2.2.3
  9.2.3 Potential for Violence
  9.2.4 Fear
  9.2.5 Post Trauma Response
    9.2.5.1 Rape Trauma Syndrome
      9.2.5.1.1 Rape Trauma
      9.2.5.1.2 Compound Reaction
      9.2.5.1.3 Silent Reaction
    9.2.5.2
  9.2.6
  9.2.7
9.3

Section VII Approved nursing diagnoses

This section contains two documents, the list of nursing diagnoses approved by the North American Nursing Diagnosis Association (Section VII A) and the approved nursing diagnoses with definitions, defining characteristics, and related factors (Section VII B). The numerical codes and Human Response Patterns from NANDA Taxonomy I were used to prepare the List of Approved Diagnostic Labels. New diagnoses are marked with a (+) for easy recognition. A new format developed by the Diagnosis Review Committee was used to reformat diagnoses approved at previous conferences. The numerical codes from NANDA Taxonomy I were used with the diagnostic label for purposes of ordering the Approved Nursing Diagnoses. Multiple diagnoses which were sufficiently developed (i.e., self-care deficits and rape-trauma syndrome) were separated into discrete diagnoses. Two diagnoses (sensory/perceptual alterations and tissue perfusion, altered) were left as multiple diagnoses with a caveat to use the appropriate numerical code to designate the specific sense or tissue. The substantiating/supportive materials for new diagnoses are included. An asterisk (*) next to a defining characteristic indicates a critical defining characteristic (must be present for the diagnosis to be made).

List of approved diagnostic labels

PATTERN 1: EXCHANGING.

1.1.2.1	Nutrition, altered: More than body requirements
1.1.2.2	Nutrition, altered: Less than body requirements
1.1.2.3	Nutrition, altered: Potential for more than body requirements
1.2.1.1	+Infection: Potential for
1.2.2.1	+Body temperature, altered: Potential
1.2.2.2	+Hypothermia
1.2.2.3	+Hyperthermia
1.2.2.4	+Thermoregulation, ineffective
1.3.1.1	Bowel elimination, altered: Constipation
1.3.1.2	Bowel elimination, altered: Diarrhea
1.3.1.3	Bowel elimination, altered: Incontinence
1.3.2	Urinary elimination, altered patterns
1.3.2.1.1	+Incontinence, stress
1.3.2.1.2	+Incontinence, reflex
1.3.2.1.3	+Incontinence, urge
1.3.2.1.4	+Incontinence, functional
1.3.2.1.5	+Incontinence, total
1.3.2.2	+Urinary retention
1.4.1.1	Tissue perfusion, altered: Renal, cerebral, cardiopulmonary, gastrointestinal, peripheral ++
1.4.1.2.1	Fluid volume excess
1.4.1.2.2.1	Fluid volume deficit: Actual (1)
1.4.1.2.2.1	Fluid volume deficit: Actual (2)
1.4.1.2.2.2	Fluid volume deficit: Potential
1.4.2.1	Cardiac output, altered: Decreased
1.5.1.1	Gas exchange, impaired
1.5.1.2	Airway clearance, ineffective
1.5.1.3	Breathing pattern, ineffective
1.6.1	Injury, potential for
1.6.1.1	Injury, potential for: Suffocating
1.6.1.2	Injury, potential for: Poisoning
1.6.1.3	Injury, potential for: Trauma
1.6.2.1.1	Skin integrity, impaired: Actual
1.6.2.1.2	Skin integrity, impaired: Potential
1.6.2.2	+Tissue integrity, impaired
1.6.2.2.1	Tissue integrity, impaired: oral mucous membrane

PATTERN 2: COMMUNICATING.

2.1.1.1	Communication, impaired: Verbal

PATTERN 3: RELATING.

3.1.1	+Social interaction, impaired
3.1.2	Social isolation
3.2.1	Role performance, altered
3.2.1.1.1	Parenting, altered: Actual
3.2.1.1.2	Parenting, altered: Potential
3.2.1.2.1	Sexual dysfunction
3.2.2	Family processes, altered
3.3	+Sexuality, altered patterns

PATTERN 4: VALUING.

4.1.1	Spiritual distress (distress of the human spirit)

PATTERN 5: CHOOSING.

5.1.1.1	Coping, ineffective individual
5.1.1.1.1	+Adjustment, impaired
5.1.2.1.1	Coping, ineffective family: Disabled
5.1.2.1.2	Coping, ineffective family: Compromised
5.1.2.2	Coping, family: Potential for growth
5.2.1.1	Noncompliance (specify)

PATTERN 6: MOVING.

6.1.1.1	Mobility, impaired physical
6.1.1.2	Activity intolerance
6.1.1.3	Activity intolerance: Potential
6.2.1	Sleep pattern disturbance
6.3.1.1	Diversional activity, deficit
6.4.1.1	Home maintenance management, impaired
6.4.2	Health maintenance, altered
6.5.1	Self-care deficit: Feeding
6.5.1.1	+Swallowing, impaired
6.5.2	Self-care deficit: Bathing/hygiene
6.5.3	Self-care deficit: Dressing/grooming
6.5.4	Self-care deficit: Toileting
6.6	+Growth and development, altered

++See NANDA Taxonomy I for numerical codes to designate specific tissue.

+New nursing diagnoses approved 1986.

PATTERN 7: PERCEIVING.

7.1.1	Self-concept, disturbance in: Body-image
7.1.2	Self-concept, disturbance in: Self-esteem
7.1.3	Self-concept, disturbance in: Personal identity
7.2	Sensory/perceptual alterations: Visual, auditory, kinesthetic, gustatory, tactile, olfactory +++
7.2.1.1	+Unilateral neglect
7.3.1	+Hopelessness
7.3.2	Powerlessness

PATTERN 8: KNOWING.

8.1.1	Knowledge deficit (specify)
8.3	Thought processes, altered

+++See NANDA Taxonomy I for numerical codes to designate specific sense(s).

PATTERN 9: FEELING.

9.1.1	Comfort, altered: Pain
9.1.1.1	+Comfort, altered: Chronic pain
9.2.1	Anxiety
9.2.2.1	Grieving, dysfunctional
9.2.2.2	Grieving, anticipatory
9.2.3	Violence, potential for: Self-directed or directed at others
9.2.4	Fear
9.2.5	+Post-trauma response
9.2.5.1.1	Rape-trauma syndrome
9.2.5.1.2	Rape-trauma syndrome: Compound reaction
9.2.5.1.3	Rape-trauma syndrome: Silent reaction

Approved nursing diagnoses classified by human response patterns

1.1.2.1 NUTRITION, ALTERED: MORE THAN BODY REQUIREMENTS

Definition

The state in which an individual is experiencing an intake of nutrients which exceeds metabolic needs.

Defining characteristics
Major

Weight 10 percent over ideal for height and frame; *weight 20% over ideal for height and frame; *triceps skin fold greater than 15 mm in men, 25 mm in women; sedentary activity level; reported or observed dysfunctional eating patterns: pairing food with other activities; concentrating food intake at end of day; eating in response to external cues such as time of day or social situation; eating in response to internal cues other than hunger, e.g., anxiety.

Related factors

Excessive intake in relation to metabolic need.

1.1.2.2 NUTRITION, ALTERED: LESS THAN BODY REQUIREMENTS

Definition

The state in which an individual experiences an intake of nutrients insufficient to meet metabolic needs.

Defining characteristics
Major

Loss of weight with adequate food intake; body weight 20 percent or more under ideal; reported inadequate food intake less than RDA (recommended daily allowance); weakness of muscles required for swallowing or mastication; report or evidence of lack of food; aversion to eating; reported altered taste sensation; satiety immediately after ingesting food; abdominal pain with or without pathology; sore, inflamed buccal cavity; capillary fragility; abdominal cramping; diarrhea or steatorrhea; hyperactive bowel sounds; lack of interest in food; perceived inability to ingest food; pale conjunctival and mucous membranes; poor muscle tone; excessive loss of hair; lack of information, misinformation; misconceptions.

Related factors

Inability to ingest or digest food or absorb nutrients due to biological, psychological, or economic factors.

1.1.2.3 NUTRITION, ALTERED: POTENTIAL FOR MORE THAN BODY REQUIREMENTS
Definition

The state in which an individual is at risk of experiencing an intake of nutrients which exceeds metabolic needs.

Risk factors

*Reported or observed obesity in one or both parents; *rapid transition across growth percentiles in infants or children; reported use of solid food as major food source before 5 months of age; observed use of food as reward or comfort measure; reported or observed higher baseline weight at beginning of each pregnancy; dysfunctional eating patterns: pairing food with other activities; concentrating food intake at end of day; eating in response to external cues such as time of day or social situation; eating in response to internal cues other than hunger, such as anxiety.

Related factors

Hereditary predisposition; excessive intake during late gestational life, early infancy, and adolescence; frequent closely spaced pregnancies; dysfunctional psychological conditioning in relation to food; membership in lower socioeconomic group.

1.2.1.1 INFECTION, POTENTIAL FOR

Definition

The state in which an individual is at increased risk for being invaded by pathogenic organisms.

Risk factors

Inadequate primary defenses (broken skin, traumatized tissue, decrease in ciliary action, stasis of body fluids, change in pH secretions, altered peristalsis); inadequate secondary defenses (e.g., decreased hemoglobin, leukopenia, suppressed inflammatory response) and immunosuppression; inadequate acquired immunity; tissue destruction and increased environmental exposure; chronic disease; invasive procedures; malnutrition; pharmaceutical agents; trauma; rupture of amniotic membranes; insufficient knowledge to avoid exposure to pathogens.

Substantiating/supportive materials

Kim, M.J. and Moritz, D.A.: Classification of nursing diagnoses: proceedings of the third and fourth national conferences, New York, 1982, McGraw-Hill.

Porth, C.: Pathophysiology, Philadelphia, 1982, Lippincott.

Groer, M. and Shekleton, M.: Basic pathophysiology: a conceptual approach, St. Louis, 1983, The C.V. Mosby Co.

Cohen, P., Pinching, A., Rees, A., and others: Infection and immunosuppression, Quarterly J. Med. **51**:1-15, 1982.

Related factors

See Risk Factors.

1.2.2.1 BODY TEMPERATURE, ALTERED: POTENTIAL

Definition

The state in which the individual is at risk for failure to maintain body temperature within normal range.

Risk factors

Extremes of age; extremes of weight; exposure to cool/cold or warm/hot environments; dehydration; inactivity or vigorous activity; medications causing vasoconstriction/vasodilation; altered metabolic rate; sedation; inappropriate clothing for environmental temperature; illness or trauma affecting temperature regulation.

Substantiating/supportive materials

Groer, M. and Shekleton, M.: Basic pathophysiology: a conceptual approach, Chapter 5, St. Louis, 1983, The C.V. Mosby Co.

Iveson-Iveson, J.: Body temperature, Nurs. Mirror **154**: 32, 1982.

Related factors

See Risk Factors.

1.2.2.2 HYPOTHERMIA

Definition

The state in which an individual's body temperature is reduced below his/her normal range.

Defining characteristics
Major

Reduction in body temperature below normal range.

Minor

Cool skin, mental confusion, decreased pulse and respiration.

Substantiating/supportive materials

Drummond, G.: Hypothermia: its causes, effects and treatment in the very young and old, Nurs. Times **75:**2116, 1979.

Guyton, A.C.: Human physiology and mechanisms of disease, 3rd ed, Philadelphia, 1982, W.B. Saunders.

Hayter, G.: Hypothermia/hyperthermia in older persons, J. Gerontol. Nurs. **6**(2):65-68, 1980.

Sawetz, E., Melnick, J.L., and Adelberg, E.A.: Review of medical microbiology, 13th ed, CA, 1970, Lange Medical.

Kim, M.J. and Moritz, D.A.: Classification of nursing diagnoses: proceedings of the third and fourth national conferences, New York, 1982, McGraw-Hill.

Related factors

Exposure to cool or cold environment; illness or trauma; inability or decreased ability to shiver; malnutrition; inadequate clothing; consumption of alcohol; medications causing vasodilation; evaporation from skin in cool environment; decreased metabolic rate; inactivity; aging.

1.2.2.3 HYPERTHERMIA

Definition

A state in which an individual's body temperature is elevated above his/her normal range.

Defining characteristics
Major

Increase in body temperature above normal range.

Minor

Flushed skin, skin warm to touch, increased respiratory rate, tachycardia, seizures/convulsions.

Substantiating/supportive materials

Francis, B.: Hot and cold therapy. J. Nurs. Care **15:**18-20, 1982.

Hayter, J.: Hypothermia/Hyperthermia in older persons. J. Gerontol. Nurs. **6**(2):65-68, 1980.

Heineman, H.S.: What to do for the patient with fever, Consultant **18:**21-24, 1978.

Lorin, M.I.: Elevated body temperature: symptomatic treatment, Consultant **20:**130-131, 1980.

McCarthy, P.L., et al.: Diagnostic styles of attending physicians, residents, and nurses in evaluating febrile children, Clin. Ped. **21:**534-537, 1982.

Wright, P.F., Thompson, J., McKee, K.T., et al.: Patterns of illness in the highly febrile young child: epidemiological, clinical, and laboratory correlates. Pediatrics **67:**694-700, 1981.

Related factors

Exposure to hot environment; vigorous activity; medications/anesthesia; inappropriate clothing; increased metabolic rate; illness or trauma; dehydration; inability or decreased ability to perspire.

1.2.2.4 THERMOREGULATION, INEFFECTIVE

Definition

The state in which an individual's temperature fluctuates between hypothermia and hyperthermia.

Defining characteristics
Major

Fluctuations in body temperature above or below the normal range. See also major and minor characteristics present in hypothermia and hyperthermia.

Substantiating/supportive materials

Drummond, G.: Hypothermia: its causes, effects, and treatment in the very young and very old. Nursing Times, Dec. 6, 2115-2116, 1979.

Groer, M. and Shekleton, M.: Basic pathophysiology: a conceptual approach, Chapter 5, St. Louis, 1983, The C.V. Mosby Co.

Related factors

Trauma or illness; immaturity; aging; fluctuating environmental temperature.

1.3.1.1. BOWEL ELIMINATION, ALTERED: CONSTIPATION

Definition

A state in which an individual experiences a change in normal bowel habits characterized by a decrease in frequency and/or passage of hard dry stools.

Defining characteristics
Major

Decreased activity level; frequency less than usual; hard forced stools; palpable mass; reported feeling of pressure in rectum; reported feeling of rectal fullness; straining at stool.

Minor

Abdominal pain; appetite impairment; back pain; headache; interference with daily living; use of laxatives.

1.3.1.2. BOWEL ELIMINATION, ALTERED: DIARRHEA

Definition

A state in which an individual experiences a change in normal bowel habits characterized by the frequent passage of loose, fluid, unformed stools.

Defining characteristics
Major

Abdominal pain; cramping; increased frequency; increased frequency of bowel sounds; loose, liquid stools; urgency.

Minor

Change in color.

1.3.1.3 BOWEL ELIMINATION, ALTERED: INCONTINENCE

Definition

A state in which an individual experiences a change in normal bowel habits characterized by involuntary passage of stool.

Defining characteristics
Major

Involuntary passage of stool.

1.3.2 URINARY ELIMINATION, ALTERED PATTERNS
Definition
The state in which the individual experiences a disturbance in urine elimination.

Defining characteristics
Major

Dysuria; frequency; hesitancy; incontinence; nocturia; retention; urgency.

Related factors

Multiple causality, including: anatomical obstruction, sensory motor impairment, urinary tract infection.

1.3.2.1.1 INCONTINENCE, STRESS

Definition

The state in which an individual experiences a loss of urine of less than 50 ml occurring with increased abdominal pressure.

Defining characteristics
Major

Reported or observed dribbling with increased abdominal pressure.

Minor

Urinary urgency; urinary frequency (more often than every 2 hours).

Substantiating/supportive materials

Dufault, K.: Urinary incontinence: United States and British nursing perspectives, J. Gerontol. Nurs. **4**(2): 28-33, 1978.
Eastwood, H.: Differential diagnosis of urinary incontinence in the elderly, Geriatric Med. Today **2**(4):19-28, 1983.

Field, M.A.: Urinary incontinence in the elderly: an overview, J. Gerontol. Nurs. **5**(1):12-19, 1979.

Voith, A.M., Madson, L.A., Smith, D.A., and others: Validation of nursing diagnosis regarding urinary incontinence, Milwaukee, 1985, Columbia Hospital.

Voith, A.M. and Smith, P.A.: Validation of the nursing diagnosis of urinary retention, Nurs. Clinics N.A. **20**:723-729, 1985.

Voith, A.M.: A conceptual framework for nursing diagnoses regarding alterations in urinary elimination, Rehab. Nurs. **11**(1):18-21, 1986.

Related factors

Degenerative changes in pelvic muscles and structural supports associated with increased age; high intra-abdominal pressure (e.g., obesity, gravid uterus); incompetent bladder outlet; overdistention between voidings; weak pelvic muscles and structural supports.

1.3.2.1.2 INCONTINENCE, REFLEX

Definition

The state in which an individual experiences an involuntary loss of urine, occurring at somewhat predictable intervals when a specific bladder volume is reached.

Defining characteristics
Major

No awareness of bladder filling; no urge to void or feelings of bladder fullness; uninhibited bladder contraction/spasm at regular intervals.

Substantiating/supportive materials

Dufault, K.: Urinary incontinence: United States and British nursing perspectives, J. Gerontol. Nurs. **4**(4): 28-33, 1978.

Eastwood, H.: Differential diagnosis of urinary incontinence in the elderly, Geriatric Med. Today **2**(4):19-28, 1983.

Field, M.A.: Urinary incontinence in the elderly: an overview, J. Gerontol. Nurs. **5**(1):12-19, 1979.

Voith, A.M., Madson, L.A., Smith, D.A., and others: Validation of nursing diagnosis regarding urinary incontinence, Milwaukee, 1985, Columbia Hospital.

Voith, A.M. and Smith, P.A.: Validation of the nursing diagnosis of urinary retention, Nurs. Clinics N. A., **20**:723-729, 1985.

Voith, A.M.: A conceptual framework for nursing diagnoses regarding alterations in urinary elimination, Rehab. Nurs. **11**(1):18-21, 1986.

Related factors

Neurological impairment (e.g., spinal cord lesion which interferes with conduction of cerebral messages above the level of the reflex arc).

1.3.2.1.3 INCONTINENCE, URGE

Definition

The state in which an individual experiences involuntary passage of urine occurring soon after a strong sense of urgency to void.

Defining characteristics
Major

Urinary urgency; frequency (voiding more often than every 2 hours); bladder contracture/spasm.

Minor

Nocturia (urination more than two times per night); voiding in small amounts (less than 100 cc) or in large amounts (more than 550 cc); inability to reach toilet on time.

Substantiating/supportive materials

Dufault, K.: Urinary incontinence: United States and British nursing perspectives, J. Gerontol. Nurs. **4**(2): 28-33, 1978.

Eastwood, H.: Differential diagnosis of urinary incontinence in the elderly, Geriatric Med. Today **2**(4):19-28, 1983.

Field, M.A.: Urinary incontinence in the elderly: an overview, J. Gerontol. Nurs. **5**(1):12-19, 1979.

Voith, A.M., Madson, L.A., Smith, D.A., and others: Validation of nursing diagnosis regarding urinary incontinence, Milwaukee, 1985, Columbia Hospital.

Voith, A.M. and Smith, P.A.: Validation of the nursing diagnosis of urinary retention, Nurs. Clinics N. A., **20**:723-729, 1985.

Voith, A.M.: A conceptual framework for nursing diagnoses regarding alterations in urinary elimination, Rehab. Nurs. **11**(1):18-21, 1986.

Related factors

Decreased bladder capacity (e.g., history of PID, abdominal surgery, indwelling urinary catheter); irritation of bladder stretch receptors causing spasm (e.g., bladder infection); alcohol; caffeine; increased fluids; increased urine concentration; overdistention of bladder.

1.3.2.1.4 INCONTINENCE, FUNCTIONAL

Definition

The state in which an individual experiences an involuntary, unpredictable passage of urine.

Defining characteristics
Major

Urge to void or bladder contractions sufficiently strong to result in loss of urine before reaching an appropriate receptacle.

Substantiating/supportive materials

Dufault, K.: Urinary incontinence: United States and British nursing perspectives, J. Gerontol. Nurs. **4**(2): 28-33, 1978.

Eastwood, H.: Differential diagnosis of urinary incontinence in the elderly, Geriatric Med. Today **2**(4):19-28, 1983.

Field, M.A.: Urinary incontinence in the elderly: an overview, J. Gerontol. Nurs. **5**(1):12-19, 1979.

Voith, A.M., Madson, L.A., Smith, D.A., and others: Validation of nursing diagnosis regarding urinary incontinence, Milwaukee, 1985, Columbia Hospital.

Voith, A.M. and Smith, P.A.: Validation of the nursing diagnosis of urinary retention, Nurs. Clinics N. A., **20:**723-729, 1985.

Voith, A.M.: A conceptual framework for nursing diagnoses regarding alterations in urinary elimination, Rehab. Nurs. **11**(1):18-21, 1986.

Related factors

Altered environment; sensory, cognitive, or mobility deficits.

1.3.2.1.5 INCONTINENCE, TOTAL

Definition

The state in which an individual experiences a continuous and unpredictable loss of urine.

Defining characteristics
Major

Constant flow of urine occurs at unpredictable times without distention or uninhibited bladder contractions/spasms; unsuccessful incontinence refractory treatments; nocturia.

Minor

Lack of perineal or bladder filling awareness; unawareness of incontinence.

Substantiating/supportive materials

Dufault, K.: Urinary incontinence: United States and British nursing perspectives, J. Gerontol. Nurs. **4**(2): 28-33, 1978.

Eastwood, H.: Differential diagnosis of urinary incontinence in the elderly, Geriatric Med. Today **2**(4):19-28, 1983.

Field, M.A.: Urinary incontinence in the elderly: an overview, J. Gerontol. Nurs. **5**(1):12-19, 1979.

Voith, A.M., Madson, L.A., Smith, D.A., and others: Validation of nursing diagnosis regarding urinary incontinence, Milwaukee, 1985, Columbia Hospital.

Voith, A.M. and Smith, P.A.: Validation of the nursing diagnosis of urinary retention, Nurs. Clinics N. A., **20:**723-729, 1985.

Voith, A.M.: A conceptual framework for nursing diagnoses regarding alterations in urinary elimination, Rehab. Nurs. **11**(1):18-21, 1986.

Related factors

Neuropathy preventing transmission of reflex indicating bladder fullness; neurological dysfunction causing triggering of micturition at unpredictable times; independent contraction of detrusor reflex due to surgery; trauma or disease affecting spinal cord nerves; anatomic (fistula).

1.3.2.2. URINARY RETENTION

Definition

The state in which the individual experiences incomplete emptying of the bladder.

Defining characteristics
Major

Bladder distention; small, frequent voiding or absence of urine output.

Minor

Sensation of bladder fullness; dribbling; residual urine; dysuria; overflow incontinence.

Substantiating/supporting materials

Dufault, K.: Urinary incontinence: United States and British nursing perspectives, J. Gerontol. Nurs. **4**(2): 28-33, 1978.

Eastwood, H.: Differential diagnosis of urinary incontinence in the elderly, Geriatric Med. Today **2**(4):19-28, 1983.

Field, M.A.: Urinary incontinence in the elderly: an overview, J. Gerontol. Nurs. **5**(1):12-19, 1979.

Voith, A.M., Madson, L.A., Smith, D.A., and others: Validation of nursing diagnosis regarding urinary incontinence, Milwaukee, 1985, Columbia Hospital.

Voith, A.M. and Smith, P.A.: Validation of the nursing diagnosis of urinary retention, Nurs. Clinics N. A., **20**:723-729, 1985.

Voith, A.M.: A conceptual framework for nursing diagnoses regarding alterations in urinary elimination, Rehab. Nurs. **11**(1):18-21, 1986.

Related factors

High urethral pressure caused by weak detrusor; inhibition of reflex arc; strong sphincter; blockage.

1.4.1.1 TISSUE PERFUSION, ALTERED: RENAL, CEREBRAL, CARDIOPULMONARY, GASTROINTESTINAL, PERIPHERAL++

Definition

The state in which an individual experiences a decrease in nutrition and oxygenation at the cellular level due to a deficit in capillary blood supply.

Defining characteristics

Major

	Estimated sensitivities & specificities	
	Chances that characteristic will be present in given diagnosis	Chances that characteristic will not be explained by any other diagnosis
Skin temperature, cold extremities	High	Low
Skin color		
Dependent, blue or purple	Moderate	Low
*Pale on elevation, color does not return on lowering of leg	High	High
*Diminished arterial pulsations	High	High
Skin quality: shining	High	Low
Lack of lanugo	High	Moderate
Round scars covered with atrophied skin		
Gangrene	Low	High
Slow-growing, dry, brittle nails	High	Moderate
Claudication	Moderate	High
Blood pressure changes in extremities		
Bruits	Moderate	Moderate
Slow healing of lesions	High	Low

++See NANDA Taxonomy I for numerical codes to designate specific tissues.

Related factors

Interruption of flow, arterial; interruption of flow, venous; exchange problems; hypovolemia; hypervolemia.

1.4.1.2.1 FLUID VOLUME EXCESS

Definition

The state in which an individual experiences increased fluid retention and edema.

Defining characteristics
Major

Edema; effusion; anasarca; weight gain; shortness of breath, orthopnea; intake greater than output; S/3 heart sound; pulmonary congestion (chest x-ray); abnormal breath sounds, rales (crackles); change in respiratory pattern; change in mental status; decreased hemoglobin and hematocrit; blood pressure changes; central venous pressure changes; pulmonary artery pressure changes; jugular vein distention; positive hepatojugular reflex; oliguria; specific gravity changes; azotemia; altered electrolytes; restlessness and anxiety.

Related factors

Compromised regulatory mechanism; excess fluid intake; excess sodium intake.

1.4.1.2.2.1 FLUID VOLUME DEFICIT: ACTUAL (1)

Definition

The state in which an individual experiences vascular, cellular, or intracellular dehydration.

Defining characteristics
Major

Dilute urine; increased urine output; sudden weight loss.

Minor

Possible weight gain; hypotension; decreased venous filling; increased pulse rate; decreased skin turgor; decreased pulse volume/pressure; increased body temperature; dry skin; dry mucous membranes; hemoconcentration; weakness; edema; thirst.

Related factors

Failure of regulatory mechanisms.

1.4.1.2.2.1 FLUID VOLUME DEFICIT: ACTUAL (2)

Definition

The state in which an individual experiences vascular, cellular, or intracellular dehydration.

Defining characteristics
Major

Decreased urine output; concentrated urine; output greater than intake; sudden weight loss; decreased venous filling; hemoconcentration; increased serum sodium.

Minor

Hypotension; thirst; increased pulse rate; decreased skin turgor; decreased pulse volume/pressure; change in mental state; increased body temperature; dry skin; dry mucous membranes; weakness.

Related factors

Active loss.

1.4.1.2.2.2 FLUID VOLUME DEFICIT: POTENTIAL

Definition

The state in which an individual is at risk of experiencing vascular, cellular, or intracellular dehydration.

Risk factors

Increased output; urinary frequency; thirst, altered intake.

Related factors

Extremes of age; extremes of weight; excessive losses through normal routes (e.g., diarrhea); loss of fluid through abnormal routes (e.g., indwelling tubes); deviations affecting access to, intake of, or absorption of fluids (e.g., physical immobility); factors influencing fluid needs (e.g., hypermetabolic state); knowledge deficiency related to fluid volume; medications (e.g., diuretics).

1.4.2.1 CARDIAC OUTPUT, ALTERED: DECREASED

Definition

A state in which the amount of blood pumped by an individual's heart is sufficiently reduced that it is inadequate to meet the needs of the body's tissues.

Defining characteristics
Major

Variations in blood pressure readings; arrhythmias; fatigue; jugular vein distention; color changes, skin and mucous membranes; oliguria; decreased peripheral pulses; cold clammy skin; rales; dyspnea, orthopnea; restlessness.

Minor

Change in mental status; shortness of breath; syncope; vertigo; edema; cough; frothy sputum; gallop rhythm; weakness.

1.5.1.1 GAS EXCHANGE, IMPAIRED

Definition

The state in which the individual experiences a decreased passage of oxygen and/or carbon dioxide between the alveoli of the lungs and the vascular system.

Defining characteristics
Major

Confusion; somnolence; restlessness; irritability; inability to move secretions; hypercapnea; hypoxia.

Related factors

Ventilation perfusion imbalance.

1.5.1.2 AIRWAY CLEARANCE, INEFFECTIVE

Definition

A state in which an individual is unable to clear secretions or obstructions from the respiratory tract to maintain airway patency.

Defining characteristics
Major

Abnormal breath sounds (rales [crackles], rhonchi [wheezes]); changes in rate or depth of respiration; tachypnea; cough, effective/ineffective, with or without sputum; cyanosis; dyspnea.

Related factors

Fatigue/decreased energy; tracheobronchial infection, obstruction, secretion; perceptual/cognitive impairment; trauma.

1.5.1.3 BREATHING PATTERN, INEFFECTIVE

Definition

The state in which an inhalation and/or exhalation pattern does not enable adequate pulmonary inflation or emptying.

Defining characteristics
Major

Dyspnea; shortness of breath; tachypnea; fremitus; abnormal arterial blood gas; cyanosis; cough; nasal flaring; respiratory depth changes; assumption of 3-point position; pursed-lip breathing/prolonged expiratory phase; increased anteroposterior diameter;

use of accessory muscles; altered chest excursion.

Related factors

Neuromuscular impairment; pain, musculoskeletal impairment; perception/cognitive impairment; anxiety; fatigue/decreased energy.

1.6.1 INJURY, POTENTIAL FOR

Definition

A state in which the individual is at risk of injury as a result of environmental conditions interacting with the individual's adaptive and defensive resources.

Risk factors

Internal. Biochemical, regulatory function: sensory dysfunction, integrative dysfunction, effector dysfunction; tissue hypoxia; malnutrition; immune-autoimmune; abnormal blood profile; leukocytosis/leukopenia; altered clotting factors; thrombocytopenia; sickle cell, Thalassemia; decreased hemoglobin; physical: broken skin, altered mobility; developmental age: physiological, psychosocial; psychological: affective, orientation.

External. Biological: immunization level of community, microorganism; chemical: pollutants, poisons, drugs (pharmaceutical agents, alcohol, caffeine, nicotine, preservatives, cosmetics and dyes, nutrients [vitamins, food types]); physical: design, structure, and arrangement of community, building, or equipment; mode of transport/transportation; people/provider: nosocomial agents; staffing patterns; cognitive, affective, and psychomotor factors.

Related factors

Interactive conditions between individual and environment which impose a risk to the defensive and adaptive resources of the individual.

Internal factors (host):

Biological; chemical; physiological; psychological perception; developmental.

External factors (environment):

Biological; chemical; physiological; psychological; people/provider.

1.6.1.1 INJURY, POTENTIAL FOR: SUFFOCATING

Definition

Accentuated risk of accidental suffocation (inadequate air available for inhalation).

Risk factors

Internal (individual). Reduced olfactory sensation; reduced motor abilities, lack of safety education; lack of safety precautions; cognitive or emotional difficulties; disease or injury process.

External (environmental). Pillow placed in an infant's crib; propped bottle placed in an infant's crib; vehicle warming in closed garage; children playing with plastic bags or inserting small objects into their mouths or noses; discarded or unused refrigerators or freezers without removed doors; children left unattended in bathtubs or pools; household gas leaks; smoking in bed; use of fuel-burning heaters not vented to outside; low-strung clothesline; pacifier hung around infant's head; person who eats large mouthfuls of food.

1.6.1.2 INJURY, POTENTIAL FOR: POISONING

Definition

Accentuated risk of accidental exposure to or ingestion of drugs or dangerous products in doses sufficient to cause poisoning.

Risk factors

Internal (individual). Reduced vision; verbalization of occupational setting without adequate safeguards; lack of safety or drug education; lack of proper precautions; cognitive or emotional difficulties; insufficient finances.

External (environmental). Large supplies of drugs in house; medicines stored in unlocked cabinets accessible to children or confused persons; dangerous products placed or stored within the reach of children or confused persons; availability of illicit drugs potentially contaminated by poisonous additives; flaking, peeling paint or plaster in presence of young children; chemical contamination of food and water; unprotected contact with heavy metals or chemicals; paint, lacquer, etc., in poorly ventilated areas or without effective protection; presence of poisonous vegetation; presence of atmospheric pollutants.

1.6.1.3 INJURY, POTENTIAL FOR: TRAUMA

Definition

Accentuated risk of accidental tissue injury (e.g., wound, burn, fracture).

Risk factors

Internal (individual). Weakness; poor vision; balancing difficulties; reduced temperature or tactile sensation; reduced large or small muscle coordination; reduced hand-eye coordination; lack of safety education; lack of safety precautions; insufficient finances to purchase safety equipment or effect repairs; cognitive or emotional difficulties; history of previous trauma.

External (environmental). Slippery floors (e.g., wet or highly waxed); snow or ice collected on stairs, walkways; unanchored rugs; bathtub without hand grip or antislip equipment; use of unsteady ladders or chairs; entering unlighted rooms; unsturdy or absent stair rails; unanchored electric wires; litter or liquid spills on floors or stairways; high beds; children playing without gates at the top of stairs; obstructed passageways; unsafe window protection in homes with young children; inappropriate call-for-aid mechanisms for bed-resting clients; pot handles facing toward front of stove; bathing in very hot water (e.g., unsupervised bathing of young children); potential igniting gas leaks; delayed lighting of gas burner or oven; experimenting with chemical or gasoline; unscreened fires or heaters; wearing plastic apron or flowing clothes around open flame; children playing with matches, candles, cigarettes; inadequately stored combustibles or corrosives (e.g., matches, oily rags, lye); highly flammable children's toys or clothing; overloaded fuse boxes; contact with rapidly moving machinery, industrial belts, or pulleys; sliding on coarse bed linen or struggling within bed restraints; faulty electrical plugs, frayed wires, or defective appliances; contact with acids or alkalis; playing with fireworks or gunpowder; contact with intense cold; overexposure to sun or sun lamps, radiotherapy; use of cracked dishware or glasses; knives stored uncovered; guns or ammunition stored unlocked; large icicles hanging from roof; exposure to dangerous machinery; children playing with sharp-edged toys; high crime neighborhood and vulnerable client; driving a mechanically unsafe vehicle; driving after partaking of alcoholic beverages or drugs; driving at excessive speeds; driving without necessary visual aids; children riding in the front seat in car; smoking in bed or near oxygen; overloaded electrical outlets; grease waste collected on stoves; use of thin or worn potholders or mitts; unrestrained babies riding in car; nonuse or misuse of necessary headgear for motorized cyclists or young children carried on adult bicycles; unsafe road or road-crossing conditions; play or work near vehicle pathways (e.g., driveways, laneways, railroad tracks); nonuse or misuse of seat restraints.

1.6.2.1.1 SKIN INTEGRITY, IMPAIRED: ACTUAL

Definition

A state in which the individual's skin is adversely altered.

Defining characteristics
Major

Disruption of skin surface; destruction of skin layers; invasion of body structures.

Related factors

External (environmental). Hyper- or hypothermia; chemical substance; mechanical factors (shearing forces, pressure, restraint); radiation; physical immobilization; humidity.
Internal (somatic). Medication: altered nutritional state (obesity, emaciation); altered metabolic state; altered circulation; altered sensation; altered pigmentation; skeletal prominence; developmental factors; immunological deficit; alterations in turgor (change in elasticity).

1.6.2.1.2 SKIN INTEGRITY, IMPAIRED: POTENTIAL

Definition

A state in which the individual's skin is at risk of being adversely altered.

Risk factors

External (environmental). Hypo- or hyperthermia; chemical substances; mechanical factors (shearing forces, pressure, restraint); radiation; physical immobilization; excretions/secretions; humidity.
Internal (somatic). Medication; alterations in nutritional state (obesity, emacia-

tion); altered metabolic state; altered circulation; altered sensation; altered pigmentation; skeletal prominence; developmental factors; alterations in skin turgor (change in elasticity); psychogenic; immunologic.

1.6.2.2 TISSUE INTEGRITY, IMPAIRED

Definition

A state in which an individual experiences damage to mucous membrane, corneal, integumentary, or subcutaneous tissue.

Defining characteristics
Major

Damaged or destroyed tissue (cornea, mucous membrane, integumentary, or subcutaneous).

Substantiating/supportive materials

Cameron, O., La Plante, J., Lenk, D., et al.: Pressure sore guidelines: nursing diagnosis and management, Detroit, 1984, Harper-Grace Hospitals.

David, J.: Tissue breakdown, Nurs. Mirror **158**, Supplement:i-xvi, 1984.

Hilderly, L.: Skin care in radiation therapy: a review of the literature, Oncology Nurs. Forum **10**(1):51-56, 1983.

Horsley, J.: Preventing decubitus ulcers, CURN Project, New York, 1981, Grune & Stratton, Inc.

Hubalik, K. and Kim, M.J.: Nursing diagnoses associated with heart failure in critical care nursing. In Kim, M.J., McFarland, G.K., and McLane, A.M., editors: Classification of nursing diagnoses: proceedings of the fifth national conference, St. Louis, 1984, The C.V. Mosby Co.

Rovee, D.T.: Effect of local wound environment on epidermal healing. In Maibach, H.L., and Rovee, D.T., editors: Epidermal wound healing, Chicago, 1972, Year Book Medical Publishers.

Rudolph, R. and Noe, J.M.: Chronic problem wounds, Boston, 1983, Little, Brown, & Co.

Sklar, C.G.: Pressure ulcer management in the neurologically impaired patient, J. Neurosurgical Nurs. **17** (1):30-36, 1985.

Related factors

Altered circulation; nutritional deficit/excess; fluid deficit/excess; knowledge deficit; impaired physical mobility; irritants, chemical (including body excretions, secretions, medications); thermal (temperature extremes); mechanical (pressure, shear, friction); radiation (including therapeutic radiation).

1.6.2.2.1 TISSUE INTEGRITY, IMPAIRED: ORAL MUCOUS MEMBRANE

Definition

The state in which an individual experiences disruptions in the tissue layers of the oral cavity.

Defining characteristics
Major

Oral pain/discomfort; coated tongue; xerostomia (dry mouth); stomatitis; oral lesions or ulcers; lack of or decreased salivation; leukoplakia; edema; hyperemia; oral plaque; desquamation; vesicles; hemorrhagic gingivitis, carious teeth; halitosis.

Related factors

Pathological conditions: oral cavity (radiation to head or neck); dehydration; trauma (chemical, e.g., acidic foods, drugs, noxious agents, alcohol; mechanical, e.g., ill-fitting dentures, braces, tubes [endotracheal/nasogastric], surgery in oral cavity); NPO for more than 24 hours; ineffective oral hygiene; mouth breathing; malnutrition; infection; lack of or decreased salivation; medication.

2.1.1.1 COMMUNICATION, IMPAIRED VERBAL

Definition

The state in which an individual experiences a decreased or absent ability to use or understand language in human interaction.

Defining characteristics
Major

*Unable to speak dominant language;
*speaks or verbalizes with difficulty; *does

not or cannot speak; stuttering; slurring; difficulty forming words or sentences; difficulty expressing thought verbally; inappropriate verbalization; dyspnea; disorientation.

Related factors

Decrease in circulation to brain; physical barrier (brain tumor, tracheostomy, intubation); anatomical defect, cleft palate; psychological barriers (psychosis, lack of stimuli); cultural differences; developmental or age related.

3.1.1 SOCIAL INTERACTION, IMPAIRED

Definition

The state in which an individual participates in an insufficient or excessive quantity or ineffective quality of social exchange.

Defining characteristics
Major

Verbalized or observed discomfort in social situations; verbalized or observed inability to receive or communicate a satisfying sense of belonging, caring, interest, or shared history; observed use of unsuccessful social interaction behaviors; dysfunctional interaction with peers, family and/or others.

Minor

Family report of change of style or pattern of interaction.

Substantiating/supportive materials

Bulechek, G. and McCloskey, J.: Nursing interventions: treatments for nursing diagnoses, Philadelphia, 1985, W.B. Saunders.
Jones, P.E. and Jakob, D.: The definition of nursing diagnoses; phase 3 and final report, Toronto, 1982, University of Toronto Faculty of Nursing.

Related factors

Knowledge/skill deficit about ways to enhance mutuality; communication barriers;

self-concept disturbance; absence of available significant others or peers; limited physical mobility; therapeutic isolation; socio-cultural dissonance; environmental barriers; altered thought processes.

3.1.2 SOCIAL ISOLATION

Definition

Aloneness experienced by the individual and perceived as imposed by others and as a negative or threatening state.

Defining characteristics
Major

Objective. Absence of supportive significant others (family friends, group); sad dull affect; inappropriate or immature interests/activities for developmental age/stage; uncommunicative, withdrawn, no eye contact; preoccupation with own thoughts, repetitive meaningless actions; projected hostility in voice, behavior; seeking to be alone, or existing in a subculture; evidence of physical/mental handicap or altered state of wellness; behavior unaccepted by dominant cultural group.

Subjective. Expressed feelings of aloneness imposed by others; expressed feelings of rejection; experienced feelings of difference from others; inadequacy in or absence of significant purpose in life; inability to meet expectations of others; insecurity in public; expressed values acceptable to the subculture but unacceptable to the dominant cultural group; expressed interests inappropriate to the developmental age/state.

Related factors

Factors contributing to the absence of satisfying personal relationships, such as: delay in accomplishing developmental tasks; immature interests; alterations in physical appearance; alterations in mental status; unaccepted social behavior; unaccepted social values; altered state of wellness; inadequate personal resources; inability to engage in satisfying personal relationships.

3.2.1 ROLE PERFORMANCE, ALTERED

Definition

Disruption in the way one perceives one's role performance.

Defining characteristics
Major

Change in self-perception of role; denial of role; change in others' perception of role; conflict in roles; change in physical capacity to resume role; lack of knowledge of role; change in usual patterns of responsibility.

3.2.1.1.1 PARENTING, ALTERED: ACTUAL

Definition

Changes in ability of nurturing figure(s) to create an environment which promotes the optimum growth and development of another human being.†

Defining characteristics
Major

Abandonment; running away; verbalization of inability to control child; incidence of physical and psychological trauma; lack of parental attachment behaviors; inappropriate visual, tactile, or auditory stimulation; negative identification of infant/child's characteristics; negative attachment of meanings to infant/child's characteristics; constant verbalization of disappointment in gender or physical characteristics of infant/child; verbalization of resentment towards infant/child; verbalization of role inadequacy; *inattention to infant/child's needs; verbal disgust at body functions of infant/child; non-

---

†It is important to state as a preface to this diagnosis that adjustment to parenting in general is a normal maturational process that elicits nursing behaviors of prevention of potential problems and health promotion.

compliance with health appointments for self or infant/child; *inappropriate caretaking behaviors (toilet training, sleep/rest, feeding); inappropriate or inconsistent discipline practices; frequent accidents; frequent illness; growth and development lag in child; *history of child abuse or abandonment by primary caretaker; verbalization of desire to have child call him/her by first name versus traditional cultural tendencies; child receives care from multiple caretakers without consideration for the needs of the infant/child; compulsive seeking of role approval from others.

Related factors

Lack of available role model; ineffective role model; physical and psychosocial abuse of nurturing figure; lack of support between/from significant other(s); unmet social/emotional maturation needs of parenting figures; interruption in bonding process (i.e., maternal, paternal, other); unrealistic expectations for self, infant, partner; perceived threat to own physical or emotional survival; mental and/or physical illness; presence of stress (financial, legal, recent crisis, cultural move); lack of knowledge; limited cognitive functioning; lack of role identity; lack of (or inappropriate) response of child to relationship; multiple pregnancies.

3.2.1.1.2 PARENTING, ALTERED: POTENTIAL

Definition

Possibility of changes in ability of nurturing figure(s) to create an environment which promotes the optimum growth and development of another human being.†

---

†It is important to state as a preface to this diagnosis that adjustment to parenting in general is a normal maturational process that elicits nursing behaviors of prevention of potential problems and health promotion.

Risk factors

Lack of parental attachment behaviors; inappropriate visual, tactile, or auditory stimulation; negative identification of infant/child's characteristics; negative attachment of meanings to infant/child's characteristics; constant verbalization of disappointment in gender or physical characteristics of infant/child; verbalization of resentment towards infant/child; verbalization of role inadequacy; *inattention to infant/child's needs; verbal disgust at body functions of infant/child; noncompliance with health appointments for self or infant/child; *inappropriate caretaking behaviors (toilet training, sleep/rest, feeding); inappropriate or inconsistent discipline practices; frequent accidents; frequent illness; growth and development lag in child; *history of child abuse or abandonment by primary caretaker; verbalized desire to have child call him/her by first name versus traditional cultural tendencies; child receives care from multiple caretakers without consideration for the needs of the infant/child; compulsive seeking of role approval from others.

Related factors

Lack of available role model; ineffective role model; physical and psychosocial abuse of nurturing figure; lack of support between/from significant other(s); unmet social/emotional maturation needs of parenting figures; interruption in bonding process (i.e., maternal, paternal, other); unrealistic expectations for self, infant, or partner; perceived threat to own physical or emotional survival; mental or physical illness; presence of stress (financial, legal, recent crisis, cultural move); lack of knowledge; limited cognitive functioning; lack of role identity; lack of (or inappropriate) response of child to relationship; multiple pregnancies.

3.2.1.2.1 SEXUAL DYSFUNCTION

Definition
The state in which an individual experiences a change in sexual function that is viewed as unsatisfying, unrewarding, or inadequate.

Defining characteristics
Major

Verbalization of problem; alterations in achieving perceived sex role; actual or perceived limitation imposed by disease and/or therapy; conflicts involving values; alteration in achieving sexual satisfaction; inability to achieve desired satisfaction; seeking confirmation of desirability; alteration in relationship with significant other; change of interest in self and others.

Related factors
Biopsychosocial alteration of sexuality: ineffectual or absent role models; physical abuse; psychosocial abuse, (e.g., harmful relationships); vulnerability; values conflict; lack of privacy; lack of significant other; altered body structure or function (pregnancy, recent childbirth, drugs, surgery, anomalies, disease process, trauma, or radiation); misinformation or lack of knowledge.

3.2.2 FAMILY PROCESSES, ALTERED

Definition
The state in which a family that normally functions effectively experiences dysfunction.

Defining characteristics
Major

Family system unable to meet physical needs of its members; family system unable to meet emotional needs of its members; family system unable to meet spiritual needs of its members; parents do not demonstrate respect for each other's views on child-rearing practices; inability to express/accept wide range of feelings; inability to express/accept feelings of members; family unable to meet security needs of its members; inability of family members to relate to each other for mutual growth and maturation; family uninvolved in community activities; inability to accept/receive help appropriately; rigidity in function and roles; family not demonstrating respect for individuality and autonomy of its members; family unable to adapt to change/deal with traumatic experience constructively; family failing to accomplish current/past developmental tasks; unhealthy family decision-making process; failure to send and receive clear messages; inappropriate boundary maintenance; inappropriate/poorly communicated family rules, rituals, or symbols; unexamined family myths; inappropriate level and direction of energy.

Related factors
Situation transition or crises; developmental transition or crisis.

3.3 SEXUALITY, ALTERED PATTERNS

Definition
The state in which an individual expresses concern regarding his/her sexuality.

Defining characteristics
Major

Reported difficulties, limitations, or changes in sexual behaviors or activities.

Substantiating/supportive materials
Broam, B.: Consensus about the marital relationship during transition to parenthood, Nurs. Research **33**:223-228, 1984.
Jones, P.E., and Jakob, D.: The definition of nursing diagnosis: phase 3 and final report, Toronto, 1982, University of Toronto Faculty of Nursing.
Roberts, C.S., and Feetham, S.L.: Assessing family functioning across three areas of relationships, Nurs. Research **31**:231-235, 1982.

Related factors

Knowledge/skill deficit about alternative responses to health-related transitions or altered body function or structure (illness or medical); lack of privacy; lack of significant other; ineffective or absent role model; conflicts with sexual orientation or variant preferences; fear of pregnancy or of acquiring sexually transmitted disease; impaired relationship with significant other.

4.1.1 SPIRITUAL DISTRESS (DISTRESS OF THE HUMAN SPIRIT)

Definition

Disruption in the life principle which pervades a person's entire being and which integrates and transcends one's biological and psychosocial nature.

Defining characteristics
Major

*Expressed concern with meaning of life/death and or belief systems; anger toward God; questioned meaning of suffering; verbalized inner conflict about beliefs; verbalized concern about relationship with deity; questioned meaning of own existence; inability to participate in usual religious practices; seeking of spiritual assistance; questioned moral/ethical implications of therapeutic regimen; gallows humor; displacement of anger toward religious representatives; description of nightmares/sleep disturbances; alteration in behavior/mood evidenced by anger, crying, withdrawal, preoccupation, anxiety, hostility, apathy, etc.

Related factors

Separation from religious/cultural ties; challenged belief and value system (e.g., due to moral/ethical implications of therapy, due to intense suffering).

5.1.1.1 COPING, INEFFECTIVE INDIVIDUAL
Definition

Impairment of adaptive behaviors and problem solving abilities of a person in meeting life's demands and roles.

Defining characteristics
Major

*Verbalization of inability to cope or inability to ask for help; inability to meet role expectations; inability to meet basic needs; *inability to solve problems; alteration in societal participation; destructive behavior toward self or others; inappropriate use of defense mechanisms; change in usual communication patterns; verbal manipulation; high illness rate; high rate of accidents.

Related factors

Situational crises; maturational crises; personal vulnerability.

5.1.1.1.1 ADJUSTMENT, IMPAIRED

Definition

The state in which the individual is unable to modify his/her life style/behavior in a manner consistent with a change in health status.

Defining characteristics
Major

Verbalization of non-acceptance of health status change; non-existent or unsuccessful ability to be involved in problem solving or goal setting.

Minor

Lack of movement toward independence; extended period of shock, disbelief, or anger regarding health status change; lack of future-oriented thinking.

Substantiating/supportive materials

Beglinger, J.E.: Coping tasks in critical care: patients and families, Dim. Critical Care Nurs. **2**(2):80-89, 1983.

Cheney, R.J.: Emotional adaptation to disability, Rehab. Nurs. **9**(5):36-37, 1984.

Gentry, W.D., et al.: Type A/B differences in coping with acute myocardial infarction: further considerations (editorial), Heart Lung **13**(3):212-214, 1983.

Miller, P., et al.: Family health and psychosocial responses to cardiovascular diseases, Health Values **7**(6):10-15, 1983.

Oberst, M.T., et al.: Going home: patient and spouse adjustment following cancer surgery, Topics Clinical Nurs. **7**(1):46-57, 1985.

Ott, C.R., et al.: A controlled randomized study of early cardiac rehabilitation: the sickness impact profile as an assessment tool, Heart Lung **12**(2):162-170, 1983.

Related factors

Disability requiring change in life style; inadequate support systems; impaired cognition; sensory overload; assault to self-esteem; altered locus of control; incomplete grieving.

somaticism; taking on illness signs of client; decisions and actions by family which are detrimental to economic or social well-being; agitation, depression, aggression, or hostility; impaired restructuring of a meaningful life for self, impaired individualization, prolonged overconcern for client; neglectful relationships with other family members; client's development of helpless, inactive dependence.

Related factors

Significant person with chronically unexpressed feelings of guilt, anxiety, hostility, despair, etc.; dissonant discrepancy of coping styles for dealing with adaptive tasks by the significant person and client or among significant people; highly ambivalent family relationships; arbitrary handling of family's resistance to treatment, which tends to solidify defensiveness as it fails to deal adequately with underlying anxiety.

5.1.2.1.1 COPING, INEFFECTIVE FAMILY: DISABLED

Definition

Behavior of significant person (family member or other primary person) that disables his or her own capacities and the client's capacities to effectively address tasks essential to either person's adaptation to the health challenge.

Defining characteristics
Major

Neglectful care of the client in regard to basic human needs or illness treatment; distortion of reality regarding the client's health problem, including extreme denial about its existence or severity; intolerance; rejection; abandonment; desertion; carrying on usual routines, disregarding client's needs; psycho-

5.1.2.1.2 COPING, INEFFECTIVE FAMILY: COMPROMISED

Definition

Insufficient, ineffective, or compromised support, comfort assistance, or encouragement, usually by a supportive primary person (family member or close friend); client may need this support to manage or master adaptive tasks related to his or her health challenge.

Defining characteristics
Major

Subjective. Client expresses or confirms a concern or complaint about significant other's response to his or her illness or disability or to other situational or developmental crises with personal reactions (e.g., fear, anticipatory grief, guilt, or anxiety); significant person describes or confirms inadequate understanding or knowledge base which interferes with effective assistive or supportive behaviors.

Objective. Significant person attempts assistive or supportive behaviors with less than satisfactory results; significant person withdraws or enters into limited or temporary personal communication with the client at the time of need; significant person displays protective behavior disproportionate (too little or too much) to the client's abilities or need for autonomy.

Related factors

Inadequate or incorrect information or understanding by a primary person; temporary preoccupation by a significant person who is trying to manage emotional conflicts and personal suffering and is unable to perceive or act effectively in regard to client's needs; temporary family disorganization and role changes; other situational or developmental crises or situations the significant person may be facing; in turn, little support provided by client for primary person; prolonged disease or disability progression that exhausts supportive capacity of significant people.

5.1.2.2 COPING, FAMILY: POTENTIAL FOR GROWTH

Definition

Effective managing of adaptive tasks by family member involved with the client's health challenge, who now is exhibiting desire and readiness for enhanced health and growth in regard to self and in relation to the client.

Defining characteristics
Major

Family member attempting to describe growth impact of crisis on his or her own values, priorities, goals, or relationships; family member moving in direction of health-promoting and enriching life-style which supports and monitors maturational processes, auditing and negotiating treatment programs, and generally choosing experiences which optimize wellness; individual expressing interest in making contact on a one-to-one basis or on a mutual-aid–group basis with another person who has experienced a similar situation.

Related factors

Needs sufficiently gratified and adaptive tasks effectively addressed to enable goals of self-actualization to surface.

5.2.1.1 NONCOMPLIANCE (SPECIFY)

Definition

A person's informed decision not to adhere to a therapeutic recommendation.

Defining characteristics
Major

*Behavior indicative of failure to adhere (by direct observation or by statements of patient or significant others); objective tests (physiological measures, detection of markers); evidence of development of complications; evidence of exacerbation of symptoms; failure to keep appointments; failure to progress.

Related factors

Patient value system: health beliefs, cultural influences, spiritual values; client-provider relationships.

6.1.1.1.1 MOBILITY, IMPAIRED PHYSICAL

Definition

A state in which the individual experiences a limitation of ability for independent physical movement.

Defining characteristics
Major

Inability to purposefully move within the physical environment, including bed mobility, transfer, and ambulation; reluctance to attempt movement; limited range of motion; decreased muscle strength, control or mass; imposed restrictions of movement, including mechanical, medical protocol; impaired coordination.

Related factors

Intolerance to activity/decreased strength and endurance; pain/discomfort; perceptual/ cognitive impairment; neuromuscular impairment; musculoskeletal impairment; depression/severe anxiety.

SUGGESTED CODE FOR FUNCTIONAL LEVEL CLASSIFICATION

0 = Completely independent.
1 = Requires use of equipment or device.
2 = Requires help from another person for assistance, supervision, or teaching.
3 = Requires help from another person and equipment device.
4 = Dependent, does not participate in activity.

6.1.1.2 ACTIVITY INTOLERANCE

Definition

A state in which an individual has insufficient physiological or psychological energy to endure or complete required or desired daily activities.

Defining characteristics
Major

*Verbal report of fatigue or weakness; abnormal heart rate or blood pressure response to activity; exertional discomfort or dyspnea; electrocardiographic changes reflecting arrhythmias or ischemia.

Related factors

Bedrest/immobility; generalized weakness; sedentary lifestyle; imbalance between oxygen supply/demand.

6.1.1.3 ACTIVITY INTOLERANCE: POTENTIAL

Definition

A state in which an individual is at risk of experiencing insufficient physiological or psychological energy to endure or complete required or desired daily activities.

Risk factors

History of previous intolerance; deconditioned status; presence of circulatory/respiratory problems; inexperience with activity.

6.2.1. SLEEP PATTERN DISTURBANCE

Definition

Disruption of sleep time causes discomfort or interferes with desired life-style.

Defining characteristics
Major

*Verbal complaints of difficulty falling asleep; *awakening earlier or later than desired; *interrupted sleep; *verbal complaints of not feeling well-rested; changes in behavior and performance (increasing irritability, restlessness, disorientation, lethargy, or listlessness); physical signs (mild fleeting nystagmus, slight hand tremor, ptosis of eyelid, expressionless face, dark circles under eyes, frequent yawning, changes in posture); thick speech with mispronunciation and incorrect words.

Related factors

Sensory alterations: internal (illness, psychological stress); external (environmental changes, social cues).

6.3.1.1. DIVERSIONAL ACTIVITY, DEFICIT

Definition

The state in which an individual experiences decreased stimulation from or interest or engagement in recreational or leisure activities.

Defining characteristics
Major

Patient's statements regarding: boredom, wish that there was something to do, wish to read, etc.; usual hobbies cannot be undertaken in hospital.

Related factors

Environmental lack of diversional activity, as in long-term hospitalization or frequent lengthy treatments.

6.4.1.1. HOME MAINTENANCE MANAGEMENT, IMPAIRED

Definition

Inability to independently maintain a safe growth-promoting immediate environment.

Defining characteristics
Major

   Subjective. *Household members express difficulty in maintaining home in comfortable fashion; *household requests assistance with home maintenance; *household members describe outstanding debts or financial crises.

   Objective. Disorderly surroundings; *unwashed or unavailable cooking equipment, clothes, or linen; *accumulation of dirt, food wastes, or hygienic wastes; offensive odors; inappropriate household temperature; *overtaxed family members (e.g., exhausted, anxious); lack of necessary equipment or aids; presence of vermin or rodents; *repeated hygienic disorders, infestations, or infections.

Related factors

Individual/family member disease or injury; insufficient family organization or planning; insufficient finances; unfamiliarity with neighborhood resources; impaired cognitive or emotional functioning; lack of knowledge; lack of role modeling; inadequate support systems.

6.4.2. HEALTH MAINTENANCE, ALTERED

Definition

Inability to identify, manage, or seek out help to maintain health.

Defining characteristics
Major

Demonstrated lack of knowledge regarding basic health practices; demonstrated lack of adaptive behaviors to internal/external environmental changes; reported or observed inability to take responsibility for meeting basic health practices in any or all functional pattern areas; history of lack of health–seeking behavior; expressed interest in improving health behaviors; reported or observed lack of equipment, financial, or other resources; reported or observed impairment of personal support systems.

Related factors

Lack of or significant alteration in communication skills (written, verbal, or gestural); lack of ability to make deliberate and thoughtful judgments; perceptual/cognitive impairment (complete/partial lack of gross or fine motor skills); ineffective individual coping; dysfunctional grieving; unachieved developmental tasks; ineffective family coping; disabling spiritual distress; lack of material resources.

6.5.1. SELF-CARE DEFICIT: FEEDING

Definition

A state in which the individual experiences an impaired ability to perform or complete feeding activities for him/herself.

Defining characteristics
Major: Self-feeding deficit (Level 0-4) *

Inability to bring food from a receptacle to the mouth.

Related factors

Intolerance to activity, decreased strength and endurance; pain/discomfort; perceptual or cognitive impairment; neuromuscular impairment; musculoskeletal impairment; depression/severe anxiety.

6.5.1.1. SWALLOWING, IMPAIRED

Definition

The state in which an individual has decreased ability to voluntarily pass fluids and/or solids from the mouth to the stomach.

Defining characteristics
Major

Observed evidence of difficulty in swallowing (e.g., stasis of food in oral cavity, coughing/choking).

Minor

Evidence of aspiration.

Substantiating/supportive materials

Gettrust, K.V., Ryan, S.C., and Engelman, D.S.: Applied nursing diagnosis: guides for comprehensive care planning, New York, 1984, John Wiley & Sons.
Larsen, G.L.: Chewing and swallowing. In Martin, N., Holt, N.B., and Hicks, D.B., editors: Comprehensive rehabilitation nursing, New York, 1981, McGraw-Hill.

Tilton, C.N. and Maloof, M.: Diagnosing the problems in stroke, Amer. J. Nurs. **82**:596-601, 1982.
Welnetz, K.: Maintaining adequate nutrition and hydration in the dysphagic ALS patient, Canadian Nurse **79**(3):30-34, 1983.

Related factors

Neuromuscular impairment (e.g., decreased or absent gag reflex, decreased strength or excursion of muscles involved in mastication, perceptual impairment, facial paralysis); mechanical obstruction (e.g., edema, tracheostomy tube, tumor); fatigue; limited awareness; reddened, irritated oropharyngeal cavity.

6.5.2. SELF-CARE DEFICIT: BATHING/HYGIENE

Definition

A state in which the individual experiences an impaired ability to perform or complete bathing/hygiene activities for him/herself.

Defining characteristics
Major: Self-bathing/hygiene deficit (Level 0-4) +

*Inability to wash body or body parts; inability to obtain or get to water source; inability to regulate water temperature or flow.

Related factors

Intolerance to activity, decreased strength and endurance; pain/discomfort; perceptual or cognitive impairment; neuromuscular impairment; musculoskeletal impairment; depression/severe anxiety.

6.5.3 SELF-CARE DEFICIT: DRESSING/GROOMING

Definition

A state in which the individual experiences an impaired ability to perform or complete

---

†For definition of code, see Mobility, impaired physical.

†For definition of code, see Mobility, Impaired Physical.

dressing and grooming activities for him/herself.

Defining characteristics
Major: self-dressing/grooming deficits (level 0-4)+

*Impaired ability to put on or take off necessary items of clothing; impaired ability to obtain or replace articles of clothing; impaired ability to fasten clothing; inability to maintain appearance at a satisfactory level.

Related factors

Intolerance to activity, decreased strength and endurance; pain/discomfort; perceptual or cognitive impairment; neuromuscular impairment; musculoskeletal impairment; depression/severe anxiety.

6.5.4. SELF-CARE DEFICIT: TOILETING

Definition

A state in which the individual experiences an impaired ability to perform or complete toileting activities for him/herself.

Defining characteristics
Major: self-toileting deficit (level 0-4)+

*Unable to get to toilet or commode; *unable to sit on or rise from toilet or commode; *unable to manipulate clothing for toileting; *unable to carry out proper toilet hygiene; unable to flush toilet or commode.

Related factors

Impaired transfer ability; impaired mobility status; intolerance to activity, decreased strength and endurance; pain/discomfort; perceptual or cognitive impairment; neuromuscular impairment; musculoskeletal impairment; depression/severe anxiety.

---

†For definition of code, see Mobility, Impaired Physical.

6.6 GROWTH AND DEVELOPMENT, ALTERED

Definition

The state in which an individual demonstrates deviations in norms from his/her age group.

Defining characteristics
Major

Delay or difficulty in performing skills (motor, social, or expressive) typical of age group; altered physical growth; inability to perform self-care or self-control activities appropriate for age.

Minor

Flat affect; listlessness, decreased responses.

Substantiating/supportive materials

Campbell, C.: Nursing diagnosis and intervention in nursing practice, New York, 1984, John Wiley & Sons.

Coviak, C.P. and Derhammer, J.: A proposal for a new nursing diagnosis: alterations in growth and development. Unpublished paper. Allendale, MI, 1983, Grand Valley State College.

Jones, P.E. and Jakob, D.: The definition of nursing diagnoses: phase 3 and final report, Toronto, 1982, University of Toronto Faculty of Nursing.

Related factors

Inadequate caretaking; indifference, inconsistent responsiveness, multiple caretakers; separation from significant others; environmental and stimulation deficiencies; effects of physical disability; prescribed dependence.

7.1.1 SELF-CONCEPT, DISTURBANCE IN: BODY-IMAGE

Definition

Disruption in the way one perceives one's body image.

Defining characteristics
Major

A or B must be present to justify the diagnosis of body image, alteration in: *A = verbal response to actual or perceived change in structure or function; *B = non-verbal response to actual or perceived change in structure or function. The following clinical manifestations may be used to validate the presence of A or B.

Objective. Missing body part; actual change in structure or function; not looking at body part; not touching body part; hiding or over-exposing body part (intentional or unintentional); trauma to nonfunctioning part; change in social involvement; change in ability to estimate spatial relationship of body to environment.

Subjective. Verbalization of change in lifestyle; fear of rejection or of reaction by others; focus on past strength, function, or appearance; negative feelings about body, and feelings of helplessness, hopelessness, or powerlessness; preoccupation with change or loss; emphasis on remaining strengths and heightened achievement; extension of body boundary to incorporate environmental objects; personalization of part or loss by name; depersonalization of part or loss by impersonal pronouns; refusal to verify actual change.

Related factors

Biophysical; cognitive/perceptual; psychosocial; cultural or spiritual.

7.1.2 SELF-CONCEPT, DISTURBANCE IN: SELF-ESTEEM
Definition

Disruption in the way one perceives one's self-esteem.

Defining characteristics
Major

Inability to accept positive reinforcement; lack of follow-through; nonparticipation in therapy; not taking responsibility for self-care (self-neglect); lack of eye contact; self-destructive behavior.

7.1.3 SELF-CONCEPT, DISTURBANCE IN: PERSONAL IDENTITY

Definition

Inability to distinguish between self and non-self.

Defining characteristics

To be developed.

7.2 SENSORY/PERCEPTUAL ALTERATIONS: VISUAL, AUDITORY, KINESTHETIC, GUSTATORY, TACTILE, OLFACTORY†††

Definition

A state in which an individual experiences a change in the amount or patterning of incoming stimuli accompanied by a diminished, exaggerated, distorted, or impaired response to such stimuli.

Defining characteristics
Major

Disoriented in time, in place, or with persons; altered abstraction; altered conceptualization; change in problem-solving abilities; reported or measured change in sensory acuity; change in behavior pattern; anxiety; apathy; change in usual response to stimuli; indication of body-image alteration; restlessness; irritability; altered communication patterns.

Minor

Complaint of fatigue; alteration in posture; change in muscular tension; inappropriate responses; hallucinations.

---

†††See NANDA Taxonomy I for numerical codes to designate specific sense(s).

Related factors

Altered environmental stimuli, excessive or insufficient; altered sensory reception, transmission, or integration; chemical alterations: endogenous (electrolyte), exogenous (drugs, etc.); psychological stress.

7.2.1.1 UNILATERAL NEGLECT

Definition

The state in which an individual is perceptually unaware of and inattentive to one side of the body.

Defining characteristics
Major

Consistent inattention to stimuli on affected side.

Minor

Inadequate self-care; positioning and/or safety precautions in regard to the affected side; lack of looking toward affected side; leaving of food on plate on affected side.

Substantiating/supportive materials

Saxton, D.F., Pelikan, P.K., Nugent, P.M., and Hyland, P.S.: The Addison-Wesley manual of nursing practice, Menlo Park, CA, 1983, Addison-Wesley.

Wolanin, M.O., and Phillips, L.A.: Confusion: prevention and care, St. Louis, 1981, The C.V. Mosby Co.

Related factors

Effects of disturbed perceptual abilities, e.g., hemianopsia; one-sided blindness; neurologic illness or trauma.

7.3.1 HOPELESSNESS

Definition

A state in which an individual sees limited or no alternatives or personal choices available and is unable to mobilize energy on his/her own behalf.

Defining characteristics
Major

Passivity, decreased verbalization; decreased affect; verbal cues (despondent content, "I can't," sighing).

Minor

Lack of initiative; decreased response to stimuli; decreased affect; turning away from speaker; closing eyes; shrugging in response to speaker; decreased appetite; increased sleep; lack of involvement in care/passivity in allowing care.

Substantiating/supportive materials

Eisman, R.: Why did Joe die? Amer. J. Nurs. **71**:501-503, 1971.

Farberiow, N.L.: Suicide prevention in the hospital, Hosp. Comm. Psych. **32**(2):99-104, 1981.

Jalowiec, A., and Powers, M.J.: Stress and coping in hypertensive and ER patients, Nurs. Research **30**:10-15, 1981.

Jourard, S.M.: Living and dying: suicide, an invitation to die, Amer. J. Nurs. **70**:269, 273-275, 1970.

Kritek, P.: Patient power and powerlessness. Supervisor Nurse, **12**(6):26-29, 32-34, 1981.

Lambert, V.A. and Lambert, C.E., Jr.: Role theory and the concept of powerlessness, J. Psychosocial Nurs. **19**(9):11-14, 1981.

Miller, C., Denner, P., and Richardson, V.: Assisting the psychosocial problems of cancer patients: a review of current research, Int. J. Nurs. Studies **13**(3):161-166, 1976.

Related factors

Prolonged activity restriction creating isolation; failing or deteriorating physiological condition; long-term stress; abandonment; lost belief in transcendent values/God.

7.3.2 POWERLESSNESS

Definition

Perception that one's own actions will not significantly affect an outcome; perceived lack of control over current situation or immediate happening.

Defining characteristics
Major

Severe. Verbal expression of having no control or influence over situation; verbal expression of having no control or influence over outcome; verbal expression of having no control over self-care; depression over physical deterioration which occurs despite patient compliance with regimens; apathy.

Moderate. Nonparticipation in care or decision making when opportunities are provided; expression of dissatisfaction and frustration over inability to perform previous tasks or activities; lack of monitoring progress; expression of doubt regarding role performance; reluctance to express true feelings, fearing alienation from care givers; passivity; inability to seek information regarding care; dependence on others that may result in irritability, resentment, anger, and guilt; lack of defense of self-care practices when challenged.

Low. Expression of uncertainty about fluctuating energy levels; passivity.

Related factors
Health care environment; interpersonal interaction; illness-related regimen; life-style of helplessness.

8.1.1 KNOWLEDGE DEFICIT (SPECIFY)

Definition
To be developed.

Defining characteristics
Major

Verbalization of problem; inaccurate follow-through of instructions: inaccurate performance on tests; inappropriate or exaggerated behaviors (e.g., hysterical, hostile, agitated, or apathetic).

Related factors
Lack of exposure; lack of recall; information misinterpretation; cognitive limitation; lack of interest in learning; unfamiliarity with information resources.

8.3 THOUGHT PROCESSES, ALTERED

Definition
A state in which an individual experiences a disruption in cognitive operations and activities.

Defining characteristics
Major

Inaccurate interpretation of environment; cognitive dissonance; distractibility; memory deficit/problems; egocentricity; hyper- or hypovigilance.

Minor

Inappropriate nonreality-based thinking.

9.1.1 COMFORT, ALTERED: PAIN

Definition
A state in which an individual experiences and reports the presence of severe discomfort or an uncomfortable sensation.

Defining characteristics
Major

Subjective. Communication (verbal or coded) of pain descriptors.

Objective. Guarding behavior, protective; self-focusing; narrowed focus (altered time perception, withdrawal from social contact, impaired thought processes); distraction behavior (moaning, crying, pacing, seeking out other people or activities, restlessness); facial mask of pain (eyes lack luster, "beaten look," fixed or scattered movement, grimace); alteration in muscle tone (may span from listless to rigid); autonomic responses not seen in chronic stable pain (diaphoresis, blood pressure and pulse change, pupillary dilatation, increased or decreased respiratory rate).

Related factors

Injuring agents (biological, chemical, physical, or psychological).

9.1.1.1 COMFORT, ALTERED: CHRONIC PAIN

Definition

A state in which the individual experiences pain that continues for more than 6 months in duration.

Defining characteristics
Major

Verbal report or observed evidence of pain experienced for more than 6 months.

Minor

Fear of reinjury; physical and social withdrawal; altered ability to continue previous activities; anorexia; weight changes; changes in sleep patterns; facial mask; guarded movements.

Substantiating/supportive materials

Carpenito, L.J.: Handbook of nursing diagnosis, New York, 1984, J.B. Lippincott.
McCaffrey, M.: Nursing management of the patient with pain, 2nd ed. Philadelphia, 1979, J.B. Lippincott.

Related factors

Chronic physical/psychosocial disability.

9.2.1 ANXIETY

Definition

A vague uneasy feeling whose source is often nonspecific or unknown to the individual.

Defining characteristics
Major

Subjective. Increased tension; apprehension; painful and persistent increased helplessness; uncertainty; fearfulness; regret; overexcitement; becoming rattled; distress; becoming jittery; feelings of inadequacy; shakiness; fear of unspecific consequences; expressed concerns about changes in life events; worry; anxiousness.

Objective. *Sympathetic stimulation: cardiovascular excitation, superficial vasoconstriction, pupil dilation; restlessness; insomnia; glancing about; poor eye contact; trembling/hand tremors; extraneous movement (foot shuffling, hand/arm movements); facial tension; voice quivering; focus on self; increased wariness; increased perspiration.

Related factors

Unconscious conflict about essential values/goals of life; threat to self-concept; threat of death; threat to or change in health status; threat to or change in role functioning; threat to or change in environment; threat to or change in interaction patterns; situational/maturational crises; interpersonal transmission/contagion; unmet needs.

9.2.2.1 GRIEVING, DYSFUNCTIONAL

Definition

To be developed.

Defining characteristics
Major

Verbal expression of distress at loss; denial of loss; expression of guilt; expression of unresolved issues; anger; sadness; crying; difficulty in expressing loss; alterations in eating habits, sleep patterns, dream patterns, activity level, or libido; idealization of lost object; reliving of past experiences; interference with life functioning; developmental regression; labile affect; alteration in concentration or pursuit of tasks.

Related factors

Actual or perceived object loss (in the broadest sense); objects may include people, possessions, jobs, status, home, ideals, and parts and processes of the body.

9.2.2.2 GRIEVING, ANTICIPATORY

Definition
To be developed.

Defining characteristics
Major

Potential loss of significant object; expression of distress at potential loss; denial of potential loss; guilt; anger; sorrow; choked feelings; change in eating habits; alteration in sleep patterns; alteration in activity level; altered libido; altered communication pattern.

9.2.3 VIOLENCE, POTENTIAL FOR: SELF-DIRECTED OR DIRECTED AT OTHERS

Definition
A state in which an individual experiences behaviors that can be physically harmful to the self or others.

Risk Factors

Body language: clenched fists, tense facial expression, rigid posture, tautness indicating effort at control; hostile threatening verbalization: boasting or prior abuse of others; increased motor activity: pacing, excitement, irritability, and agitation; overt and aggressive acts: goal-directed destruction of objects in environment; possession of destructive means: gun, knife, or other weapon; rage; self–destructive behavior, active aggressive suicidal acts; suspicion of others, paranoid ideation, delusions, and hallucinations; substance abuse/withdrawal; increasing anxiety level; fear of self or others; inability to verbalize feelings; repetition of verbalizations: continued complaints, requests, or demands; anger; provocative behavior: argumentative behavior, dissatisfaction, overreaction, hypersensitivity: vulnerable self-esteem; depression (specifically active, aggressive, suicidal acts).

Related factors

Antisocial character; evidence of battering (women); catatonic excitement; evidence of child abuse; manic excitement; organic brain syndrome; panic states; rage reactions; suicidal behavior; temporal lobe epilepsy; toxic reactions to medication.

9.2.4 FEAR

Definition

Feeling of dread related to an identifiable source which the person validates.

Defining characteristics
Major

Ability to identify object of fear.

9.2.5 POST-TRAUMA RESPONSE

Definition

The state of an individual experiencing a sustained painful response to unexpected extraordinary life events.

Defining characteristics
Major

Reexperience of the traumatic event which may be identified in cognitive, affective, or sensory motor activities (flashbacks, intrusive thoughts, repetitive dreams or nightmares, excessive verbalization of the traumatic event, or verbalization of survival guilt or guilt about behavior required for survival).

Minor

Psychic/emotional numbness (impaired interpretation of reality, confusion, dissociation or amnesia, vagueness about traumatic event, or constricted affect); altered life style (self-destructiveness, such as substance abuse, suicide attempt, or other acting-out behavior, difficulty with interpersonal relationships, development of phobia regarding trauma, poor impulse control/irritability, and explosiveness).

Substantiating/supportive materials

Burgess, A., and Holstrom, L.L.: Rape-trauma syndrome. Am. J. Psychiatry, **131**:981-986, 1974.

Green, B., et al.: A conceptual framework for post-traumatic stress syndromes among survivor groups. In Figley, C.R., (Editor): Trauma and its wake. New York, 1984, Brunner/Mazel.

Holstrom, L.L. and Burgess, A.W.: Development of diagnostic categories: sexual trauma. Am. J. Nursing, **75**:1286-1291, 1975.

Horowitz, M.J.: Psychological response to serious life events. In Hamilton, V., and Warburton, M.D., (Editors): Human stress and cognition: New York, 1979, J. Wiley & Sons.

Lipkin, O.J., et al: Vietnam veterans and post-traumatic stress disorder. Hosp. Comm. Psych. **33**:908-912, 1982.

Related factors

Disasters, wars, epidemics, rape, assault, torture, catastrophic illness, or accident.

9.2.5.1.1 RAPE-TRAUMA SYNDROME

Definition

Forced, violent sexual penetration against the victim's will and consent. The trauma syndrome that develops from this attack or attempted attack includes an acute phase of disorganization of the victim's life-style and a long-term process of reorganization of life-style.**

Defining characteristics
Major

Acute phase. Emotional reactions (anger, embarrassment, fear of physical violence and death, humiliation, revenge, and self-blame); multiple physical symptoms (gastrointestinal irritability, genitourinary discomfort,

---

** This syndrome includes the following subcomponents: Rape-Trauma, Compound Reaction, and Silent Reaction. In this text each appears as a separate diagnosis.

muscle tension, and sleep pattern disturbance).

Long-term phase. Changes in life-style (changes in residence); dealing with repetitive nightmares and phobias; seeking family support; seeking social network support).

9.2.5.1.2 RAPE-TRAUMA SYNDROME: COMPOUND REACTION

Definition

Forced, violent sexual penetration against the victim's will and consent. The trauma syndrome that develops from this attack or attempted attack includes an acute phase of disorganization of the victim's life-style and a long-term process of reorganization of life-style.**

Defining characteristics
Major

Acute phase. Emotional reactions (anger, embarrassment, fear of physical violence and death, humiliation, revenge, and self-blame); multiple physical symptoms (gastrointestinal irritability, genitourinary discomfort, muscle tension, and sleep pattern disturbance); reactivated symptoms of previous conditions (i.e., physical illness, psychiatric illness); reliance on alcohol or drugs.

Long-term phase. Changes in life-style (changes in residence); dealing with repetitive nightmares and phobias; seeking family support; seeking social network support).

9.2.5.1.3 RAPE-TRAUMA SYNDROME: SILENT REACTION
Definition

Forced, violent sexual penetration against the victim's will and consent. The trauma syndrome that develops from this attack or

---

** This syndrome includes the following three subcomponents: Rape-Trauma, Compound Reaction, and Silent Reaction. In this text each appears as a separate diagnosis.

attempted attack includes an acute phase of disorganization of the victim's life-style and a long-term process of reorganization of life-style.**

Defining characteristics
Major

Abrupt changes in relationships with men; increase in nightmares; increased anxiety during interview (i.e., blocking of associations, long periods of silence, minor stuttering, and physical distress); pronounced changes in sexual behavior; no verbalization of the occurrence of rape; sudden onset of phobic reactions.

**This syndrome includes the following three subcomponents: Rape-Trauma, Compound Reaction, and Silent Reaction. In this text each appears as a separate diagnosis.

REFERENCES

Hurley, M.E.: Classification of nursing diagnoses: proceedings of the sixth conference, St. Louis, 1986, The C.V. Mosby Co.

Kim, M.J., McFarland, G.K., and McLane, A.M., editors: Classification of nursing diagnoses: proceedings of the fifth national conference, St. Louis, 1984, The C.V. Mosby Co.

Kim, M.J., McFarland, G.K., and McLane, A.M., editors: Pocket guide to nursing diagnoses, St. Louis, 1984, The C.V. Mosby Co.

Kim, M.J., and Moritz, D.A., editors: Classification of nusing diagnoses: proceedings of the third and fourth national conferences, New York, 1982, McGraw-Hill Book Co.

Nanda business meeting

Report of the President

The North American Nursing Diagnosis Association, Inc., is an organization of professional nurses whose purpose, according to Association Bylaws, is to develop, refine, and promote a taxonomy of nursing diagnostic terminology of general use to professional nurses. During the past biennium, the Association has made significant progress in each of these areas. This was possible because of the voluntary work of the Officers, Directors, committee members, and all who have contributed to the work of the Association. The Executive Director, Karen Murphy, and her staff are to be commended for their interest and commitment to the organization and the NANDA Office.

The Officers and Directors extended their appreciation to Ann Becker (Missouri) and Mary Hurley (New Jersey), whose terms as Directors expired in 1985. Newly elected Directors, Lynda Juall Carpenito (New Jersey) and Mi Ja Kim (Illinois), were welcomed.

Acting on behalf of the membership, the Officers and Directors in their four meetings during the biennium accomplished a significant amount of work associated with NANDA's purposes and organization. This report addresses their actions and deliberations.

FIVE-YEAR GOALS FOR THE ASSOCIATION

Officers and Directors established five-year goals for the association. These were published in the newsletter and are reported in the Ad Hoc Master Planning Committee Report. Committees will develop yearly plans related to these goals.

Membership in the Association

The Association has nearly doubled its membership during 1984–86. Currently, there are 1200 members and 9 associate members.

Incorporation of the Association

Incorporation of the North American Nursing Diagnosis Association under the tax code 501(c) 6 was attained on February 28, 1985. As required by the provisions of this tax classification, previous financial ties to St. Louis University were terminated. Details of incorporation are included in the Treasurer's Report.

Bylaws of the Association

The Officers and Directors proposed changes in the bylaws which were submitted to the General Assembly of the Members in March 1986. Proposed changes are in areas required for incorporation, dues, financial administration, officers and duties, nominating committee, and regional affairs.

Yearly audit of the Association

The Officers and Directors approved a yearly audit of NANDA financial accounts in May 1985 (see Treasurer's Report).

Fiscal year of the Association

The Officers and Directors approved July 1–June 30 as the fiscal year for the Association.

NANDA office location

An invitation from Sigma Theta Tau to relocate the NANDA office at a Center for Nursing in Indiana was declined. The NANDA office will remain at St. Louis University School of Nursing, and NANDA will donate funds to an endowed scholarship fund established at the School.

NANDA scholarship

With incorporation, NANDA established new relationships with St. Louis University. The School of Nursing will continue to provide space for the NANDA office. Beginning in fiscal year 1986, NANDA will donate $1500 to a NANDA Endowed Scholarship Fund that will establish a scholarship to be given to a senior or graduate student. In 1985 a one-time, $5000 donation to the Fund was made in recognition of the previous assistance St. Louis University has provided to the Association. A letter of appreciation for the contributions of St. Louis University School of Nursing since 1972 was sent to Dean Joan Hrubetz.

NANDA archives

Archivists are being consulted on organization of historical materials accumulated since 1973.

Standing committee activities and membership

The central purposes and functions of NANDA stated in the bylaws were the focus of committee activities. As may be seen in Committee Reports, significant achievements have been made. The increased interest throughout North America in use of nursing diagnoses in direct care, quality assurance, standards, computerized information systems, statistical reporting, and reimbursement has been an incentive to committee members to continue the development, refinement, and promotion of diagnostic terminology.

Committee members are appointed by the chair with approval of the President for a period of a year. This appointment is renewable each year—providing membership is renewed—with a maximum service of four years. The Officers and Directors have deliberated on methods to increase membership participation in activities of the Association. An Ad Hoc Committee was established in December 1985 to review and recommend any necessary revisions in the organizational structure of the Association, including provisions for committees and committee membership in the NANDA bylaws, policies, and procedures. Mi Ja Kim (Illinois) and Joyce Shoemaker (Alabama) are co-chairs of this committee.

Methods have been considered for disseminating information to the membership regarding activities of the Officers/Directors and Committees. In 1985, the *Newsletter* began to carry "Board Briefs," a research column will be instituted shortly by the Research Committee; and the Diagnosis Review, Taxonomy, Public Relations, and Program Committees have informed the membership about committee activities through the *Newsletter*. Other committees will be preparing items for the *Newsletter* during 1986-1988. A new format was designed for the *Newsletter* by Mary Sampel, Editor (Missouri), and many positive comments from the membership have been received.

Regional affairs

There has been widespread regional interest in nursing diagnosis, and numerous local, state, or regional groups have been formed or extended. Some groups have sought clarification of their relationship with NANDA and networks with other groups in the United States and Canada. An Ad Hoc Committee on Regional Group Relations, chaired by Laura Rossi (Massachusetts), was appointed (see Program Committee Report).

Interorganizational liaisons

NANDA continues to maintain a formal liaison with the American Nurses Association through the Cabinet on Practice. A recent letter from President Cole stated that the ANA has written to the World Health Organization indicating its willingness to "assist with the review of Chapter XVI, XVII, and XIX of the draft ICD-10 and to request consideration of an International Classification of Nursing to be included in the Family of Classifications of the tenth or future revisions of the International Classification of Diseases." The work of NANDA is cited in the letter to the World Health Organization. The NANDA President will participate in a meeting in the Spring of 1986 to (1) plan a response to the decision of WHO and (2) "decide how to coordinate this activity among the nursing communities in the United States and Canada."

As reported in the *American Nurse* (1983), the former ANA Steering Committee on Classifications for Nursing Practice Phenomena recommended policy in matters related to classification systems and maintained a collaborative relationship with NANDA. The letter to WHO is an outgrowth of the work of that committee. Dr. Virginia Saba is the ANA representative to the International Classification of Diseases (ICD-10) Revision Conference.

In response to our request, there will be a NANDA-sponsored program at the 1986 ANA Biennial Convention in Anaheim, California. The program will be June 18, from 8 to 10 am. This will be the seventh consecutive year that

NANDA has presented a program at the ANA Convention.

A liaison with the Canadian Nurses Association was sought in 1984 and is currently under study by that organization.

NANDA became a member of the Nursing Organization Liaison Forum (NOLF) in response to an invitation from ANA in 1984. This Forum provides opportunities for networking among specialty organizations. The Board declined the invitation to join the Nurses Coalition for Legislative Action because lobbying for legislation was not within the purposes and goals of NANDA. No action was taken to establish a formal liaison with specialty organizations in addition to that provided by NOLF.

International affairs

An Ad Hoc International Affairs Committee was established by the Board in May 1985. Winnifred Mills (Alberta, Canada) and Gertrude McFarland (Virginia) are co-chairs of the committee (see Committee Report).

It was not possible to present a program at the International Council of Nurses in 1985; this will be pursued for the next ICN meeting in 1989.

Theorist Group of NANDA

Sister Callista Roy, Chairperson of the Theorist Group, believes that the task of this group is completed; however, theory issues still need to be addressed by the Association. The structure of the relationship between the Theorist Group and NANDA was referred to the Taxonomy Committee.

Ad hoc master planning committee

Marjory Gordon (Massachusetts), Chairperson
Derry Ann Moritz (Connecticut), Chair, Public Relations
Joyce Shoemaker (Alabama), Chair, Nominations
Phyllis Kritek (Wisconsin), Chair, Diagnosis Review and Taxonomy
Lynda Carpenito (New Jersey), Chair, Membership
Gertrude McFarland (Virginia), Chair, Research
Audrey McLane (Wisconsin), Chair, Program
Winnifred Mills (Alberta, Canada), Co-Chair, Ad Hoc International
Mi Ja Kim (Illinois), Director
Kristine Gebbie (Oregon), Treasurer
Jane Lancour (Wisconsin), Secretary

The Ad Hoc Master Planning Committee was established by the President to develop goals for implementing the purposes of the Association and provide a framework for Committee activities. The committee has met twice.

A survey of Sixth Conference participants' perceptions regarding the goals of NANDA and the purposes and functions of the Association specified in the bylaws was used to generate a set of five-year goals in 1985. The following goals and subgoals for 1990 were published in the *Newsletter* for solicitation of comments from the membership:

1. Increased number of published nursing diagnoses that met NANDA's criteria (which will include reliability, validity, format, and a process and criteria for acceptance of diagnoses).
   a. To promote the validity and reliability of accepted and to-be-developed nursing diagnoses.
   b. To develop guidelines for development and refinement of nursing diagnoses.
   c. To develop criteria for acceptance of nursing diagnoses.
   d. To stimulate development of research models for clinical study of nursing diagnoses.

2. The NANDA Taxonomy (classification system) and nursing diagnoses will be accepted for common use by at least one national nursing organization or accepted by one funding organization.
   a. To increase visibility of NANDA to all major nursing organizations.
   b. To promote research that will demonstrate the utility of nursing diagnosis in practice and education.
   c. To establish collaborative relationships with other health care organizations.

3. The organizational structure of NANDA will facilitate the achievement of the organization's purpose and functions (in a timely manner).
   a. To critically evaluate committee functions/outcomes.
   b. To maintain financial reserves sufficient to support a minimum of 12 months of Association activities.
   c. To expand the budget to include funding for projects consistent with the organizations goals.
   d. To resolve the question of the relationship between NANDA and other nursing diagnosis groups.

4. The membership of NANDA will be 1500, 75 percent of whom will have attended a major NANDA conference or participated in a major activity of NANDA.

As is evident in standing committee reports, methods for attaining these goals and subgoals have begun to be implemented. The above goals will continue to be used by committee chairpersons as one focus for committee activities. Further deliberations of this committee during 1986 to 1988 will be focused on (1) methods to implement the goals through standing committee activities and (2) further consideration of the specified functions of NANDA in the bylaws: conducting conferences, publishing documents, facilitating research, and serving as an information resource.

Report of the treasurer

The Treasurer's report consists of three fiscal documents:

The audited statement for the year ended June 20, 1985

The Balance sheet for the period July 1, 1985, to December 31, 1985

The Budget for the current fiscal year July 1, 1986, to June 30, 1986

The Board will consider and adopt a budget for 1986-1987 at its March meeting. I would be pleased to answer any questions the membership may have.

NORTH AMERICAN NURSING DIAGNOSIS ASSOCIATION STATEMENT OF REVENUE, EXPENSE, AND CHANGES IN FUND BALANCE-CASH BASIS, YEAR ENDED JUNE 30, 1985*

Revenue and support

Dues	$18,280
Newsletter	3,719
Royalties	10,693
Donation	14,300
Conference	170
Interest	555
Miscellaneous	110
TOTAL REVENUE AND SUPPORT	$47,827

Expenses

Program services

Newsletter	$ 2,746
Conference	704
	$ 3,468

Board and committee expense

Board travel	$11,269
Board telephone	67

Board postage	29
Committee travel	3,452
Committee telephone	675
Committee postage	19
	$15,511

General and administrative

Salaries	$16,337
Employment taxes	1,146
Telephone	1,010
Postage	1,659
Duplicating	720
Supplies	954
Professional services	1,272
Miscellaneous office	1,446
Bank charges	99
	$24,643

Equipment purchased	$ 2,545
TOTAL EXPENSE	$46,168
EXCESS REVENUE OVER EXPENSE	$ 1,660
Fund balance, beginning of year	$22,661
Fund balance, end of year	$67,321

NORTH AMERICAN NURSING DIAGNOSIS ASSOCIATION BUDGET, 1985 to 1986

Income

Dues	$ 19,000
Newsletter	3,750
Royalties	5,000
Conference	80,000
Interest	600
Donations	5,000
Reserve	67,320
TOTAL INCOME	$180,670

Expenses

Salaries	$ 18,000
Payroll taxes	1,200

*This statement of assets and fund balance was examined in accordance with generally accepted auditing standards by Betty Sano, CPA. She found that it represents fairly the assets of NANDA and its revenue, expenses, and changes in fund balance.

Staff development	500	Conference	45,700
Telephone	1,000	Newsletter	3,400
Postage	2,000	Promotional	2,000
Miscellaneous office expense	200	Board expenses	12,000
Office supplies	800	Committee expenses	23,285
Office services (temporary secretarial)	1,000	Proceedings	6,000
MasterCard/Visa	1,000	Research grants	750
Legal and accounting	1,200	TOTAL EXPENSES	$122,885
Computer center	850	EXPECTED END-OF-YEAR BALANCE	$ 57,735
Equipment	500		

Executive director's report

MEMBERSHIP ADMINISTRATION

The North American Nursing Diagnosis Association has grown from approximately 700 members in 1984, to over 1200 in 1986. Additionally, we have over 700 nonmember subscribers to the *Nursing Diagnosis Newsletter*, which is published quarterly.

The "What Is NANDA?" brochure, developed by the Public Relations and Membership Committees, and the promotional poster have been distributed to 40 groups for exhibit at local nursing diagnosis programs in 1985-1986.

The Membership Application was revised, and now includes a nursing diagnosis activity and interest survey. We have made the membership mailing list available to seven persons or companies whose purpose was related to promoting nursing or nursing diagnosis.

A logo for NANDA was designed shortly after the 1984 conference, and the *Newsletter* design was upgraded wih the Winter '85 edition. The *Newsletter* was made a membership benefit beginning in 1985. Its scope and volume have grown considerably since the last conference; and new feature columns are planned, including a Research Column, and listing New Diagnoses under consideration by the Diagnosis Review Committee.

EQUIPMENT

The membership and subscription lists are maintained on NANDA's computer, which has access to the St. Louis University VAX System. This system was selected because we are able to maintain our own personal computer (a Digital Rainbow 100+), and we added a line to the VAX to increase memory capacity. Some records are maintained, and word processing is done on the Executive Director's IBM PC.

PERSONNEL

NANDA has two parttime employees. The secretary and executive director each work an average of 20 hours per week, varying from less than 10 to more than 40 hours a week, depending on the work load. Temporary secretarial assistance is hired on occasion. Demands of the growing Association may require expanding the personnel in the near future.

FINANCIAL ADMINISTRATION

Upon advice of the Board, and with the assistance of a lawyer and CPA, NANDA incorporated and became financially independent. Money reserves from the St. Louis University account were transferred to an interest-bearing checking account and a Certificate of Deposit. The CPA has set up a bookkeeping system consistent with the standards of accounting procedure. Our accounts were audited and found to be in good order.

Program committee report

Audrey M. McLane, Wisconsin, Chairperson
Ann Becker, Missouri
Mi Ja Kim, Illinois
Mary Ann Kelly, South Carolina
Laura Rossi, Massachusetts

There were two Program Committee meetings to plan the Seventh National Conference. In addition, a joint committee composed of members of the Program and Research Committees, Audrey McLane, Mi Ja Kim, and Gertrude McFarland, met to make the final selections of abstracts for the conference.

One hundred and thirty abstracts were submitted for the scientific sessions. Each abstract was sent to three doctorally prepared NANDA members for blind review. With one exception, the reviewers were nonboard members. The final blind review and the selection of abstracts for paper or poster sessions were done by the joint committee.

Mary Ann Kelly assumed the responsibility for planning the meetings of the Special Interest Groups held in conjunction with the Seventh Conference. Laura Rossi assumed the responsibility for planning the Regional Group Meetings held in conjunction with the conference.

REGIONAL GROUP RELATIONS (AD HOC COMMITTEE)

An Ad Hoc Committee on Regional Group Relations was established at the direction of the Board. Laura Rossi, Boston, Massachusetts, served as chairperson and Audrey M. McLane, Milwaukee, Wisconsin, served as the Board representative. Two additional members, Peggy McComb, Portland, Oregon, and Linda Cooper, Toronto, Ontario, were appointed by the chairperson.

The committee met and made the following recommendations to the Board:

1. Identify existing regional groups and geographical areas served.
2. Develop criteria to differentiate local and regional groups.
3. Establish guidelines for local group formation including resources.
4. Plan programs for Regional Group leaders at biennial conferences.
5. Develop a mechanism for registering groups within NANDA.

In addition, the committee developed the following:

1. Definition, purpose, and functions of regional groups.
2. Definition, purpose, and functions of local groups.
3. A list of suggestions for local groups in formation stages.

REGIONAL AFFAIRS COMMITTEE

At its December meeting, the Board of Directors authorized continuation of the Ad Hoc Committee on Regional Groups and recommended a bylaws change to establish a standing committee on Regional Affairs. The ad hoc committee will meet just prior to the Seventh Conference on March 7, 1986.

Publications committee report

Kristine M. Gebbie, Oregon, Chairperson
Mary Hurley, New Jersey
Dorothy Jones, Massachusetts
Mary Sampel, Missouri
Joyce Shoemaker, Alabama

Since the last General Assembly, the Publications Committee has done work in three areas:

1. Proceedings

   The proceedings of the sixth Conference on Classification of Nursing Diagnosis, edited by Mary Hurley and published by The C.V. Mosby Company, are just now reaching print. The Committee is committed to shortening the time between conference and publication data as much as possible. The process of selection of editor and publisher has become more formalized. The policy of the Committee, confirmed by the Board, is to minimize the addition of specially prepared materials, and emphasize advance preparation of manuscripts whenever possible.

2. Newsletter

   Mary Sampel has continued to edit the NANDA *Newsletter*, which is now in a new, more formal layout. The committee has provided guidance on policies regarding reports of articles and books, announcements of programs, and letters to the editor. The Committee is pleased with the progress of the newsletter.

3. Journal

   The Committee has explored the possibility of a commercially published journal devoted to nursing diagnosis and related topics. While the decision to date has been that we are not ready for such a move, it seems timely to take the necessary first steps, such as potential readership survey. After discussions with several interested publishers, it is the decision of the Committee, confirmed by the Board, to conduct this survey independently. Results will be reviewed carefully prior to proceeding with a publisher or deciding to put such a journal on hold for the time being.

The NANDA Publications Committee has enjoyed the opportunity to serve NANDA members in the past two years, and members would be happy to meet with any interested persons to discuss committee activities in greater detail.

Public relations committee report

Derry Ann Moritz, Connecticut, Chairperson
Carol Baer, Massachusetts
Kristine Gebbie, Oregon
Barbara McGuire, British Columbia
Dee-J Putzier, Oregon
Marylouise Welch, Connecticut

Corresponding members:
Joseph Burley, Mississippi
Vickie Chambers, New York
Marie Price, Ontario
Constance Welzel, New York
Jackie Wylie, Michigan

Advisor: Joanne Bennett, New York

Committee activities were primarily conducted via seven conference calls and liaison telephone conference or travel.

Target journals and organizations for PR efforts were explored. Journals in Canada and the United States have been identified, and restricted numbers have been selected for advertising (owing to cost). Press releases regarding the Seventh Conference were and will be sent to numerous journals and organizations. It is planned that the many specialty groups currently represented in NANDA be contacted as sources for PR. A Speakers' Guide and Information Sheet are available to enhance PR efforts.

Promotion of NANDA at local, state, regional, and national conferences via posters and brochures has occurred. Forty "PR Packets" have been requested for display, and many are used at several programs.

Forwarding of press releases to specialty organizations and journals has occurred in order to promote the conference activities. Some regional groups or specialties have secured their own press coverage. It has evolved that the function of this committee relates to mass coverage for NANDA events such as the biennial conference, proceedings publication, and organizational changes.

Although comprehensive data have not been compiled, impressions are that the greatest yield of new members and conference participants comes via the *Newsletter*, word of mouth, and local conference attendance.

The intent to have materials on NANDA in each formally organized nursing group by October 1985 was partially achieved. Specialty groups and state organizations have been contacted about the availability of NANDA materials, and asked to notify headquarters when they wish to receive such materials. This allows organizations to determine receipt of materials at their own discretion.

A logo was approved by the Board April 1985 and was professionally reproduced immediately thereafter. Theme colors of burgundy on grey for promotional materials was selected by the PR Committee and endorsed by the Board.

On-going effort to accomplish news coverage beyond the nursing media has resulted in initial prospects of interest from one medical journal.

Liaison members were established between the PR Committee and Membership (Dee-J Putzier), Program (JoAnne Bennett), and Publications (Kristine Gebbie). These liaisons serve to avoid duplication of activities and to provide PR support.

GOALS FOR 1986-1988

Support for Program Committee via:
Preparation of press packet
Securing of news media coverage of conference and speakers
Covering (for news releases):
Program content, Awards, SIG's and Regional Group Meetings, Business Meeting, Paper and Poster Presentations

LONG-TERM GOALS

Collaborate with Publications Committee in 1986 Proceedings publicity.

Reinstitute efforts to articulate with other health professionals regarding nursing diagnosis and NANDA.

Promote nursing diagnosis in lay publications and nonnursing health publications.

Encourage members of NANDA to submit possible articles of interest to the lay public to PR Committee (with Publications Committee) for editorial assistance.

Increase membership involvement in PR goal achievement via:

1. Developing a mechanism whereby NANDA members with expertise and membership in specialty organizations can serve as links to those organizations.
2. Developing a mechanism for earmarking conference which NANDA members may be attending (e.g., via work with data from membership) to request NANDA publicity.
3. Sending annual reminder to specialty and state/regional organizations of NANDA's available materials.

Research committee report

Gertrude K. McFarland, Virginia, Chairperson
Betty Chang, California
Phyllis Jones, Ontario
Mi Ja Kim, Illinois
Joanne McCloskey, Iowa
Elizabeth McFarlane, District of Columbia

Some new members have been added to our Research Committee since the last National Conference. The Committee has conducted its business by correspondence, telephone, and meetings held during the last National Conference, during the interim in Chicago, and prior to and during the Seventh Conference.

The Committee has developed and revised goals and implemented an Action Plan. The following have been accomplished:

Participated in the final selection process for research papers and poster presentations for the Seventh Conference.

Planned and initiated news items and a Research Column for the *Newsletter*. The first Research Column has been developed for the Spring 1986 edition.

Is planning to submit an abstract to the ANA Council of Nurse Researchers.

Developed, for Board action, comprehensive application review and selection process for nursing diagnosis research proposals submitted to NANDA for funding. The purpose of these grants is to provide seed money for research endeavors concerning nursing diagnosis.

Developed and proposed, for Board action, plans for an international conference designed to promote nursing diagnosis research by developing useful research methodologies and models.

Diagnosis review committee report

Phyllis Kritek, Wisconsin, Chairperson
Lynda Juall Carpenito, New Jersey
Cynthia Dougherty, Washington
Kristine Gebbie, Oregon
Dorothea Fox Jakob, Ontario
Julie Rovtar Marshall, Illinois
Derry Ann Moritz, Connecticut
Maureen Shekleton, Illinois

1. The Diagnosis Review Committee (DRC) conducted extensive business since the Sixth Conference, through mail communication and review, four conference call meetings, and one 2-day in-person meeting.
2. The DRC completed all tasks proposed at the Sixth National Conference, utilizing the assumptions reported to and accepted by the General Assembly at that time.
3. The following tasks and activities were completed:
   a. Development, review, revision, approval, and dissemination of
      1. "Development/Submission Guidelines for Proposed New Nursing, Diagnoses"
      2. "Diagnosis Review Cycle" description and policies
      3. Diagnosis Proposal and Evaluation formats and forms
      4. Publication policy statements and protocols, with consent forms
      5. Review process sequences: Appropriate protocols, record keeping documents, and policies
      6. Calls for and application mechanisms for Clinical/Technical Review Task Force members
      7. Newsletter utilization procedures for DRC
   b. The first formal revue cycle of NANDA was initiated and completed to the point of General Assembly review and comment.
      1. Policies and procedures for all stages of cycle review were developed and to the degree feasible, implemented
      2. From prior submissions to NANDA that predated these policies and protocols, those submissions that met minimal guidelines for review of proposed *new* diagnosis were selected for the first review cycle
      3. Fifty-seven proposals were "grandfathered" through the first review cycle in this fashion
      4. DRC members served as primary reviewers, five Clinical/Technical Review Task Force members were selected for each diagnosis; prior volunteers were utilized
      5. Twenty-two proposed new diagnoses were approved for submission to the General Assembly for review and comment and NANDA membership voting
      6. Conceptually overlapping proposed diagnoses were, to the degree possible, reviewed by the same persons
      7. All stages of the process were evaluated for problems and, where possible, corrected.
   c. The second formal review cycle of NANDA was initiated
      1. As of January 1, 1986, all proposed new diagnoses were included in this new review cycle
      2. The policies, procedures, and protocols developed based on cycle I evaluation were implemented
      3. Improved Clinical/Technical Review Task Force membership procedures were developed and implemented
      4. Mechanisms to facilitate coordination between DRC and the Central Office were created and implemented, including coding, mailing, documentation, and fiscal accountability mechanisms
      5. Additional developmental needs in terms of the review process were identified and efforts at solutions initiated.
   d. A DRC budget was developed and submitted to the NANDA Board
   e. A review of previously approved

NANDA diagnoses was conducted to determine their incongruence with new policies and procedures; a proposed minimum refinement of prior work to facilitate subsequent refinement was proposed for General Assembly review and comment. Minimum refinement involves acceptance of definitions of all extant diagnoses to assure a common starting point for further developments.

4. DRC will address the following future activities:
   a. Clarification of interface with the Taxonomy Committee
   b. Further review and refinement of DRC policies and procedures
   c. The creation of Special Task Forces to deal with specific problems generic to the diagnosis development process, such as diagnoses that appear to overlap with medical diagnoses
   d. Diagnoses revision procedures.

Taxonomy committee report

Phyllis B. Kritek, Wisconsin, Chairperson
Susan Fowler, Wisconsin
Lois Hoskins, District of Columbia
Mary Hurley, New Jersey
Mary Kerr, Pennsylvania
Winnifred Mills, Alberta
Barbara Rottkamp, New York
Judy Warren, South Carolina

1. The Taxonomy Committee (TC) conducted its business since the Sixth Conference through mail communications and two conference call meetings.
2. The TC completed all tasks proposed at the Sixth National Conference, utilizing the assumptions reported to and accepted by the General Assembly at that time.
3. The following tasks and activities were completed:
   a. TC review of taxonomy work to date, including previous conference work on taxonomies, Theorist Group work, the Fifth Conference Taxonomy Group work, extant published literature, the ANA Classification Group work, and the current NANDA alphabetic list, including its advantages and disadvantages.
   b. TC recommendation to NANDA Board that the initial taxonomy developed by the Fifth Conference Taxonomy Group be reviewed, critiqued, revised, and forwarded to the Board and General Assembly as the official NANDA Taxonomy.
   c. Solicitation of review and critique of the proposed taxonomy by several groups: Fifth Conference Taxonomy Group, Sixth Conference Taxonomy Volunteers, NANDA Board, and TC.
   d. Content analysis of critique and review responses; incorporation of majority report recommendations into a revised taxonomy.
   e. Preparation of revised taxonomy for Board and General Assembly review and action; delineation of procedures for same.
4. A TC budget was developed and submitted to the NANDA Board.
5. TC will address the following future activities:
   a. Clarification of interface with Diagnosis Review Committee.
   b. Development of a possible consensus conference to refine the first taxonomy (if approved) to be presented at the Eighth Conference as the second taxonomy.
   c. Development of guidelines for on-going taxonomy revisions.
   d. Further refinement of nature and policies of taxonomy committee.
   e. Develop improved publicity mechanisms for the taxonomy.
   f. Devise mechanism to work more collaboratively with other groups developing classification schemata.
6. *Recommendation:* The Taxonomy Committee recommends that the General Assembly, by a positive vote, indicate endorsement of the NANDA Nursing Diagnosis Taxonomy I as presented and discussed at this Conference during Taxonomy Sessions I and II.

Membership committee report

Lynda Juall Carpenito, New Jersey,
 Chairperson
Winnifred Mills, Alberta, Canada
Peggy McComb, Oregon
Mary Lee Kirkland, South Carolina
Christine Miaskowski, New York
Andrea Bircher, Oklahoma

As the newly appointed chairperson (December 1985), I will convene a meeting of this committee at the Seventh National Conference to establish goals.

ACTIVITIES TO DATE

1. 1200+ members as of December 1985.
2. The *Newsletter* subscription is now included in the membership fee.
3. The membership registration information has been updated and is retrievable from the computer.

GOAL

To explore mechanisms for increasing membership throughout North America.

MECHANISM TO ACHIEVE GOAL

1. Establish a liaison for membership in each regional group.
2. Provide regional groups with material for potential members, e.g., the *Newsletter*.
3. Produce overhead transparencies which could be loaned or sold (at cost) to groups to share information about NANDA in their regions.

Ad Hoc Committee on International Affairs

Gertrude K. McFarland, Co-chairperson,
  Maryland
Winnifred Mills, Co-chairperson, Alberta,
  Canada
Josephine Flaherty, Ontario, Canada
Helen Glass, Manitoba
Virginia Saba, District of Columbia
Karin von Schilling, Ontario, Canada

Subcommittee Members:
Jeanette Clough, Massachusetts
Beatrice Turkoski, Wisconsin

The Ad Hoc Committee on International Relations was established following NANDA Board discussions in 1984. Two board members, Gertrude McFarland and Winnifred Mills, agreed to be co-chairs of the committee. Goals were presented to the board in May 1985, and include outreach, first to other English-speaking countries and then elsewhere in the world. Since that time, contact lists (outside North America) have been developed, and additional members were added to the committee. Liaison has been established with the European Region of WHO, and letters introducing NANDA will be sent to specific contact persons in Australia, New Zealand, and the members of ICN. We are aware that one nursing diagnosis handbook has been translated into French, and we anticipate additional translations of nursing diagnosis information into other languages in the future.

At the March 8, 1986, Board meeting, the following motion was carried and now comes before the General Assembly:

That the board bring to the General Assembly the following motion: that over the next two years NANDA explore the implications of establishing formal international status including budgetary implications, name change, and other relevant issues with the possibility of a bylaws change at the next general assembly.

Approved motions from NANDA General Assembly, Seventh National Conference, 1986

Motion 1

Moved acceptance of Treasurer's report.

Motion 2

Moved acceptance of Program Committee report.

Motion 3

Moved acceptance of Publication Committee report.

Motion 4

Moved acceptance of Public Relations report.

Motion 5

Moved acceptance of Research Committee report.

Motion 6

Moved acceptance of Diagnosis Review Committee report.

Motion 7

Moved that the General Assembly, by a positive Vote, indicate endorsement of the NANDA Taxonomy I as distributed at the Seventh NANDA Conference.

Motion 8

Moved that the Taxonomy Committee take under consideration the recommendations, discussion, and suggestions made by participants of the Seventh NANDA Conference during Taxonomy Session I and II and the Taxonomy Special Interest Group Meeting and use these in its development of NANDA Taxonomy II. 2nd.

Amendment to the motion

Moved to insert "written recommendations by members sent to the Taxonomy Committee" between the words "Special Interest Group Meeting" and the word "and."

Motion 9

Moved to accept the report of the Ad Hoc Committee on Regional Affairs.

Motion 10

Moved to accept the report of the Ad Hoc Committee on International Affairs.

Motion 11

Moved that over the next two years, NANDA explore the implications of establishing formal international status, including budgetary implications, name change, and other relevant issues, with the possibility of a bylaw change at the next General Assembly.

Motion 12*

Moved adoption of the proposed Amendment I, which amends Section 3 of Article 1, the restrictions governing NANDA's tax status.

Motion 13*

Moved adoption of the second set of proposed amendments, Article III of the Bylaws.

Motion 14*

Moved adoption of the proposed amendments to Article IV, regarding the officers and duties of officers.

Motion 15*

Moved adoption of the proposed amendment to Article V, board of directors.

Motion 16*

Moved adoption of the proposed amendment to Article V, deleting Section E, the Nominations Committee.

Motion 17*

Moved adoption of the proposed amendment to Article VI by the addition of a Section H on Regional Affairs.

Motion 18*

Moved adoption of the proposed amendment to Article VII on "Elections."

Motion 19*

Moved adoption of the proposed amendment to Article IX, "Meetings." 2nd.

Amendments to the amendment

Moved to strike the word "whatever" in Article IX.

Moved to amend the amendment in Article IX, under A, "with regard to any special meeting, each director will be sent written notice at least ten days prior to the date of the meeting" should be corrected to say "each member shall be sent written notice."

---

*See Appendix H: NANDA Bylaws.

Motion 20

Moved that the General Assembly approve the Board's action to set dues at $25.00 per year, effective with the 1987 membership year.

Motion 21

Moved that the Board of Directors establish a Resolutions Committee.

Motion 22

Moved that the Taxonomy Committee present any proposed document called "NANDA Taxonomy II" that includes any revisions from NANDA Taxonomy I, and present them to the membership at least ninety days prior to the Eighth NANDA Conference in 1988; and set aside time prior to an endorsement of NANDA Taxonomy II for discussion and debate by the General Assembly. 2nd.

Amendment to the motion

Moved to strike "ninety days" and insert "thirty days."

Motion 23

Moved that NANDA go on record as supporting the concept that only registered, professional nurses be responsible and accountable for identifying the nursing diagnoses for their patient population.

Awards ceremony

TASK FORCE MEMBERS:
Ann Becker, Mary Hurley,
Joyce Shoemaker

At the Sixth Conference, NANDA recognized the contributions of several persons in the area of nursing diagnosis. At the Board meeting which followed, a motion was passed appointing a task force to explore the concept of a biennial award ceremony in conjunction with the conference. The task force looked at several issues including eligibility, criteria, identification of nominees, and process. At the May 1985 board meeting, the task force recommended that the board establish an Awards Committee. This proposal was accepted.

The task force made recommendations on several issues as part of the proposal. Four awards categories were explored and three were recommended. To briefly define the specific categories, lifetime membership will be given to each President at the end of her/his term of office. There is an Honorary membership category for persons actively involved in nursing diagnosis and/or the goals and objectives of the Association but who cannot, for whatever reason, fulfill the requirements for membership. Unique Contribution is the name of the third category and is purposely general. It is expected to be the most frequent award distributed. As the criteria for this category are developed and refined, the membership will be provided with the mechanism by which to gain recognition for their achievements. It would be difficult and unwielding to have many specific categories, and the task force believes that criteria for the category, Unique Contribution, can be developed and applied fairly while judging a wide variety of activities. A fourth category, Board Member Service Award, was not recommended because it was felt that a significant contribution on the board could be recognized through one of the other categories.

At present, we have identified two mechanisms for nominating candidates. The first is board recommendation and the second is membership recommendations through the *Newsletter*.

The Award Ceremony at this Seventh Conference was held in conjunction with a dinner and the keynote address on the first evening of the conference. Eleanor Borkowski, M. Lucy Feild, and Audrey M. McLane received Unique Contribution Awards, and Karen Murphy received an Honorary Membership Award. To honor these individuals, each received a plaque with the name of the award, the person's name, and the year. In addition, each person will have her name placed on a plaque that remains in the NANDA office.

AWARD FOR UNIQUE CONTRIBUTION TO THE ADVANCEMENT OF NURSING DIAGNOSIS ELEANOR BORKOWSKI

Eleanor Borkowski has demonstrated the unique ability to identify a very special need and then to organize the resources to meet that need. She has been employed at San Bernadino County Medical Center in California since September 1979. During that time, she has advanced from Assistant Director of Education to Director of Education, and to her current position as Assistant Director of Nurses. In each of these roles, she has maintained awareness of the need for nursing diagnosis in clinical practice, and she has provided the necessary peer support for implementing nursing diagnosis in her agency.

As an active member of the North American Nursing Diagnosis Association, Eleanor has been committed to the concept of Regional Organization so that nurses in all areas and levels of practice can share in the work of our group. In line with this belief, she was instrumental in the creation of the Southern California Nursing Diagnosis Association. As its first president, she used her organizational skills to build membership to more than 400 in the first year and to more than 500 after one and a half years. Her creative leadership also facilitated the development of a traveling education program on nursing diagnosis. This program is an 8-hour workshop aimed at the instruction of staff nurses—consistent with Eleanor's belief that the staff nurse level is critical to the implementation of nursing diagnosis in clinical practice. The program is currently being marketed to health care institutions.

As a leading force in Southern California, Eleanor has enriched the quality of nursing practice in her state and she has contributed uniquely to the goals of our organization. It is an honor to present her with this award this evening.

AWARD FOR UNIQUE CONTRIBUTIONS TO THE ADVANCEMENT OF NURSING DIAGNOSIS M. LUCY FEILD

Lucy Feild has contributed to the advancement of nursing diagnosis for a number of years, and she is well known regionally and nationally for her efforts. She has provided leadership in the Massachusetts Conference Group for the Classification of Nursing Diagnoses since 1976. In her role as Assistant Professor of Nursing at Boston University during the years 1978-1981, she influenced curriculum change to incorporate the use of the clinical judgment process and the application of nursing diagnosis in complex patient care situations. In her current position as a clinical nurse specialist at Brigham and Women's Hospital in Boston, she has chaired the Nursing Process Task Force that has developed and implemented a plan for a hospitalwide clinical decision-making course. She is the recipient of a professional recognition Award for Excellence in Nursing Practice at Peter Bent Brigham Hospital in 1979; and an award from the Massachusetts Nurses' Association in 1980 in Recognition of Service that contributed to the improvement of nursing practice.

Lucy has presented more than sixty papers and workshops on the topic of nursing diagnosis throughout the United States, and she is credited with a number of publications on nursing diagnosis. As a member of the ANA Council of Medical-Surgical Nursing Practice, she co-authored a widely acclaimed position paper that compares the ANA Standards of Practice with the Social Policy Statement and proposed dynamic revolutionary changes in education and practice reflecting the pivotal role of nursing diagnosis.

As a teacher, clinician, and scholar, Lucy Feild has represented nursing in the best possible manner, and she has provided leadership consistent with the goals of our organization. It is an honor to present her with this award.

AWARD FOR UNIQUE CONTRIBUTION TO NURSING DIAGNOSIS DR. AUDREY M. McLANE

Dr. Audrey M. McLane has been an active and influential force in the national effort to promote the classification of nursing diagnoses since the 1970s. She was a member of the Task Force of the National Group on Classification of Nursing Diagnoses from 1978 to 1983. When the initial NANDA elections were held, she was elected to the Board of Directors, an office she continues to hold. In addition to her many board responsibilities, she has chaired the Program Committee and coordinated the highly successful Sixth and Seventh Conferences.

Dr. McLane has presented papers at the last three conferences, and she has served as co-editor of the Proceedings of the Fifth Conference. She also co-edited the *Pocket Guide to Nursing Diagnoses*, which received the American Journal of Nursing Book of the Year Award. She has authored papers in Mosby's reference, *Clinical Nursing*, and in the *Nursing Clinics of North America*. She has presented papers related to nursing diagnosis at the ANA Convention, the AACN National Teaching Institute, and the Midwest Nursing Research Society. Her research interests have focused on clinical testing of diagnoses as well as on the implementation and utilization of nursing diagnoses.

In addition to her national activities, Dr. McLane has been involved in activities related to nursing diagnosis in regional and local professional organizations. She is an active member of the Wisconsin Nurses's Association and has been a member of the Steering Committee of its Nursing Diagnosis Interest Group. She has also been a Convenor (1981-1984) of the Nursing Diagnosis Research Group of the Midwest Nursing Research Society, and she holds membership on the Steering Committee of the Midwest Nursing Diagnosis Task Force.

Clearly, Dr. McLane's commitment to nursing diagnosis has pervaded all aspects of her professional life. Through her local, regional, and national activities, she has been a vital force in bringing us to where we are today. She is truly deserving of this award for her Unique Contribution to the work of classification of nursing diagnoses.

HONORARY MEMBERSHIP AWARD
KAREN K. MURPHY

Karen Murphy became involved in the activities of our organization at about the time planning for the Third National Conference on Classification of Nursing Diagnoses had begun. For that conference and for all the succeeding ones, Karen has been responsible for the administrative functions entailed in making our conferences the smashing successes they have been. Because of her creativity, ability to coordinate, and attention to detail, we are gathered together for another successful happening—our Seventh Conference.

With the establishment of the North American Nursing Diagnosis Association in 1983, the Board of Directors identified a need for an Executive Director. Karen was the person chosen to fill that position because of the several years of invaluable assistance she has provided to us prior to the formalization of our organization. Since her appointment, she has facilitated the incorporation of our Association. She has also paid our bills, monitored our budget, handled our correspondence, managed our telephones, fielded our inquiries, made travel and hotel arrangements for board and committee meetings, arranged conference calls, computerized our membership list, negotiated with publishers, handled election ballots, staffed the board meetings, and facilitated the work of our committees. She has also been our chief worrier as we have experienced our growing pains!

Karen is not a nurse and therefore is not eligible for regular membership. Without her, however, NANDA, would not be where it is today. So it is fitting that she be awarded this Honorary Membership this evening.

Appendix D **Summary and future directions**

AUDREY M. McLANE, Ph.D., R.N.

One of the most interesting and exciting facets of the Seventh Conference on Classification of Nursing Diagnoses was the realization by the 615 participants that they were creating nursing history. Each conference has been an historical event but the Seventh was marked by a sense of anticipation as well. That is to say, not only nursing's history, but also one of many alternative futures for nursing was in the making. With this in mind, then, it is important that any attempt to summarize and suggest future directions from the Seventh Conference be done in such a manner as to demonstrate the continuity of these proceedings with earlier conferences.

The number of research papers presented at each biennial conference has increased substantially. In the summary of the proceedings of the Third and Fourth Conference, Mi Ja Kim (1982) acknowledged the inclusion of 10 research papers from the two conferences. A total of 25 research papers were presented at the Fifth Conference (Kim, McFarland, and McLane, 1984). These included 11 papers from the scientific sessions, 3 papers presented to groups working on specific diagnosis, and 11 research poster presentations. Forty research papers were included in the proceedings of the Sixth Conference, as were 22 paper and 18 poster presentations (Hurley, 1986). During the Seventh Conference, 74 research reports were presented, in addition to 16 papers and 58 poster presentations. Manuscripts from 47 of the presentations and abstracts from the remaining 27 are included in these proceedings. The increase in quantity of papers has been accompanied by a concomitant improvement in the quality of research. However, the need for more research models for validating nursing diagnoses was expressed repeatedly by participants. The picture that emerges is one of a continuing evolution of the scientific bases for the approved diagnoses and gradual attainment of some of the goals envisioned by members of the original National Task Force on Classification of Nursing Diagnoses.

The relationship of the work of the Nurse Theorists to the activities of biennial conferences has been of continuing interest. In the proceedings of the Third and Fourth conferences, Kim elaborated on the dynamic relationship between the National Group (now known as NANDA) and the Nurse Theorists as they began their work to elicit an organizing principle for a taxonomy from the approved diagnoses. While the complexity of this endeavor created concern among the members, Kim was very optimistic about the future and expressed confidence in the leaderhip of the Nurse Theorist Group under Sister Callista Roy. Kim said: "We trust her leaderhip in this key position will bring the success of achieving the original goal" (Kim, 1982, p. 381). During this conference, participants have seen the achievement of the goal initiated by the Nurse Theorists and brought to fruition by the Taxonomy Committee under the direction of Phyllis Kritek. The endorsement of the Human Response Patterns as the organizing framework for NANDA's Taxonomy was truly an historic moment in the life of this organization. The members of the Board of Directors, the Taxonomy Committee, and the Program Committee made every effort to provide a program that not only permitted but required an examination and critique of the pertinent issues involved in endorsing a taxonomy. Two taxonomy information sessions and the business meeting provided opportunities for discussion and debate of the proposed taxonomy. A careful examination of the invited papers and the committee reports provides additional evidence of the care taken to assure that the General Assembly was fully informed prior to a vote to endorse NANDA Taxonomy I.

The papers presented by invited speakers Myrtle Aydelotte, Margaret Newman, Myra Levine, and Marjory Gordon represent not just papers conceived and developed for this conference, but the culmination of years of creative and critical thinking and integration of their ideas with the work and goals of NANDA. These papers influenced the participants' thinking during the conference by raising specific questions about nursing's theoretical orientation, by heightening their awareness of the many unresolved issues in creating taxonomies, and by delineating some of the unresolved issues in diagnostic development and validation.

Margaret Newman, whose contributions to the earlier work of the Nurse Theorists were substantial, emphasized the crucial importance of identifying sequential patterns that evolve over time. She sees nursing at the forefront of pattern recognition and suggests that the key to nursing diagnosis is not outside ourselves (about the client) but is rather to be found in information "continuously available to us within our pattern of interaction with the client" (Newman, 1986). Like the initial report of the Nurse Theorists, the full impact of Newman's conceptualizations on the work of NANDA will be known only *a posteriori.*

The critique by Myra Levine of the term, human response, the human response patterns, and the words used to label diagnoses was incisive. She expressed concern about the philosophical issues "hidden in the jargon" of human responses. She called for a moratorium on the acceptance of diagnostic labels and urged nurses at local meetings to use the processes adopted by participants at the First and Second Conferences "to develop a true taxonomy of nursing" (Levine, 1986). The process relies on nurses' recalling signs and symptoms of patient problems, a form of consensual validity. Gordon pointed out that the majority of the current diagnostic categories were developed in that way.

Some issues currently under discussion in nursing diagnosis were reviewed by Marjory Gordon. Two neglected areas of research, reliability of defining characteristics and epidemiologic studies, were viewed as critical. She expressed the need for explicit guidelines for using qualitative and quantitative research methods to stimulate clinical research. The consolidation of the work on classification by various groups was also seen as necessary for comparisons across settings.

Myrtle Aydelotte's appraisal of the state of the art of nursing taxonomies appeared harsh (her words), but the questions she raised demonstrated a real optimism about the future of nursing diagnosis. For example, she expressed concern

that "who is qualified to diagnose" was not discussed in the literature. This issue has been debated rather heatedly at local, state, and regional conferences. Perhaps a national debate is needed. The other question raised by Aydelotte—When will the work of NANDA be officially endorsed and legitimized by the American Nurses' Association (ANA)—requires continuation and further development of the on-going collaboration between NANDA and ANA.

Discussion and debate about individual diagnoses at biennial conferences has always served as a magnet to bring together that critical mass of clinicians, theorists, and researchers so necessary for progress in a discipline. Consideration of individual diagnoses was absent from the Sixth Conference as the Diagnostic Review Committee worked out policies and procedures for submission, technical review, general assembly reveiew, and voting by the membership. Nine new diagnoses were approved at the Fifth National Conference for clinical testing and use. Participants in the Seventh Conference had the first opportunity, as members of the General Assembly, to be part of a new review process adopted in the NANDA Bylaws. Review and comment by the General Assembly represent one step in the multilevel refinement and review process that influences the profession at large to "take seriously" the work of NANDA. This detailed process will certainly undergo some refinements as NANDA pursues its goals. However, it is important at this time to acknowledge the contribution of the Diagnostic Review Committee under the leadership of Phyllis Kritek for developing the basic structure for the activity that represents the central focus of this organization.

The papers presented by Joyce Fitzpatrick and Anayis Derdiarian on the question of etiology can also be viewed in an historical context. In a review of the literature included in the proceedings of the Fifth Conference, McLane and Fehring (1984) pointed out that the importance of locating probable cause(s), etiologies, has been a recurring theme in the literature of nursing diagnoses. Etiological concerns have been expressed at every conference despite the wide acceptance of the PES format (Problem, Etiology, Signs/Symptoms) suggested by Gordon. In a paper at the Fifth National Conference, Garyfallia Forsyth phrased it well when she said that etiology was one of the "troublesome issues." She developed a fine presentation of the historic and philosophic evolution of scientific theory, and presented a conceptualization of etiology with its value implications to nursing science. Joyce Fitzpatrick's paper, presented at this conference, is a further elucidation of the complex conceptual concerns underlying the notion of etiology—and, of course, eventually the broader notion of causality. Anayis Derdiarian focused on the practical relevance of etiology and emphasized the importance of gathering validating data for etiological factors as well as for defining characteristics. Both papers, Fitzpatrick's and Derdiarian's, add substantially to understanding the complexity and importance of the etiology issue—but the issue remains unresolved. As theories are proposed to explain various phenomena, and as research-based protocols are developed to test interventions for a given diagnosis at multiple sites, then new insights may be gained that will keep the issue of etiology alive for the forseeable future.

Recognition of the limitations of a medical data base for the generation of nursing diagnoses has led to a proliferation of nursing data bases and a subsequent quest for one common data base for nursing. An evening forum, with presentations by Laura Rossi and Joyce Taylor, provided opportunity for lively discussion and debate about the merits of Levine's conservation principles (Taylor) and Gordon's functional health patterns (Rossi) as frameworks for organizing data for nursing diagnoses. Many questions were raised about the compatibility of these and other nursing data bases with NANDA's human response patterns.

The systematic testing of interventions for each diagnosis that was brought to the fore in this conference by Steven Hayes has its own historical antecedents. Kim, in the proceedings of the Third Conference, recommended that research studies be conducted to "identify effective nursing therapies for each nursing diagnosis and to document the quality of nursing care" (Kim, 1982, p. 382). During the Sixth Conference, Harriet Werley, Distinguished Professor of Nursing who is recognized internationally for her contributions to nursing research, challenged the General Assembly to place more emphasis on the testing of treatments for nursing diagnoses. One poster presentation by Ellen Wilson at the Sixth Conference and one by Marlene Reimer at the Seventh could be classified as intervention papers. The excellent paper and workshop conducted by Steven Hayes at this conference should generate an exponential increase in research on specific nursing interventions. Time series designs with their underlying theme of repeated measures may have even more far-reaching effects on the quality of care, if clinicians incorporate repeated measurement as an ongoing part of nursing practice. Incorporation of continuous measurement and evaluation as essential components of practice would forever lay to rest the "cookbook—standardized care plan" approach to solving patient problems. Use of repeated measures to evaluate interventions (practice decisions) would result in patient/family records that would be gold mines for research, models for teaching, and data for assuring quality of care. Regional Nursing Diagnoses Groups could take the lead in developing and testing nursing interventions.

Kristine Gebbie addressed four questions related to fee-based reimbursement for nursing diagnoses: Why hasn't it happened; why is the system sought; what is the potential for political support; and what are the prerequisites? Gebbie's responses to these questions were unexpected and unique. They represent the kind of practical, insightful, and forthright thinking NANDA has come to expect from a nurse who raised the initial question that led to the First National Conference on classification of nursing diagnoses (Gebbie and Lavin, 1975).

Harriet Werley brought to the Seventh Conference the product of another historic conference, the National Invitational Conference on Nursing's Minimum Data Set (NMDS). Several members of NANDA's Board and members at large were among those invited to participate in that historic conference. NMDS includes three categories: nursing care, demographics, and service elements. Since nursing diagnosis is one of the four elements in the category of nursing care, Werley emphasized the importance of continued support for the nursing diagnosis movement (including the testing of interventions); promotion of nursing diagnosis research programs; and inclusion of nursing in the International Classification of Diseases (ICD-10) Revision. Werley's last point is consistent with NANDA's ongoing interest in exploring existing classification systems for their compatibility with nursing diagnoses. Major nomenclatures and classification systems used by health care institutions were discussed at the Second National Conference (Gebbie, 1976, pp. 141-146).

The sheer volume of research presentations makes an adequate summary impossible. Diagnostic validation, with 7 formal paper presentations, and diagnostic reasoning, with 4 formal paper presentations, had the largest number of studies presented during the scientific sessions. Diagnostic validation had the largest total number of paper/poster presentation (N=37). Models for research in these two areas may account for the quality (number of papers in scientific sessions) and quantity (total number in a category). For example, the classic paper by Gordon and Sweeney (1979), Fehring's (1986) presentation at the Sixth Conference, and Tanner's (1982) initial presentation at the Third Conference and continuing work on diagnostic reasoning have received widespread recognition. The few studies in the other categories (described in the preface) suggest the importance of developing models for research in these areas. Additional methodologies are also needed for clinical validation and diagnostic reasoning studies, despite the apparent amount of activity in the two areas.

Future directions for nursing diagnosis and NANDA as an organization were addressed by many speakers and participants during the four-day conference. Those which seem most important include: further elaboration of the taxonomy through identification of additional human response patterns; refinement of diagnoses approved prior to formalization of the process; development of explicit guidelines for applying qualitative and quantitative methods for studying nursing diagnoses; exploration of consolidation of diagnostic classification systems; support for nursing participation in the next revision of the International Classification of Diseases; support for funding for nursing research; development of a formal relationship with regional nursing diagnosis groups; and continuation of collaboration with ANA.

The new standing committee on Regional Affairs has as its major goal the development of a formal relationship between NANDA and the Regional Groups. These groups have not been formally recognized for the tremendous contributions they make to both implementation of and research on nursing diagnoses. The groups carry on the work of the conference in the intervening 24 months, and their regional networking gives them a base for collaborative research endeavors. NANDA has great expectations for their future contributions as individuals and as groups.

A clearer vision of the possible futures for nursing diagnosis and NANDA can be gained by taking the time to study the proceedings of this conference and the other six conferences. The history of NANDA's collective and individual efforts to explicate the nature of nursing points the way to the future. There have been very clear messages in the past, and there were clearer messages at this conference about what nursing's future could be. But, it is up to each nurse to help create that future. At the Second Conference (speaking above the din of hammering in a very old hotel undergoing renovation in downtown St. Louis to a group of participants, less than one quarter the size of this group), Sr. Callista Roy stated with the clear voice of conviction and commitment that Nursing Diagnoses tells the world who we are, what we do, and how we relate to others. There is no other statement, said in so few words, that communicates the importance of the work of the members of NANDA and the general assembly at the biennial conferences. For many nurses, Roy's statement was and is a partial answer to a very troublesome question—what is nursing?

REFERENCES

Gebbie, K.M., editor: Summary of the Second National Conference: classification of nursing diagnoses. St. Louis, 1976, Clearinghouse, National Group for Classification of Nursing Diagnoses.

Gebbie, K.M., and Lavin, M.A., editors: Classification of nursing diagnoses: proceedings of the First National Conference, St. Louis, 1975, The C.V. Mosby Co.

Hurley, M., editor: Classification of the nursing diagnoses: proceedings of the Sixth Conference, St. Louis, 1986, The C.V. Mosby Co.

Kim, M.J., McFarland, G.K., and McLane, A.M., editors: Classification of nursing diagnoses: proceedings of the Fifth National Conference, St. Louis, 1984, The C.V. Mosby Co.

Kim, J.J., and Moritz, D.A., editors: Classification of nursing diagnoses: proceedings of the Third and Fourth National Conferences, New York, 1982, McGraw-Hill Book Co.

Regional Group meetings

Laura Rossi, Chairperson of the Ad Hoc Committee on Regional Groups, coordinated the Regional Group meetings at the Seventh Conference. The members of the Ad Hoc Committee are: Laura Rossi, chairperson (Massachusetts); Audrey M. McLane, board representative (Wisconsin); Peggy McComb (Oregon); and Linda Cooper (Ontario, Canada).

The Ad Hoc Committee on Regional Groups was charged with the responsibility of exploring issues related to the development of a structural relationship between regional groups and NANDA, and between the regional groups and local groups. A survey was mailed to the representatives from groups that were *known* to exist. There is no complete data base concerning the existence of geographic areas covered by Regional Groups.

The results of the survey revealed enthusiasm for such an effort to be undertaken, but there was caution/concern expressed about disruption of existing group structures at the local and regional levels. For these reasons, the following recommendations were made and partially undertaken at the Seventh Conference:

1. Identification of regional groups and geographic areas.
2. Distinguishing between local and regional groups.
3. Supporting the establishment of the Regional Affairs Committee as a standing committee of NANDA to: address regional issues; to promote further exploration of a regional structure; and to encourage increased communication between NANDA and the Regional Groups.

The Regional Groups met on the first day of the conference to discuss their responses to the Ad Hoc Committee Recommendations. A second meeting was held by the regional group leaders after the General Assembly approved a bylaws change to establish a standing committee on Regional Affairs. There was a consensus among the regional group leaders that a major thrust must be made in the direction of a better definition of the roles and responsibilities of the Regional Groups within NANDA.

There are an enormous number of resources and creative activities in the Regional Groups. The activities include beginning networking and implementation meetings, monthly educational meetings, and sophisticated efforts to encourage research. The Midwest Nursing Diagnosis Task Force was recognized for allocating funds for the support of nursing research. The first award will be made at its biennial conference in Spring 1987.

Eight regional groups met at the conference. The following list includes the name of each group and its chairperson.

Bay Area Nursing Diagnosis Association
Chairperson: Gail Marculescu

Southern California Nursing Diagnosis Association
Chairperson: Eleanor Borkowski

Southern Regional Nursing Diagnosis Conference Group
Chairperson: Mary Ann Kelly

Mid-Atlantic Nursing Diagnosis Group
Chairperson: Lynda Carpenito

Mid-America Regional Nursing Diagnosis Conference Group
Chairperson: Marion Resler

Massachusetts & Northeast Regional Groups
Chairpersons: Elizabeth Hiltunen
Lenore Boles
Beverly Bartlett

Midwest Nursing Diagnosis Task Force
Chairperson: Kenneth Cianfrani

Northwest Regional Nursing Diagnosis Group
Chairperson: Peggy McComb

Special Interest Group meetings

The purposes of the SIG Special Group meetings at NANDA's Seventh Conference were:

1. To share information not otherwise reported at the Conference.

   Research: Completed, in progress, tool development, and requests for assistance (subjects, co-investigators, location of tools, etc.).

   Implementation: Status of ongoing use, plans for beginning, documentation methods, and requests for assistance.

   New Diagnoses: Identified and developed or partially developed, title identified or suggested, and requests for assistance in developing.

2. To develop networking in an area of interest.

   Report area of interest or regional networking group.

   Request participation in group to be formed.

Eleven SIGs met at the Seventh Conference. The group reports, designated leader, and recorder are included in the following section.

Agency implementation/quality/assurance
Leader: Carol Blankenship
Recorder: Diane Aideuis

Computerization
Leader: Christine Galante
Recorder: Kathleen Bloom

Critical care
Leader: Cynthia Dougherty
Recorder: Colleen M. O'Brien

Curriculum/educational implementation
Leader: Carol Christensen
Recorder: Mary Kontz

Direct pay for nursing service
Leader: Linda Grilley
Recorder: Jesse Greene

Long-term care
Leader: Joan Caley
Recorder: Marie Maguire

Mental health
Leader: Margaret McComb
Recorder: Lynda Hallinan

Nurse practitioners and family health
Leader: Dorothy Jones
Recorder: Sabrina Richer

Research
Leader: Kay Avant
Recorder: Theresa Glydenvand

Taxonomy
Leader: Judith J. Warren
Recorder: Regina Maibusch

Wellness
Leader: Sue Popkess-Vawter
Recorder: Linda Cooper

AGENCY IMPLEMENTATION/ QUALITY ASSURANCE

There were 71 participants in this group's meeting. The main topics of concern included:

1. Improvement of diagnostic reasoning as key to successful implementation.
2. The use of clinical judgment, the use of thinking process, and the need for academic preparation with continued update among practitioners.
3. Nursing care plans—need to be creative, avoid duplication, review with physicians for their information, consider what are independent nursing care plans. There is a need for guidelines to increase the standards of care. The need for many to identify the difference of the medical order sheet as separate from the nursing care plan.
4. Computerization coming from standardized care plans; nursing protocols preprinted on care plans.
5. Discussion of dependent, interdependent, and independent nursing functions.
6. Protocols—need supplemental guides for patient teaching.
7. The group would like assistance/direction from NANDA in terms of implementation of nursing diagnoses and documentation of use through patient care records.
8. Recognition of nursing diagnosis by physicians and other health care professionals.

Solution: inservice/educate other professionals, joint physician/nursing departmental committees.

9. Aspects of quality assurance include: committee structure to include representation from all nursing departments, development of outcome criteria/standards, monitor functions, and peer review/audit.

10. Advancement from quality assurance to identifying and carrying through with research issues.

COMPUTERIZATION

There were 70 participants present. Main issues discussed were:

1. Teaching nursing students about computers; what resources are available for teaching computer courses related to nursing? Three available books by Sweeney, Saba, and Ball and Hannah.

2. Nursing information systems now in use:
   a. Use of HBO system
   b. Ulticare system
   c. Technicon
   d. Spectra 2000 Medical Information System
   e. COMA system
   f. NIH system

3. Utilization of computers for research; Kathy Bloom (Jacksonville, Florida) offered to send information on two packages to interested participants.

CRITICAL CARE

There were 69 in attendance at this meeting. Main issues discussed included:

1. A new diagnosis, "Inability to Wean from Ventilator," was proposed

2. Inclusion of collaborative problems in the care plan—the group concluded that we do not have all labels needed for nursing practice

3. Identification of the commonly termed phenomenon "ICU psychosis" as a nursing problem amenable to independent nursing theapy—the group concluded that there is a need to be creative in generating diagnostic labels and not just rely on "approved" diagnoses.

4. "Potential" nursing diagnoses and related etiological factors; group consensus was that nurses' influence the outcome of risk factors by more than simply monitoring and reporting to the physician.

5. The direction of influence in NANDA should be from the membership up.

6. Nurses need to generate working diagnoses and report these to NANDA.

7. How to communicate the benefits of nursing to the public

8. Need to clarify and make explicit the relationship between NANDA and AACN.

CURRICULUM/EDUCATIONAL IMPLEMENTATION

There were 72 participants at this meeting. The main topics included:

1. A one-year implementation project looking at application of nursing diagnosis at the associate degree level (Laboure' College, Boston, Massachusetts); there are 123 learning packages integrating nursing diagnosis. There was discussion of interests in levels and placement in the curriculum of nursing diagnoses, and whether learning activity packages are helpful for more experienced nurses learning nursing diagnoses?

2. Interests in networking among diploma program faculty.

3. Collaborative problems as an alternative to nursing diagnoses; methods to differentiate nursing diagnoses (from collaborative problems).

4. Use of defining characteristics to differentiate between specific diagnoses that appear to overlap.

5. Implementation of nursing diagnosis in a baccalaureate curriculum (Loyola University, Chicago).

6. Implementation of nursing diagnosis in a diploma program.

7. Implementation of nursing diagnoses using preprinted standardized care plans, report of project at Research Medical Center, Kansas City, Missouri. Recommendation to develop minimal Quality Assurance Standards.

DIRECT PAY FOR NURSING SERVICE

There were 20 participants in attendance. Topics discussed were:

1. Relationship between nursing diagnoses and patient acuity (DRGs).
2. Research study in an extended care facility examining relationships between nursing diagnoses and resource utilization, such as staffing patterns, patient census/classification.
3. Implementation report on use of nursing diagnosis in a hospice.
4. Home health care—the relationships among reimbursement, nursing diagnosis, and skilled nursing requirements.
5. Issue of costing out nursing resources when there's a fine line between dependent/interdependent/independent nursing practices.

LONG-TERM CARE

There were 17 participants in this special interest group. Issues that evolved from the discussion were:

1. Confusion concerning the two diagnostic labels, "Alteration in Activities of Daily Living" and "Alterations in Self Care." Suggestion that Alteration in ADL has a broader perspective to deal with than discharge, home management, and recreation needs and that Alteration in Self Care be more specific, based on functional assessment.
2. Concerns that nursing as a part of the multidisciplinary health team may lose some of its uniqueness. Some facilities use nursing diagnosis taxonomy on the interdisciplinary care plan, but do not require this of other health professionals. In some institutions, the entire health team has adopted M. Gordon's Functional Health Patterns. Who can make the diagnoses? Who can be accountable? Who plans/carries out interventions?
3. There is a need for a firm link between extended care facilities and acute care settings through the use of nursing diagnoses; valuable information is lost concerning patient needs/care when the patient is transferred from one setting to another.
4. Administrative concerns regarding resource allocation methods. Some felt that RUGS

does not measure patient care needs accurately.

5. The need for a nursing diagnosis addressing the constant vigilance a caregiver provides in the home setting with a chronically ill individual, resulting in the caregiver's "burnout syndrome." Suggestions for diagnostic labels: "Alteration in Home Health Management," "Compromised Coping," "Hypervigilance."

MENTAL HEALTH

There were 24 participants in this session. The group discussed such issues as implementation of nursing diagnosis in multidisciplinary settings and how nursing differs from the practice of other professionals in the mental health arena; choosing nursing diagnoses in the psychiatric setting; computerization of nursing diagnosis; prioritization of nursing diagnoses; assigning a sixth Axis to DSM III revision to incorporate the nursing role, and the need for a taxonomy of assets. The group asks NANDA to address the need for positive language in the proposed taxonomy, to investigate and possibly represent the nursing standpoint in the proposed DSM III revision, and to consider the addition of a mental health component to the category "exchanging."

NURSE PRACTITIONER/ FAMILY HEALTH

There were 29 present in this special interest group. Topics that were discussed in this meeting were:

1. Difficulty implementing the nurse practitioner role (when the role is not as a physician's assistant).
2. Difficulty implementing nursing diagnoses in a primary care setting or specialty areas (e.g., in a diabetic clinic).
3. Growth and development needs aren't addressed (i.e., where do you include premenstrual syndrome, pregnancy?).
4. The diagnosis of "Family Coping" seems too broad; there is a need to separate or break it down more.
5. Difficulty in differentiating among "anxiety," "coping," and "fear" in diagnostic labels.

6. Questions about knowing if we have identified a correct nursing diagnosis.
7. The Wellness Center as a working model for nursing.
8. A quality assurance tool dealing with family structure and related nursing diagnoses.
9. Need to consider qualifiers.
10. Ways to network after the Seventh Conference.

RESEARCH

There were 90 participants present in this session.

Research completed

Focus began on research that has been completed. Joie Whitney, University of Washington (Seattle) shared a research project which used the Carnavelli model as an assessment form for identifying new nursing diagnoses for psychiatric patients. Diagnoses that repeated over the population of six patients were: somatization, postoverdose syndrome, and emancipation. This project was funded by a GRSG grant. Lorraine Walker, University of Texas (Austin) reported on a research project she had completed which focused on observing mother/baby interaction. She cited that a major problem in doing qualitative nursing research is the lack of sound methodology to guide nursing diagnosis research. Lorraine suggested that a goal of this group might be to develop material to provide guidance in methodology for nursing diagnosis research. Sharon L. Merritt, Southern Illinois University (Edwardsville), reminded those present that the MNRS is sponsoring a symposium to focus on methodologies. This will be held in St. Louis, April 5-7, 1987.

Research in progress

The session next focused on nursing diagnosis research in progress. Virginia Aukamp (Doctoral Candidate) Decatur, Illinois, shared work she is doing on her doctoral dissertation. Virginia has done a field study and now is in the clinical setting validating the nursing diagnoses of Knowledge Deficit and Anxiety in the third trimester of pregnancy. She is identifying the defining characteristics for both of these diagnoses and in addition is trying to validate whether nurses are assessing these diagnoses correctly. Virginia shared

her frustration over the lack of direction in nursing diagnoses methodology. Mary Lou Kiley, University Hospital at Cleveland (Ohio) reported on the development of a data base in nursing diagnosis in the clinical setting. Her institution is using nursing diagnosis to measure nursing need. Patients are assessed daily, and these assessments are recorded daily on portable computer terminals. These data are used to validate the patients' need for nursing care. They are building a data base of 25,000 to 30,000 cases per year. Nursing diagnosis is used as a basis for their classification system and is correlated to DRG and length of stay. Mary Ann Anderson, Weber State College (Ogden, Utah) shared that in their AD program, Linda Carpenito helped them to develop a nursing diagnosis—based curriculum. She reported that while nursing students were educated in nursing diagnosis, none of the hospitals in the area had implemented. She reported on the follow-up they are involved in to encourage the implementation of nursing diagnosis. Sue Baird Holmes, St. Joseph Hospital (Milwaukee, Wisconsin) reported on the second phase of development of the Baird Body Image Tool. This tool uses a Likert scale format to validate the defining characteristics of the nursing diagnosis, Body Image Disturbance. Devamma Purushotham (Windsor, Ontario) shared the work she has done on her doctoral dissertation in the area of nursing diagnosis and its relation to nursing education. The focus of her study was that of looking at and comparing the abilities of the baccalaureate and diploma nursing students to assess and make nursing diagnoses. Rosemary McKeighan (Iowa City) reported that she is testing the efficacy of software developed to teach students to make nursing diagnoses. This data base can be manipulated to pull out the nursing diagnosis as well. She invited others to use and test this software.

Implementation

The purpose of this portion of the session was to share information on the implementation of nursing diagnosis research. Mary Lou Kiley, University Hospitals at Cleveland (Ohio), reported that they have implemented the NANDA Nursing Diagnosis list in their institution. In addition they have also implemented 12 new diagnoses. These diagnoses have been submitted to

NANDA for progression through the review cycle. Carol Hudgings, Hospital Corporation of America (Nashville, Tennessee), shared with the group that she is currently working on developing a computerized distributive system for nursing. They requested assistance in obtaining data on frameworks, etiologies, and outcomes. Jo Ann Maklebust, Harper Hospital (Michigan), reported that she has proposed a change in the nursing diagnosis of Impaired Skin Integrity to Impaired Tissue Integrity. She noted that the nursing diagnosis related to oral mucous membranes could be subsumed under this new diagnosis. She also reported that MINDA is offering grants of up to $1,000 for those doing nursing diagnosis research in Michigan. She is also looking at the process of how a nursing diagnosis is written. Pauline Dion (Massachusetts) shared that she is presenting a poster session on this topic, and Marie Gould (Maryland) reported she has had an article accepted for publication in this area.

Networking

Mary Venn (Wisconsin) reported that she would like to network with individuals in the area of validating defining characteristics for nursing diagnoses. Karen Budd (Ohio) shared that she has developed the tool "Indicators of Health" and would like to network individuals interested in a wellness focus.

New diagnoses

This portion of the session provided time to share research being done on new nursing diagnoses. Mary V. Hanley, Nurse Consultant (Boston), reported on work she is doing on two pulmonary diagnoses: impaired airway maintenance and impaired pulmonary host defenses. Her work in the diagnosis impaired pulmonary host defenses focuses on risk identification and prevention. She is also working with the steering committee of the American Thoracic Society to develop standards in this area.

TAXONOMY

There were 52 participants involved in this meeting. The taxonomy interest group met to discuss the proposed endorsement of Nursing Diagnosis Taxonomy I. Discussions concerned six major topics: taxonomic structure, the level of the diagnostic statement, needed taxonomic research, the place of development and wellness diagnoses, general issues pertaining to implementation, and the Taxonomy Committee's structure and purpose. Each of these concerns will be summarized.

The taxonomic structure was discussed and four general concerns were noted. First, the qualifiers need to be reexamined. There seems to be an inconsistent use of qualifiers at different levels of the taxonomy while other useful qualifiers are left out. One concern was how to deal with the time issue. Perhaps "resolving:" should be added to the qualifiers list. There seems to be a need, also, to address amount and purpose in the diagnostic statement, and qualifiers may be a way to solve this problem. Finally, some qualifiers that were discussed at the Sixth Conference seem to have disappeared. What happened to the "readiness for growth" proposed by Dorothea Jakob? There was consensus that the Taxonomy Committee should reexamine all the qualifiers with the possibility that recommendations be made to rename some of them. Second, the group was concerned that the taxonomy had not been tested in a pilot project. It is true that NANDA has not funded nor designed any implementation or research project; however, several hospitals and one book (Gettrust et al., 1984) have organized the diagnoses under the pattern of human responses. They report that the taxonomic structure has clinical usefulness for them. Committee members present stated that this was of concern to them, but until a taxonomic structure was endorsed by NANDA, a formal testing of the structure was beyond the Bylaws' charge to the committee. Then there was concern that many nurses felt "locked into the taxonomy as a worksheet." Diagnostic labels could come only from the "holes" in the taxonomy. It was reaffirmed that practice generated the diagnoses and not the taxonomic structure. The structure, or taxonomic trees, was a method of visualizing relationships among the labels not one of forcing a fit to reality. Third, some of the old diagnoses may need to be revised or redefined in light of the proposed taxonomy. Kritek cautioned the group not to worry at this time about perfection at that level, but to focus on conceptual relationships and identification of new diagnoses. Nursing has used the "current stuff" (definitions for the diagnoses) for about a hundred years without getting traumatized by not being perfect. Fourth, the categories of the taxonomy are disjunctive instead of mutually exclusive, and there seems to be many overlaps between the categories. The domain of nursing, which is being classified, is intellectually complex and the task of classifying/conceptualizing will probably become more difficult. In developing the structure, it is difficult "to see what is not there" or "to see the holes." Yet, it is this task that is exciting—the identification of the phenomena of concern for nursing. There was much discussion concerning whether the taxonomic categories should be disjunctive or mutually exclusive. Is the holistic nature of nursing causing some of this overlap, and should that nature be considered in determining the characteristics of the taxonomic structure? The Taxonomy Committee members stated that they intend to invite a consultant on taxonomic structure to assist them in grappling with this issue.

The second major topic of discussion was the question: "What levels of the diagnostic taxonomy should the practicing nurse be interested in?" Dr. Kritek affirmed that the clinically useful level is of most interest. An example of one that may not be useful is alteration in communication. This particular diagnosis seems to be too broad. There must be many different clinically useful diagnoses under this category since nurses do very different things for clients who have physical problems as opposed to psychologic or social problems. If this is true, then there needs to be some guidelines developed for using the taxonomy to get at the clinically useful diagnoses. If there is agreement on clinically useful diagnoses, what are the categories at the other levels called? Are they still diagnoses or diagnostic categories or . . . ?

This discussion led to the question of what kind of research is needed to refine the taxonomy—the third major topic of the meeting. Is the next step concept analysis or concept exploration? There was concern with the approach as there is still much descriptive research that needs to be done on each diagnosis and the taxonomy structure. The endorsement of the taxonomy is necessary to this research task since research cannot focus on the alphabet, it needs patterns. But what is a pattern? Does it occur at only one level

of the taxonomy or are all levels patterns? Perhaps the word "pattern" should be eliminated when discussing the taxonomy. However, one thing that has occurred as a result of the taxonomy and the nice fit with patterns of human responses is that they have moved nursing further away from the body systems review (the medical model). Finally, as with the level of diagnosis, research needs to be at a practical or useful level. It is too soon to select or impose one particular model of research to explicate the taxonomic structure.

The fourth major topic of concern was the place of the diagnoses concerning client development and wellness. These two areas are gaining in importance as nursing practice assumes a greater role in health promotion and disease risk-factor reduction. Yet, there is no place in the taxonomy for these practice areas. The diagnoses in the taxonomy are all problem-focused. Where would the diagnoses concerning development or wellness fit? Concerning the issue of development, the group discussed two options. First, development may be a separate pattern of human responses: "developing." Developmental concerns appear to be a very large domain that may make intervention complex and problematic. Such intervention may affect all patterns of human responses. This leads to a discussion of the second option that development may be an alteration in (some activity) related to developmental delay in cognitive, motor, emotional, nutritional, function? This etiologic approach might be a better way to handle the pervasiveness of the influence of development on all the patterns.

Several nurses who work with children and their families or expectant families were concerned about the problem-focus of the taxonomy. They did not feel that the current diagnoses were adequate to label their phenomena of concern. It was reaffirmed that nursing is still in the early stages of developing nursing diagnoses and taxonomic structure. Perfection is not present, and there are many diagnostic areas that are just beginning to be developed. Caution needs to be given, though; there should not be an effort to develop nursing diagnoses for each medical specialty, i.e., pediatrics, obstetrics, psychiatry, and so forth. The discussion then focused on the problem of who was the object of the diagnosis—the fetus, the neonate, the pregnant mother, or the family. How does one separate the patient role from the parent role or the family role? There was no answer, but the group felt this was an important area for further study.

The fifth major topic discussed was general issues pertaining to implementation. There were three issues. First, practicing nurses must work with the nursing domain, the medical domain, and the psychological domain. Often nursing diagnoses do not fit with the last two domains. How is this handled? Nurses must function in all three areas, the last two involved interdependent and dependent roles and actions. Nursing diagnoses are used in the nursing domain and involve independent and interdependent roles and actions. Nurses do not need nursing diagnoses to parallel medical or psychological diagnoses. Our phenomenon of concern is patterns of human responses, not disease processes. The second issue concerned the interrelationships of the nine patterns of the first level of the taxonomy. A problem in one pattern may affect the other eight patterns. For example, how much effect does alteration in verbal communication have on choosing? How does one find the "root" of the problem? It requires complex knowledge and high-level analytic skills. It is, also, essential in setting priorities among diagnoses. The third issue was a request to return to the work session format of the early NANDA conferences. Members of the NANDA board who were present stated that at this time there is no interest in returning to that activity. The work sessions need to occur prior to the national conferences either in NANDA's committees or in the regional/local groups. Another option is to have research on taxonomy conferences to conduct this type of nurturing and growth process, but NANDA is now concerned with the work and business of naming phenomena and placing diagnoses into the taxonomy. The organization has grown and matured in function from the early days.

The sixth and last major topic of discussion was the Taxonomy Committee's structure and purpose. The first concern was why did the Committee select theorists' work over Gordon's? There are many taxonomic structures that could have been selected—Omaha's format, ANA's format, Gordon's format, and others. NANDA had asked the theorists for assistance in developing a taxonomic structure, and now that structure needs endorsement so it can be tested. The testing may either demonstrate a good fit or the need to develop/select another structure. Second, does the Committee initiate work to develop nursing diagnoses? The Committee felt that it would be presumptuous of the Committee to say they had the knowledge to identify all the needed diagnoses and to develop them for use. It is not the purpose of the Committee to identify diagnoses, but to develop and refine the taxonomic structure. Diagnoses need to come from the experience of practicing nurses. If the Committee identifies the diagnoses, then the development and acceptance of the diagnoses are no longer a consensus effort of the NANDA membership. Third, are there criteria for the development of diagnostic categories and diagnostic labels? When nurses submit new labels should they identify the level of abstraction to facilitate placement in the taxonomic structure? There are guidelines for the submission of new diagnoses. These were developed by the Diagnosis Review Committee. Currently, there are no guidelines for the placement of the diagnoses into the taxonomy. This will be a task for the Taxonomy Committee to address prior to the next conference. Fourth, will information concerning the taxonomy be published in a timely fashion? Two years is a long time to wait for publication of the Proceedings. Suggestions were made for a column in the NANDA Newsletter. Dr. Kritek stated that in the past there had been copyright problems but that these had been handled. The Committee will be encouraged and will be encouraging others to publish their ideas and research in other publications to engage in an active dialogue in the literature. From this dialogue, a sounder taxonomic structure should emerge. A second suggestion was that NANDA serve as a data base and assist in providing information and names of people to assist in networking. The Committee members responded positively to both suggestions and will discuss their implementation.

The meeting of the taxonomy group provided a positive forum for the discussion of problems and concerns about the proposed Nursing Diagnosis Taxonomy I. The committee members received a lot of feedback and information to use in their work of refining the proposed structure upon its endorsement by the attending members of NANDA.

WELLNESS

Thirty-five nurses participated in this group meeting. Topics which were discussed included:

1. Report of the work done by a subcommittee to define "Wellness" (Barbara Pokorny).
2. Bibliography computer research related to Wellness (Sue Popkess Vawter).
3. Possible mechanisms for this group to communicate between conferences.
4. Victoria Meissner voiced identified difficulty in labeling nursing diagnoses to deal with the basically healthy child who needs assistance with the mastery of developmental tasks (e.g., toilet training). Possible solution: Incorporate "effective," "functional" as possible qualifiers in the statement.
5. Jan Pierce requested assistance to develop a clinically useful diagnosis/tool for normal labor and delivery—mother and neonate. There is an article in February 1986 Maternal Child Nurse Journal.
6. Suzanne McGuiness is developing standard care plans for labor and delivery and the neonate.

REFERENCE

Gettrust, K.V., Ryan, S.C., and Engelman, D.S.: Applied nursing diagnosis: guidelines for comprehensive care planning, New York, 1985, John Wiley & Sons.

Appendix G   Acknowledgement of other contributions to the Seventh Conference

The chairperson and members of the Program Committee, executive officers of NANDA, and the Board of Directors extend their appreciation to the following NANDA members who volunteered their time and expertise to do blind reviews of the abstracts received for paper and poster presentations.

ABSTRACT REVIEWERS

Dr. Janet Awtrey
Dr. Andrea Bircher
Dr. Kenneth Cianfrani
Dr. Patricia Clunn
Dr. Richard Fehring
Dr. Frances Fickess
Dr. Sheila Fredette
Dr. June Gray
Dr. Edward Halloran
Dr. Lois Hoskins
Dr. Dorothy Jones
Dr. Mary Ann Kelly
Dr. Nancy Lackey
Dr. Joanne McCloskey
Dr. Elizabeth McFarlane
Dr. Helen Niskala
Dr. Myrna Pickard
Dr. Sue Ellen Pinkerton
Dr. Devamma Purushotaham
Dr. Evelyn Redding
Dr. Barbara Rottkamp
Dr. Virginia Saba
Dr. Joyce Shoemaker

Dr. Ruth Stollenwerk
Dr. Roberta Thiry
Dr. Rosemary Wang
Dr. Shirley Ziegler

DIAGNOSIS REVIEWED BUT NOT APPROVED BY NANDA MEMBERS
Deconditioning (not approved)

Definition
A state in which the physical work capacity of an individual is reduced.

Defining characteristics
Major
Weakness
Dizziness
Shortness of breath
Lethargy
Muscle atrophy
Decreased endurance
Minor
Lightheadedness
Lethargy
Diaphoresis
Syncope
Palpitation
Shortness of breath
Orthostatic hypotension

RELATED FACTORS
Prolonged inactivity in contrast to an individual's normal level.

SUBSTANTIATING/SUPPORTIVE MATERIALS

Fitzgerald, P.A., and Mansfield, L.W.: Cardiac response to selected activities in hospitalized patients, Circulation **46**(4), 11-24, 1972.

Hutelmyer, C.: Rehabilitation of the cardiac patient. In W.C. McGurn, editor: People with cardiac problems: nursing concepts, Philadelphia, 1981, Lippincott.

Selye, H.: Stress without distress, Philadelphia, 1974, Lippincott.

Sivarajan, E.S.: Cardiac rehabilitation: activity and exercise program. In Underhill, et al., editors: Cardiac nursing, Philadelphia, 1982, Lippincott.

Wagner, E., and Williams, P.S.: Rehabilitation after myocardial infarction. In Andreoli, K.G., et al., editors: Comprehensive cardiac care, St. Louis, 1983, The C.V. Mosby Co.

ARTICLE I TITLE, PURPOSE AND FUNCTION

Section 1. Title. The name of this association shall be the North American Nursing Diagnosis Association, Inc.

Section 2. Purpose. This association is organized to develop, refine and promote a taxonomy of nursing diagnostic terminology of general use to professional nurses.

Section 3. Restrictions. The association qualifies as a tax exempt organization within the meaning of section 501 (c) (6) of the U.S. Internal Revenue Code. The affairs of the association shall be conducted in such a manner as to qualify for tax exemption under that provision.

Section 4. Equal Rights. The purposes of this association shall be unrestricted by consideration of nationality, race, creed, life style, color, sex, or age.

Section 5. Functions. The function of the association shall be to develop and promote a taxonomy of nursing diagnoses, including but not limited to:

a) conducting conferences
b) publishing documents
c) facilitating research
d) serving as an information resource

ARTICLE II MEMBERSHIP

Section 1. Member. A member is one:

a) who has been granted a license to practice as a registered nurse and who does not have a license under suspension or revocation, or
b) whose dues are not delinquent.

Section 2. Associate Member. An associate member is one who does not qualify as a member, who shares an interest in the purposes of the association and whose dues are not delinquent. Associate members do not have a vote, but may actively participate in all other affairs of the association.

Section 3. The presentation to this association of completed application, as required by association policy or Bylaws, together with annual dues shall establish them as a member or associate member of this association.

Section 4. Membership Year. The membership year shall be a period of 12 consecutive months, beginning January 1 of each calendar year.

ARTICLE III FINANCIAL ADMINISTRATION

Section 1. Fiscal Year. The fiscal year of this association shall commence on the first day of July of each year.

Section 2. Dues. The dues of this association shall be set by. the Board of Directors with the approval of two-thirds of the General Assembly. Any member who fails to pay the dues within four (4) months after they become payable shall be dropped from the membership rolls.

Section 3. Change of Dues. No monies shall be refunded nor additional monies collected when a change of dues category is made within a membership year.

Section 4. Budget. A budget for each year shall be adopted by the Board of Directors prior to the beginning of the fiscal year.

Section 5. Executive Director's Duties. The Executive Director shall have the authority to direct and maintain the headquarters of the association; insure that all funds, physical assets and other property of the organization are safeguarded and administrated, as directed by the Board of Directors.

ARTICLE IV OFFICERS AND DUTIES OF OFFICERS

Section 1. The officers of this association shall be a president, a vice-president, a secretary, and a treasurer who shall be elected as hereinafter provided.

Section 2. Duties. The officers of the association shall constitute an executive committee, and are authorized to transact the business of the association between meetings of the Board, and assist the president as needed. They shall also perform the duties usually performed by such officers as specified in these Bylaws or as designated by the Board.

Section 3. Term of office. The term of office

for all officers shall commence at the beginning of the association's fiscal year and shall continue until the expiration of their respective terms of office or until their successors are elected. No officer shall be eligible to serve more than two consecutive terms in the same office. A member who has served more than half a term shall be deemed to have served a term. The term of office shall be four years.

Section 4. President. The president shall be chairman of the Board of Directors; shall be an ex officio member of all committees and task forces except the Nominating Committee; shall preside at all meetings of this association; appoint special committees or task forces as outlined by these Bylaws or the Board; serve as the association's representative; and perform all other duties of the office.

Section 5. Vice-president. The Vice-president shall assume the duties of the president in case of that officer's absence or inability to serve.

Section 6. Secretary. The secretary shall keep minutes of all proceedings of this association and the Board; shall report at meetings of this association or Board; shall be familiar with procedures of the headquarters of this association relating to notification of elections or appointments, notices of time and place of meetings, records of members, and policies of the Board and the association. The secretary shall perform such other duties as may be assigned by the Board.

Section 7. Treasurer. The treasurer shall have custody of the funds and securities of this association; shall see that full and accurate financial reports are made to the Board and association meetings. The treasurer shall perform such other duties as may be assigned by the Board.

Section 8. Compensation. Elected offices shall not receive any compensation for their services as such but may be reimbursed for their expenses.

ARTICLE V BOARD OF DIRECTORS

Section 1. Composition. The Board of Directors of the association shall be the officers plus seven directors, who shall be elected as hereinafter provided.

Section 2. Term of office. The term of office for all directors shall commence at the beginning of the association's fiscal year, and shall continue until the expiration of their respective terms of office or until their successors are elected. No Board member shall be eligible to serve more than two consecutive terms. A member who has served more than half a term shall be deemed to have served a term. The term of office shall be four years.

Section 3. Meetings. The Board of Directors shall meet at least annually during the fiscal year of the association.

Section 4. Special meetings. Special meetings of the Board may be called by the president on 10 days notice to each member and shall be called by the president on like notice upon the written request of four or more members of the Board.

Section 5. Automatic vacancy of office. If any member of the Board is absent from two regular meetings in succession, unless excused by the Board for valid reasons, the office shall automatically become vacant and the vacancy shall be filled as provided in these Bylaws.

Section 6. Powers of the Board. The Board of Directors shall have power and authority over the affairs and business of this association between regular association meetings, except that of modifying any action taken by the members. It shall perform the duties prescribed in these Bylaws and such others as may be delegated to it by the association. The Board in addition shall:

a) appoint an executive director and fix compensation for the position. The executive director shall serve at the pleasure of the Board with duties and responsibilities conferred by the Board.

b) establish administrative policies governing the affairs of the association.

c) develop a master plan allowing the accomplishment of the association's purposes and for the growth and prosperity of the association.

d) transact the general business of the association.

e) report business transacted at regular meetings of the association and give an annual report to the membership and at regular meetings of the association.

f) act as custodian of the property, securities and records of the association; select a place for deposit of the funds of the association; provide for the audit of the books of the association; provide for bonding of association officials as it may deem necessary and provide for payment of authorized expenses.

g) establish and dissolve committees, task forces and appointments for such to accomplish the purposes of this association.

h) have the power to fill vacancies except the offices of president and vice-president.

i) decide on the date and place of association meetings.

j) perform such other duties as may be assigned elsewhere in these Bylaws or by the association.

Section 6. Retiring Members. All retiring members of the Board shall deliver to the association within one month all association properties in their possession.

ARTICLE VI COMMITTEES

Section 1. Committee appointments. The association may have standing committees. Each committee shall be chaired by a member of the Board as appointed by the president. The appointed chair shall name additional members with attention to geographic and clinical practice distribution with concurrence by the president. The size of the committee shall be determined by the Board. Committees shall report to the Board and to meetings of the association as requested or as required by these Bylaws.

Section 2. Committees. The association may have, but shall not be limited to, the following committees:

a) Program Committee. The Program Committee shall plan the general assembly meetings of the association and provide consultation to regional groups and special interest groups desiring to conduct programs of interest to members of the association.

b) Publications Committee. The Publications Committee shall oversee the publications of the association including but not limited to a regular newsletter, official proceedings of the general assembly, and nursing diagnoses. Recommendations for the editors of these documents shall be submitted to the Board.

c) Membership Committee. The Membership Committee shall provide for distribution of information for those eligible and interested in association membership. The Committee

shall review and accept applications with concurrence of the Board.

d) Diagnosis Review Committee. The Diagnosis Review Committee shall review proposed diagnoses and recommend acceptance/modification/rejection to the Board. The Committee shall appoint specialized clinical/technical review task forces in specific clinical areas to review diagnoses prior to Committee action; shall designate the format for submission of proposed diagnoses or changes to existing diagnoses; and following meetings of the general assembly shall prepare proposed diagnoses in final form as recommended for membership voting.

e) Research Committee. The Research Committee shall promote conducting research studies and review research papers for the publications of the Association.

f) Public Relations Committee. The Public Relations Committee shall promote the relationship with other nursing and health professionals and keep the association abreast of their trend and pertinent activities. The committee shall serve as the advocate/spokesman for general affairs of the Association.

g) Taxonomy Committee. The Taxonomy Committee shall develop and regularly review a taxonomic system for the diagnoses, and submit to the Board for review and action; promote its (taxonomy) use, and promote collaboration with groups supporting other established health-related taxonomies.

h) Regional Affairs. The committee shall promote the involvement of members in affairs of the association through activities and communication at a local or regional level, and provide a mechanism for bringing issues of regional concerns to the attention of the Board and the Association.

Section 3. Term of office. The term of office shall be four (4) years. One-half of each of the Committees shall be appointed every two years.

Section 4. Automatic vacancy of office. If any member of a committee is absent from two regular meetings in succession, unless excused by the Board for valid reasons, the office shall automatically become vacant and the vacancy shall be filled as provided in these Bylaws.

Section 5. Retiring members. All retiring members of the Committees shall deliver to the association within one month all association properties in their possession.

ARTICLE VII ELECTIONS

Section 1. Nominating Committee. The President shall appoint a chair and one (1) member to a Nomination Committee. No member of the committee may be a member of the Board of Directors. In addition, three (3) members shall be elected by the memberhsip during the regular elections. All terms shall be four (4) years.

Section 2. Ballot and Election. All elections shall be in accordance with written Board policy and these Bylaws. An election is constituted by a plurality of voting members and in case of a tie, the choice shall be by lot.

Section 3. Tellers. The president shall appoint tellers one month in advance of elections, who shall serve as inspectors of the election.

ARTICLE VIII GENERAL ASSEMBLY

Section 1. Composition. The composition of the General Assembly shall be the voting members and associate members who are in attendance at the meetings of the association.

Section 2. Authority. The General Assembly shall approve policies and Bylaws to govern the association; shall review and comment on proposed diagnoses for the Diagnosis Review Committee's actions prior to the submission to the membership for acceptance.

ARTICLE IX MEETINGS

Section 1. Regular meetings. Regular meetings of the General Assembly shall be at least once every thirty (30) months.

a) With regard to regular meetings, receipt of a copy of a written notice setting the time and place of each regular meeting shall be deemed sufficient notice of the meeting. With regard to any special meeting, each member shall be sent written notice at least ten (10) days prior to the date of the meeting. Said notice shall set forth the time and place of the meeting. It shall not be required that any such notice set forth the purpose for which the meeting is being called.

b) Waiver of Notice. Whenever any notice is required to be given under the provision of these By-Laws or under the provisions of the Articles of Incorporation or under the provisions of the laws of the State of Missouri a waiver thereof in writing, signed by the person or persons entitled to such notice, whether before or after the time stated therein, shall be deemed equivalent to the giving of such notice. Further, the notice may be published in the Association's newsletter, which is mailed to all members, and the notice therein shall be deemed to meet any notice requirements.

Section 2. Special meetings. Special meetings of the General Assembly may be called by the president upon majority vote of the Board or upon the written request of five (5) members each from twenty states.

ARTICLE X QUORUM

Section 1. General Assembly. Twenty percent of the voting membership of the association shall constitute a quorum at any regular or special meeting of the General Assembly.

Section 2. Board of Directors. A majority of the members of the Board shall constitute a quorum at any meeting of the Board.

ARTICLE XI PARLIAMENTARY AUTHORITY

The rules contained in "Robert's Rules of Order, Newly Revised" shall govern meetings of this association in all cases to which they are applicable and in which they are not inconsistent with these Bylaws.

ARTICLE XII AMENDMENTS

Section 1. Amendments. Amendments to these Bylaws must be submitted to the Board prior to submission to the General Assembly.

Section 2. Previous notice. These Bylaws may be amended at any regular or special meeting of the General Assembly by a two-thirds vote of the members present and voting, provided the proposed amendments have been sent to all members at least two months prior to the meeting.

Section 3. No notice. These Bylaws may be amended without previous notice at any regular or special meeting of the General Assembly by a ninety nine percent vote of those members present and voting.

ARTICLE XIII DISSOLUTION

The association may be dissolved by a two-thirds vote of the members upon recommendation of the General Assembly. Upon dissolution after payment of all liabilities, the remaining assets shall be distributed to any nursing organization provided that no distribution shall be made to any organization not then covered by Section 501 (c) (3) of the Internal Revenue Service Code of 1954 or the corresponding provisions of any future federal or applicable tax law.

The North American Nursing Diagnosis Association adopted its bylaws in April, 1982. The organization replaced the National Group for the Classification of Nursing Diagnosis which was established in 1973. The organization incorporated in February, 1985, and the bylaws were amended in March, 1986.

Appendix I Participants in Seventh Conference

Mary Abraham
Cleveland, OH

Marilyn Abraham
Alcester, SD

Marsha Adams
Centreville, AL

Frenita Agbayani
Matteson, IL

Dianna Aideuis
Chapel Hill, NC

Pam Allen
Springfield, IL

Rebecca Ambrosini
Connelsville, PA

Janice Ander
Hanover Park, IL

Joan Andersen
Philadelphia, PA

Mary Ann Anderson
Sunset, UT

Minnie Anderson
Indianapolis, IN

Mary Anderson
Dayton, OH

Laura Ashcraft
Benton, AZ

Laura Aukamp
Macon, IL

Kay Avant
Waco, TX

Myrtle Aydelotte
Iowa City, IA

Linda Baas
Cincinnati, OH

Carol Baer
Medford, MA

Sarah Bahlke
Kalamazoo, MI

Laurie Baker
New York, NY

Cynthia Balin
Orlando, FL

Juanita Balke
Grosse Pointe, MI

Karen Ballard
Builderland, NY

Linda Banks
Des Moines, IA

Jamie Banks
Sheridan, WY

Vivian Barry
Chicago, IL

Beverly Bartlett
Granby, MA

Marilyn Bayne
Timonium, MD

Ann Becker
St. Louis, MO

Ruth Becker
Detroit, MI

Doris Bell
Florissant, MO

Gwethalyn Bello
Ann Arbor, MI

Karen Bennett
Willowbrook, IL

JoAnne Bennett
New York, NY

Katherine Berry
Richmond, VA

Debra Berry
Carson City, MI

Ruth Beyer
Janesville, WI

Kathleen Beyerman
Somerville, MA

Mary Biebel
Milwaukee, WI

Barbara Biehler
Bloomington, IL

Andrea Bircher
Oklahoma City, OK

Virginia Blackmer
Franklin, NH

Carol Blankenship
Johnson City, TN

Wanda Blaser
Topeka, KS

Virginia Blom
Sioux City, IA

Kathleen Bloom
Jacksonville, FL

Lynn Bobel
Novi, MI

Lenore Boles
Norwalk, CT

Victoria Borces
Miami Beach, FL

Eleanor Borkowski
Redlands, CA

Susan Boultbee
Gilford, NH

Precilla Boykin
Fairfax, VA

Lucy Brand
Thompsonville, MI

Nancy Breidenbach
Dayton, OH

Ruth Ann Brintnall
Grand Rapids, MI

Margaret Briody
Rochester, NY

Genee Brukwitzki
Mequon, WI

Mary Bruskewitz
Brown Deer, WI

Karen Budd
Lakewood, OH

Gloria Bulechek
Solon, IA

Roberta Bumann
Winona, MI

Barbara Burke
Dearborn, MI

Joseph Burley
Ocean Springs, MS

Catherine Burns
Sherwood, OR

Joan Caley
Vancouver, WA

Lucy Callaghan
Overland Park, KS

Connie Campbell
Chicago, IL

Kimberly Campbell-Voytal
Atlanta, GA

Elizabeth Cannizzaro
New Alexandria, PA

Janice Cantrall
Burlington, KY

Martha Carlson
Champaign, IL

Rose Caroll-Johnson
Los Angeles, CA

Lynda Carpenito
Mickelton, NJ

Suzanne Cascino
Chicago, IL

Carol Cattaneo
Mission, KS

Jeanette Chambers
Columbus, OH

Patricia Chambers
Dayton, OH

Mary Champagne
Stanford, NC

Sheron Chishold
Petoskey, MI

Linda Chmielewski
Sauk Rapids, MN

Carol Christiansen
Gainesville, FL

Diane Christopherson
Reading, MA

Michele M. Chu
S. San Francisco, CA

Kenneth Cianfrani
Gurnee, IL

Carla Clark
Phoenix, AZ

Pru Cleghorn
Edwardsville, IL

Jeanette Clough
Wakefield, MA

Pat Cole
Des Moines, IA

Marga Coler
Storrs, CT

Luna Collado
Orlando Park, IL

Ann Collard
Wellesley, MA

Phyllis Collier
Edina, MN

Shirley Connelly
Roseville, MN

Linda Cooper
Toronto, Ontario

Lynn Cooper-Pace
Nepean, Ontario

Jan Corder
Monroe, LA

Nancy Coulter
Pacific Palisades, CA

Cynthia Coviak
Ada, MI

Carrie Craft
Jeffersontown, KY

Martha Craft
Solon, IA

Carol Craft
St. Louis, MO

Emily Cramer
Columbus, OH

Susan Creager
Mattawan, MI

Nancy Creason
Champaign, IL

Patricia Cremins
Milton, MA

Carolyn Critz
Monroe, LA

Betty Croonquist
Kandiyohi, MN

Joan Crosley
Babylon, NY

Emma Jean Cross
Edwardsville, IL

Janet Cuddigan
Omaha, NB

Janice Curry
Cincinnati, OH

Carol Daisy
Glastonbury, CT

Joanne Dalton
Duxbury, MA

Lynne Dapice
South Burlington, VT

Joseph Davie
San Diego, CA

Kay Davis
Stony Brook, NY

Gail Davis
Denton, TX

Carol Delage
St. Paul, MN

Andrea Depew
Champaign, IL

Anayis Derdiarian
Sherman Oaks, CA

Carol Dickel
Davenport, IA

Kaye Dietrich
Kiel, WI

Jacqueline Dietz
Chicago, IL

Ann Dillon
New Lenox, IL

Kathryn Dillow
Rantoul, IL

Pauline Dion
Williamstown, MA

Janet Dobrzyn
Van Nuys, CA

Rita Dodd
Chatham, IL

Marilynn Doenges
Colorado Springs, CO

Mary Dokmanovich
San Diego, CA

Susan Donnelly
East Corinth, VT

Cynthia Dougherty
Seattle, WA

Therese Dowd
Lincoln, NB

Lynda Dowling
Olathe, KS

Brigid Doyle
San Francisco, CA

Diane Drevs
Moville, IA

Marilyn Dubree
Nashville, TN

T. Audean Duespohl
Pittsburgh, PA

Lee Duke
Centerville, UT

Joyce Dungan
Evansville, IN

Joan Dunn
Grand Island, NY

Joan Duslak
Downers Grove, IL

Jennifer Early
Des Moines, IA

Sharon Eddy
Columbus, OH

Jacqueline Edgecomb
Portland, ME

Paula Elmer
Monroe, WI

Diane Engelman
Milwaukee, WI

Teresa Fadden
Milwaukee, WI

Carolyn Fallica
Wallham, MA

Jill Fargo
Milwaukee, WI

Dodie Farny
Denver, CO

Richard Fehring
Wauwatosa, WI

Luanne Fendrich
Peoria, IL

Mildred Fenske
Knoxville, TN

Melba Figgins
Martin, TX

Ann Fitzgerald
Omaha, NB

Joan Fitzmaurice
Newtonville, MA

Joyce Fitzpatrick
Cleveland, OH

Donnie Floyd
Little Rock, AR

Nancy Flynn
Havertown, PA

Joan Foley
Milwaukee, WI

Judith Forde
Kalamazoo, MI

Susan Fowler
Eau Claire, WI

Ann Frank
Milwaukee, WI

Diana Frankfurth
Greendale, WI

Sheila Fredette
Fitchburg, MA

Cecilia Freeman
Menomonee Falls, WI

Margaret Freundl
Beavercreek, OH

Gail Furney
Cuyahoga Falls, OH

Susan Galanes
Matteson, IL

Christine Galante
Temple Hills, MD

Susan Gardner
Cedar City, UT

Ellen Garneau
Meredith, NH

Gramatice Garofallou
Bronx, NY

Kathrine Garthe
Northport, MI

Patricia Gault
Minneapolis, MN

Kristine Gebbie
Portland, OR

Michele Geiger-Bronsky
Huntington Beach, CA

Georges Gentry
South Gate, CA

Elizabeth Gerety
Boring, OR

Barbara Gibb
Milwaukee, WI

Nancy Gilliland
Wilmington, NC

Orpha Glick
Iowa City, IA

Nelda Godfrey
Liberty, MO

Elaine Goehner
Pasadena, CA

Adelita Gonzales
Dallas, TX

Marjory Gordon
Brighton, MA

Marie Gould
Laurel, MD

Angelynn Grabau
Lincoln, NB

Theresa Graf
Rockville Centre, NY

Jesse E. Greene
Pendleton, SC

William Greenfield
Pembroke Pines, FL

Lessie Griffith
Salinas, CA

Linda Grilley
Wausau, WI

Casimir Grochowski
Midwest City, OK

Phyllis Gruizenga
Paw Paw, MI

Pauline Guay
North Andover, MA

Mary Grace Gundran
Melrose Park, IL

Teresa Gyldenvand
West Des Moines, IA

Barbara Haas
Yarmouth, ME

Kathryn Hafford
Amelia, Virginia

Mary Martha Hall
Houston, TX

Linda Hallinan
Sumter, SC

Edward Halloran
Shaker Heights, OH

Barbara Hammer
Marshalltown, IA

Doris Hancock
Louisville, KY

Mary Hanley
West Roxbury, MA

RuthAnn Harp
North Little Rock, AR

Renee Harris
Cleveland, OH

Bonnie Hartley
Toronto, Ontario

Donna Hartweg
Bloomington, IL

Steven Hayes
Reno, NV

Debra Heidrich
Cleveland, OH

Barbara Helmer
St. Louis, MO

Sylvia Hennessey
Thomaston, CT

Beth Hepola
Bellaire, TX

Mary Hermann
Newburgh, IN

Bridget Hier
Royal Oak, MI

Katharyne Higgins
Masbury, OH

Doris Hill
Chicago, IL

Kathleen Hillegas
Ann Arbor, MI

Sharon Hilton
Santa Anna, CA

Elizabeth Hiltunen
Ipswich, MA

Cindsley Hindsley
Wahiawa, HI

Irma Lou Hirsch
Kansas City, MO

Teresa Hitzeman
Ossian, IN

Jacqueline Hjelm
Eau Claire, WI

Helen Hogan
Farmerville, LA

Rosemarie Hogan
Cleveland, OH

Sue Holmes
Milwaukee, WI

Beth Honkamp
St. Cloud, MN

Constance Hoover
Hinsdale, IL

Karen Hoover
Hinsdale, IL

Martha Horst
Dalton, OH

Barbara Hoshiko
University Heights, OH

Lois Hoskins
Silver Spring, MD

Melanie Hotz
Washington, PA

Marguerite Hotz
Milwaukee, WI

Carol Hudgings
Nashville, TN

Kathy Huls-Sours
Eau Claire, WI

Mary Hurley
Saddle Brook, NJ

Donna Ignatavicius
Baltimore, MD

Beatrice Iho
Rochester, MI

Patricia Iyer
Stockton, NJ

Esther Jacobs
Skokie, IL

Dorothea Jakob
Toronto, Ontario

Janice Janken
Providence, RI

Patricia Jarosz
Troy, MI

Mary Jeffries
Honolulu, HI

Debra Jenkins
Decatur, IL

Jean Jenny
Nepean, Ontario

Betty Johnson
Oak Park, IL

Shayna Johnson
Sioux Falls, SD

JoAnne Johnson
Cincinnati, OH

Sharon Johnson
Wayne, PA

Mildred Jones
Fairfax, VA

Phyllis Jones
Toronto, Ontario

Dorothy Jones
Braintree, MA

Kay Judge
Mitchell, SD

Sherrie Justice
Toledo, OH

Beatrice Kalisch
Saline, MI

Annette Kaminsky
Milwaukee, WI

Janet Kasno
Southfield, MI

Mary Ann Kelly
Seneca, SC

Carol Kemper
Cincinnati, OH

Eileen Kenkel-Rossi
Milwaukee, WI

Donna Kennedy
Granby, MA

Mary Kerry
Gibsonia, PA

Christine Kessel
Dubuque, IA

Mary Lou Kiley
South Euclid, OH

Mi Ja Kim
Des Plaines, IL

Chie Kimoto
Los Angeles, CA

Terrie Kirkpatrick
Greenville, SC

Audrey Klopp
Brookfield, IL

Rita Knoop
Troy, OH

Mary Kolbe
Lincoln, NB

Mary Kontz
Miami, FL

Laura Koppenhoefer
Normal, IL

Sue Kovats-Bell
Kalamazoo, MI

Doris Kowalski
Galesburg, IL

Vicki Kraus
Iowa City, IA

Patricia Kraynick
Whitefish Bay, WI

Phyllis Kritek
Whitefish Bay, WI

Patricia Kucharski
Gales Ferry, CT

Fern Kulman
Colonia, NJ

Joan Kulpa
Peoria, IL

Lynda Kushnir-Pekrul
Regina, Saskatchewan

Nancy Lackey
Urerland Park, KS

Susan Lampe
Minneapolis, MN

Jane Lancour
Wauwatosa, WI

Norma Lang
Milwaukee, WI

Regina Lange
Rock Island, IL

Teddy Langford
Lubbock, TX

Paul Langlois
Chicago, IL

June Larson
Vermillion, SD

Sandra Laski
Chantilly, VA

Pamela Lawrence
Oil City, PA

Linda Lazure
Omaha, NB

Helena Lee
Milwaukee, WI

Anne LeGresley
Brookline, MA

Gail Lennan
Portage, MI

Mary Lenny
Maryville, TN

Ruth Leo
Grove City, PA

Cindy Lessow
Phoenix, AZ

Leva Lessure
Evansville, IN

Rona Levin
Westbury, NY

Myra Levine
Chicago, IL

Janice Lewis
Countryside, IL

Peggy Lindsay
Hesperia, CA

Deloris Long
Chicago, IL

Kay Lopez
New Orleans, LA

Cecile Loreck
Milwaukee, WI

Mariann Lovell
Xenia, OH

Barb Lowes
Cape Girardeau, MO

Ilene Lubkin
Danville, CA

Annette Lueckenotte
Normal, IL

Margaret Lunney
Staten Island, NY

Rose Lusk
Troy, IL

Louette Lutjens
Plainell, MI

Brenda Lyon
Nineveh, IN

Meridean Maas
Liscomb, IA

Suzanne MacAvoy
Ridgefield, CT

Linda Madden
Lexington, KY

Eunice Madsen
Murfreesboro, TN

Lou Ann Madson
Shorewood, WI

Margaret Magnussen
Albuquerque, NM

Jeane Maguire
Vienna, VA

Marie Maguire
Elkorn, WI

Barbara Maher
Harvey, LA

Regina Maibusch
Milwaukee, WI

Jo Ann Maklebust
Livonia, MI

Carol Mandle
Lexington, MA

Ann Manton
Westwood, MA

Gail Marculescu
Sunnyvale, CA

Patricia Martin
Beavercreek, OH

Karen Martin
Omaha, NB

Jean Martinson
Minneapolis, MN

Jean Masunaga
Fremont, CA

Joscelyn Matthewman
Mississauga, Ontario

Nancy Matulich
New Orleans, LA

Carol Matz
Boyertown, PA

Peggy Mayfield
Fort Worth, TX

Lucille McCarty
Erie, PA

JoAnne McCloskey
Iowa City, IA

Margaret McComb
Portland, Oregon

Eleanor McConnell
Hillsborough, NC

Kathleen McCormick
Gaithersburg, MD

Ann McCourt
North Easton, MA

Kyra McCoy
Portland, OR

Bonnie McDonald
Iowa City, IA

Sandra McDonald
Marion, IA

Mary McDowell
Richmond, KY

Mary McElroy
Columbus, OH

Gertrude McFarland
Clifton, VA

Elizabeth McFarlane
Burke, VA

Suzanne McGuiness
Columbus, OH

Ann McGuire
St. Louis, MO

Barbara McGuire
Vancouver, British Columbia

Joanne Ingalls McKay
Oak Park, IL

Rosemary McKeighen
Oxford, IA

Beverly McKenna
Bellevue, WA

Joyce McKinney
East St. Louis, IL

Audrey McLane
Milwaukee, WI

Jacqueline McNally
Metairie, LA

Marie McQueen
Philadelphia, PA

Peg Mehmert
Davenport, IA

Victoria Meissner
Sunland, CA

Karen Metzger
Falmouth, ME

Emmy Miller
Richmond, VA

Penny Miller
Pittsburg, PA

Winnifred Mills
Edmonton, Alberta

Stephanie Minerath
Ann Arbor, MI

Mary Moberg
St. Paul, MN

Linda Mondoux
Northville, MI

Martha Montgomery
Detroit, MI

Sue Moorhead
Davenport, IA

Mary Moorhouse
Colorado Springs, CO

Karen Morgan
Jefferson City, MO

Derry Ann Moritz
New Haven, CT

Elizabeth Mottet
San Diego, CA

Sharon Moudry
Minneapolis, MN

Judith Mueller
Redway, CA

Terry Mullen
Palmer, MA

Marlene Mullin
Royal Oak, MI

Dawneane Munn
Lincoln, NB

Clara Muret
Muskogee, OK

Margaret Murphy
Wellesley Hills, MA

Judith Myers
St. Louis, MO

Charlotte Naschinski
Silver Spring, MD

Joanne Nattrass
Decatur, IL

Marie Neaton
Ann Arbor, MI

Lois Newman
Witchita, KS

Margaret Newman
St. Paul, MN

Naomi Nibbelink
Topeka, KS

Mary Niemeyer
Ann Arbor, MI

Kathryn Niesen
Houston, MN

Judy Nixon
Winnipeg, Manitoba

Lucyanne Nolan
Martinez, GA

Mary Nordtverdt
Pierre, SD

Joan Norris
Omaha, NB

Laura Nosek
Solon, OH

Colleen O'Brien
Denmark, WI

Evelyn O'Connor
New Bern, NC

Jean O'Neil
Watertown, MA

Eileen Sjoberg O'Neill
Ashburnham, MA

Trinidad Ortega
Addison, IL

Elizabeth Outlaw
Stamford, CT

Susan Copeland Owen
Plymouth, MI

Karen Padrick
Portland, Oregon

Rhonda Panfilli
Dearborn, MI

P. Pantojas
Stony Brook, NY

Mary Paquette
Pacific Palisades, CA

Elinor Parsons
West Chicago, IL

Ann Patterson
Nashville, TN

Cheryl Patterson
Seven Hills, OH

Queen Patterson
Hazel Crest, IL

Melinda Paull
Kalamazoo, MI

Carol Pavlish
Prior Lake, MN

Ruth Payton
Ruper Marlboro, MD

Marilyn Peasley
Marshalltown, IA

Audrey Peeso
Augusta, WI

Virginia Pellegrinelli
Erie, PA

Mabel Penney
St. Paul, MN

Sherry Perkins
Dallas, TX

Ann Perry
St. Louis, MO

Dorothy Petersen
Sioux Falls, SD

Harriet Pfotenhauer
Richmond, KY

Jan Pierce
Davenport, IA

Marguerite Pike
Westmont, IL

Norma Pinnell
Godfrey, IL

Nancy Pogue
St. Joseph, IL

Patricia Pohl
Chicago, IL

Bernadette Pohlmann
Hanover Park, IL

Barbara Pokorny
Niantic, CT

Carolyn Pontius
Akron, Ohio

Sue Popkess-Vawter
Prairie Village, KS

Eileen Porter
Oshkosh, WI

Pat Potter
Overland, MO

Marie Price
Bruce Mines, Ontario

Nancy Prince
Ann Arbor, MI

Virginia Prout
West Roxbury, MA

Rose Puerto
Hindsdale, IL

Lucille Pulliam
Avondale, PA

Devamma Purushotham
Windsor, Ontario

Dee-J Putzier
Beaverton, OR

Precilla Quillen
Oxford, OH

Linda Rabinowitz
Dallas, TX

Kay Rademacher
St. Clair Shores, MI

Lina Rahal
Blainville, Montreal

Deborah Raines
Arlington, VA

Marilyn Rantz
Delavan, WI

Cheryl Ratliff
Leawood, KS

Marlene Reimer
Calgary, Alberta

Charla Renner
Bloomington, IL

Marion Resler
St. Louis, MO

Tamera Rice
Irving, CA

Paula Rich
Philadelphia, PA

Lee Richard
Highland Park, IL

Ruth Dryer Richard
Highland Park, IL

Marilyn Richardson
Oxford, OH

Sabrina Richer
Rochester, MI

Mary Ridgeway
Albuquerque, NM

Elvi Rigby
Marshfield, MA

Mary Riner
Jefferson City, MO

Mary Riordan
Brookline, MA

Cynthia Roberts
Evansville, IN

Lisa Rodriguez
Kenner, LA

Paul Roland
Oxford, MA

Beverly Ross
Indianapolis, IN

Jo Ellen Ross
Iowa City, IA

Laura Rossi
Medway, MA

Barbara Rottkamp
Westbury, NY

Carolyn Rundle
Janesville, WI

Judith Runk
Royal Oak, MI

Wanda Ruthven
Fremont, CA

Alice Ryan
Erie, PA

Susan Ryan
Wauwatosa, WI

Vivianne Saba
Montreal, Quebec

Mary Sampel
Ballwin, MO

Diane Sanders
Seattle, WA

Monica Sanger
Hartford, WI

Shannon Sayles
Arlington, VA

Carol Schaefer
Eau Claire, WI

Theresa Schaefer
Houston, TX

Diane Schank
Hinsdale, IL

Barbara Scheffer
Ann Arbor, MI

Penny Schoenmehl
Delmar, CA

Carolyn Schultz
Johnstown, PA

Pat Schultz
Newport, KY

Jill Schumacher
Portland, OR

Stephanie Scinta
Bettendorf, IA

Leann Scroggins
Rochester, MN

Marita Sension
Chenoa, IL

Elaine Serra
Irvine, CA

Constance Settlemyer
Arnold, PA

Karen Sexton
Paris, KY

Mary Shannahan
Tallahassee, FL

Rebecca Shaw
Peoria, IL

Maureen Shekleton
Glen Ellyn, IL

Kathleen Sheppard
Katy, TX

Joyce Shoemaker
Huntsville, AL

Laura Shore
Richmond, VA

Mary Sieggreen
Northville, MI

Susan Simmons-Alling
Bethesda, MD

Peggy Singer
Natick, MA

Luella Sinha
Winnepeg, Manitoba

Margie Sipe
Wellesley, MA

Donna Skouse
Kansas City, MO

Carol Smejkal
Wauwatosa, WI

Donna Smith
Lincoln, NB

Carol Soares-O'Hearn
Waltham, MA

Debbie Soholt
Aberdeen, SD

June Soto
Rego Park, NY

Sheila Southwell
Denver, CO

Martha Spier
St. Louis, MO

Judith Spilker
Cincinnati, OH

Debra Spunt
Baltimore, MD

Rose Squires
Phoenix, AZ

Margaret Stafford
Northlake, IL

Harriet Strakey
Quinton, VA

Drue Steele
Dayton, OH

Maribeth Stein
Bellevue, WA

Brenda Stevenson
Dayton, OH

Paula Steward
Country Club Hill, IL

Patricia Stieren
Springfield, IL

Dorothy Stitzlein
Loudonbille, OH

Betty Stock
St. Louis, MO

Barbara Stocks
Havelock, NC

Ann Stoewer
Dayton, OH

Barbara Strohl-Denn
Detroit, MI

Mary Strong
Topeka, KS

Kathy Strong
West Bend, WI

Rosemarie Suhayda
Woodridge, IL

Sharon Summers
Overland Park, KS

Alice Swan
Roseville, MN

Margaret Swinford
Cincinnati, OH

Carol Szymczak
Milwaukee, WI

Betsy Talbot
Cedar City, UT

Fe Tamparong
Santa Ana, CA

Barbara Taptich
Mercerville, NJ

Joyce Taylor
San Francisco, CA

Susan Taylor
Columbia, MO

Clark Taylor
Lake Park, FL

Lynne Thelan
LaJolla, CA

Roberta Thiry
Pittsburg, KS

Joan Thompson
Cedar City, UT

Marita Titler
Alburnett, IA

Lauren Tofias
Streetsville, Ontario

Virginia Tolentino
Westmont, IL

Eleanor Toney
Champaign, IL

Sally Traylor
Urbana, IL

Jill Triick
Grand Rapids, MI

Sally Tripp
Amherst, MA

Gail Tumulty
River Ridge, LA

Beatrice Turkoski
Milwaukee, WI

Martha Turner
Upper Marlboro, MD

Laura Upchurch
Fisher, IL

Linda Urden
San Diego, CA

Roberta Urick
Clarkston, MI

Danielle Valois
Bellefeville, Quebec

Margie Van Meter
Ann Arbor, MI

Dorothy Varchol
Milford, OH

Barbara Vassallo
Willingboro, NJ

Maria Vasselman
Commack, NY

Beth Vaughan-Wrobel
Fayetteville, AR

Mary Venn
Eau Claire, WI

Carol Viamontes
Bridgewater, NJ

Karen Vincent
Randolph, MA

Anne Marie Voith
Glendale, WI

Jacqueline Wachowski
Milwaukee, WI

Sharon Wahl
Omaha, NB

Jeanette Waits
Jackson, MS

Patricia Waldron
Bridgeview, IL

Shirley Walker
Champaign, IL

Lorraine Walker
Austin, TX

Jane Wall
West Allis, WI

Christine Walsh
Erie, PA

Rosemary Wang
Barrington, NH

Cathy Rogers Ward
Los Angeles, CA

Sandra Ward
Little Rock, AR

Christine Ward
Weatherford, OK

Judith Warren
Charleston, SC

Lora Wasko
Belleville, IL

Joanne Wattrass
Decatur, IL

Judith Weatherall
Champaign, IL

Carolyn Weber
Wichita, KS

Janet Weber
Perkins, MO

Nancy Weinberg
Metairie, LA

Marylouise Welch
West Hartford, CT

Harriet Werley
Milwaukee, WI

Una Beth Westfall
Portland, OR

J.L. Vance Wheller
Anaheim, CA

Joan White
Forest Park, IL

Roger Whiting
Chippewa Falls, WI

Georgia Whitley
Plainfield, IL

Joie Whitney
Seattle, WA

Paul Wibbenmeyer
Chicago, IL

Hildegarde Wieckowski
Milwaukee, WI

Jill Wiley
Wattsburg, PA

Roxanne Wilson
Sartell, MN

Sharon Wilson
Ft. McMurray, Alberta

Sharon Witmer
Stanton, CA

Francine Wojton
Lakewood, OH

Anne Woodtli
Tucson, AZ

Marian Worthy
Springfield, IL

Linda Wray
Richmond, KY

Jackie Wylie
Kalamazoo, MI

Lillian Yeager
Louisville, KY

Karen York
Dayton, OH

Florence Young
Mayfield Heights, OH

Cassandra Zak
Holland, OH

Irene Zbuckvich
Valencia, PA

Dorothy Zelenski
Johnstown, PA

Shirley Ziegler
Lewisville, TX

Karin Zuehls
W. Burlington, IA

Index

T indicates table